CBS—Quick Medical Examination Review Series

# GENERAL SURGERY

## FIFTEENTH EDITION

**Edited by :**
**DR. M.S. BHATIA** (MD, Dip. WPA, MNAMS)
Professor & Head, Department of Psychiatry
University College of Medical Sciences
&
Guru Teg Bahadur Hospital,
Dilshad Garden, Delhi - 110095

**Previously at :**
Maulana Azad Medical College and Associated Hospitals, New Delhi
&
Lady Hardinge Medical College and Associated Hospitals, New Delhi

**Contributing Editor :**
**DR. NIRMALJIT KAUR** (MD)
Senior Specialist, Department of Microbiology
Dr. R.M.L. Hospital
New Delhi-110001
**Previously at :**
LHMC & Smt. S.K. Hospital, New Delhi

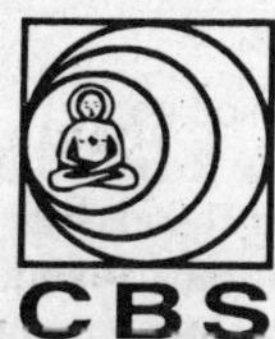


**CBS Publishers & Distributors Pvt. Ltd.**
New Delhi • Bengaluru • Chennai • Kochi • Kolkata • Mumbai
Hyderabad • Nagpur • Patna • Pune • Vijayawada

**DEDICATED TO**
**READERS WHO READ, UNDERSTAND**
**&**
**RECIPROCATE**

**ISBN: 978-81-239-1856-3**

First Edition: 1992
Second Edition: 1993
Third Edition: 1994
Fourth Edition: 1995
Fifth Edition: 1996
Sixth Edition: 1997
Seventh Edition: 1998
Eighth Edition: 1999
Ninth Edition: 2000
Tenth Edition: 2001
Eleventh Edition: 2002
Twelfth Edition: 2003
Thirteenth Edition: 2004
Fourteenth Edition: 2005
Fifteenth Edition: 2010
**Reprint: 2018**



Published by **Satish Kumar Jain** and produced by **Varun Jain** for
**CBS Publishers & Distributors Pvt. Ltd.**,
4819/XI Prahlad Street, 24 Ansari Road, Daryaganj, New Delhi - 110002
delhi@cbspd.com, cbspubs@airtelmail.in • www.cbspd.com
Ph.: 23289259, 23266861, 23266867 • Fax: 011-23243014

*Corporate Office:* 204 FIE, Industrial Area, Patparganj, Delhi - 110 092
Ph: 49344934 • Fax: 011-49344935
E-mail: publishing@cbspd.com • publicity@cbspd.com

*Branches:*
- ***Bengaluru:*** 2975, 17th Cross, K.R. Road, Bansankari 2nd Stage, Bengaluru - 70 • Ph: +91-80-26771678/79 • Fax: +91-80-26771680 E-mail: cbsbng@gmail.com, bangalore@cbspd.com
- ***Chennai:*** No. 7, Subbaraya Street, Shenoy Nagar, Chennai - 600030 Ph: +91-44-26681266, 26680620 • Fax: +91-44-42032115 E-mail: chennai@cbspd.com
- ***Kochi:*** Ashana House, 39/1904, A.M. Thomas Road, Valanjambalam, Ernakulum, Kochi • Ph: +91-484-4059061-65 Fax: +91-484-4059065 • E-mail: cochin@cbspd.com
- ***Kolkata:*** 6-B, Ground Floor, Rameshwar Shaw Road, Kolkata - 700014 Ph: +91-33-22891126/7/8 • E-mail: kolkata@cbspd.com
- ***Mumbai:*** 83-C, Dr. E. Moses Road, Worli, Mumbai - 400018 Ph: +91-9833017933, 022-24902340/41 • E-mail: mumbai@cbspd.com

*Representatives:*
- Hyderabad: 0-9885175004
- Nagpur: 0-9021734563
- Patna: 0-9334159340
- Pune: 0-9623451994
- Jharkhand: 0-9811541605
- Uttarakhand: 0-9716462459

*Printed at:* J.S. Offset Printers, Delhi (India)

# PREFACE

Life is a continuous learning process. Human beings are born to learn and gain knowledge. Education is a means to acquire knowledge and skills that an individual desires to practise. Examinations are the means to evaluate the knowledge. Though no method of evaluation is without flaw, the process of standardization has resulted in a multiple choice system of examination. This system satisfies the basic qualities of a measuring instrument viz., validity, reliability and objectivity.

Recently, a number of books have been published about these examinations but the **best book still remains that which covers the maximum number of questions, which had been asked in that particular examination,** because the chance of repetition of these questions from so-called **"Question Bank"** remains very high. Recently, it has been observed that many **"Question Banks"** have overlapped. So, it is best to do a book which is complete and covers the **"Question Banks"** of maximum number of examinations. This book is being forwarded in this direction.

This book is designed as a supplement to the standard textbooks. It includes the **Referenced - MCQ's** (of previous years papers) of various PG Medical Entrance and Services Examinations **speciality-wise and Chapter-wise** arranged. The students while preparing the text or just before the examination can quickly go through this book. This will help in detecting the areas of weakness in understanding the text and thus, will improve the skills with multiple choice system of examination. It is a favourite book for **"Paper-setters".**

The importance of doing MCQ's alongwith text has increased tremendously because, recently, it has become a tendency to frame MCQ's usually not covered by the standard textbooks followed at undergraduate level. **"Quick Medical Text Review Series"** (in 20 subjectwise books from same publishers) can be a useful adjuant to this book.

Beware of the **Fraudulent Books** available in the market, which covers a part of copied **'Question Bank'** from this book, and also, based on **'Constructed'** rather than **'Original'** Question Book. It is suggested not to waste time on these books. Every MCQ matters a lot in a highly competitive exams.

I request the readers not to forget to send their opinions, as also suggestions and contributions if any, about all aspects of this book. It will be of invaluable help in enhancing the utility of the book in future.

All suggestions are welcome and will be duly acknowledged in future editions.

**— Editors**

A book of the Readers, for the Readers, by the Readers

## NOTE

The MCQ's of multiple response type (i.e. with **more than one correct answer** have been omitted in this Edition. Kindly refer to separate books **(PGI MD Entrance Examination & DNB Entrance Examination)** by the same author and Publishers.

## ADVICE

Read carefully the suggestions in the beginning of this book.

Prepare text from books suggested in the beginning and go through **Referenced MCQ's** of this book. Don't waste time in **inexperienced, incomplete and fraudulent courses & books for PG Medical Entrance Examinations.**

# ABOUT THE BOOK

This book has been compiled with the main aim to help the students to **quickly revise the Chapter-wise up-to-date referenced questions** asked in various entrance examinations (Years indicated in the brackets).

**Quick Medical Examinations Review Series** contains Speciality-wise 45,000 MCQ's based on up-to-date papers from 1978 onwards.

The important examinations covered in this book (with code word in the bracket) are :

| | *Examinations* | *Code used* |
|---|---|---|
| ***(A)*** | ***All India level*** | |
| 1. | All India Postgraduate Entrance Examination | (AI) |
| 2. | AIIMS MD Entrance Examination | (AIIMS) |
| 3. | PGI MD Entrance Examination | (PGI) |
| 4. | Combined Medical Services Examination by UPSC | (UPSC) |
| 5. | Civil Services Entrance Examination, Part-I (Medicine) | (CS) |
| 6. | Army Medical Corps Entrance Examination | (AMC) |
| 7. | Diplomate of National Board Entrance Examination | (DNB) |
| 8. | NIMHANS PG Entrance Examination | (NIMHANS) |
| 9. | Sanjay Gandhi PG Institute Entrance Examination | (SGPGI) |
| 10. | CIP Ranchi PG Entrance Examination | (CIP) |
| 11. | Manipal Academy of Higher Education PG Entrance Examination | (Manipal/MAHE) |
| 12. | Sree Chitra Tirunal Institute for Medical Science & Technology | (SCTIMST) |
| 13. | Command Hospital, Bangalore | (CH) |
| 14. | Bhabha Atomic Research Centre | (BARC) |
| 15. | Institute of Aerospace Medicine | (IAM) |
| ***(B)*** | ***State level*** | |
| 16. | Delhi MD Entrance Examination | (Delhi) |
| 17. | Bihar MD Entrance Examination | (Bihar) |
| 18. | JIPMER PG Entrance Examination | (JIPMER) |
| 19. | CMC PG Entrance Examination | (CMC) |
| 20. | Rohtak PG Entrance Examination | (Rohtak) |
| 21. | MP State PG Entrance Examination | (MP) |
| 22. | AP State MD Entrance Examination | (AP) |
| 23. | TN State MD Entrance Examination | (TN) |
| 24. | Karnataka Postgraduate Medical Entrance Examination | (Karnataka) |
| 25. | Maharashtra PG Entrance Examination | (Maharashtra) |
| 26. | Kerala State MD Entrance Examination | (Kerala) |
| 27. | Rajasthan Postgraduate Entrance Examination | (Rajasthan) |
| 28. | PG Entrance Examination, Varanasi | (BHU) |
| 29. | Burdwan University | (BU) |
| 30. | Combined Entrance Examination for PG Courses, U.P. | (UP) |
| 31. | Punjab State PG Entrance Examination | (Punjab) |
| 32. | Aligarh Muslim University PG Entrance Examination | (AMU) |
| 33. | Nizam's Institute Entrance Examination, Hyderabad | (Nizam's) |
| 34. | Postgraduate Admission Test, Orissa | (Orissa) |
| 35. | Calcutta University Public Service Commission | (CUPSC) |
| 36. | TN Public Service Commission | (TNPSC) |
| 37. | Calcutta PG Entrance Examination | (Calcutta) |
| ***(C)*** | ***Foreign*** | |
| | PLAB, FCGP, GMC, FLEX, USMLE, MRCP, FRCS, MRCOG, etc. | |

## Sources of Errors (General Surgery)

**Example 1** : **The risk factor for development of hepatocellular carcinoma include :** **Karnataka 1994**

A. Hepatitis-B
B. Aflatoxin
C. Sclerosing cholangitis
D. Primary biliary cirrhosis

**Answer** : Both "A" and "B" (Harrison's Principles of Internal Medicines) (Karnataka PG Entrance is a single response exam).

**Example 2** : **Indication of surgery in chronic pancreatitis is :** **AIIMS 1985**

A. Pain
B. Diabetes mellitus
C. Risk of malignancy
D. Jaundice

**Answer** : Both "A" and "D" (Bailey & Love's Short Practice of Surgery,)

**Example 3** : **Ulcerative colitis is associated with the following, except : AI 1989**

A. Toxic megacolon
B. Massive bleeding
C. Perforation
D. Stricture of the colon

**Answer** : 'None of the above' as all of the above choices are true (i.e. they are seen as complications of ulcerative colitis —Fibrous stricture - 6%, Massive haemorrhage - 3% Toxic dilatation - 1.5% and Perforation - 1%) (Bailey & Love Short Practice of Surgery,)

**Example 4** : **Hereditary factors are important in causation of :** **Delhi 1993**

A. Retinoblastoma
B. Carcinoma breast
C. Bronchogenic carcinoma
D. Carcinoma pancreas

**Answer** : Both "A" and "B" are correct as genetic factors are important in both (in Retinoblastoma—deletion of Band 13 & 14 and in Ca breast — risk is two to three fold increased as compared to the general population (Harrison's Principles of Internal Medicine,)

**Example 5** : **The most frequent site of carcinoma in oesophagus is :** **Delhi 1984, 87**

A. Upper-one-third
B. Middle-one-third
C. Lower-one-third
D. Anywhere

**Answer** : Choice "(B)" Harrison's Principles of Internal Medicine
Choice "(B)" Robbin's Pathologic Basis of Disease
Choice "(C)" Davidson's Principles and Practice of Medicine
Choice "(C)" Bailey and Love's Short Practice of Surgery
**N.B.** (In females, it is most common in upper third (Bailey & Love).

**Advice**

Questions with inaccurate language (structuring) or wrong choices should better be left unattempted.

# IMPORTANT GENERAL SURGERY TEXT FOR MCQ's

| | |
|---|---|
| **General Topics** | Wound healing (signs of inflammation, factors affecting), Suturing (Primary and Secondary), Keloid, Tumours (TNM classification, Malignant melanoma, Basal cell carcinoma), Ulcers (edges in specific disorders), Haemorrhage (Types, Management), Fluids and electrolytes (Acidosis, Alkalosis, Composition of fluids used), Gangrene, Lymphangitis, Pre & Post-operative care, Post-operative Complications, Special medical problems. |
| **Burns & Plastic Surgery** | Burns (degrees, management), Grafts, Plastic surgery. |
| **Neurosurgery** | Head injury (Glasgow coma scale, Management), Haematoma (Subdural, Extradural, Lucid interval), Brain Tumours (Secondaries, Primaries, Calcification, Effects) Aneurysms, Abscesses, Hydrocephalus, Spine (Tumours, Injuries), Nerves (Regeneration, Suturing). |
| **Maxillofacial Surgery** | Cleft lip, and Palate, Lefort classification of Jaw injuries, Jaw swellings (classification, dentigerous cyst), Tongue (Carcinoma), Salivary glands (Ducts, Swellings, Tumors). |
| **Neck & Breast** | Branchial cyst, Cystic hygroma, Carotid body tumour, Block dissection (Crile's), Thyroid (Function tests, Swellings, Tumours, Wayne's index, Postoperative Complications, Thyroglossal cysts), Breast swellings, cancer & surgery. |
| **Cardiothoracic Surgery** | Thorax (injuries, effusions, haemorrhage, management), Bypass Surgery, Surgery for valvular lesions. |
| **Gastrosurgery** | **Oesophagus** (Achlasia, Congenital anomalies, Hiatus hernia, Carcinoma, Rupture), **Stomach** (Blood and lymphatic supply, Investigations Peptic ulcer, Tumors), Duodenum (Achlasia, diverticulum), Liver (Hepatomegaly, Tumours, Cirrhosis, Abscess). Spleen (Splenomegaly, Splenectomy), Gall bladder (Cholelithiasis, Cholecystitis, Cholecystectomy, Congenital bile duct anomalies, Charcot triad), Pancreas (Pancreatitis, Tumours), Others (Appendicitis, Carcinoid, Intestinal obstruction, Crohn's disease, Ulcerative colitis, Diverticulitis, Ca Colon and rectum, Haemorrhoids, Anal Fistula, Fissure, Rectal Prolapse, Meckel's diverticulum. |
| **Hernia** | Terminology, Types, Inguinal, Umbilical, Femoral (contents, surgery), Incisional. |
| **Genitourinary Surgery** | Polycystic kidney, Horseshoe kidney, Pyonephrosis, Renal calculi and Tumours (Wilm's, Grawitz's), Bladder (calculi, Diverticulum, Cancer, Rupture of bladder and urethra), Prostate (BHP, Carcinoma), Testes (Torsion, Hydrocele, Tumours) |
| **Miscellaneous** | Transplantation, Named signs, Tests, and Operations |

# IMPORTANT TIPS OF GENERAL SURGERY

## Read

| | |
|---|---|
| * Imaging in acute abdomen | Bailey & Love's **Short Practice of Surgery** |
| * Imaging in Trauma | Bailey & Love's **Short Practice of Surgery** |
| * Hypertrophic scar versus keloid | Bailey & Love's **Short Practice of Surgery** |
| * Composition of commonly used intravenous fluids | Bailey & Love's **Short Practice of Surgery** |
| * Surgical dressings | Bailey & Love's **Short Practice of Surgery** |
| * Antiseptics used in surgery | Bailey & Love's **Short Practice of Surgery** |
| * Risk factors for deep vein thrombosis & venous thromboembolism | Bailey & Love's **Short Practice of Surgery** |
| * D/D of swollen limb | Bailey & Love's **Short Practice of Surgery** |
| * Classification of shock, Glasgow coma scale & revised Trauma scale | Bailey & Love's **Short Practice of Surgery** |
| * Do's & Don't in Missile Injuries | Bailey & Love's **Short Practice of Surgery** |
| * Classification of Nerve injuries | Bailey & Love's **Short Practice of Surgery** |
| * Timing of treatment for cleft lip & cleft palate | Bailey & Love's **Short Practice of Surgery** |
| * Adverse factor influencing healing | Bailey & Love's **Short Practice of Surgery** |
| * Types of Suture material | Bailey & Love's **Short Practice of Surgery** |
| * Treatment of oesophagus perforation | Bailey & Love's **Short Practice of Surgery** |
| * Classification of oesophageal motility disorder | Bailey & Love's **Short Practice of Surgery** |
| * Peptides & Neuropeptides in stomach | Bailey & Love's **Short Practice of Surgery** |
| * Tests for liver function | Bailey & Love's **Short Practice of Surgery** |
| * D/D of splenomegaly | Bailey & Love's **Short Practice of Surgery** |
| * Ranson & Glasgow scales for prognosis in acute peritonitis | Bailey & Love's **Short Practice of Surgery** |
| * Uses of Lap. surgery | Bailey & Love's **Short Practice of Surgery** |
| * Pseudobstruction of intestines | Bailey & Love's **Short Practice of Surgery** |
| * Anuria & retention | Bailey & Love's **Short Practice of Surgery** |
| * Treatment of incontinence | Bailey & Love's **Short Practice of Surgery** |
| * Arterial ulcer versus venous ulcer | **Manipal Manual of Surgery** |
| * Buerger's disease versus Atherosclerosis | **Manipal Manual of Surgery** |
| * Dry gangrene versus wet gangrene | **Manipal Manual of Surgery** |
| * Tests for varicose veins | **Manipal Manual of Surgery** |
| * Chronic gastric ulcer versus duodenal ulcer | **Manipal Manual of Surgery** |

| | |
|---|---|
| * Hydatid cyst of liver | **Manipal Manual of Surgery** |
| * Portal hypertension | **Manipal Manual of Surgery** |
| * Rupture of spleen & splenectomy | **Manipal Manual of Surgery** |
| * D/D of peritonitis | **Manipal Manual of Surgery** |
| * Difference between TB, Crohn's & ulcerative colitis | **Manipal Manual of Surgery** |
| * Intestinal obstruction - D/D | **Manipal Manual of Surgery** |
| * Bleeding per rectum | **Manipal Manual of Surgery** |
| * D/D of Renal mass | **Manipal Manual of Surgery** |
| * Seminoma versus teratoma | **Manipal Manual of Surgery** |
| * D/D of hematuria | **Manipal Manual of Surgery** |
| * Everything about peptic ulcer | Bailey & Love's **Short Practice of Surgery** |
| * Tumors of Esophagus | **Current Surgical Diagnosis & Treatment** |
| * Symptoms and treatment of Ca rectum | Bailey & Love's **Short Practice of Surgery** |
| * About Carcinoma breast | **Current Surgical Diagnosis & Treatment** |
| * About Named Signs, and Syndromes | Bhatia's **Quick Medical Text Review Series, Surgery** |
| * About symptoms, complications and treatment of Ulcerative colitis & Crohn's disease | Bailey & Love's **Short Practice of Surgery** |
| * Mediastinal tumors | Bailey & Love's **Short Practice of Surgery** |
| * Everything about Hernia (Inguinal & femoral-complications & treatment) | Bailey & Love's **Short Practice of Surgery** |
| * Eponyms | Bhatia's **Quick Medical Text Review Series, Surgery** |
| * About Milestones in History | Bhatia's **Quick Medical Text Review Series, Surgery** |
| * About Appendicitis (Symptoms Signs D/D, complications & treatment) | Bailey & Love's **Short Practice of Surgery,** |
| * About carcinoma and benign Hypertrophy of Prostate | Bailey & Love's **Short Practice of Surgery** |
| * About Intestinal obstruction | Bailey & Love's **Short Practice of Surgery** |
| * About Testicular disease (ectopic, undescended, varicocele, hydrocele, tumors) | Bailey & Love's **Short Practice of Surgery** |
| * About Gall stones | **Current Surgical Diagnosis & Treatment** |
| * About Intraperitoneal abscess | Bailey & Love's **Short Practice of Surgery** |
| * About Suture Materials | Bhatia's **Quick Medical Text Review Series, Surgery** |
| * About Pancreatitis & Ca Pancreas | Bailey & Love's **Short Practice of Surgery** |
| * About Carcinoid syndrome | **Current Surgical Diagnosis & Treatment** |
| * About Glasgow Coma scale | Bhatia's **Quick Medical Text Review Series, Surgery** |
| * About Skin grafts | Bhatia's **Quick Medical Text Review Series, Surgery** |
| * About Achalasia cardia | Bailey & Love's **Short Practice of Surgery** |

| | |
|---|---|
| * About Child's Criteria | Bhatia's **Quick Medical Text Review Series, Surgery** |
| * About Pyloric stenosis | Bailey & Love's **Short Practice of Surgery** |
| * About retention of urine & Ca urinary bladder | Bailey & Love's **Short Practice of Surgery** |
| * About Portal Hypertension & Splenectomy | **Current Surgical Diagnosis & Treatment** |
| * About Hirschsprung's Disease | Bailey & Love's **Short Practice of Surgery** |
| * About Intravenous fluids | Bhatia's **Quick Medical Text Review Series, Surgery** |
| * One must know about Commonest sites of lesions and Important Points | Bhatia's **Quick Medical Text Review Series, Surgery** |

# CONTENTS

# 1

# IMPORTANT TEXT OF GENERAL TOPICS

## CAUSES OF RAYNAUD'S SYNDROME

**Primary**

* Constitutional disturbance of the finger circulation (e.g. hereditary cold fingers, acrocyanosis).
* Raynaud's disease (Lewis' 'local fault' in the digital arteries).

**Secondary**

* Connective tissue disorders (e.g. systemic sclerosis, systemic lupus erythematosus, polyarteritis nodosa, rheumatoid arthritis dermatomyositis, polymyositis).
* Atherosclerosis
* Thromboangitis obliterans
* Cold injury (e.g. frosbite)
* Occupation disorder (hypothenar hammer syndrome, vibration white finger syndrome)
* Haematological disease (e.g. polycythemia vera)
* Drugs (e.g. ergot, beta-blockers, contraceptive pill)
* Malignant disease
* Others (e.g. serum hepatitis, chronic renal failure).

## SUTURE MATERIALS

**Types of Suture materials :**

**Absorbable**

* Plain catgut—natural monofilament
* Chronic catgut—natural monofilament
* Polyglycolic acid—synthetic braided (Dexon)
* Polyglactin—synthetic braided (Vicryl)
* Polydioxanone—synthetic monofilament (PDS)

**Non-absorbable**

* Silk—natural braided
* Linen—natural braided
* Stainless steel wire—monofilament or braided
* Nylon—synthetic, usually monofilament (Ethilon)
* Polyester—synthetic monofilament (Prolene)
* Polytetrafluoroethylene (PTEF)—synthetic, extended/teased' monofilament (Goretex).

## SUTURE MATERIALS & ABSORPTION

*ABSORBABLE :*

* Plain catgut — 5-70 days
* Chronic catgut — 20-90 days
* Vicryl polyglactin (braided) — 40-90 days
* PDS polydioxanone (Monifilament) — 90-200 days

# MCQ's OF GENERAL TOPICS

## 1-A. Wounds, Suturing, Keloids, Infections, Cysts

**1. Human bite infection at a metacarpophalangeal joint is apt to : AMU 1987**
A. Involve the palm
B. Spread along lumbrical canals
C. Cause suppurative arthritis
D. Involve tendon sheaths
E. All of the above

**2. When is the maximum collagen content of wound tissue noted : Rohtak 1987**
A. Between 3rd to 5th day
B. Between 6th to 7th day
C. 17th to 21st day
D. 24-30 days

**3. The "golden period" for treatment of open wounds is — hours. AMU 1986**
A. 4 B. 6
C. 12 D. 16
E. 20

**4. A patient with an open wound presenting 10 hours after injury should be : PGI 1984; Delhi 1989**
A. Debrided and closed per primum
B. Closed per primum
C. Debrided and closed per secundum
D. Closed per primum debrided and antibiotics

**5. Which of the mycoses is characterized by cervico-facial lesions, abdominal cutaneous fistulae and periappendiceal absceses : UPSC 1986**
A. Blastomycosis B. Actinomycosis
C. Coccidioidomycosis D. Histoplasmosis
E. Moniliasis

**6. Most common infection of the hand is : UPSC 1984**
A. Acute paronychia B. Felcon
C. Web space infection D. Palmar abscess

**7. Leucine aminopeptidase is elevated in obstruction of : AIIMS 1985**
A. Ureter B. Urethra
C. Common bile duct D. Spermatic cord

**8. Hidradenitis suppurative is found to occur in: AIIMS 1986**
A. Axilla B. Circumanal
C. Scalp D. Groin

**9. Bee venom can be neutralised by applying: AMC 1986**
A. Soda bicarbonate B. Vinegar
C. Lemon juice D. Dilute HCL

**10. The most dangerous injury is : AMC 1987**
A. Snake bite B. Scorpion bite
C. Wasp sting D. Human bites

**11. The best site for intramuscular injection is : AMC 1981**
A. Deltoid
B. Anterolateral part of thigh
C. Upper-outer segment of buttocks
D. Upper-inner segment of buttocks

**12. The worst position for scars is : AIIMS 1986**
A. Back B. Shoulder
C. Sternum D. Abdomen

**13. The best scars are formed in———. AMC 1983**
A. Infants B. Children
C. Adults D. Very old people

**14. Commonest cause of cellulitis is : Delhi 1985, 90**
A. Staphylococcus B. Streptococcus
C. E. coli D. Hemophilus

**15. Hyperbaric oxygen is useful in all except : PGI 1983**
A. Tetanus B. Gas gangrene
C. Frostbite D Vincent's angina

**16. Commonest form of actinomycosis is : AIIMS 1983**
A. Facio cervical B. Thoracic
C. Liver D. Right iliac fossa

**17. Globi are seen in ________leprosy. AMC 1983, 89**
A. Tuberculoid B. Lepromatous
C. Borderline lepromatous D. Borderline tuberculoid

| Ans. | | | | | | | | | |
|---|---|---|---|---|---|---|---|---|---|
| 1. E | 2. B | 3. B | 4. C | 5. B | 6. A | 7. C | 8. A | 9. A | 10. D |
| 11. C | 12. C | 13. D | 14. B | 15. D | 16. A | 17. B | | | |

**18. Which of the following organ does not have draining lymph node : TN 1993**
A. Tonsil B. Kidney
C. Liver D. Spleen

**19. In which site is a wound least likely to heal : AI 1993**
A. Dorsal thorax B. Eyelid
C. Upper arm D. Face

**20. Commonest cause of metabolic acidosis in surgical patient is : AI 1993**
A. Enteric fistula
B. Acute circulatory failure
C. Pancreatic fistula
D. Adrenal insufficiency

**21. Smooth muscles are not pain sensitive to : AI 1993**
A. Cutting with knife B. Distension
C. Stretching D. Torsion

**22. Healing is delayed in deficiency of all except : AI 1993**
A. Vitamin-C B. Zn
C. Cu D. Ca++

**23. If there is pus collection in the hand the Rx of choice is : Delhi 1992**
A. Drainage after localization
B. Only antibiotics
C. Drainage irrespective of localization of site
D. Plastering

**24. Oriental sore in commonest on : AIIMS 1986**
A. Genitalia B. Face
C. Chest D. Back

**25. Which of the following is absolutely essential for healing of surgical wound : Delhi 1985**
A. Vitamin-D B. Vitamin-C
C. Carbohydrate D. Balanced diet

**26. The most common abdominal mass in a neonate is : UP 1996**
A. Hydronephrotic kidney
B. Congenital megacolon
C. Wilms tumour
D. Polycystic kidney

**27. Treatment of choice for necrotizing fascitis is : Delhi 1997**
A. Intravenous ciprofloxacin
B. Fasciotomy
C. Metronidazole with broad spectrum antibiotics
D. Anti-gas gangrene serum

**28. Hydatid cyst in the left lobe of the liver in a young man should be : UP 1996**
A. Aspirated percutaneously
B. Removed with the left lobe
C. Excised after injecting it with a scolicidal agent
D. Treated with mebendazole

**29. Fresh clean wounds have no resistance to infection from surface contamination for first ——hours. AMC 1986**
A. 6 B. 12
C. 12 D. 24

**30. All are distension cysts except : WB 1998**
A. Cystic hygroma B. Thyroglossal cyst
C. Epididymal cyst D. Follicular cyst

**31. Bullet wounds near major blood vessels should be explored only if : AMC 1985**
A. The extremity is cold
B. The fingers or toes are paralysed
C. The pulse is weakened
D. There is no pulse
E. In all cases regardless of physical findings

**32. Scalene fat pad biopsy obtains nodes from : AIIMS 1986**
A. Deep cervical chain B. Supraclavicular area
C. Jugular chain D. Carotid sheath chain
E. Superior mediastinum

**33. Most commonly affected peripheral nerve in leprosy is : DNB 1988**
A. Ulnar B. Radial
C. Median D. Lateral popliteal

**34. Moon's molars are seen in : PGI 1981**
A. Syphilis B. Leprosy
C. Amyloidosis D. Actinomycosis

**35. Scrum pox is seen among______players. AIIMS 1983**
A. Football B. Hockey
C. Rugby D. Chess

**36. Which of the following is incorrect regarding carbuncle : UPSC 1983**
A. Staphylococcal infection
B. Diabetes present
C. Males more common
D. Common before age of 40

**37. Sebaceous cyst does not occur in the ———. PGI 1983**
A. Scalp B. Scrotum
C. Back D. Sole

| Ans. | | | | | | | | | |
|---|---|---|---|---|---|---|---|---|---|
| 18. D | 19. A | 20. B | 21. A | 22. D | 23. A | 24. B | 25. B | 26. C | 27. C |
| 28. C | 29. A | 30. C | 31. E | 32. E | 33. A | 34. A | 35. C | 36. D | 37. D |

**38. Which of the following part of the body is not affected by leprosy : AIIMS 1987**
A. Testes B. Ovary
C. Nasal mucosa D. Axilla

**39. What is malignant hydatid disease : AIIMS 1987**
A. Malignant change in hydatid cyst
B. Infection with E. multilocularis
C. Hydatid disease in immunocompromised host
D. None of the above

**40. Hypertrophic scar is : AMC 1986, 87**
A. More common in abdomen
B. Red and become thick white later on
C. Same as keloid
D. None of the above

**41. Cellulitis is infection of : UPSC 1983; AMC 1986**
A. Hair follicles B. Subcutaneous spaces
C. Nailbed D. Any of the above

**42. All of the following interferes with healing except : UPSC 1982; ESI 1985**
A. Jaundice B. Diabetes mellitus
C. Tension D. None of the above

**43. In Filariasis, Elephantiasis is because of : UPSC 1983, 87**
A. Perilymphatic fibrosis
B. Obstruction of lymphatics by adult worm
C. Obstruction and lymphangitis
D. Lymph node inflammation

**44. A ruptured nerve with untidy wound is best sutured in : Delhi 1989**
A. 6 hours B. 1—2 weeks
C. 2—3 weeks D. 4 weeks

**45. Fresh infected incised wound is best treated: Delhi 1986**
A. Washing
B. Washing and debridement
C. Antiserum
D. Antibiotics

**46. Regarding management of lacerated wound which is incorrect : AMC 1987**
A. Damaged skin should be excised
B. Rent in deep fascia meticulously sutured
C. Bad muscle should be removed
D. Fracture should be reduced

**47. Lymph nodes draining a syphilitic chance of the genitalia area are: TN 1990**
A. Bulky B. Firm
C. Soft D. Cystic

**48. Epidermal (Sebaceous) cysts are essentially characterised by one of the following : AIIMS 1987**
A. Punctum
B. Contents consisting of epithelial debris
C. Sebaceous material
D. Intravascular space

**49. Which of the following refers to 'Enzymatic debrima of the wound' : DNB 1988**
A. Hydrogen peroxide B. Streptokinase
C. Hyaluronidase D. None of the above

**50. The normal tensile strength of tissue at the site of wound is gained after : AMC 1985**
A. One week of wound healing
B. Two weeks of wound healing
C. Two months of wound healing
D. Two years of wound healing

**51. A malignant pustule is : UPSC 1987**
A. An infected secondary deposit in the skin
B. A rapidly spreading rodent ulcer
C. An infected molluscum sebaceum
D. Anthrax of the skin

**52. Regarding wound healing which is not true: Delhi 1984**
A. Impaired by radiation
B. Impaired by haematoma
C. Impaired by infection
D. Stimulated by steriods

**53. An antibioma is : DNB 1990**
A. An all powerful antibiotic
B. An antibiotic contaminant
C. A malignant tumour caused by antibiotics
D. An excess mass of fibrous tissue around a small abscess persistantly treated by antibiotics

**54. Commonest cause of wound infection is : Kerala 1996**
A. Staph. aureus
B. Streptococcus pyogenes
C. Pseudomonas
D. E. coli
E. Anaerobes

**55. True about actinomycosis is : Kerala 1996**
A. Does not affect intestine
B. Is caused by fungus
C. Not susceptible to any antibiotics
D. Treatment of choice is amputation
E. Does not affect lymph nodes

| Ans. | | | | | | | | | |
|---|---|---|---|---|---|---|---|---|---|
| 38. B | 39. B | 40. B | 41. B | 42. D | 43. C | 44. D | 45. B | 46. B | 47. C |
| 48. A | 49. C | 50. D | 51. D | 52. D | 53. D | 54. A | 55. B | | |

**56. A patient with grossly contaminated wound presents 12 hours after an accident. His wound should be managed by : UPSC 1996**

A. Through cleaning and primary repair.
B. Through cleaning with debridement of all dead and devitalised tissue without primary closure.
C. Primary closure over a drain.
D. Covering the defect with split skin graft after cleaning.

**57. Consider the following abscesses : UPSC 1996**

1. Scalp abscess 2. Parotid abscess
3. Ischiorectal abscess 4. Inguinal abscess

Among these, one should not wait for fluctuation to develop in the case of :

A. 1 and 2 B. 2 and 3
C. 3 and 4 D. 1 and 4

**W58. Regarding Ludwig's angina, all are true except : AMC 1986**

A. It is streptococcal infection
B. It is an infection of cellular tissue
C. Administration of antibiotics in early stages
D. All of the above

**59. A boil is : AMC 1984**

A. Any abscess of the skin
B. The same as a carbuncle
C. An acute infection of hair follicle
D. An infection of a hair follicle by demodex folliculorum

**60. Contraindications of surgical removal of tuberculous lymphadenitis are : AIIMS 1983**

A. Active tuberculosis elsewhere in the body
B. Discharging sinuses
C. Lymph nodes present in more than one plane
D. Lots of periadenitis
E. All of the above

**61. Operative control of bleeding from wounds of scalp is best done by : PGI 1983**

A. Direct pressure applied to the skin
B. Diathermy to bleeding vessels
C. Eversion
D. Applying several forceps to the bleeding points

**62. A mycotic aneurysm from the aetiological point of view should be related only to : TN 1998**

A. Bacterial infection B. Fungal infection
C. The retinal vessels D. The tympanic artery

**63. Elephantiasis chirurgens is : AMU 1985**

A. Caused due to classical filariasis
B. Is a complication of radial mastectomy
C. It is more common in obese patients
D. A and B
E. B and C

**64. A patient presenting with a pulp abscess of the finger should be treated principally with : Delhi 1982**

A. Penicillin B. Chloramphenicol
C. Incision D. Poulticing

**65. Frost bite affects : Rajasthan 1998**

A. Lip B. Tongue
C. Nose & ear D. Trunk

**66. When performing primary treatment of untidy hand injuries it is essential : AIIMS 1986**

A. To obtain skin closure
B. To repair divided nerves
C. To repair divided tendons
D. To repair divided tendons and nerves

**67. Which of the following is a distension cyst : Kerala 1998**

A. Cystic hygroma B. Bartholin's cyst
C. Sebaceous cyst D. Thyroglossal cyst

**68. Dissecting aneurysm of aorta are common in : AIIMS 1985**

A. Atherosclerosis B. Marfan's syndrome
C. Pulseless disease D. Buergers disease

**69. To what category does the surgical wound belong : Karnataka 1998**

A. Dirty B. Contaminated
C. Non-sterile D. Clean

**70. Pyrexia due to wound infection commonly occurs after : AMU 1987**

A. Third post-operation day
B. Fifth post-operation day
C. Seventh post-operation day
D. Second post-operation day

**71. In wound debridement, the best criterion for determining viability of the tissse is : TN 1989**

A. Tenseness of enveloping fascia
B. Ability to bleed freely when cut
C. Contractility of muscle
D. Colour changes of muscle.

**72. Which of the following is not regained even after complete healing of the wounds : UPSC 1987**

A. Blood supply B. Tensile strength
C. Elasticity D. Nerve supply

**73. Which of the following lays down collagen during wound healing : UPSC 1988**

A. Blood vessel around the wound
B. Epithelial cells
C. Endothelial cells
D. Fibroblasts

| Ans. | 56. B | 57. D | 58. NONE | 59. C | 60. E | 61. C | 62. A | 63. E | 64. C | 65. C |
|---|---|---|---|---|---|---|---|---|---|---|
| | 66. A | 67. A | 68. B | 69. D | 70. B | 71. B | 72. C | 73. D | | |

**74. Furuncle and carbuncle are differentiated by : PGI 1984**

A. Presence of coagulase + ve organisms in the furuncle.
B. Presence of multiple drainage sites in carbuncle.
C. Both are the names of single pathological conditions.
D. None of the above.

**75. Morphine given for injury is primarily : UPSC 1991**

A. A sedative B. An analgesic
C. A diaphoretic D. An emetic

**76. Chronic thick walled pyogenic abscess may be due to the following except : PGI 1982**

A. Presence of a foreign body
B. Prolonged antibiotic therapy
C. Virulent strains of organism
D. Inadequate drainage

**77. Following are true of erysipelas except : AIIMS 1982**

A. Streptococcal infection
B. Contagious and infectious
C. Margins are raised
D. Common in tropics

**78. The following tumours in human being are believed to be of viral origin except : AIIMS 1985 ; PGI 1994**

A. Hodgkin's disease
B. Hepatocarcinoma
C. Nasopharyngeal carcinoma
D. Uterine cervical carcinoma

**79. Following clinical states predispose to carbuncle formation except : AIIMS 1987, 89**

A. Diabetes mellitus B. Uraemia
C. Jaundice D. Steroid therapy

**80. Which of the following is not a staphylococcal infection : AIIMS 1983; PGI 1986**

A. Furuncle B. Carbuncle
C. Impetigo D. Sebaceous cyst

**81. The most common cranial nerves involved in leprosy (neutiric type) are : PGI 1987**

A. V, VI B. V, VII
C. VI, VII D. IV, V
E. VI, VIII

**82. A farmer with ulcer induratė on leg with multiple sinuses discharging granules, most likely diagnosis is: AIIMS 1994**

A. Mycetoma B. Scrofuloderma
C. Lupus vulgaris D. Actinomycosis

**83. Bacterigras is highly effective against: DNB 1989**

A. Staph. aureus infection
B. Streptococcal infection
C. Pseudomonas infection
D. Candidiasis

**84. The contaminated wound is treated by all except : PGI 1982; AMC 1987, 88**

A. Primary closure
B. Haemostasis
C. Injection tetanus toxoid
D. Debridement

**85. Which of the following characterise a Dermoid Cyst: Karnataka 1996**

A. Cheesy material
B. Presence of chorionic epithelium
C. Tooth
D. Air

**86. All of the following are functions of endocyst of hydatid cyst, except : Delhi 1991, 94**

A. Secretion of hydatid fluid
B. Formation of ectrocyst
C. Formation of pericyst
D. Formation of Brood capsule

**87. In Ludwig's angina, the danger is : AMC 1983, 84, 87**

A. Cardiac arrythmias B. Convulsions
C. Glottic oedema D. Pulmonary oedema

**88. Injuries to extensor tendon of hand is treated by : AI 1994**

A. Primary suturing B. Secondary suturing
C. Excision D. Only plaster

**89. The most frequent source of Gram negative infection is from the : Karnataka 1993**

A. Respiratory system
B. Genitourinary system
C. Gastrointestinal system
D. Soft tissue infections

**90. The phase of preparation in wound healing when there is no recordable tensile strength lasts for : Karnataka 1993**

A. 1—4 days B. 4—10 days
C. 10—20 days D. More than 20 days

**91. The most important factor in maintenance of oxygen supply and delivery to the wound is : Karnataka 1993**

A. Blood volume B. Blood Viscosity
C. Pulmonary function D. Cardiac function

| Ans. | 74. B | 75. B | 76. C | 77. D | 78. A | 79. C | 80. D | 81. B | 82. A | 83. A |
|---|---|---|---|---|---|---|---|---|---|---|
| | 84. C | 85. C | 86. C | 87. C | 88. A | 89. B | 90. C | 91. C | | |

**92. Life and limb threatening infections are found in : UPSC 1994**

I. Necrotising fascitis
II. Clostridial gangrene
III. Progressive synergitic bacterial gangrene
IV. Phlegmasia cerulea dolens

A. I, II and III B. I, II and IV
C. I, III and IV D. II, III and IV are correct

**93. Wound contraction is caused by : PGI 1993**

A. Fibroblasts B. Myofibroblasts
C. Smooth muscle fibres D. Macrophages

**94. Keloid is best treated by : UPSC 1995**

A. Intrakeloidal injection of triamcinolone
B. Wide excision and skin grafting
C. Wide excision and suturing
D. Deep X-ray therapy

**95. A carbuncle is ideally treated by : UPSC 1995**

A. Incision and drainage
B. Cruciate incision and deroofing
C. Antibiotics alone
D. Wide excision

**96. Epitheloid granulomas are characteristic of : Rajasthan 1989**

A. TB
B. Sarcoidosis
C. Eosinophilic granuloma
D. Mycosis fungoides

**97. Wound healing is delayed in all of the following, except : Delhi 1994; Rajasthan 1994**

A. Elderly individual B. Newborn baby
C. Uraemic patient D. Jaundiced patient

**98. Necrotising granuloma is seen in : Delhi 1996**

A. TB B. Sarcoidosis
C. Syphilis D. Brucellosis

**99. Which of the following statement is true about Vincent's angina : Delhi 1997**

A. Caused by anaeobic, gram negative organisms.
B. Tonsillar infection occurs mainly.
C. Treatment is with penicillin and metronidazole.
D. All of the above.

**100. The condition in which disruption of a post-operative abdominal wound is likely to occur in : Orissa 1999**

A. When sutured with alloy steel wire
B. Hypoproteinemia
C. Vitamin-A deficiency
D. Vitamin-D deficiency

**101. In the healing of a clean wound the maximum immediate strength of the wound is reached by : Orissa 1999**

A. 2-3 days B. 4-7 days
C. 10-12 days D. 13-18 days

**102. A localised area of redness and swelling with several discharging sinuses is most likely : Orissa 1999**

A. A pyogenic granuloma
B. A sinus
C. An abscess
D. A carbuncle

**103. Regarding prophylactic Antibiotics all are true except : Kerala 2000**

A. Maximal blood and tissue levels should be achieved at Incision before contamination occurs.
B. Empiric choice of antibiotics depends on the expected spectrum of organisms likely to be encountered.
C. Newer wide spectrum antibiotics should be used.
D. Intravenous administration at the time of induction of anaesthesia is optimal.
E. In long operations antibiotics may be repeated 8 and 16 hours later.

**104. I.V. antibiotics for prophylaxis should best be given : DNB 2001**

A. Post-operatively B. Night before surgery
C. With premedication D. Any time

**105. Revised Trauma Score accounts for : UPSC 2001**

A. Respiratory rate, pulse rate and systolic blood pressure.
B. Pulse rate and respiratory rate.
C. Systolic blood pressure and pulse rate.
D. Respiratory rate and systolic blood pressure.

**106. Which one of the following is not included in the treatment of malignant melanoma : UPSC 2005**

A. Radiation B. Surgical excision
C. Chemotherapy D. Immunotherapy

**107. Most likely cause of infection with use of silk sutures is : Delhi 2001**

A. Non-absorbable
B. Cuts through the tissues
C. Bacteria lodge in the interstices
D. Foreign body reaction

**108. Material used in Lepstein's operation : CMC 2001**

A. Steel wire B. Polyethelene mesh
C. Cotton thread D. Catgut

| Ans. | | | | | | | | | |
|---|---|---|---|---|---|---|---|---|---|
| 92. B | 93. B | 94. B | 95. C | 96. D | 97. B | 98. A | 99. D | 100. B | 101. C |
| 102. C | 103. B | 104. B | 105. D | 106. A | 107. C | 108. A | | | |

**109. Complete restoration of tensile strength of the wound compatible to normal tissue takes as long as : UPSC 2002**

A. Two weeks B. Six weeks
C. Six months D. 2 years

**110. Revised Trauma score by Champion include the following except : UPSC 2002**

A. Glasgow coma scale B. Systolic blood pressure
C. Respiratory rate D. Pulse rate

**111. Which one of the following preservatives is used while packing catgut suture : AIIMS 2002**

A. Isopropyl alcohol B. Colloidal iodine
C. Glutaraldehyde D. Hydrogen peroxide

**112. Blackening and tattooing of skin and clothing can be best demonstrated by : AI 2003**

A. Luminol spray B. Infrared photography
C. Ultraviolet light D. Magnifying lens

**113. Which one of the following is not true about carbuncle : UPSC 2003**

A. It is an infective gangrene of the subcutaneous tissue.
B. The most common site is nape of the neck.
C. Appearance is cribriform.
D. The patient is always diabetic.

**114. Which one of the following is not correct regarding chylolymphatic cyst : UPSC 2003**

A. It does not contain chyle very frequently.
B. Enucleation is impossible because its blood supply is same as that of the adjacent intestine.
C. It is the most common mesenteric cyst.
D. It is line by endothelium and has no efferent lymphatic communications.

**115. The most important step in the management of untidy wound is : UPSC 2003**

A. Primary suturing B. Wound excision
C. Antiseptic dressing D. Immediate skin grafting

**116. Following the primary wound closure, epithelialization is complete : UPSC 2003**

A. Within 12 hours B. Within 24 to 48 hours
C. Within 3 to 5 days D. After 7 days

**117. Early stage of trauma is characterised by : AI 2003**

A. Catabolism B. Anabolism
C. Glycogenesis D. Gluconeogenesis

**118. Bed sore is an example of : AI 2003**

A. Tropical ulcer B. Trophic ulcer
C. Venous ulcer D. Post-thrombotic ulcer

**119. Regarding gas gangrene, one of the following is correct: AI 2004**

A. It is due to Clostridium Botulinum infection.
B. Clostridial species are gram-negative spore forming anaerobes.
C. The clinical features are due to the release of protein endotoxin.
D. Gas is invariably present in the muscle compartments.

**120. Which one of the following preservatives is used while packing catgut suture: AI 2004**

A. Isopropyl alcohol B. Colloidal Iodine
C. Glutaraldehyde D. Hydrogen peroxide

**121. Chronically lymphoedematous limb is predisposed to all of the following except: AI 2004**

A. Thickening of the skin
B. Recurrent soft tissue infections
C. Marjolin's ulcer
D. Sarcoma

**122. The most common malignant tumor of adult males in India is: AI 2004**

A. Oropharyngeal carcinoma
B. Gastric carcinoma
C. Colo-rectal carcinoma
D. Lung cancer

**123. The management of fat embolism includes all of the following except: AI 2004**

A. Oxygen
B. Heparinization
C. Low Molecular weight dextran
D. Pulmonary Embolectomy

**124. First treatment of rupture of varicose veins at the ankle should be : AI 2004**

A. Rest in prone position of patient
B. Application of a tourniquet proximally
C. Application of a tourniquet distally
D. Direct Pressure and Elevation

**125. Pancreatitis, pituitary tumor and phaeochromocytoma may be associated with : AI 2004**

A. Medullary carcinoma of the thyroid
B. Papillary carcinoma of the thyroid
C. Anaplastic carcinoma of the thyroid
D. Follicular carcinoma of the thyroid

**126. Persistent vomiting most likely causes : AI 2004**

A. Hyperkalaemia B. Acidic urine excretion
C. Hypochloraemia D. Hyperventilation

**Ans.** 109. C 110. D 111. A 112. B 113. D 114. B 115. B 116. B 117. A 118. B
119. D 120. A 121. C 122. A 123. D 124. D 125. A 126. C

**127. A 70 years old male who has been chewing tobacco for the past 50 years presents with a six months history of a large, fungating, soft papillary lesions in the oral cavity. The lesion has penetrated into the mandible. Lymph nodes are not palpable. Two biopsies taken from the lesion proper show benign appearing papillomatosis with hyperkeratosis and acanthosis infiltrating the subjacent tissues. The most likely diagnosis is: AI 2004**

A. Squamous cell papilloma
B. Squamous cell carcinoma
C. Verrucous carcinoma
D. Malignant mixed tumor

**128. Regarding gas gangrene, one of the following is correct: AI 2004**

A. It is due to Clostridium Botulinum infection.
B. Clostridial species are gram-negative spore forming anaerobes.
C. The clinical features are due to the release of protein endotoxin.
D. Gas is invariably present in the muscle compartment.

**129. Which one of the following preservatives is used while packing catgut suture : AI 2004**

A. Isopropyl alcohol
B. Colloidal Iodine
C. Glutaraldehyde
D. Hydrogen peroxide

**130. Which one of the following is NOT a principle followed in the management of missile injuries : UPSC 2004**

A. Excision of all dead tissues
B. Removal of foreign bodies
C. Removal of fragments of bone
D. Leaving the wound open

**131. An open wound contracts by : Karnataka 2005**

A. Stretching of surround tissues
B. Epithelial growth
C. Skin Grafting
D. Fibroblast proliferation

**132. Surgically used suture material polydioxanone (PDS) : COMEDK-2005**

A. Is non-absorbable and remains encapsulated.
B. Undergoes hydrolysis and complete absorption.
C. Undergoes phagocytosis and enzymatic engradation.
D. Is specifically used for heart valves or synthetic grafts.

**Ans.** **127. C** **128. D** **129. A** **130. C** **131. B** **132. B**

# 1-B. TUMORS, ULCERS

**1. Single pigmented naevi on the hand may be premalignant. They should be : AMU 1987**
A. Left alone B. Cauterized
C. Fulgurated D. Irradiated
E. Excised

**2. A blue-green discharge from an ulcer indicates infection with : AIIMS 1985**
A. Candida albicans
B. Staphylococcus aureus
C. Streptococcus viridans
D. Pseudomonas pyocyaneus
E. None of the above

**3. Maximum normal adult level of alpha fetoprotein is less than———— . DNB 1991**
A. 10 ng/ml B. 12 ng/ml
C. 14 ng/ml D. 16 ng/ml

**4. Hutchinson's freckle is a type of : DNB 1990**
A. Haemangioma B. Fibroma
C. Melanoma D. Lipoma

**5. Raised level of carcinoma-embryonic antigen is seen in : DNB 1990; PGI 1993**
A. Ca.Breast B. Lung Cancer
C. Ovarian Cancer D. Ca. colon

**6. Lesion most likely to undergo malignancy is : TN 1993**
A. Intradermal naevus B. Junctional naevus
C. Actinic dermatitis D. Dermal naevi

**7. Mode of spread of Sarcoma is : TN 1993**
A. Lymphatics B. Blood vessels
C. Nerves D. Direct invasion

**8. Ulcer is defined as : TN 1993**
A. Pus discharging
B. Granulated wound
C. Indurated lesion
D. Discontinuity in the epithelium

**9. Following are causes of non-healing ulcers except : TN 1993**
A. Varicose veins B. CCF
C. Infaction D. Chronic smoking

**10. ↑ incidence with U.V. light exposure causes : Delhi 1992**
A. Basal Cell Ca. B. Sq. cell Ca.
C. Adeno Ca. D. None of the above

**11. Bowen's disease of the skin is : DNB 1989**
A. A type of dermatitis
B. A tumour of sweat glands
C. A premalignant intradermal condition
D. None of the above

**12. Dercum's disease is commonest on : AIIMS 1984**
A. Face B. Arm
C. Back D. Thigh

**13. In internal organs, haemangioma is most commonly seen in : AMU 1980**
A. Liver B. Spleen
C. Kidney D. Heart

**14. Implantation dermoid in the skin is commonly lined by : BHU 1987**
A. Epidermis B. Dermis
C. Sweat gland D. Sebaceous gland
E. None of the above

**15. Which of the following is not true about basal cell carcinoma : Delhi 1997**
A. Most common site is upper part of face.
B. Faster growing malignancy than Sq. cell carcinoma.
C. Lymphatic spread uncommon.
D. Prolonged exposure to sunlight is a predisposing factor.

**16. The term "chemodectoma" denotes a tumour involving the : AIIMS 1985**
A. Adrenal gland B. Pituitary
C. Carotid bodies D. Spinal cord
E. Heart

**17. Melanoma should be excised with a margin of : UPSC 1988**
A. 2 cm B. 5 cm
C. 7 cm D. 10 cm
E. None of the above

| Ans. | 1. E | 2. D | 3. A | 4. C | 5. D | 6. D | 7. B | 8. D | 9. D | 10. A |
|---|---|---|---|---|---|---|---|---|---|---|
| | 11. C | 12. C | 13. A | 14. C | 15. B | 16. C | 17. B | | | |

**18. Strawberry angioma in a child is treated by : Delhi 1984**

A. Masterly inactivity
B. Injection of sclerosants
C. Injection of hot water
D. Excision and skin grafting

**19. The commonest malignancy in man over the age of sixty-five is : AMC 1984**

A. Multiple myeloma
B. Oropharyngeal carcinoma
C. Prostatic carcinoma
D. Carcinoma rectum

**20. Alpha feto protein levels are raised in all except : PGI 1985, 88**

A. Embryonic cell carcinoma
B. Endodermal sinus tumour
C. Hepatoma
D. Fetus

**21. The term universal tumour refers to : AIIMS 1984**

A. Adenoma B. Papilloma
C. Fibroma D. Lipoma

**22. Plexiform neurofibromatosis commonly affects the —— nerve. AIIMS 1983**

A. 7th B. 5th
C. 6th D. 8th

**23. Recurrent fibroid refers to fibrosarcoma arising in : PGI 1983**

A. Uterus B. Scar tissue
C. Ovary D. Muscle

**24. Commonest site for rodent ulcer is : PGI 1982**

A. Inner canthus B. Outer canthus
C. Angle of mouth D. Cheek

**25. Squamous cell carcinoma can arise from: AIIMS 1983**

A. Long standing venous ulcers
B. Chronic lupus vulgaris
C. Rodent ulcer
D. All of the above

**26. Treatment of choice in Giant cell reparative granuloma is : AIIMS 1992**

A. Curettage B. Wide excision
C. Excision D. Radiotherapy

**27. Sebaceous cyst is a : TN 1996**

A. Distension cyst B. Retention cyst
C. Implantation dermoid D. Mucous cyst

**28. Carcinosarcoma is seen in : PGI 1993**

A. Liver B. Uterus
C. Breast D. Skin

**29. An ulcer on the finger with axillary lymphadenopathy suggests infection with : JIPMER 1993**

A. Nocardia B. Coccidoides
C. Sporothrix D. Histoplasma

**30. Prognosis in malignant melanoma is indicated by : JIPMER 1998**

A. Depth of invasion B. Giant cells
C. Colour of lesion D. Site of lesion

**31. Malignant cell in Hodgkin's lymphoma is : PGI 1983**

A. Reed Sternberg cell B. Lymphocytes
C. Histiocytes D. Reticulum cells

**32. Rodent ulcer is : UPSC 1983; AMC 1986**

A. Squamous cell carcinoma
B. Basal cell carcinoma
C. TB ulcer
D. Ulcer in Hodgkin's

**33. The TNM classification for malignancies is a : Bihar 1998**

A. Clinical classification
B. Clinicoradiological classification
C. Histological classification
D. Radiological classification

**W34. All of the following metastasize to lymph nodes in neck, except : AI 1996**

A. Ca. tongue B. Ca. pharynx
C. Ca. cheek D. Ca. vocal cords

**35. The malignant tumours that spread by predominantly by vascular permeation is : PGI 1981**

A. Carcinoma of the breast
B. Lymphosarcoma
C. Renal cell carcinoma
D. Basal cell carcinoma

**36. True about leukoplakia : Delhi 1989**

A. Is premalignant
B. Aspergillus infection
C. Gonorrhoea is a rare cause
D. Smoking is a rare cause

**37. Which of the following is premalignant : Delhi 1986**

A. Angular stomatitis
B. Leukoplaqia vulva
C. Glandular hypertrophy of stomach
D. All of the above

**38. Margins of squamous cell carcinoma are : Delhi 1986**

A. Inverted B. Everted
C. Rolled D. Undermined

| Ans. | | | | | | | | | | |
|---|---|---|---|---|---|---|---|---|---|---|
| | 18. A | 19. C | 20. B | 21. D | 22. B | 23. D | 24. A | 25. D | 26. B | 27. B |
| | 28. B | 29. C | 30. A | 31. A | 32. B | 33. A | 34. NONE | 35. C | 36. A | 37. B |
| | 38. B | | | | | | | | | |

**39. Keloid is common in : Delhi 1986**
A. Dark people B. Pregnancy
C. Tuberculosis D. All of the above

**40. All of the following are benign tumors except : AI 1996**
A. Chondroma B. Chordoma
C. Synovioma D. Neurolemma

**41. Ultimate difference in benign and malignant tumours is : Delhi 1985**
A. Local infilteration B. Metastasis
C. Mitotic Figures D. Death

**42. Apudomas can arise from the following except: PGI 1987**
A. Pancreas B. Skin
C. Intestine D. Lymphnodes

**43. Steriod therapy is useful in one of the following haemangioma : AMU 1986**
A. Cavernous B. Capillary
C. Strawberry D. Haemangiomas of adult

**44. A tuberculous ulcer has: AP 1990**
A. Shelving edge B. A rolled adge
C. An undermined edge D. An everted edge

**45. Implantation dermoid is useful noticed in cases of : DNB 1989**
A. Pricking due to blunt needle
B. Pricking due to sharp needle
C. Amputation stump
D. Incised wound
E. None of the above

**46. A lustreless black lesion under the great toe nail of a 50 years old patient, noticed for three months is likely to be : UPSC 1985**
A. Sub-lingual haematoma
B. Glomus tumour
C. Malignant melanoma
D. Chronic paronychia

**47. Secondaries are not seen in : Rajasthan 1998**
A. Breast B. Brain
C. Lung D. Testis

**48. A decubitus ulcer is : AMC 1987**
A. A venous ulcer
B. An ulcer in the region of the elbow
C. A pressure sore
D. An ulcer of the tongue

**49. Neuroblastoma may arise at any of following sites except : AMU 1990**
A. Posterior mediastinum B. Adrenals
C. Cervical region D. Brain

**50. Which of the following neoplasms has a definite tendency to run in families : MAHE 1994**
A. Astrocytoma
B. Carcinoma of the prostate
C. Multiple adenomatous polyps of the colon
D. Osteogenic sarcoma

**51. The treatment of a malignant melanoma should include all of the following except : MAHE 1994**
A. Wide excision of the tumour.
B. En bloc removal of the adjacent, involved lymph nodes.
C. Immediate excision of any enlarging lymph node in the post-operative period.
D. Post-operative radiotherapy to the surgical area and the adjacent lymph nodes.

**52. Grossly visible venous invasion is a characteristic feature of carcinoma of the : MAHE 1995**
A. Breast B. Colon
C. Kidney D. Ovary

**53. The following tumor has multicentric origin : TN 1989**
A. Basal cell carcinoma
B. Malignant melanoma
C. Squamous cell carcinoma
D. Lymphatic leukemia

**54. All of the following regarding rodent ulcers are correct excepts : UPSC 1985**
A. No lymph nodal involvement
B. Common on face
C. It is radiosensitive
D. Epithelial pearl formation is seen

**55. Regarding glomus tumour, which of the following is not true : AMU 1986, 92; DNB 1996**
A. It is a red/purple nodule under digital nail
B. It is painless
C. It resembles a naevus
D. Histologically, it is angiomyoneuroma

**56. The floor of a tuberculous ulcer will be seen to contain : UPSC 1985**
A. Apple jelly granulation
B. A wash-leather slough
C. Strawberry granulations
D. Fat

**57. Commonest cancer in males in India is of : UPSC 1984; AIIMS 1985, 86, 89**
A. Bronchus B. Stomach
C. Head and neck area D. Urinary bladder

| Ans. | | | | | | | | | |
|---|---|---|---|---|---|---|---|---|---|
| 39. A | 40. B | 41. B | 42. D | 43. C | 44. C | 45. A | 46. C | 47. D | 48. C |
| 49. D | 50. C | 51. D | 52. C | 53. D | 54. D | 55. B | 56. A | 57. C | |

**58. In which of the following, metastasis disappears if primary is removed surgically : AIIMS 1985**
A. Colon B. Kidney
C. Melanoma D. Lung

**59. Common cause of enlargement of inguinal lymph nodes is : PGI 1985; AIIMS 1985**
A. Melanoma foot
B. Carcinoma prostate
C. Adenocarcinoma rectum
D. Carcinoma cervix

**60. The best result in treatment of capillary naevus have been achieved by : AIIMS 1987, 88**
A. Using full thickness of skin graft
B. Dermabrasion
C. Tatooing
D. Argon laser treatment

**61. Familial tendency is seen in following except : JIPMER 1997**
A. Ca breast B. Ca stomach
C. Ca colon D. Ca larynx

**62. Metastatic carcinomatous lymph nodes are : UPSC 1986**
A. Soft and matted B. Soft and fluctuant
C. Very hard D. None of the above

**63. Commonest benign soft tumor is : AIIMS 1990**
A. Lipoma B. Leiomyoma
C. Hamartoma D. Fibroma

**64. Commonest site of lymphangiosarcoma is : Delhi 1998**
A. Retroperitoneum
B. Post-mastectomy edema of arm
C. Liver
D. Spleen

**65. Trophic ulcer is seen in all except: PGI 1983, 90**
A. Subacute combined degeneration
B. Leprosy
C. Syringomyelia
D. Disc prolapse
E. None of the above

**66. Prophylactic LN resection is done in : AIIMS 1998**
A. Liposarcoma
B. Fibrosarcoma
C. Embryonal rhabdomyosarcoma
D. Leiomyosarcoma

**67. All are features of Gummatous ulcer except : AP 1996**
A. Punched out edges B. Syphilitic in nature
C. Wash leather slough D. Erythematous base

**68. The most common cause of death in Kaposi's sarcoma is : Karnataka 1997**
A. Dissemination
B. AIDS
C. Massive pulmonary haemorrhage
D. Diabetes mellitus

**69. Which is not a neoplasm : Kerala 1997**
A. Pott's puffy tumour B. Sarcoma
C. Carcinoma D. Papilloma

**70. The commonest neoplasm in an adult is : Kerala 1997**
A. Sarcoma B. Papilloma
C. Teratoma D. Carcinoma

**71. Glomus tumor is usually found around finger nails or: DNB 1989**
A. Tongue B. Eye
C. Ears D. Umbilicus

**72. The edge of a basal cell carcinoma is : Karnataka 1987**
A. Sloping B. Everted
C. Undermined D. None of the above

**73. Treatment of Desmoid tumor is : AIIMS 1993**
A. Surgery B. Radiotherapy
C. Radio + chemotherapy D. Conservative treatment

**74. Which is not a tumor marker : AIIMS 1994**
A. Beta-2 macroglobulin
B. CEA
C. Alpha fetoprotein
D. HCG

**75. Match list-I with II and select in correct answer using the codes give below the lists : UPSC 1994**

| List-I (Types of ulcers) | List-II (Features of ulcers) |
|---|---|
| I. Carcinomatous ulcer | (i) Slightly raised edges with minute venules to the edge |
| II. Rodent ulcer | (ii) Everted and indurated edges |
| III. Chronic venous ulcer | (iii) Undermined edges |
| IV. Tuberculous ulcer | (iv) Slopping edges |
| | (v) Punched out edges and painless |

A. I (v) II (iii) III (i) IV (ii)
B. I (iv) II (ii) III (v) IV (i)
C. I (ii) II (i) III (iv) IV (iii)
D. I (ii) II (iv) III (i) IV (iii)

| Ans. | 58. C | 59. A | 60. A | 61. D | 62. D | 63. A | 64. B | 65. A | 66. C | 67. A |
|---|---|---|---|---|---|---|---|---|---|---|
| | 68. C | 69. A | 70. A | 71. C | 72. D | 73. A | 74. A | 75. C | | |

**76. Match List-I with List-II and select the correct answer using the codes given below the lists : UPSC 1994**

| List-I (Tumour markers) | List-II (Diseases) |
|---|---|
| I. Calcitonin | (i) Secondaries liver |
| II. Alphafoetoprotein | (ii) Medullary carcinoma thyroid |
| III. Carcinoembryonic antigen | (iii) Malignant teratoma of yolk sac |
| IV. Alkaline phosphatase | (iv) Seminoma |
| | (v) Carcinoma colon |

A. I (i) II (ii) III (iii) IV (iv)
B. I (ii) II (iii) III (v) IV (i)
C. I (i) II (iii) III (iv) IV (ii)
D. I (ii) II (i) III (v) IV (iv)

**77. A 32-years old mother of three children had noticed a dark discolouration under her right thumb nail for the past six months. The nail finally came off and was replaced by a draining ulcerated area with enlarged nodes appearing in the axilla. The most likely diagnosis is : UPSC 1994**
A. Melanoma
B. Phalangeal osteomyelitis
C. Sublingual haematoma
D. Glomus tumour

**78. Not a premalignant ulcer : Kerala 1994**
A. Bazin's ulcer
B. Paget's disease of nipple
C. Marjolin's ulcer
D. Lupus vulgaris

**79. Following are signs of internal malignancy except : PGI 1997**
A. Tuberous sclerosis B. Acanthosis nigricans
C. Dermatomyositis D. All of the above

**80. Sq. cell carcinoma is associated with : PGI 1997**
A. Bowen's disease B. Seborrhoeic keratosis
C. Lichen planus D. Pemphigus vulgaris

**81. The following organs have the lining of stratified squamous epithelium except : PGI 1994**
A. Ureter B. Pharynx
C. Vagina D. Oesophagus

**82. Most common site for lipoma to become malignant is : PGI 1994**
A. Neck B. Retroperitoneum
C. Legs D. Viscera

**83. Which of the following neurofibroma is potentially threatening : PGI 1994**
A. Multiple neurofibromatosis
B. Acoustic neuroma
C. Plexiform neurofibromatosis
D. Generalised neurofibroma

**84. Evidence of early malignant change in a pigmented mole is : Delhi 1991, DNB 1994**
A. Itching B. Rapid increase in size
C. Satellite nodules D. All of the above

**85. Which of the following is not a feature of Marjolin's ulcer : Delhi 1984, 87; JIPMER 1992**
A. Slow growth B. Found on previous scar
C. Early metastatis D. Painless

**86. Glomus tumor is found in : Delhi 1996**
A. Adrenal gland B. Finger nails
C. Liver D. Pituitary

**87. Carcinoma not metastases to brain is of : Delhi 1996**
A. Nasopharynx B. Breast
C. Lungs D. Liver

**88. True about chemodectoma is all, except : Rohtak 1996**
A. Lingual nerve palsy is often seen
B. Origin from carotid
C. Distant metastasis is rare
D. Radioresistant

**89. Generalized lymphadenopathy is seen in following except : AMC 1993, 94**
A. CLL
B. CML
C. Hodgkin's lymphoma
D. Non-Hodgkin's lymphoma

**90. In Hodgkin's lymphoma, most commonly affected lymph nodes are : AMC 1993; DNB 1995**
A. Axillary B. Cervical
C. Mediastinal D. Abdominal

**91. Which of the following metastasises to lymph nodes : AI 1997**
A. Histiocytoma
B. Angiosarcoma
C. Fibrosarcoma
D. Cavernous haemangioma

**92. CEA is increased in all except: AP 1999**
A. Lung Ca B. Melanoma
C. Pancreatic Ca D. Colorectal Ca

**93. Most common site of malignant melanoma in males is : Kerala 1999**
A. Trunk B. Lower limb
C. Toe D. Back

| Ans. | | | | | | | | | |
|---|---|---|---|---|---|---|---|---|---|
| 76. D | 77. A | 78. A | 79. A | 80. A | 81. A | 82. B | 83. B | 84. D | 85. C |
| 86. B | 87. A | 88. A | 89. B | 90. B | 91. B | 92. B | 93. A | | |

**94. All are true about malignant melanoma except : Kerala 1999**

A. Spontaneous regression
B. More in males
C. More common in albinism
D. Hentige maligna is least malignant

**95. Which one of the following statements is true in respect of stage-III pressure sore: UPSC 2000**

A. Partial thickness skin loss that involves the epidermis and or dermis.
B. Full thickness skin loss and or necrosis of subcutaneous tissue that may extend to, but not through underlying fascia.
C. Full thickness skin loss associated with extensive destruction, tissue necrosis of muscle, bone or tendon.
D. Non-blanchable erythema of intact skin.

**96. Neurofibromatosis-I is associated with all except : PGI 2000**

A. Sphenoid bone aplasia B. Acoustic neuroma
C. Deafness D. Tectal glioma

**97. Neurofibromatosis is associated with : PGI 2000**

A. Phaeochromocytoma B. Pancreatic adenoma
C. Thyroid carcinoma D. Prostatic carcinoma

**98. Consider the following principles: UPSC 2001**

1. Maintenance of nutrition
2. Debridement
3. Rotation flap

Principles involved in the treatment of decubitus ulcer would include :

A. 1, 2 and 3 B. 1 and 2
C. 2 and 3 D. 1 and 3

**99. Most with carcinoma in farmers, reaches & fisherman is : Rohtak 2001**

A. Transitional cell Ca of bladder
B. Melanoma of skin
C. Squamous cell Ca of skin
D. Basal cell carcinoma

**100. Male with solitary nodule Rt side of neck with B/L inguinal LAP with no systemic symptoms : Rohtak 2001**

A. IIIA B. IB
C. IIA D. IIIB

**101. The most common site of lentigo maligna is : AIIMS 2001**

A. Face B. Trunk
C. Palms D. Soles

**102. The nevus that would be persistent throughout life is : AIIMS 2001**

A. Strawberry angioma B. Portwine stain
C. Salmon patch D. Cavernous hemangioma

**103. A 35 years old woman presents with 1x1.5 cm size mass in the upper and outer quadrant of right breast. Her mother dies of ovarian cancer 10 years ago. The most appropriate molecular investigation is : AIIMS 2002**

A. p53 oncogene
B. Her-2 neuoncogene
C. BRCA-1 and 2 oncogene
D. Myc oncogene

**104. Isolated limb perfusion in melanoma is done with : MAHE 2001**

A. Dacarbazine B. Methotrexate
C. Melphalan D. Procarbazine

**105. The most premalignant lesion among the following is : AI 2002**

A. Leukoplakia B. Erythroplakia
C. Metaplasia D. Dysplasia

**106. Sentinel lymph node biopsy in an important part of the management of which of the following conditions : AI 2002**

A. Carcinoma prostate B. Carcinoma breast
C. Carcinoma lung D. Carcinoma nosopharyn

**107. Tongue ulcer with everted edges is : Maharashtra 2000**

A. Aphthous ulcer B. Tubercular
C. Malignant D. Dental

**108. Tumor marker for endodermal sinus tumor is : CMC 2001**

A. CEA
B. AFP
C. Beta-HCG
D. Placental alkaline phophatase

**109. Match list-I (disease conditions) and List-II (tumor markers) and select the correct answer using the codes given below the list : Karnataka 2004**

| List-I | List-II |
|---|---|
| A. Cancer breast | 1. CEA |
| B. Teratoma testis | 2. HER-2 |
| C. Cancer colon | 3. HCG |
| D. Medullary thyroid cancer | 4. Calcification |

Codes :

A. A:2, B:3, C:1, D:4 B. A:4, B:1, C:3, D:2
C. A:2, B:1, C:3, D:4 D. A:4, B:3, C:1, D:2

**110. In the acronym "SWELLING" used for the history and examination of a lump or swelling, letter 'N' stands for: Karnataka 2004**

A Nodes B Noise (Thrill/bruit)
C Numbness D Neurological effects

| Ans. | 94. B | 95. B | 96. B | 97. A | 98. A | 99. C | 100. A | 101. A | 102. B | 103. C |
|---|---|---|---|---|---|---|---|---|---|---|
| | 104. C | 105. B | 106. B | 107. C | 108. B | 109. A | 110. B | | | |

# 1. C. HAEMORRHAGE, SHOCK, FLUIDS, ELECTROLYTES

1. **The mortality rate associated with fat embolism is : AIIMS 1985**
   A. 20-30% B. 30-40%
   C. 60-70% D. 80-90%
   E. 100%
2. **Commonest cause of arteriovenous fistula is : BHU 1986**
   A. Neoplastic invasion B. Congenital
   C. Infection D. Penetrating injury
   E. None of the above
3. **Which of the following is better indicator of need for transfusion : AIIMS 1985**
   A. Urine output B. Haematocrit
   C. Colour of skin D. Clinical examination
4. **Which of the following cations or anions are significantly bound to proteins: AIIMS 1986**
   A. Magnesium B. Calcium
   C. Sodium D. Potassium
5. **The most common cause of defective haemostasis is : Rohtak 1986**
   A. Increased fibrinogen B. Anticoagulants
   C. Factor-VIII deficiency D. Factor-II deficiency
   E. Thrombocytopenia
6. **Fresh frozen plasma may be utilized in which of the following deficiencies : Rohtak 1995**
   A. Classical heamophilia
   B. von Willebrand's disease
   C. Factor-V Deficiency
   D. All of the above
   E. None of the above
7. **Which of the following bacteriae appears most frequently in endotoxic shock : Rohtak 1986**
   A. B. proteuss B. Pseudomonas
   C. Klebsiella D. Staphylococcus aureus
   E. E. coli.
8. **The antibiotic(s) of choice in gram negative septicaemia and endotoxic shock is (are) : AMU 1985**
   A. Tetracycline
   B. Staphcillin and Penicillin
   C. Penicillin and Chloromycetin
   D. Kanamycin or Colymycin
   E. Staphcillin, Kanamycin or Colymycin
9. **The priority system in emergency care of a patient dictates that which of the following should be performed first : BHU 1986**
   A. Control of massive haemorrhage
   B. Initial treatment of shock with vasopressor
   C. Diagnosis testing plus evaluation
   D. Insertion an adequate airway
10. **Deficiency of following elements is seen with Hyperalimentation exept : JIPMER 1993**
    A. Zinc B. Calcium
    C. Phosphates D. Megnesium
11. **Commonest cause of metabolic acidosis in surgical patient is : AI 1993**
    A. Enteric fistula
    B. Acute circulatory failure
    C. Pancreatic fistula
    D. Adrenal insufficiency
12. **A white leg is due to : UPSC 1983**
    A. Lymphatic obstruction.
    B. Femoral vein thrombosis + Lymphatic obstruction.
    C. Vena Cava Thrombosis + Lymphatic Obstruction.
    D. None of the above.
13. **Hyponatremia is characterized by all, except : UPSC 1986**
    A. Mental confusion B. Nausea and vomitting
    C. Weakness D. Low blood pressure
    E. Inhibition of ADH
14. **Which is not a sign of increasing blood loss: AMU 1986**
    A. Increasing Pulse rate
    B. Restlessness
    C. Increasing the pallor
    D. Shallow slow respiration

| Ans. | 1. C | 2. D | 3. A | 4. B | 5. E | 6. A | 7. E | 8. E | 9. D | 10. B |
|---|---|---|---|---|---|---|---|---|---|---|
| | 11. B | 12. B | 13. E | 14. D | | | | | | |

**15. The weight of the patients subsisting entirely on parenteral fluids should: AIIMS 1986**

A. Gain 100 - 200 gm per day.
B. Keep Weight steady
C. Loose 100 -200 gm per day
D. Loose 300 - 500 gm per day

**16. Following blood which is ready for transfusion is to remain for four hours in a warm environment because it : UPSC 1986**

A. Reduces shock
B. Increase shock
C. Favours subsequent hepatitis
D. Encourages bacterial proliferation and septicemia

**17. Excessive nasogastric suction may cause : UPSC1984**

A. Hypokalaemia B. Renal failure
C. Metabolic alkalosis D. All of the above.

**18. BMR in an adult and newborn are about ——ml. of $0_2$/kg/minute respectively : AIIMS 1983**

A. 2-3; 5-8 B. 5-8; 2-3
C. 2-4; 1-2 D. 5-8; 1-2

**19. In an adult, full term infant and preterm baby, blood volumes are ———ml\kg of body weight respectively. AIIMS 1984**

A. 70, 80, 90 B. 90, 80, 70
C. 80, 90, 70 D. 90, 70, 90

**20. Signs of hypocalcemia starts appearing when serum levels of ionized calcium falls below: Rohtak 1985**

A. 8 B. 7
C. 6 D. 4

**21. Hypoglycemia in full term and preterm babies is defined as blood glucose levels below ———mg/dl respectively. AIIMS 1986**

A. 40, 20 B. 20, 40
C. 20, 10 D. 30, 50

**22. Fluid therapy in a patient of shock should begin with : UP 1996**

A. Blood transfusion B. Crystalloid infusion
C. Plasma transfusion D. Lomodex infusion

**23. An intravenous infusion for a patient following gastrectomy should include the following anion : UP 1996**

A. Bicarbonate B. Lactate
C. Phosphate D. Chloride

**24. Stored plasma is deficient in : DNB 1990**

A. Factors 7 and 8 B. Factors 8 and 9
C. Factors 5 and 8 D. Factors 7 and 9
E. None of the above

**25. Hypokalemia is frequently responsible for which of the following : Rohtak 1986**

A. Shortened P-R interval, decrease in P-wave altitude
B. Alkaline urine
C. Paralytic ileus
D. Hyperreflexia
E. Oliguria

**26. Hypocalcemia is frequently found in which of the following states : Rohtak 1986**

A. Hypoprotinaemia B. Hypoxic acidosis
C. Acute pancreatitis D. Magnesium depletion
E. All of the above

**27. The most effective simple screening test for 'bleeders' is : AMU 1987**

A. Peripheral blood smear
B. Whole blood clotting time
C. P.T.T. plus quick test
D. Clot retraction
E. Only A and C

**28. In polycthaemia vera, the most common post-operative complication following major surgery is : AMU 1987**

A. Thrombosis B. Gastric ulcer
C. Diabetes insipidus D. Haemorrhage
E. Renal failure

**29. Coumarin reversal can best be performed with: Rohtak 1986**

A. Blood transfusion B. Vitamin $K_1$
C. Vitamin $K_2$ D. Protamine sulphate
E. Fibrinogen infusion

**30. Which of the following routes of cortisol acetate replacement is least effective : PGI 1984**

A. Intramuscular B. Intravenous
C. Oral D. Rectal suppository

**31. Protein loss after severe trauma occurs because of all of the following, except : AIIMS 1984**

A. Starvation B. Increased catabilism
C. Bed rest D. Fever
E. None of the above

**32. Treatment of septic shock often requires which of the following : BHU 1985**

A. Volume replacement B. Phenoxy benzamine
C. Antibiotics D. Chlorpromazine
E. All of the above

| Ans. | | | | | | | | | | |
|---|---|---|---|---|---|---|---|---|---|---|
| | 15. C | 16. D | 17. D | 18. A | 19. A | 20. D | 21. A | 22. B | 23. D | 24. C |
| | 25. C | 26. E | 27. E | 28. A | 29. B | 30. A | 31. E | 32. E | | |

**33. The disadvantages of elemental diets in children include : PGI 1986**

A. Hypertonic dehydration
B. Lower caloric input than intravenous alimentation
C. Dumping syndrome
D. High nitrogen input
E. All of the above

**34. Complications of total intravenous nutrition include which of the following : AIIMS 1985**

A. Sepsis
B. Pulmonary embolus
C. Hyperosmolar coma
D. Aortic valve endocarditis
E. All of the above

**35. In an acute situation where bleeding is massive and there is no time to type and cross match blood, which of the following should be utilised : PGI 1986**

A. Type AB Rh positive blood
B. O Rh positive
C. O Rh negative
D. A Rh negative
E. Ringer's lactate

**36. Which of the following vitamins appear to be essential in postoperative parenteral therapy : PGI 1986**

A. Vitamin-C B. Vitamin-B
C. Vitamin-D and A D. Vitamin-D
E. Thiamine

**37. Sudden hypovolemia due to haemorrhage is responsible for release of : PGI 1984**

A. Aldosterone B. Tryptophan
C. Testosterone D. Serotonin
E. Thyroxine

**38. Which of the following events occur in acute progressive hypoxema : AMU 1986**

A. Cardiac Failure
B. Excess lactate accumulation
C. Markedly depressed PAO2
D. Respiratory Alkalosis
E. All of the above

**39. Which does not occur in the first week of IV hyperalimentation: PGI 1988; AI 1989**

A. Weight gain B. Uremia
C. Jaundice D. Ketosis

**40. Hypovolemic shock manifest when the percentage of blood loss exceeds : AIIMS 1986; AI 1989**

A. 10% B. 15%
C. 25% D. 30%
E. 40%

**41. Blood clot of the size of clenched fist is roughly equal to : Delhi 1983**

A. 250 ml B. 350 ml
C. 500 ml D. 600 ml

**42. Blood platelets in stored blood do not remain functional after —— hrs. AIIMS 1986**

A. 24 B. 48
C. 72 D. 96

**43. Half life of factor 8 is : AIIMS 1982**

A. 7 hours B. 18 hours
C. 34 hours D. 48 hours

**44. In patients subsisting entirely on parenteral fluids, there is daily weight loss of ——. PGI 1981**

A. 50 gm B. 150 gm
C. 200 gm D. 250 gm

**45. Neurogenic shock is seen in : AMC 1988; JIPMER 1992**

A. Head injury B. Anaesthesia
C. Septicemia D. Peritonitis

**46. Following are used in embolism except : JIPMER 1992**

A. I.V. Heparin
B. Corticosteroids
C. Hyperbaric oxygen
D. Streptokinase

**47. Investigation of choice for diagnosis of deep vein Thrombosis is : AIIMS 1992**

A. Homan's sign B. Doppler
C. Isotope scan D. Venogram

**48. Unilateral hypertrophy and local gigantism is commonly caused by : AIIMS 1992**

A. Neurofibromatosis B. A.V. Fistula
C. Bone tumor D. Lipomatosis

**49. Characteristic ECG feature of Hyperkalemia is : AIIMS 1992, 95, 97**

A. U-Waves B. Narrow QRS complex
C. Tall T-waves D. Short PR interval

**50. Highest concentration of potassium is seen in : AIIMS 1992, 97**

A. Duodenum B. Jejunum
C. Ileum D. Colon

**51. Pulsating varicose vein in a young adult is due to : AIIMS 1992**

A. Deep vein thrombosis
B. Arteriovenous fistula
C. Sapheno femoral incompetence
D. Abdominal tumor

| Ans. | | | | | | | | | |
|---|---|---|---|---|---|---|---|---|---|
| 33. E | 34. E | 35. C | 36. E | 37. A | 38. E | 39. A | 40. B | 41. C | 42. A |
| 43. A | 44. B | 45. B | 46. D | 47. B | 48. B | 49. C | 50. A | 51. B | |

**52. Gastric tetany is due to : PGI 1993**
A. Calcium absorption
B. Increased calcium sequestration
C. Increased intestinal acidity
D. Vagal hyperactivity

**53. The minimum amount of proteins needed for positive nitrogen balance is : PGI 1983, 85**
A. 20-30 gm/day B. 35-40 gm/day
C. 50 gm/day D. 60 gm/day

**54. Hypochloremic alkalosis is a complication of : Delhi 1986**
A. Congenital pyloric stenosis
B. Vomiting
C. Haematemesis
D. Aspirin intoxication

**55. Reactionary haemorrhage is seen : DNB 1987**
A. At the time of operation
B. Within 12 hours operation
C. After more than 10 days
D. After more than one month

**56. All of the following condition are associated with increase in fixed acids in blood except: DNB 1989**
A. Starvation
B. Renal insufficiency
C. Release of claped aorta in the surgery of abdominal aneurysm
D. Cortisone excess

**57. Third space refers to : AP 1990**
A. Extracellular space B. Intracellular space
C. Transcellular space D. Intravascular space

**58. Secondary haemorrhage occurs : AMU 1987**
A. Immediately after operation
B. Within one day of operation
C. Within one-to-two weeks of operation
D. Within six months of operation

**59. Shock due to endotoxins produces all of the following except : AMC 1986**
A. Oliguria B. Low cardiac out put
C. Metabolic acidosis D. Hypokalemia

**60. Haematochezia means passage of ———. TN 1996**
A. Bloody stools B. Tarry stools
C. Bloody urine D. Bloody bile

**61. All of the following are surgical indications of whole blood transfusion except : PGI 1982**
A. During major operative procedure
B. Preoperatively in cases of severe chronic anemia
C. In haemophilic patients before surgery
D. Following severe burns

**62. Respiratory arrest due to respiratory alkalosis is corrected by : UPSC 1985**
A. Immediate tracheostomy
B. Insufflation with Oxygen
C. Insufflation with Carbon dioxide
D. Insufflation with Nitrous oxide

**63. Darrow's solution does not contain : AP 1989**
A. Sodium chloride B. Potassium chloride
C. Sodium bicarbonate D. Molar sodium lactate

**64. In the immediate post-operative period, body potassium is : AMU 1986**
A. Exchanged with calcium
B. Exchanged with magnesium
C. Retained in body
D. Excreted excessively

**65. In the acutely shocked patient, attainment of which of the following is most likely to show adequacy of perfusion of vital organs: AIIMS 1983**
A. Normal urine output
B. Normal arterial oxygen tension
C. Normal bicarbonate levels in the blood
D. Normal arterial blood pressure

**66. Cryoprecipitate is a rich source of : AIIMS 1985**
A. Thromboplastin B. Factor-VIII
C. Factor-X D. Factor-VII

**67. 20 mEq (mmol) of potassium chloride in 500 ml of 5% dextrose solution is given intravenously to treat : AIIMS 1984**
A. Metabolic alkalosis B. Respiratory alkalosis
C. Metabolic acidosis D. Respiratory acidosis

**68. A 45-kg patient presents with BP-70/50 mmHg, Na+ = 115 meq/1. Na+ deficit is to be corrected to 135 meq/L. How many litres of isotonic saline is needed for the patient : CMC 1998**
A. 13 L B. 18 L
C. 23 L D. 27 L

**69. A useful; though temporary improvement in a patient's ischaemic foot can be attained by giving intravenously : Delhi 1984**
A. 10% Mannitol B. 10% Dextrose
C. Dextran 40 D. Dextran 100

**70. Total amounts of fluids to be given within first 24 hours in a patient of 70 kg weight & 40% burns according to Parkland's formula is : PGI 1986**
A. 11,200 cc B. 7,600 cc
C. 7,000 cc D. 5,500 cc

**Ans.** 52. A 53. B 54. A 55. B 56. D 57. A 58. C 59. D 60. A 61. B
62. C 63. C 64. D 65. A 66. B 67. A 68. C 69. C 70. A

**71. In compatible blood transfusion, all are seen except : AIIMS 1986**

A. Bleeding from the wound
B. Thrombophlebitis at the injection site
C. Renal failure
D. Pyrexial reaction

**72. Continued severe pain may cause following except : PGI 1987**

A. Cardiac arrythmias B. ↓ Renal blood flow
C. Nausea and vomiting D. Respiratory failure

**73. In operation theatre tourniquets are used for all of the following conditions except : PGI 1982**

A. To control haemorrhage temporarily while exploration and repair has been done.
B. For some amputations.
C. For amputation in arterio sclerotic gangrene.
D. In order to obtain a bloodless field.

**74. An overdose of Heparin is treated by : DNB 1989**

A. Prostaglandins B. Phenindione
C. Protamine sulphate D. Prostigmine

**75. Maximum tourniquet time for the upper limb is : Delhi 1986**

A. 1/2 hour B. 1 hour
C. 1.5 hours D. 2 hours
E. 2.5 hours

**76. While suspecting a blood transfusion reaction, one should : AMU 1988**

A. Continuing transfusion blood and reasses the patient when whole unit of blood has been transfused.
B. Continue transfusion of blood and inject anti-histaminics and steroids.
C. Withdraw the blood transfusion immediately and give injectable antihistaminics and steroids.
D. Inject calcium gluconate immediately.

**77. Extracellular fluids losses are often extensive in all, except : UPSC 1986**

A. Hepatic coma B. Peritonitis
C. Intestinal obstruction D. Pancreatitis

**78. Of the following which is not the sign of increasing blood loss : AIIMS 1984**

A. Shallow slow breathing
B. Increase pulse rate
C. Increased pallor
D. Restlessness

**79. Which of the following would least likely to occur as an untowards reaction to heparin : AIIMS 1985**

A. Osteoporosis B. Haemorrhage
C. Hypernatremia D. Respiratory distress

**80. The fully developed picture of hypovolemic shock is characterized by the following except : AIIMS 1985**

A. Bradycardia
B. Oliguria
C. Mental dullness
D. Peripheral vasoconstriction

**81. The maximum life of a transfused R.B.C.is: DNB 1989**

A. One hour B. One day
C. 15 days D. 50 days
E. 100 days

**82. Haemorrhage is usually well tolerated in a healthy adult upto a maximum of : CSE 1996**

A. 500 ml B. 750 ml
C. 5% of blood volume D. 10% of blood volume

**83. Consider the following statements regarding haemorrhagic shock : CSE 1997**

1. Normal haematocrit suggests minor bleeding
2. Peripheral vasoconstriction is characteristic
3. Anxiety and sweating are often presents

**Of these statements :**

A. 1 and 2 are correct B. 1 and 3 are correct
C. 2 and 3 are correct D. 1, 2 and 3 are correct

**84. In a patient on anticoagulant therapy, the INR is maintained at : UPSC 2001**

A. 1.5 to 2.5 times the normal
B. 2.5 to 3.5 times the normal
C. 3.5 to 4.5 times the normal
D. 4.5 to 5.5 times the normal

**85. The percentage of the circulating blood volume in the venous system and splanchnic vessels is normally between : AMU 1988**

A. 20-30% B. 40-45%
C. 60-70% D. None of the above

**86. After haemorrhage, lost plasma proteins are replaced by : DNB 1989**

A. The small intestine B. The liver
C. The spleen D. The muscles

**87. Eusol is a : UPSC 1985**

A. Solution of Eugenol.
B. Solution derived from boric acid and bleaching powder.
C. Saline intravenous solution designed for the Europen common market.
D. A type of carbolic acid.

| Ans. | | | | | | | | | |
|---|---|---|---|---|---|---|---|---|---|
| 71. B | 72. D | 73. C | 74. C | 75. C | 76. C | 77. A | 78. A | 79. C | 80. A |
| 81. E | 82. B | 83. C | 84. B | 85. C | 86. B | 87. B | | | |

**88. Albumin infusion for parenteral use is restricted because : AMU 1989**
A. It is costly
B. Carcinogenic
C. Does not raise oncotic pressure
D. Useful in Pyloric stenosis

**89. The fluid of choice in hypovolemic shock is : AIIMS 1984, 86**
A. Ringer lactate
B. Low molecular weight dextran
C. Uncrossed 'O' blood
D. 5% Dextrose

**90. Ringer lactate contains : AIIMS 1985, 86**
A. $Na^+$, $K^+$
B. $Na^+$, $K^+$, $Cl^-$
C. $Na^+$, only
D. $Na^+$, $K^+$, $Cl^-$, $Ca^+$

**91. Stripping of varicose veins of the leg saphenous system is indicated in varicosities with : AIIMS 1985**
A. Deep vein thrombosis
B. Venous ulcer
C. Pregnancy
D. Episodes of thrombophlebitis

**92. The anti-coagulant solution commonly used to store blood is : AIIMS 1986, 87**
A. Heparin
B. EDTA
C. Na-citrate
D. Acid citrate dextrose

**93. Blood transfusion reaction during surgery is mediated by : JIPMER 1997**
A. Pyrexia
B. Hemetemesis
C. Excessive haemorrhage from the wound site
D. Hypertension

**94. All are complications of IV lipid infusion except : AIIMS 1987**
A. Lactic acidosis
B. Ketosis
C. Deterioraton of LFT
D. Thrombocytopenia

**95. In a acute trauma, adequate urine output is : AMC 1985; PGI 1989**
A. 10-15 cc/hour
B. 20-30 cc/hour
C. 30-45 cc/hour
D. 20-25 cc/hour

**96. The decreased in hematocrit is vital if it is less than : AIIMS 1986**
A. 40%
B. 25%
C. 30%
D. 20%

**97. The best method to control severe external haemorrhage is : AIIMS 1983; AMC 1987**
A. Pressure by finger
B. Haemostasis
C. Tourniquet to artery
D. Tourniquet to vein

**98. Mannitol is useful in all of the following except : Karnataka 1996**
A. Tumorogenic edema
B. Vasculogenic edema
C. Hepatic encephalopathy
D. Intracranial haemorrhage

**99. The highest concentration of potassium is in : AIIMS 1985**
A. Plasma
B. Isotonic saline
C. Ringer lactate
D. Darrow's solution

**100. In a patient with shock, which of the following is not seen in late stage : AIIMS 1983, 88; AMC 1987**
A. Peripheral vasoconstriction
B. Bradycardia
C. Hypotension
D. Oliguria

**101. Fluid replacement is indicated in following types of shock except : NIMHANS 1997**
A. Hypovolemic shock
B. Anaphylactic shock
C. Haemorrhagic shock
D. Cardiogenic shock

**102. Crush syndrome is best treated by : AIIMS 1993**
A. Maintaining high urine output
B. Hydrocortisone
C. Acidification of urine
D. 20% Dextrose

**103. The most common hemostatic defect encountered in surgery is : Karnataka 1993**
A. Christmas disease
B. Hemophilia
C. Fibrinolysis
D. Thrombocytopenia

**104. The volume of the various fluid compartments of the body depends on : Karnataka 1993**
A. Body size
B. Weight
C. Sex
D. All of the above

**105. The principal buffers of the extra-cellular fluid space are : Karnataka 1993**
A. Proteins
B. Phosphates
C. Bicarbonate carbonic acid
D. All of the above

**106. Spontaneous bleeding usually occurs with a platelet count of : Karnataka 1993**
A. Less than 50,000 $mm^3$
B. 50,000—75,000/$mm^3$
C. 75,000—1,00,000/$mm^3$
D. 1,00,000—1,50,000/$mm^3$

**Ans.** **88. A** **89. A** **90. D** **91. B** **92. D** **93. C** **94. D** **95. C** **96. D** **97. A**
**98. D** **99. D** **100. B** **101. D** **102. A** **103. D** **104. D** **105. D** **106. A**

**107. Hypochloraemic alkalosis, hypokalemia and paradoxic aciduria occurs in : Karnataka 1993**

A. Salicylate poisoning
B. Hypertrophic pyloric stenosis
C. Diuretic therapy
D. Burns with dehydration

**108. Which one of the following factors does not play a role in fluid retention after injury : UPSC 1994**

A. Antidiuretic hormone B. Capillary permeability
C. Renin D. Hyperglycemia

**109. How long (hours) must a vessel 1-3.5 mm in diameter be ligated to produce haemostasis : DNB 1989**

A. 12 B. 24
C. 48 D. 96

**110. Commonest artery for cannulation is : PGI 1997**

A. Radial B. Ulnar
C. Brachial D. Femoral

**111. The number of calories provided by 3 litres of 5% dextrose solution are : Delhi 1992**

A. 600 calories B. 1000 calories
C. 1600 calories D. 2000 calories

**112. The most important cause of sodium depletion seen in surgical practice is : Delhi 1992, 94**

A. Small intestinal obstruction
B. Severe diarrhoea
C. Adrenocortical insufficiency
D. Bronchial carcinoma

**13. Consider the following statements : UPSC 1997**

The ratio of ankle to brachial systolic pressure reflects :

I. Viability of the diseased limb
II. Non-viable limb
III. Blood flow in the ischaemic areas of skin
IV. Haemodynamic status in relatively large vessels

A. I, II, III B. II, III, IV
C. I, II, IV D. I, III, IV

**114. All of the following are causes of increased coagulability of blood except : PGI 1988**

A. Infections B. After burns
C. Visceral carcinoma D. After haemorrhage

**115. Most excessive bleeding occurs when an artery is : PGI 1995**

A. Completely severed
B. Partially severed
C. Ends are trapped within fracture bone ends
D. Thrombosed

**116. Central venous pressure monitoring is helpful in : UPSC 1997**

A. Regulating the speed and amount of fluid infusion.
B. Regulating the dose of noradrenaline.
C. Deciding the need for plasma infusion.
D. Deciding the requirement for blood transfusion.

**117. The effect of prolonged ascorbic acid depletion in a healing wound is : Orissa 1999**

A. An increase in collagen and reticulum
B. No increase in collagen formation
C. Lack of collagen and reticulum
D. No change in reticulum

**118. By which route is the administration of replacement fluid is preferred : Orissa 1999**

A. Oral B. Intravenous
C. Intramuscular D. Subcutaneous

**119. Consider the following sign(s) : CSE 1999**

1. Increasing pallor
2. Restlessness
3. Air hunger
4. Water-hammer pulse

Haemorrhagic shock due to acute blood loss includes :

A. 1 and 4 B. 1 and 2
C. 1, 2 and 3 D. 2, 3 and 4

**120. The best treatment in a patient with dehydration repeated vomiting and having metabolic alkalosis is : AIIMS 1999**

A. $NH_4Cl$ B. I.V. saline
C. I.V. potassium D. I.V. saline + potassium

**121. 0.5 Lt. blood loss in 30 min. in normal healthy man produces : AIIMS 1999**

A. Increased H.R. with low B.P.
B. Prominently increased H.R.
C. Low B.P., low H.R.
D. Normal B.P. with slightly raised H.R.

**122. Ankle brachial pressure index > 1 is seen in : Kerala 1999**

A. Partial obstruction
B. Impending gangrene
C. Normal lower limb vessels
D. Complete obstruction

**123. MC cause of acute hyponatremia in surgical patients : Kerala 1999**

A. Intestinal obstruction
B. SIADH
C. Appendicitis
D. Cholecystitis

| Ans. | 107. B | 108. A | 109. D | 110. A | 111. A | 112. A | 113. A | 114. B | 115. C | 116. A |
|---|---|---|---|---|---|---|---|---|---|---|
| | 117. C | 118. C | 119. C | 120. A | 121. A | 122. C | 123. A | | | |

**124. Butchers thigh true is : MAHE 1999**

A. Injury to femoral vessels when using a butchers knife
B. Tear of vastus lateralis
C. Tear of Gluteus maximus
D. Sciatic nerve injury Pa

**W125. Consider the following statements:**
**Static nutritional assessment of the preoperative patient consists of: UPSC 2000**

1. Anthropometry
2. Measurement of plasma proteins
3. Estimation of nitrogen balance
4. Estimation of methyl histidine excretion

**Which of the above statements are correct:**

A. 1 and 2 B. 1 and 3
C. 2 and 4 D. 2 and 3

**126. Consider the following statements : UPSC 2000**

During normovolemic haemodilution using plasma volume substitute, gelatine is used :

1. Initially at a higher volume (1.5-2.0 times the volume loss are infused).
2. Because it increases the optimization of fibronectin.
3. Because there is not antithrombotic effects.
4. Because reinfusions are needed more frequently.

Which of these statements are correct :

A. 1, 2 and 3 B. 2, 3 and 4
C. 1, 3 and 4 D. 1, 2 and 4

**127. External haemorrhage is initially best controlled by: JIPMER 2000**

A. Tourniquet B. Elevation of limb
C. Pressure at the site D. Operative treatment

**128. The following transfusion should be given to a patient with obstructive jaundice who is to be operated: JIPMER 2000**

A. Fresh frozen plasma transfusion
B. Whole blood
C. Cryoprecipitate
D. Buffy coated blood

**129. Found in crush syndrome are all except : UP 1999**

A. Cardiac tamponade
B. Myoglobinuria
C. Oligemic shock
D. Dialysis may be life saving in uremia

**130. The following regarding the causes of immediate death following trauma are true except : Kerala 2000**

A. Extensive trauma to the brain
B. Rupture of major air ways
C. Injury to major blood vessels
D. Massive blood loss into the chest
E. Extensive injury to the heart

**131. A Case of blunt trauma, in shock, not responding to IV crystalloids require : AI 2001**

A. Immediate laparotomy
B. Blood transfusion
C. Albumin transfusion
D. Abdominal compression

**132. By definition, what percentage loss of blood is termed as severe haemorrhagic shock : DNB 2001**

A. Below 20 B. 20-40
C. Above 40 D. More than 60

**133. Most common haematological abnormality seen in massive blood transfusion is : Kerala 2001**

A. Dilutional thrombocytopenia
B. Depletion of factor 5
C. Depletion of factor 8
D. All

**134. A person brought to ER with h/o accident 36 hrs back in shock, which is the best method for fluid replacement in this case : Kerala 2001**

A. PCV & ESR B. CVP
C. Pulse & BP D. Clinical assessment

**135. Intra-operative hypothermia is caused by all except : MAHE 2001**

A. Vasoconstriction B. Vasodilation
C. I/V fluids D. None

**136. True regarding the following statements in all except : SGPGI 2002**

A. 500 ml of normal saline contains 77 mEq of Na+.
B. 50 ml 25% dextrose gives 50 kcal of energy.
C. 20 ml 15% potassium chloride contains 40 meq of K+.
D. 10 ml of calcium chloride contains 9 meq of Ca++.

**137. Hypovolemia due to severe blood loss is replenished in emergency by : BHU 2002**

A. Ringer lactate
B. Normal saline
C. Colloid
D. Only by blood after matching

**138. Butchers thigh would refer to : MAHE 2003**

A. Lipodystrophy of subcutaneous tissue.
B. Section of femoral vessels during boning.
C. Rupture of vastus lateralis.
D. Fracture of femur.

**139. Which of the following ions is lost in a patient with severe vomiting : UP 2003**

A. Sodium B. Potassium
C. Chloride D. Hydrogen ions

**Ans.** **124. A** **125. ALL** **126. A** **127. C** **128. A** **129. A** **130. A** **131. A** **132. C** **133. A**
**134. B** **135. C** **136. B** **137. C** **138. B** **139. D**

# 1-D. ANEURYSMS, VARICOSE VEINS, THROMBOEMBOLISM, GANGRENE, LYMPHANGITIS

1. **The etiologic agents of gas gangrene are large Gram positive anaerobic rods that posses a central or subterminal spore. Which of the following cause gas gangrene in man : AIIMS 1984**
   A. Clotridium perfringens
   B. C. novyi
   C. C. septicum
   D. C. histolyticum
   E. All of the following
2. **The most effective arterial substitute for small vessel bypass is : BHU 1986**
   A. Woven Dacron B. Autologous vein
   C. Bovine beterograft D. All of the above
   E. None of the above
3. **Lumbar sympathectomy in Buerger's disease is done for : JIPMER 1993**
   A. Rest pain
   B. Intermittent claudication
   C. Skin ulceration
   D. Gangrene foot
4. **Following are used in the treatment of superficial venous thrombosis except : AIIMS 1992**
   A. Rest and elevation
   B. Treat associated malignancy
   C. Immediate anticoagulation
   D. Analgesics
5. **Migratory Thrombophlebitis is a feature of : AI 1993**
   A. Pancreatitis B. Varicose veins
   C. Pancreatic Ca D. Buerger's disease
6. **Trendelenburg test for varicose veins tests the potency of : Delhi 1992; TN 1993**
   A. Sapheno femoral junction
   B. Deep perforators below knee
   C. Dorsal Tibial Vein
   D. Popliteal vein only
7. **Which of the following would be most likely to be contraindicated in any peripheral arterial disease : PGI 1984.**
   A. Alcohol B. High fat diet
   C. Purines D. Tobacco
8. **Which of the following is most important in the treatment of gas gangrene : AMC 1985**
   A. Penicillin therapy
   B. Anti-gas gangrene serum
   C. Hyperbaric oxygen
   D. Surgical debridement
   E. Blood transfusion
9. **All of the following are true about tetanus, except: UPSC 1985**
   A. There is loss of consciousness during convulsions.
   B. Trismus is the first sign to appear.
   C. Sedative drugs are used to control the convulsions.
   D. Toxins of tetanus do not travel along muscle or tissue planes.
   E. In early stage use of human A.T.S. is very effective.
10. **The best method for diagnosis of Deep vein Thrombosis is : Delhi 1989; Rohtak 1986; JIPMER 1992**
    A. $I^{131}$ Fibrinogen studies
    B. Plethysmography
    C. Contrast phlebography
    D. Doppler examination
11. **The management of traumatic peripheral vein injuries in the lower extremity popliteal injuries should include : AIIMS 1986**
    A. Ligation
    B. End-to-end anastomosis if technically possible
    C. Bypass with autologous vein graft
    D. All of the above
    E. None of the above

**Ans.** 1. E 2. B 3. A 4. C 5. C 6. A 7. D 8. D 9. A 10. D 11. D

**12. Predicting the success rate of an amputation can be done most successfully by : AMC 1989**

A. Doppler studies of vessels above and below operative side.
B. Measurement of skin-blood flow by fluorence comparison of amputation site to normal reference site.
C. Angiography.
D. Thermography.
E. All of the above.

**13. The most ominous kind of pain with peripheral vascular disease is : PGI 1984**

A. Abrupt, constant pain due to arterial occlusion.
B. Intermittent muscle pain due to arterial spasm.
C. Rest pain usually due to tissue necrosis and ischemic neuritis.
D. Burning type of pain due to skin ulceration.
E. Numb type of pain with digital gangrene.

**14. The most serious form of clostridial infection is : PGI 1984**

A. Simple contamination
B. Anaerobic cellulitis
C. Anaerobic myonecrosis
D. Putrefaction
E. All of the above are equal

**15. The commonest cause of aneurysm formation is : UPSC 1982, 83; AMC 1986, 87**

A. Gun shot injury B. Syphilis
C. Congenital factors D. Atherosclerosis

**16. The Cimino shunt is an arterivenous fistula : UPSC 1986**

A. External at the ankle B. External at the wrist
C. Internal at the thigh D. Internal at the wrist

**17. Intermittent claudication is caused by : UPSC 1985**

A. Venous occlusion B. Arterial insufficiency
C. Neural compression D. Muscular dystrophy

**18. The vessels most commonly involved in Thrombo angitis obliterans is : AIIMS 1992**

A. Femoro-popliteal
B. Ilio-femoral
C. Aorto-iliac
D. Anterior and posterior tibial

**19. Lerische syndrome is due to obstruction of: JIPMER 1992**

A. Aortic and iliac arteries
B. Bilateral iliac arteries
C. Both
D. None

**20. Milrory's disease is : JIPMER 1992**

A. Edema due to filariasis
B. Congenital lymphedema
C. Lymphedema following surgery
D. Post-cellulitic lymphedema

**21. Treatment of choice in acute lymphangitis is : AIIMS 1992**

A. Cotrimoxazole B. Cephalexin
C. Erythromycin D. Penicillin

**22. Most common complication of varicose vein stripping is: AIIMS 1992**

A. Infection B. Haemorrhage
C. Ecchymosis D. Thromboembolism

**23. A knitted Dacron artery graft : AIIMS 1984**

A. It not porous
B. Is eventually dissolves by tissue reaction
C. Never gets infected
D. Can be easily incised and the opening resutured

**24. Commonest variety of aneurysm is : Delhi 1983**

A. Fusiform B. Saccular
C. Mycotic D. Dissecting

**25. For aortic graft the best material available is : Delhi 1992**

A. Dacron B. Artery
C. Vein D. None

**26. Predisposition to thromboangitis obliterans is : Delhi 1989**

A. Immobility B. Obesity
C. Atherosclerosis D. Smoking

**27. Diagnosis of abdominal aneurysm : Delhi 1989**

A. Hollowedness in left loin region
B. Fluid thrill or pulsatile mass
C. Visible peristalsis
D. Absence of pulsations in limbs

**28. CCK fistula is between : Delhi 1986**

A. Axillary vein and Axillary artery
B. Profunda femoris and Saphenous vein
C. Operation for Portal Hypertension
D. In aneurysm

**29. Best treatment for established gangrene is : Delhi 1985**

A. Local debridement
B. Antigas gangrene serum
C. Penicillin
D. Amputation

**30. A properly operated varicose vein has a recurrence rate of : Delhi 1984**

A. About 10% B. About 25%
C. About 50% D. Over 60%

| Ans. | | | | | | | | | |
|---|---|---|---|---|---|---|---|---|---|
| 12. B | 13. A | 14. C | 15. D | 16. D | 17. B | 18. D | 19. A | 20. B | 21. D |
| 22. C | 23. D | 24. A | 25. A | 26. D | 27. B | 28. B | 29. D | 30. A | |

31. **All are true incase of Raynaud's disease except: AIIMS 1984**
A. Is a vasospatic condition
B. Bilateral and symmetrical involvement of hands
C. Common in young females
D. The radial pulse is always absent

32. **All of the following statements are true regarding saphenous, except : PGI 1986**
A. Swelling disappears completely when the patient lies down.
B. Unlike hernia there is no impulse felt on coughing.
C. Venous hun can be heard.
D. Fluid thrill is felt when saphenous vein is tapped.

33. **Acute lymphangitis : AMC 1985**
A. Is a common feature of mild bacterial infection
B. Is usually due to streptococcus viridans
C. May by-pass the lymph nodes immediately proximal to the site of infection
D. Should be investigated by emergency lymphangiography.
E. Should be incised without delay and culture swabs taken.

34. **An influence for good in managing a patient with intermittent claudication is : TN 1989**
A. Exercise B. Smoking
C. Sugar D. Steroids

35. **The term 'venous pump' refers to : AMC 1987**
A. The apparatus used for rapid transfusion of blood.
B. Part of autotransfusion apparatus.
C. Musculofascial anatomy and physiology of the calf.
D. The presence of valves in the inferior vena cava.

36. **Thromboendarterectomy is : UPSC 1992**
A. The ideal operation for Buerger's disease
B. The ideal operation for Raynaud's disease
C. Used for carotid artery stenosis
D. The same operation as embolectomy

37. **Rest pain is felt commonly at: UPSC 1989**
A. Great toe B. Foot
C. Calf D. Knee

38. **Operations for varicose veins are best accomplished by : AIIMS 1984, 86**
A. Stripping
B. Multiple subcutaneous ligatures
C. Subfascial ligatures
D. Division and ligation at the sites of a bad leak from the deep to the superficial venous system

39. **The appropriate management of thrombophlebitis of superficial veins is : AIIMS 1984**
A. Supportive bandages and ambulation
B. Supportive bandages and strict bed rest
C. Anticoagulants and bed rest
D. Anticoagulants and ambulation

40. **The best indicator of ischemia is : Kerala 1998**
A. Colour change
B. Colour change and oedema
C. Skin changes
D. Hair loss

41. **DVT is seen in following except : AIIMS 1998**
A. Subungual melanoma B. Lower limb trauma
C. Cushing's syndrome D. Surgery in hip/pelvis

42. **Trendelenburg test is not useful in the diagnosis of : AIIMS 1985, 86**
A. Deep vein thrombosis
B. Valvular incompetence of perforators near knee
C. Saphenous vein to femoral vein junction
D. Wheather saphenous vein ligation is useful or not

43. **Which of the following material is most useful in surgery of popliteal artery block : AIIMS 1984**
A. Gastrex
B. Saphenous vein
C. Autogenous umbilical vein
D. Internal iliac artery

44. **Amputated limb is preserved in : AIIMS 1985, 86**
A. Dry cold B. Cold saline
C. Ringer lactate D. At room temperature

45. **Frost bite of a limb is best treated by : AIIMS 1985, 86**
A. Graduated warming
B. Rapid warming
C. Amputation
D. Lumbar sympathectomy

46. **Amputation is not indicated in : AIIMS 1985, 86**
A. Maduromycosis B. Chronic osteomyelitis
C. Buerger's disease D. Gas gangrene

47. **Which of the following is not a feature of the arterio-venous fistula of a limb : AIIMS 1985, 86**
A. Pain and gangrene
B. Increased in length of limb
C. Congestive heart failure
D. Recurrent bleeding

| Ans. | | | | | | | | | |
|---|---|---|---|---|---|---|---|---|---|
| **31. D** | **32. B** | **33. C** | **34. A** | **35. C** | **36. C** | **37. B** | **38. D** | **39. A** | **40. B** |
| **41. A** | **42. A** | **43. B** | **44. A** | **45. A** | **46. B** | **47. D** | | | |

**48. Which of the following are features of fat embolism except : AIIMS 1986, 87**

A. Lipemia with purpura
B. Dysponea with bacterial pulmonary infiltrate
C. Pulmonary infarction
D. Clouding of consciousness

**49. What is not a feature of aortoiliac obstruction : AIIMS 1987**

A. Poor collaterals
B. Extensive along Ext. iliac artery
C. No palpation of distal pulses
D. Surgery has good prognosis

**50. Differentiation of primary and secondary lymphoedema by lymphangiography is by : DNB 1988; AIIMS 1987**

A. Dilated portions of lymph nodes
B. Back flow
C. Absent lymphatics
D. Foaming pattern of lymph nodes

**51. Portocaval anastomosis is seen in all except : AIIMS 1987**

A. Lower end of oesophagus
B. Around umbilicus
C. Rectum and anal canal
D. Liver

**52. Which of the following measures are taken to prevent post-operative thromboembolism: CSE 1998**

1. Use of elastic stockings and exercise
2. Early ambulation
3. Prophylactic anti-coagulant therapy

**Select the correct answer using the codes given below:**
**Codes :**

A. 1, 2 and 3 B. 1 and 2
C. 2 and 3 D. 1 and 3

**53. Commenest cause of lymphedema in india is : AIIMS 1990**

A. Filariasis B. Radiation
C. Surgery D. Bacterial infection

**54. Following are complications of lymphedema except : PGI 1983, 1990**

A. Thickening of skin
B. Lymphangitis
C. Hypoproteinemia
D. Lymphosarcomatous change

**55. Propagation of the thrombus occurs in thrombosis of : AIIMS 1988; PGI 1989**

A. Vein B. Artery
C. Aorta D. Aneurysm

**56. Commonest cause of thrombophlebitis in upper extrimities is : PGI 1989**

A. Trauma B. Infection
C. Intravenous infusion D. Varicosites

**57. Gangrene great toe is seen in : PGI 1990**

A. Monkeberg's medial sclerosis
B. Atherosclerosis obliterans
C. Infective endocarditis
D. Myocardial infarction

**58. In Buerger's disease, characteristics are all, except : PGI 1990**

A. Above 50 years of age group
B. Episodic exacerbations and remissions
C. Only in males
D. Smokers
E. Neurovascular bundle is involved

**59. The duration of heparin therapy in deep vein thrombosis is : WB 1996**

A. 7-10 days B. 15-20 days
C. 3-4 days D. 1 month

**60. Causative factors in embolization of major arteries are all except: PGI 1986**

A. Mural thrombus following myocardial infarction
B. Ventricular aneurysm
C. Cardiac myxoma
D. Patent ventricular septal defects

**61. Hypotension in a case of gas gangrene is best treated by : JIPMER 1987**

A. Ringer lactate B. Normal saline
C. Plasma D. Whole blood

**62. All of the following are seen in deep vein thrombosis, except : AI 1990**

A. Pain B. Discolouration
C. Swelling D. Claudication

**63. Commonest site of thromboangitis obliterans is : AI 1990**

A. Femoral artery B. Popliteal artery
C. Iliac artery D. Pelvic vessels

**64. Congenital A-V fistulas in the thigh will be associated with all except: PGI 1989**

A. Increased cardiac output
B. Increased skin temperature
C. Gigantism of limb
D. Superficial for venous engorgment

**65. Preferred material for femoropopliteal bypass is: PGI 1989**

A. Dacron B. PTFE
C. Saphenous vein D. Gortex

**Ans.** 48. C 49. A 50. C 51. D 52. A 53. A 54. C 55. A 56. C 57. B
58. A 59. A 60. D 61. D 62. D 63. B 64. B 65. C

66. **The reliable sign of deep vein thrombosis is : Karnataka 1989**
A. Swelling of limb distally
B. Positive Homan's sign
C. Tenderness
D. Dilation of superficial veins

67. **Surgery in varicose vein is contraindicated in : AIIMS 1993**
A. Multiple incompetent perforators
B. Deep vein thrombosis
C. Varicose vein with leg Ulcer
D. All of the above

68. **Investigation of choice in Varicose vein : Kerala 1997**
A. Plethysmography B. Doppler studies
C. Venogram D. CT scan

69. **In the case of a person in whom the varicose veins have ruptured at the ankle, the first treatment would consist of : UPSC 1994**
A. Keeping the patient in a sitting position.
B. Application of a tourniquet proximally.
C. Application of two tourniquets, one proximally and the other distally.
D. Applying direct pressure over the bleeding point.

70. **Which one of the following is not an indication for sympathectomy for ischaemia of the lower limb : UPSC 1994**
A. Claudication
B. Rest pain
C. Ischaemic ulcers
D. Secondary Raynaud's phenomenon

71. **Which of the following is not a risk factor for deep venous thrombosis : UPSC 1995**
A. Duration of surgery more than 30 minutes
B. Prior history of venous thrombosis
C. Age less than forty years
D. Obesity

72. **What percentage of amputated limbs, produce phatom limb pain : Rajasthan 1991**
A. <1% B. 5%
C. 10% D. 35%

73. **Inferior vena cava thrombosis is associated with collaterals with upper trunk. Cause is at : AI 1997**
A. Thoraco abdominal vessels
B. Paraumbilical veins
C. Sup. rectal veins
D. Inf. mesenteric veins

74. **Trendelenburg sign is due to paralysis of : AI 1997**
A. Sup. Gluteal nerve B. Inf. Gluteal nerve
C. Obturator nerve D. Femoral nerve

75. **The most common vein to get thrombosed is the : AIIMS 1999**
A. Long saphenous B. Short saphenous
C. Femoral D. Posterior tibial

76. **Aortic aneurysm now-a-days is commonly due to : MAHE 1999**
A. Atherosclerosis B. Trauma
C. Syphilis D. Congenital

77. **Vicryl, the commonly used suture material is a : UPSC 2000**
A. Homopolymer of polydioxanone
B. Co-polymer of glycolide and lectide
C. Homopolymer of glycolide
D. Homopolymer of lectide

78. **A 42-years old man with previously good health complains of pain in the legs on walking 400 yards. The pain begins in the calf, but spreads to involve the thigh and both buttocks. It disappears on standing for a few minutes. He also suffers from impotence. His legs appear completely normal to inspection. His further treatment would involve : UPSC 2000**
A. Administration of drugs for symptomatic relief
B. Femoropopliteal bypass
C. Aortoiliac bypass
D. Ileo femoral angioplasty

79. **Venocaval occlusion is contraindicated in all except : JIPMER 2000**
A. Septic emboli
B. Femoropopliteal thrombosis
C. Pulmonary emboli
D. Contraindication to anti-coagulants

80. **Grade-I lymphoedema is: JIPMER 2000**
A. Pitting oedema upto ankle
B. Non-pitting oedema upto ankle
C. Pitting oedema upto knee
D. Non-pitting oedema upto knee

81. **Peripheral arterial occlusion (sudden onset) is characterized by all except : PGI 2000**
A. Paresthesia B. Rubor
C. Pallor D. Pain

| Ans. | 66. B | 67. B | 68. C | 69. D | 70. A | 71. C | 72. D | 73. A | 74. A | 75. A |
|---|---|---|---|---|---|---|---|---|---|---|
| | 76. A | 77. B | 78. D | 79. C | 80. C | 81. B | | | | |

**82. Abdominal Aneurysm is characterized by all except : PGI 2000**

A. Elective surgery complication should be < 5% in 30 days.
B. Emergency surgery complication < 10%.
C. Rarely asymptomatic before rupture.
D. Bigger the size it is more prone to rupture.

**83. All of the following are correct about axillary vein thrombosis except : AI 2001**

A. Cervical rib may cause
B. Can be treated with IV anticoagulant
C. Embolectomy done in all cases
D. Can be precipitated by overuse of muscle

**84. An obese patient develops acute oedematous lower limb followings a pelvic surgery. Deep vein thrombosis is suspected. The most useful initial investigation in this case would be: UPSC 2001**

A. Doppler imaging B. Fibrinogen uptake
C. Venography D. Plethysmography

**85. Consider the following statements : UPSC 2001**

Immediate treatment of deep vein thrombosis involves
1. Heparinisation
2. Graduated compression stocking
3. Tissue plasminogen activator

Which of the above statements are correct :
A. 1, 2 and 3 B. 1 and 2
C. 2 and 3 D. 1 and 3

**86. Diabetic gangrene is due in : Rohtak 2001**

A. Decreased distal rèsistance
B. Peripheral neuritis
C. Arteriosclerosis
D. All of the above

**87. Most common complication of aortic aneurysm repair : MAHE 2001**

A. Renal B. Respiratory
C. Metabolic D. Cardiac

**88. A patient presents following road traffic accident with swelling in right inguinal region. Peripheral pulses are normal in the lower limb. On exploration external femoral vein was found to be torn. Treatment of choice is : Delhi 2001**

A. Ligate the two ends of external femoral vein.
B. End-to-end anastomosis of vein.
C. Ligate the femoral artery along with the vein.
D. Repair the vein by a Dacron graft.

**89. All of the following are correct regarding AV fistula except : AI 2001**

A. Arterialisation of the veins
B. Proximal compression causes increase in heart rate
C. Causes arrhythima
D. Cause LV enlargement and LVF

**90. A patient presented with pulsatile varicose veins. The cause is most likely to be : AIIMS 2001**

A. Right ventricular failure
B. Incompetence of the tricuspid valve
C. DVT
D. Klippel-Trenuayay syndrome

**91. All the following are true about claudication except : SGPGI 2002**

A. It appears as a cramp like pain.
B. It can occur on sitting for a long time in a cramped-up position
C. If it occurs in upper limb it is known as writers spasm.
D. It is relieved on taking rest.

**92. Visceral aneurysm is most common in : JIPMER 2002**

A. Splenic-A B. Lt gastric-A
C. Hepatic-A D. Renal-A.

**93. All are seen in thromboangitis obliterans except : AI 2002**

A. Intermittent claudication
B. Migratory superficial thrombophlebitis
C. Raynaud's phenomenon
D. Absent popliteal pulsation

**94. A 59 years old woman had a left femoral venous thrombosis during a pregnancy 30 years ago. The left greater saphenous vein had been stripped at age 21. She now presents with a large non-healing ulceration over the medical calf, which has progress despite bedrest, elevation and use of a suppor stocking. Descending phlebo-graphy of the left leg demonstrates a patient deep venous system with free flow of dye from the groin to foot. The first profunda femoris valve is competent. Appropriate management might include which of the following : AI 2002**

A. Division of the superficial femoral vein in the groin and transplantation of its vein in the below the level of the complement profound valve.
B. Saphenous venous crossover graft win anastomosis of the end of the right saphenous vein into the side of the left common femoral vein.
C. Left iliofemoral venous thromboectomy with creation of a temporary arteriovenous fistula.
D. Subfascial ligation of perforating veins in the left calf.

Ans. 82. B 83. C 84. A 85. D 86. D 87. B 88. A 89. B 90. D 91. C
92. A 93. D 94. A

**95. Injection sclerotherapy for varicose veins is by using: AIIMS 1984**

A. Phenol
B. Absolute alcohol
C. 70% alcohol
D. Ethanolamine oleate

**96. A person suffering from varicose veins of the right lower limb is found to be bleeding profusely from the leg while working. The immediate action required : UPSC 2002**

A. Shift him immediately to the hospital
B. Apply a tourniquet to the thigh
C. Lower the limb and apply pressure bandage
D. Elevate the limb and apply pressure bandage

**97. True about iliac artery aneurysm are all, except : CIP 2001**

A. Manifest as G.I bleeding
B. Isolated aneurysm
C. Continuation of aortic aneurysm
D. Ruptures into sigmoid colon
E. Pulsatile in feeling can be felt by L/R

**98. If a patient with Raynaud's disease immersed his hands in cold water, the hand will : AI 2003**

A. Became red B. Remain unchanged
C. Turn white D. Became Blue

**99. Pseudoclaudication is due to the compression of : AI 2003**

A. Femoral artery B. Femoral nerve
C. Cauda equina D. Popliteal artery

**100. A newborn boy had a soft, fluctuant, tobulated mass on the posterior part of the neck, extending into axilla. The clinical diagnosis is: UPSC 2004**

A. Spring water cyst B. Myelocele
C. Cystic Hygroma D. Bronchial cyst

**101. Match List-I with List-II and select the correct answer using the codes given below the Lists : UPSC 2004**

| List-I | List-II |
|---|---|
| a. Azoospermia | 1. Female inguinal canal |
| b. Gynaecomastia | 2. Indirect inguinal hernia |
| c. Nuck's hernia | 3. Infertility |
| d. Bubonocele | 4. Young males |

**Codes:**

A. a3 b1 c4 d2 B. a2 b4 c1 d3
C. a3 b4 c1 d2 D. a2 b1 c4 d3

**102. Examples of indirect traumatic gangrene are all, except: Karnataka 2004**

A Use of local anaesthetic with adrenaline and tourniquet for digits.
B Pressure of fractured bone on main artery to a limb.
C Thrombosis of large artery following injury.
D That resulting from crush or pressure injury.

**103. Axillary vein thrombosis is NOT a complication of: Karnataka 2004**

A. Thoracic outlet syndrome
B. Simple mastectomy
C. Excessive upper limb exercise
D. Strap-hangers

**104. All hernias involving bowel that reach the stage of vascular compromise, do cause symptoms & signs of intestinal obstruction, except : Karnataka 2005**

A. Sciatic hernia B. Littre's hernia
C. Cloquet's hernia D. Seraffini's hernia

**Ans.** **95. D** **96. D** **97. B** **98. C** **99. D** **100. C** **101. C** **102. D** **103. B** **104. B**

# 1-E. MISCELLANEOUS

1. **Secondary amyloidosis occurs in all except : AIIMS 1982**
   A. Chronic osteomyelitis
   B. Rheumatoid arthritis
   C. Leprosy
   D. Syphilis
2. **The most reliable investigation in amyloid disease is: AIIMS 1982**
   A. Rectal biopsy B. Immunoglobulin assay
   C. Ultrasound D. Urine examination
3. **The preferred airway in acutely unconscious adult patient is : AIIMS 1985**
   A. Tracheostomy
   B. Cuffed endotracheal tube
   C. Uncuffed endotracheal tube
   D. Ambu bag over oral and nasal passage
4. **The most frequent cause of wound infection in trauma cases is : PGI 1982**
   A. Streptococcus B. Staphylococcus
   C. E. Coli D. Pseudomonas
   E. None of the Above
5. **The most significant finding indicating a venomous snake bite is : AIIMS 1986**
   A. Excruciating Pain
   B. Severe Local Oedema
   C. Paralysis of Extremity
   D. Uncontrolled Bleeding
   E. Hypotension
6. **The greatest concentration of anaerobic bacteria within the body is : AMU 1986**
   A. Lung B. Colon
   C. Mouth D. Vagina
   E. Gall bladder
7. **Pitting edema indicates an excess of ——— litres of fluid in tissue spaces. Delhi 1982**
   A. 2.5 B. 3.5
   C. 4.5 D. 5.5
8. **Congenital constriction ring of the leg is treated by : AIIMS 1982, 84**
   A. Excision and resuturing
   B. Excision and skin grafting
   C. Multiple Z plasty
   D. Dermo-fat grafts
9. **Keratoacanthoma is : AIIMS 1984, 85**
   A. A type of basal cell carcinoma
   B. Infected sebaceous cyst
   C. Self-healing nodular lesion with central ulceration
   D. Premalignant disease
10. **Matastatic calcification is not seen in : Delhi 1986**
    A. Kidney Tubules
    B. Fundal Glands of stomach
    C. Alveoli of lungs
    D. Media of Monkeberg degeneration
11. **Clinically a saphena varix is most likely to be confused with: AMU 1987**
    A. Baker's Cyst B. Femoral Hernia
    C. A spermatocele D. A soft sore
12. **Cock's peculiar tumour is synonymous with : UPSC 1987**
    A. Rodent ulcer of the nose
    B. Local osteomyelitis of the cranium
    C. Chronic infection of a sebaceous cyst
    D. Keratin horn of the heel
13. **Sarcoidosis is also known as —— syndrome. DNB 1992**
    A. Scheie's B. Schafer's
    C. Schaumann's D. Schmidt's
14. **A Pott's puffy tumour is : UPSC 1984**
    A. A growth around fracture ankle.
    B. Tuberculosis of spine.
    C. Localised pitting oedema of the scalp with underlying osteomyelitis of part of scalp.
    D. Any of the above.

**Ans.** 1. D 2. A 3. B 4. B 5. A 6. B 7. C 8. C 9. C 10. D 11. B 12. C 13. C 14. C

**15. Match List-I with List-II and select the correct answer using the codes given below the lists :** **UPSC 1996**

| *List-I (Diseases)* | | *List-II (Laboratory test)* |
|---|---|---|
| A. Chorio-carcinoma | 1. | Frei's test |
| B. Hodgkin's disease | 2. | Casoni's test |
| C. Hydatid disease | 3. | Gordon's biological test |
| D. Lymphogranuloma inguinal | 4. | Aschheim Zondek's test |

**Codes :**

| | A | B | C | D |
|---|---|---|---|---|
| A. | 4 | 3 | 2 | 1 |
| B. | 3 | 1 | 2 | 4 |
| C. | 2 | 1 | 3 | 4 |
| D. | 4 | 2 | 3 | 1 |

**16. A port wine stain is :** **UPSC 1985**
A. A premalignant lesion of the skin
B. A type of Melanoma
C. A type of bruishing of the skin
D. A type of haemangioma

**17. Hypothermia induced by an extracorporeal system of cooling is slowest in :** **TN 1987**
A. Muscle B. Brain
C. Rectum D. Oesophagus

**18. Volkman's ischaemic contracture is due to :** **Rajasthan 1998**
A. Trauma B. Brachial artery rupture
C. Tight bandage D. Clostridial infection

**19. Ganglion contains :** **AMC 1983**
A. Mucous material B. Water
C. Blood D. All of the above

**20. An hamartoma is :** **AMC 1987**
A. Any collection of blood clot
B. A haemorrhagic cyst of the thigh
C. A developmental malformation
D. A tumour of muscle

**W21. Ischaemia means :** **PGI 1982**
A. Pain in the ischial tuberosities
B. Anaemia due to malignant secondaries in the ischial part of the pelvis
C. Is alkaline
D. Is never dangerous

**22. Volkman's ischaemic contracture :** **UPSC 1984**
A. Affects the palmar fascia.
B. Develops at the ankle in a case of chronic venous ulcer.
C. Follows ischaemia of the forearm muscles.
D. Is due to excessive scarring of the skin of the arm following a burn.

**23. Pseudo-ainhum is caused by :** **TN 1996**
A. Neural leprosy
B. Syringomyelia
C. Palmoplantar keratoderma
D. All of the above

**24. Viscera are sensitive to :** **AMC 1984**
A. Distension B. Cutting
C. Pain D. Heat

**25. Trench foot is :** **AMC 1987**
A. Sudden infected skin of the foot following the digging of a trench in wet weather.
B. An ischaemic condition of the foot following exposure to damp and cold in tight footwear.
C. Gas gangrene of the foot.
D. Chilblains of the toes.

**26. Purpura may rarely cause :** **AMU 1990**
A. Intussusception B. Volvulus
C. Arterial fibrilation D. Hernia

**27. Salmon patch usually disappears by age :** **UPSC 1985**
A. One month B. One year
C. Puberty D. None of the above

**28. In-growing toe nail is a type of :** **AIIMS 1984**
A. Congenital abnormality
B. Neoplastic process
C. Foreign body reaction
D. Degenerative process

**29. Haemochromatosis usually leads to :** **AIIMS 1985**
A. Carcinoma of liver B. Carcinoma of kidney
C. Carcinoma of lung D. Carcinoma of skin

**30. Hunterian ligation is applied in :** **AMC 1986**
A. Varicose vein leg B. AV fistulae
C. Popliteal aneurysm D. Haemorrhoidectomy

**31. Icterus Praecox :** **TN 1989**
A. Is a form of haemolytic disease of the new born due to ABO blood group incompatibility.
B. Is the other name for the physiological jaundice seen in premature infants.
C. Is haemolytic disease of the newborn due to Rhincompatibility.
D. Is the term applied for any jaundice associated with haemolysis.

**Ans.** **15. A** **16. D** **17. A** **18. C** **19. A** **20. C** **21. NONE** **22. C** **23. D** **24. A**
**25. B** **26. A** **27. B** **28. C** **29. A** **30. C** **31. A**

**32. Irradiation affects wound healing mainly by all of the following except : Delhi 1983**
A. Altering the ability of cells to multiply
B. Producing thrombosis of blood vessels
C. Delays the formation of collagen and callus
D. None of the above

**33. Tendons in tendon repair are immobilized in plaster of Paris for about ——— weeks in flexor tendons and ——— weeks for extensor tendons : AIIMS 1984**
A. 3, 4 B. 4, 3
C. 4, 6 D. 6, 4

**34. Lobster-claw hand is due to : AIIMS 1988**
A. Absence of middle finger
B. Absence of little finger
C. Absence of thumb
D. Supernumerary digits

**35. Constriction rings around a finger is best treated : AIIMS 1988**
A. Within first year of life
B. At 3 years of age
C. At 6 years of age
D. At 8 years of age

**36. Clinodactyly is best treated with : DNB 1990**
A. 'Banjo' splint B. 'Colles' plaster
C. Surgical correction D. No treatment

**37. Clinodactyly (sideways deviation of the fingers) most often involves : DNB 1990**
A. Middle finger B. Thumb
C. Ring finger D. Little finger

**38. Camptodactyly (Congenital flexion of fingers) most commonly involves : AI 1990**
A. Ring finger B. Little finger
C. Thumb D. Index finger

**39. The early sign of Sudeck's atrophy is : AIIMS 1985**
A. Swelling of the whole hand
B. Swelling of the fingers
C. Osteoporosis
D. Shooting pain

**40. Which of the following is least painful : AIIMS 1986**
A. Retropharyngeal abscess
B. Abscess of intralobar fissure of lung
C. Stenosing tenovaginitis
D. Nail bed infection

**41. The capillary haemangiomas are : AMC 1983**
A. Salmon patch B. Port wine stain
C. Strawberry angioma D. All of the above
E. None of the above

**42. Alpha sympathetic blockers are not useful in : AIIMS 1984**
A. Hypotension B. Hypovolemia
C. Phaeochromocytoma D. Buerger's disease

**43. Impotence caused by irradiation is : AIIMS 1984; UPSC 1987**
A. Partial
B. Complete
C. Only impairs erection
D. Only impairs ejaculation

**44. Doppler ultrasonography cannot differentiate between : AIIMS 1984**
A. Fresh and old clot
B. Arterial and venous occlusion
C. Large and small artery thrombosis
D. Progress or regress of thrombosis

**45. A patient undergoes a left scalene node biopsy in the surgical OPD. One hour later he develops cyanosis, dyspnoea and marked tachycardia. The manoeuvre most likely to improve his condition is : CSE 1997**
A. Blood transfusion
B. IV fluids
C. Endotracheal intubation
D. Chest tube insertion on the left side

**46. The commonest site for amyloid deposit among the following is : AIIMS 1985, 86**
A. Lungs B. Large bowel
C. Heart D. Tongue

**47. Which of the following is not a part of Hutchinson's triad : AIIMS 1985, 86**
A. Hutchinson's teeth B. Deafness
C. Retinitis pigmentosa D. Interstitial keratitis

**48. Treatment of choice in Dupuytren's contracture is : AIIMS 1985, 86**
A. Splintage and stretching
B. Local palmar fasciectomy
C. Radical fasciectomy
D. Injection of local anaesthetics

**49. Chronic lymphoedema may lead to all of the following complications except : AIIMS 1986, 87**
A. Recurrent infection B. Lymphangioma
C. Solid oedema D. Marjolin ulcer

**50. Dupuytren's contracture of the hand commonly starts in : UPSC 1986; AMC 1987; AIIMS 1987**
A. Thumb B. Index finger
C. Middle finger D. Ring finger

**Ans.** 32. C 33. B 34. A 35. A 36. D 37. D 38. D 39. A 40. B 41. D
42. A 43. B 44. A 45. D 46. B 47. C 48. B 49. D 50. D

51. **False statement about "ranula" is : Delhi 1998**
A. It is a pseudocyst
B. Lined by epithelium
C. Arises from sublingual gland
D. Appears as translucent bluish swelling

52. **Rise of 1-2°F temperature on paralysed side is : AIIMS 1983, 85**
A. Kocher Cushing sign B. Victor Horsley's sign
C. Guerin's sign D. Coleman's sign

53. **The following muscles increase the arch of the foot by their sole action except : PGI 1990**
A. Tibialis anterior and posterior.
B. Extensor hallucis longus and extensor dig. longus.
C. Peroneus longus and peroneus brevis.
D. Flexor digitorum longus and flexor hallucis longus.

54. **Investigation of choice in a 48 year old with progressive lymphnode enlargement of lift posterior cervical region is : AI 1999**
A. X-ray soft tissue nectic B. FNAC
C. Tuberculin test D. C.T. scan neck

55. **Heat application is contraindicated in : AMC 1987**
A. Trophic ulcer in a paraplegic
B. Obstructive venous drainage
C. Non-inflammatory oedema
D. All of the above

56. **In Dupuytren's contracture, the defect lies in: Delhi 1982, 83, 84; AIIMS 1983, 87; AMC 1984, 89; PGI 1988**
A. Tendon B. Nerve
C. Palmar fascia D. Palmar skin

57. **The commonest cause of fever within 48 hours of surgery is : AIIMS 1981**
A. Atelectasis B. Wound infection
C. Aspiration D. None of the above

58. **All are true regarding Erythromelalgia except : PGI 1993, 94**
A. It is painful
B. Involves the extremities only
C. Marked cutaneous vasoconstriction
D. Redness and mottling of skin are characteristic feature

59. **Maximum excavation is seen in : PGI 1994**
A. Scrofuloderma B. Lupus Vulgaris
C. TB of kidney D. TB of Thyroid

60. **Commonest cause of unilateral pedal oedema in India is : AI 1990; Delhi 1993; UPSC 1993**
A. Filariasis B. Post-traumatic
C. Deep vein thrombosis D. Osteosarcoma

61. **Which of the following is not a sign of cervical cord compression : Delhi 1992, 94**
A. Rising blood pressure
B. Tachycardia
C. Slowing respiration
D. Deterioration in level of consciousness

62. **Virchow's lymph node is located in : Delhi 1994**
A. Axilla
B. Inguinal region
C. Popliteal region
D. Left supraclavicular space

63. **Transillumination is negative in : PGI 1995**
A. Polymicrogyria B. Hydrocele
C. Cystic hygroma D. All of the above

64. **Lymph flow is —— ml/hour. Rohtak 1995**
A. 50 B. 85
C. 120 D. 200

65. **Common presentation of Zenker's diverticulum : AIIMS 1996**
A. Dysphagia
B. Gastroesophageal reflux
C. Aspiration pneumonia
D. Wheezing

66. **An 11 years old child has a lesion that starts clearing from the centre is : AI 1997**
A. Cavernous haemangioma
B. Strawberry angioma
C. Portwine stain
D. All of the above

67. **Acral lentiginous disease, good prognosis is denoted by : AI 1997**
A. Less size B. Duration of growth
C. Lymphadenopathy D. Colour

68. **Left Supraclavicular Lymphnode is enlarged in : Karnataka 1999**
A. Malignancy B. Syphilis
C. Kala Azar D. Sore throat

69. **A boy presented with a bluish swelling on his left upper eye lid which appeared at 3 months & disappeared at 1 year, most likely cause is : AI 2000**
A. Capillary hemangioma
B. Sebaceous cyst
C. Chalazion
D. Dermoid cyst

70. **Found in rhabdomyolysis is all except : UP 1999**
A. Kidney damage/ARF B. Increased CPK
C. Hypervolemia D. Myoglobinuria

| Ans. | | | | | | | | | |
|---|---|---|---|---|---|---|---|---|---|
| 51. B | 52. B | 53. D | 54. B | 55. D | 56. C | 57. A | 58. B | 59. A | 60. A |
| 61. B | 62. D | 63. A | 64. C | 65. B | 66. B | 67. A | 68. A | 69. A | 70. C |

**71. Degloving injury is : Kerala 2000**
A. Surgeon made wound B. Lacerated wound
C. Blunt injury D. Avulsion injury
E. Abrasive wound

**72. All the following are cutaneous horns except : Kerala 2000**
A. Nail horns B. Cicatrix horns
C. Sebaceous horns D. Wart or corn horns
E. Molluscum horns

**73. Liver Biopsy (Needle biopsy) is contraindicated in all, except : TNPSC 2000**
A. Right pleural space infection
B. Lax ascitis
C. Septic cholangitis
D. P.T. prolonged by 3 seconds

**74. Malignant cells in the peritoneum are due to : MAHE 2001**
A. Gravity B. Capillary permeability
C. Angiogenesis D. All of the above

**75. In a surgery post-op ward, a patient developed wound infection within 48 hours of his surgery. Subsequently 3 other patients developed similar infections in the ward. The most effective way of preventing these are : AIIMS 2001**
A. Fumigation of the ward
B. Wash OT instruments with 1% perchlorate
C. Hand-washing of all staff personnel
D. Prophylactic antibiotics

**76. A patient had increased pulsations of the lower limb veins and local gigantum of the leg. The most probable etiology is : AIIMS 2001**
A. Tumor
B. AV fistula
C. Incompetence of the saphenofemoral junction
D. Varicose veins

**77. Psoas sheath is contiguous with : JIPMER 2002**
A. External oblique muscle
B. Transversalis fascia
C. Transversus abdominis
D. Rectus abdominis

**78. A patient is admitted to the hospital with burns. The young intern doing a saphenous cut down noted that the patient developed pain and paresthesia along the dorsomedial aspect of the leg following the procedure. The nerve most likely to have been involved is : AI 2002**
A. Saphenous nerve
B. Sural nerve
C. Superficial peroneal nerve
D. Deep peroneal nerve

**79. First surgeon to get a noble prize was : BHU 2002**
A. J. Lister B. William Halsted
C. Theodore Kocher D. Billroth

**80. White persistent patch in mouth indicates : Maharashtra 2002**
A. Mucormycosis B. Streptococcal infection
C. Erythroplakia D. All of the above

**81. A 15 years old healthy boy with no major medical problem complaints that he breaks out with blocky areas of erythema that are pruritic over skin of his arm, leg, trunk, everytime within an hour of eating sea foods. The clinical features are suggestive of : AI 2003**
A. Localised immune-complex deposition
B. Cell mediated hypersensitivity
C. Localized anaphylaxis
D. Release of complement C3b

**82. Which one at the following is not correct about ainhum : UPSC 2003**
A. It occurs in Negro males who have a tendency to move barefoot.
B. It starts as a fissure at the interphalangeal joint of finger and later fibroses to form a fibrous band.
C. It is treated initially by 'Z' plasty and later on by amputation.
D. It encircles the digit and causes avascular necrosis.

**83. Which of the following is not precancerous : CUPGME-2003**
A. Tylosis B. Bowen's disease
C. Erythroleucoplakia D. None of the above

**84. The following swellings are transilluminant except : UPSC 2004**
A. Meningocele B. Hydrocele
C. Thyroglossal cyst D. Lipoma

**85. Who said these words : "To study the phenomenon of disease without books is to sail an unchartered sea, while to study books without patients is not to go to sea at all": Karnataka 2004**
A. Hamilton Bailey B. Sir Robert Hutchinson.
C. Sir William Osler D. J.B. Murphy

**86. In triage green colour indicates : COMEDK 2005**
A. Ambulatory patients
B. Dead or moribund patients
C. High priority treatment or transfer
D. Medium priority or transfer

**87. The commonest cause of water intoxication in surgical patients is due to : COMEDK 2005**
A. Colorectal wash with plain water.
B. Syndrome of inappropriate secretion of ADH.
C. Irrigation during transurethral resection of prostate.
D. Excessive infusion of 5% glucose.

| Ans. | | | | | | | | | |
|---|---|---|---|---|---|---|---|---|---|
| 71. D | 72. E | 73. B | 74. A | 75. C | 76. B | 77. B | 78. A | 79. A | 80. B |
| 81. C | 82. B | 83. A | 84. D | 85. C | 86. A | 87. D | | | |

**88. SEPS is done for :** **AI 2009**
A. Arteries B. Veins
C. Lymphatics D. A-V fistula

**89. MC cause of superficial thrombophiebitis :** **AI 2009**
A. IV injection B. DVT
C. HT D. Trauma

**90. Abdominal aortic aneurysm (AAA) ruptures most commonly :** **AI 2009**
A. Ant B. Post
C. Lat D. Non

**91. Pt. presents with puched out lesion on x-ray with Serum Na-144, K+-4.5, Ca-12, Globulin-8.4, alls 5.4, what will be next investigation to do o?** **AI 2009**
A. Serum protein electrophortic studies
B. Alk PO4 levels
C. Bone scan
D. ESR

**92. Best material for below inguinal arterial graft :** **AI 2009**
A. Saphenous upside down
B. PTFE
C. Dacron Carmustine
D. Teflon

**93. A man with blunt injury abdomen after road side accident has BP of 100/80 mm Hg, pulse 120bpm. Respiration stablized through airway. Next best step in the management is :** **AI 2009**
A. Immediate blood Transfusion
B. Blood for cross matching + IV fluids
C. Ventilate the patient
D. Rush to the OT

**94. Entrapment neuropathies commonly affect the folloeing nerves except :** **AI 2009**
A. Tibal
B. Femoral
C. Lateral cutaneous nerve of thigh
D. Median N

**95. Smoking doesn't cause which cancer :** **AI 2009**
A. Larynx B. Nasopharynx
C. Esophagus D. Bladder

**96. Pseudoclaudication seen due to :** **AI 2009**
A. Femoral artery B. Popliteal artery
C. Lumbar canal stenosis D. Radial artery

**97. Prognostic factors for lymphoma are all except :** **AI 2009**
A. Stage of disease
B. Nunmer of extralymphatic sites involved
C. LDH
D. Hemoglobin

**98. Lumber sympathectomy is of value in the management of all except :** **AI 2009**
A. Arteriovenous fistula
B. Distal ischemia
C. Intermittent claudication
D. Anhidrosis

**99. Which of the following is a marker for GIST :** **AIIMS 2009**
A. CD 117
B. CD 34
C. CD 36
D. CD 135

**100. Which of the following is a delayed obsorbable synthetic suture material ?** **Delhi 2009**
A. Chronic catgut B. Vicryl
C. Silk D. Nylon

**101. Risk factor for the development of critical limb ischemia include all except :** **Delhi 2009**
A. Diabetes
B. Hyperlipidemia
C. Moderate alcohol intake
D. Hyperhomocysteinemia

**102. All of the following are indicators of adequacy of pre-operative resuscitation except :** **Delhi 2009**
A. C-reactive protein level
B. Conciousness level
C. Urine output
D. Hematocrit level

**Ans.** 88. B 89. A 90. C 91. A 92. A 93. B 94. B 95. B 96. C 97. D
98. D 99. A 100. B 101. C 102. A

# EXPLANATIONS OF GENERAL TOPICS

## 1(A)—WOUNDS, SUTURING, KELOIDS, INFECTIONS, CYSTS

1. Ans.— E. All of the above
2. Ans.— B. Between 6th to 7th day
3. Ans.— B. 6
4. Ans.— C. Debrided and closed per secundum
5. Ans.— B. Actinomycosis
6. Ans.— A. Acute paronychia

   After this, bacterial infection sets in.
7. Ans.— C. Common bile duct
8. Ans.— A. Axilla
9. Ans.— A. Soda bicarbonate
10. Ans.— D. Human bites
11. Ans.— C. Upper-outer segment of buttocks
12. Ans.— C. Sternum
13. Ans.— D. Very old people
14. Ans.— B. Streptococcus
15. Ans.— D Vincent's angina
16. Ans.— A. Facio cervical

    Infection is subcuticular and under the eponychium, arises from a hangnail, careless nail pairing or an unsterile manicure instrument. Differential diagnosis is herpetic whitlow. Flucloxacillin or operation (of eponychium stripping) are used.
17. Ans.— B. Lepromatous
18. Ans.— D. Spleen
19. Ans.— A. Dorsal thorax

    This is common site of keloid formation especially on sternum.
20. Ans.— B. Acute circulatory failure
21. Ans.— A. Cutting with knife
22. Ans.— D. Ca++

    Vitamin-C is required for synthesis of ground substance. Vitamin-D is required for new bone formation. Vitamin-A is for epithelialization. In deficiency, healing is poor.
23. Ans.— A. Drainage after localization
24. Ans.— B. Face
25. Ans.— B. Vitamin-C
26. Ans.—C. Wilms tumour

    Answer is Wilm's tumor among choices, but otherwise Neuroblastoma is most common solid tumor of infancy and childhood and by for the most common in newborn.
27. Ans.— C. Metronidazole with broad spectrum antibiotics.
28. Ans.— C. Excised after injecting it with a scolicidal agent.
29. Ans.— A. 6
30. Ans.— C. Epididymal cyst

    Epididymal cysts are retention cysts.
31. Ans.— E. In all cases regardless of physical findings.
32. Ans.— E. Superior mediastinum
33. Ans.— A. Ulnar
34. Ans.— A. Syphilis
35. Ans.— C. Rugby
36. Ans.— D. Common before age of 40
37. Ans.— D. Sole
38. Ans.— B. Ovary
39. Ans.— B. Infection with E. multilocularis
40. Ans.— B. Red and become thick white later on.
41. Ans.— B. Subcutaneous spaces
42. Ans.— D. None of the above
43. Ans.— C. Obstruction and lymphangitis
44. Ans.— D. 4 weeks
45. Ans.— B. Washing and debridement

46. Ans.— B. Rent in deep fascia meticulously sutured.
47. Ans.— C. Soft
48. Ans.— A. Punctum
49. Ans.— C. Hyaluronidase
50. Ans.— D. Two years of wound healing
51. Ans.— D. Anthrax of the skin
52. Ans.— D. Stimulated by steriods.
53. Ans.— D. An excess mass of fibrous tissue around a small abscess persistantly treated by antibiotics.
54. Ans.— A. Staph. aureus
It is a normal commensal of skin.
55. Ans.— B. Is caused by fungus
56. Ans.— B. Through cleaning with debridement of all dead and devitalised tissue without primary closure.
57. Ans.— D. 1 and 4
58. Ans.— NONE
Question is wrong. Choice 'D' should have been 'None of the above'.
59. Ans.— C. An acute infection of hair follicle
60. Ans.— E. All of the above
61. Ans.— C. Eversion
62. Ans.— A. Bacterial infection
63. Ans.— E. B and C
64. Ans.— C. Incision
65. Ans.— C. Nose & ear
66. Ans.— A. To obtain skin closure
67. Ans.— A. Cystic hygroma
Cystic teratomas and cystadenomas are distension cysts.
68. Ans.— B. Marfan's syndrome
69. Ans.— D. Clean
70. Ans.— B. Fifth post-operation day
71. Ans.— B. Ability to bleed freely when cut
72. Ans.— C. Elasticity
73. Ans.— D. Fibroblasts
74. Ans.— B. Presence of multiple drainage sites in carbuncle.
75. Ans.— B. An analgesic
76. Ans.— C. Virulent strains of organism
77. Ans.— D. Common in tropics
78. Ans.— A. Hodgkin's disease
79. Ans.— C. Jaundice
It is a staphylococcal infection.
80. Ans.— D. Sebaceous cyst
81. Ans.— B. V, VII
82. Ans.— A. Mycetoma
83. Ans.— A. Staph. aureus infection
84. Ans.— C. Injection tetanus toxoid
85. Ans.— C. Tooth
86. Ans.— C. Formation of pericyst
87. Ans.— C. Glottic oedema
88. Ans.— A. Primary suturing
89. Ans.— B. Genitourinary system
90. Ans.— C. 10—20 days
91. Ans.— C. Pulmonary function
92. Ans.— B. I, II and IV
93. Ans.— B. Myofibroblasts
94. Ans.— B. Wide excision and skin grafting
95. Ans.— C. Antibiotics alone
Flucloxacillin is used.
96. Ans.— D. Mycosis fungoides
97. Ans.— B. Newborn baby
98. Ans.— A. TB
99. Ans.— D. All of the above
100. Ans.— B. Hypoproteinemia
101. Ans.— C. 10-12 days
102. Ans.— C. An abscess
It is caused by staphylococcus aureus. DM, uremia and steroid therapy are predispositions.
103. Ans.— B. Empiric choice of antibiotics depends on the expected spectrum of organisms likely to be encountered.
104. Ans.— B. Night before surgery
105. Ans.— D. Respiratory rate and systolic blood pressure.
106. Ans.— A. Radiation
107. Ans.— C. Bacteria lodge in the interstices
108. Ans.— A. Steel wire
109. Ans.— C. Six months

110. Ans.— D. **Pulse rate**

111. Ans.— A. **Isopropyl alcohol**

112. Ans.— B. **Infrared photography**

113. Ans.— D. **The patient is always diabetic**

Carbuncle is an infective gangrene of the subcutaneous tissue. It often occurs in the nape of the neck. Subcutaneous tissue becomes painful and hard, and the overlying skin is red. Unless prompt treatment is started to abort the lesion. Extension occurs after a few days and areas of softening appears; skin sloughs and discharges pus. Generally, there is one central large slough, surrounded by a rosette of smaller areas of necrosis.

114. Ans.— B. **Enucleation is impossible because its blood supply is same as that of the adjacent intestine.**

There are 4 types of mesenteric cysts viz. chylolymphatic, enterogenous, urogenital remnant and dermoid (teratomastous) cyst. Chylolymphatic cyst is the most common variety of mesenteric cysts and it probably arises in congenitally misplaced lymphatic tissue that has no efferent communication with the lymphatic system. Enucleation is possible without the necessity of resection of gut.

115. Ans.— B. **Wound excision**

The untidy wounds result from crushing, tearing, avulsion, vascular injuries or burns and contain devitalized tissue. Skin wound are often multiple and irregular. Tendons, arteries and nerves may be exposed; might be injured in continuity; but are not divided. Fractures are common and may be multi-fragmentary. Such wound should not be closed primarily. The correct management of untidy wounds is wound excision (excision of all devitalized tissue to create a tidy wound). Once the untidy wound has been converted to a tidy wound by the process of wound excision, it can be safely closed or allowed to heal by second intention.

116. Ans.— B. **Within 24 to 48 hours**

The epithelial defect in an incised wound is initially plugged with fibrin & the epidermis turns downwards over the edge of the underlying dermis; at 24 hours basal cells are mobilizing on the under surface of the epidermis and by 48 hours the advancing epithelial edge has undergone cellular hypertrophy and mitosis. The epithelium migrates but stops when it meets the opposite advancing epithelium.

117. Ans.— A. **Catabolism**

After trauma following changes are seen :

* Increased Oxygen consumption
* Negative Nitrogen Balance
* Increased caloric consumption
* Metabolic changes - Lipolysis, Glycogenolysis, Gluconeogenesis.
* Hormonal changes-increased (GH, NA, Adrinaline, Glucagon).

118. Ans.— B. **Trophic ulcer**

Trophic ulcer is due to Pressure Necrosis:

* e.g. -Bedsores and perforating ulcers
* MC site Heel, (In General)
* MC site Buttock and back of heel (when pt is ambulatory)

Tropical ulcer - It seems to be due to Vincents organism (Bacteroids fusiformis). It is characterized by papule pustule and a surrounding zone of inflammation.

119. Ans.— D. **Gas is invariably present in the muscle compartments.**

120. Ans.— A. **Isopropyl alcohol**

121. Ans.— C. **Marjolin's ulcer**

Lymphoedema :

- Due to impairment of the flow of lymph from an extremity.
- Primary lymphodema may be secondary to agenesis, hypoplasia or obstruction of lymphatic vessels.
- It may be associated with Turner's syndrome, Noonan syndrome Yellow nain syndrome intestinal lymphangiectasia syndrome and lymphangiomyomatosis.
- Familial lymphedenoma developing before 1 year of age is called Milroy's disease.
- Painless edema is pitting initially and becomes brawney and non-pitting with time.
- The most common cause of secondary lymphoedema world-wide is filariasis.

- There may be episodes of lymphangitis and cellulitis.
- Hypertrophy of limb results with markedly thickened skin and subcutaneous tissue.
- Rarely, lymphangiosarcoma or angiosarcoma may develop. This neoplastic transformation of blood vessels and lymphatis is called the "Stewart-Treves Syndrome".

122. Ans.— A. Oropharyngeal carcinoma
123. Ans.— D. Pulmonary Embolectomy
124. Ans.— D. Direct Pressure and Elevation
125. Ans.— A. Medullary carcinoma of the thyroid

Pancreatitis and pituitary tumor create the confusion, but there is no better option than medullary carcinoma.

126. Ans.— C. Hypochloraemia
127. Ans.— C. Verrucous carcinoma

Carcinoma in people indulge in chewing the betal nut and keep the quid of it in the cheek, is often called Verrucous carcinoma (Tobacco Chewer's carcinoma).

- Such cancers are initially soft, nonindurated papillary growths which later ulcerate.
- The lesion gradually invades and destroys the underlying soft tissues and bone.
- There may be leukoplakia to start with and this ultimately turns into malignancy.
- Spread to regional lymph nodes may occur but distant metastasis is rare.

128. Ans.— D. Gas is invariably present in the muscle compartment.
129. Ans.— A. Isopropyl alcohol
130. Ans.— C. Removal of fragments of bone
131. Ans.— B. Epithelial growth
132. Ans.— B. Undergoes hydrolysis and complete absorption.

## 1(B)—TUMORS ULCERS

1. Ans.— E. Excised
2. Ans.— D. Pseudomonas pyocyaneus
3. Ans.— A. 10 ng/ml

It is raised in testicular and liver tumors.

4. Ans.— C. Melanoma
5. Ans.— D. Ca. colon
6. Ans.— D. Dermal naevi
7. Ans.— B. Blood vessels
8. Ans.— D. Discontinuity in the epithelium
9. Ans.— D. Chronic smoking
10. Ans.— A. Basal Cell Ca
11. Ans.— C. A premalignant intradermal condition.
12. Ans.— C. Back
13. Ans.— A. Liver

It is usually the cavernous type. It is small, solitary and well defined and is found incidentally either as a hypoechoic mass on USG.

14. Ans.— C. Sweat gland
15. Ans.— B. Faster growing malignancy than Sq. cell carcinoma.
16. Ans.— C. Carotid bodies
17. Ans.— B. 5 cm
18. Ans.— A. Masterly inactivity
19. Ans.— C. Prostatic carcinoma
20. Ans.— B. Endodermal sinus tumour
21. Ans.— D. Lipoma
22. Ans.— B. 5th
23. Ans.— D. Muscle
24. Ans.— A. Inner canthus

Basal cell carcinoma or rodent ulcer is most common malignant tumor of eyelids. It is more common in lower eyelids.

25. Ans.— D. All of the above
26. Ans.— B. Wide excision
27. Ans.— B. Retention cyst
28. Ans.— B. Uterus
29. Ans.— C. Sporothrix
30. Ans.— A. Depth of invasion
31. Ans.— A. Reed Sternberg cell

32. Ans.— B. Basal cell carcinoma

33. Ans.— A. Clinical classification

34. Ans.— NONE

Question is wrongly framed.

35. Ans.— C. Renal cell carcinoma

36. Ans.— A. Is premalignant

37. Ans.— B. Leukoplakia vulva

38. Ans.— B. Everted

39. Ans.— A. Dark people

Keloid is an extreme overgrowth of scar tissue that may represent the most extreme form of hypertrophy. It is common in Afro-caribbean patients at many sites including ear lobes after piercing.

40. Ans.— B. Chordoma

41. Ans.— B. Metastasis

42. Ans.— D. Lymphnodes

43. Ans.— C. Strawberry

44. Ans.— C. An undermined edge

45. Ans.— A. Pricking due to blunt needle

Implantation dermoids arise from squamous epithelium which has been driven beneath the skin by a penetrating wound. They are classically found in the fingers of women who sew assiduously.

It is also called bed sore. It is chronic wound following tissue necrosis from pressure or shearing from contact with a supporting surface.

46. Ans.— C. Malignant melanoma

47. Ans.— D. Testis

48. Ans.— C. A pressure sore

49. Ans.— D. Brain

50. Ans.— C. Multiple adenomatous polyps of the colon.

51. Ans.— D. Post-operative radiotherapy to the surgical area and the adjacent lymph nodes.

52. Ans.— C. Kidney

53. Ans.— D. Lymphatic leukemia

54. Ans.— D. Epithelial pearl formation is seen

55. Ans.— B. It is painless

56. Ans.— A. Apple jelly granulation

57. Ans.— C. Head and neck area

58. Ans.— C. Melanoma

59. Ans.— A. Melnoma foot

60. Ans.— A. Using full thickness of skin graft

61. Ans.— D. Ca larynx

62. Ans.— D. None of the above

The Pelvic and calf veins are more commonly affected. It causes painful congestion and edema of leg. White leg or Blue leg may develop. Venous gangrene can also occur.

63. Ans.— A. Lipoma

64. Ans.— B. Post- mastectomy edema of arm

65. Ans.— A. Subacute combined degeneration

66. Ans.— C. Embryonal rhabdomyosarcoma

67. Ans.— A. Punched out edges

68. Ans.— C. Massive pulmonary haemorrhage

69. Ans.— A. Pott's puffy tumour

70. Ans.— A. Sarcoma

71. Ans.— C. Ears

It is also called glomangioma, composed of a tortous arteriole.

72. Ans.— D. None of the above

73. Ans.— A. Surgery

74. Ans.— A. Beta-2 macroglobulin

75. Ans.— C. I (ii) II (i) III (iv) IV (iii)

76. Ans.— D. I (ii) II (i) III (v) IV (iv)

77. Ans.— A. Melanoma

78. Ans.— A. Bazin's ulcer

79. Ans.— A. Tuberous sclerosis

80. Ans.— A. Bowen's disease

81. Ans.— A. Ureter

82. Ans.— B. Retroperitoneum

83. Ans.— B. Acoustic neuroma

84. Ans.— D. All of the above

85. Ans.— C. Early metastasis

86. Ans.— B. Finger nails

87. Ans.— A. Nasopharynx

88. Ans.— A. Lingual nerve palsy is often seen

89. Ans.— B. CML

90. Ans.— B. Cervical

91. Ans.— B. Angiosarcoma

Angiosarcoma of skin occurs in elderly males. The lesions occur most commonly on scalp or face. It metastasises to cervical LN or lungs.

92. Ans.— B. Melanoma

93. Ans.— A. Trunk

94. Ans.— B. More in males

95. Ans.— B. Full thickness skin loss and or necrosis of subcutaneous tissue that may extend to, but not through underlying fascia.

96. Ans.— B. Acoustic neuroma

97. Ans.— A. Phaeochromocytoma

98. Ans.— A. 1, 2 and 3

99. Ans.— C. Squamous cell Ca of skin

100. Ans.— A. III A

101. Ans.— A. Face

102. Ans.— B. Portwine stain

103. Ans.— C. BRCA-1 and 2 oncogene

104. Ans.— C. Melphalan

105. Ans.— B. Erythroplakia

Erythroplakia is defined as any lesion of oral mucosa which presents as bright red velvety plaques which cannot be characterized clinically or pathologically as any other recognisable condition. The incidence of malignant change in erythroplakia is 17-fold higher than in leucoplakia.

106. Ans.— B. Carcinoma breast

A Tru-Cut needle biopsy is required for confirming and staging Ca breast.

107. Ans.— C. Malignant

108. Ans.— B. AFP

109. Ans.— A. A2, B:3, C:1, D:4

110. Ans.— B. Noise (Thrill/bruit).

## 1(C)—HAEMORRHAGE, SHOCK, FLUIDS, ELECTROLYTES

1. Ans.— C. 60-70%

2. Ans.— D. Penetrating injury

3. Ans.— A. Urine output

4. Ans.— B. Calcium

5. Ans.— E. Thrombocytopenia

6. Ans.— A. Classical heamophilia

7. Ans.— E. E. coli.

8. Ans.— E. Staphcillin, Kanamycin or Colymycin

9. Ans.— D. Insertion an adequate airway

10. Ans.— B. Calcium

11. Ans.— B. Acute circulatory failure

12. Ans.— B. Femoral vein thrombosis + Lymphatic obstruction

13. Ans.— E. Inhibition of ADH

14. Ans.— D. Shallow slow respiration

15. Ans.— C. Loose 100 -200 gms per day

16. Ans.— D. Encourages bacterial proliferation and septicemia.

17. Ans.— D. All of the above.

18. Ans.— A. 2-3; 5-8

19. Ans.— A. 70, 80, 90

20. Ans.— D. 4

21. Ans.— A. 40, 20

22. Ans.— B. Crystalloid infusion

23. Ans.— D. Chloride

24. Ans.— C. Factors 5 and 8

25. Ans.— C. Paralytic ileus

26. Ans.— E. All of the above

27. Ans. E. Only A and C

28. Ans.— A. Thrombosis

29. Ans.— B. Vitamin $K_1$

30. Ans.— A. Intramuscular

31. Ans.— E. None of the above

32. Ans.— E. All of the above

33. Ans.— E. All of the above

34. Ans.— E. All of the above

35. Ans.— C. O Rh negative

36. Ans.— E. Thiamine

No treatment is required.

37. Ans.— A. Aldosterone

38. Ans.— E. All of the above

39. Ans.— A. Weight gain

40. Ans.— B. 15%

41. Ans.— C. 500 ml
Salmon Patch (stork bite) present at birth, disappears by 1 year of age, Portwine stain (naevus flammeus) present at birth requires excision and grafting, straw berry angioma (appear at 1-3 weeks after birth) should be allowed to undergo natural involution.

42. Ans.— A. 24

43. Ans.— A. 7 hours

44. Ans.— B. 150 gm

45. Ans.— B. Anaesthesia

46. Ans.— D. Streptokinase
Rectal biopsy is used for diagnosis

47. Ans.— B. Doppler

48. Ans.— B. A.V. Fistula

49. Ans.— C. Tall T-waves

50. Ans.— A. Duodenum

51. Ans.— B. Arteriovenous fistula
Ranula is extravasation cyst arising from a damaged sublinguial gland so named because of the likeness of swelling to belly of a little frog.

52. Ans.— A. Calcium absorption

53. Ans.— B. 35-40 gm/day

54. Ans.— A. Congenital pyloric stenosis

55. Ans.— B. Within 12 hours of operation

56. Ans.— D. Cortisone excess

57. Ans.— A. Extracellular space

58. Ans.— C. Within one-to-two weeks of operation

59. Ans.— D. Hypokalemia

60. Ans.— A. Bloody stools

61. Ans.— B. Preoperatively in cases of severe chronic anemia.

62. Ans.— C. Insufflation with Carbon dioxide

63. Ans.— C. Sodium bicarbonate

64. Ans.— D. Excreted excessively

65. Ans.— A. Normal urine output

66. Ans.— B. Factor-VIII

67. Ans.— A. Metabolic alkalosis

68. Ans.— C. 23 L

69. Ans.— C. Dextran 40

70. Ans.— A. 11,200 cc

71. Ans.— B. Thrombophlebitis at the injection site

72. Ans.— D. Respiratory failure

73. Ans.— C. For amputation in arterio sclerotic gangrene.

74. Ans.— C. Protamine sulphate

75. Ans.— C. 1.5 hours

76. Ans.— C. Withdraw the blood transfusion immediately and give injectable antihistaminics and steroids.

77. Ans.— A. Hepatic coma

78. Ans.— A. Shallow slow breathing

79. Ans.— C. Hypernatremia

80. Ans.— A. Bradycardia
Tachycardia to maintain cardiac output is seen.

81. Ans.— E. 100 days

82. Ans.— B. 750 ml

83. Ans.— C. 2 and 3 are correct

84. Ans.— B. 2.5 to 3.5 times the normal

85. Ans.— C. 60-70%

86. Ans.— B. The liver

87. Ans.— B. Solution derived from boric acid and bleaching powder.

88. Ans.— A. It is costly

89. Ans.— A. Ringer lactate

90. Ans.— D. $Na^+$, $K^+$, $Cl^-$, $Ca^+$

91. Ans.— B. Venous ulcer

92. Ans.— D. Acid citrate dextrose

93. Ans.— C. Excessive haemorrhage from the wound site.

94. Ans.— D. Thrombocytopenia

95. Ans.— C. 30-45 cc/hour

96. Ans.— D. 20%

97. Ans.— A. Pressure by finger

98. Ans.— D. Intracranial haemorrhage

99. Ans.— D. Darrow's solution

100. Ans.— B. Bradycardia

101. Ans.— D. Cardiogenic shock

102. Ans.— A. **Maintaining high urine output**

103. Ans.— D. **Thrombocytopenia**

104. Ans.— D. **All of the above**

105. Ans.— D. **All of the above**

106. Ans.— A. **Less than 50,000 mm$^3$**

107. Ans.— B. **Hypertrophic pyloric stenosis**

108. Ans.— A. **Antidiuretic hormone**

109. Ans.— D. **96**

110. Ans.— A. **Radial**

111. Ans.— A. **600 calories**

112. Ans.— A. **Small intestinal obstruction**

113. Ans.— A. **I, II, III**

114. Ans.— B. **After burns**

115. Ans.— C. **Ends are trapped within fracture bone ends.**

116. Ans.— A. **Regulating the speed and amount of fluid infusion.**

117. Ans.— C. **Lack of collagen and reticulum**

118. Ans.— C. **Intramuscular**

119. Ans.— C. **1, 2 and 3**

120. Ans.— A. **$NH_4Cl$**

121. Ans.— A. **Increased H.R. with low B.P.**

122. Ans.— C. **Normal lower limb vessels**

123. Ans.— A. **Intestinal obstruction**

124. Ans.— A. **Injury to femoral vessels when using a butchers knife.**

125. Ans.— **All**

126. Ans.— A. **1, 2 and 3**

127. Ans.— C. **Pressure at the site**

128. Ans.— A. **Fresh frozen plasma transfusion**

129. Ans.— A. **Cardiac tamponade**

130. Ans.— A. **Extensive trauma to the brain**

131. Ans.— A. **Immediate laparotomy**

132. Ans.— C. **Above 40**

133. Ans.— A. **Dilutional thrombocytopenia**

134. Ans.— B. **CVP**

135. Ans.— C. **I/V fluids**

136. Ans.— B. **50 ml 25% dextrose gives 50 kcal of energy.**

137. Ans.— C. **Colloid**

138. Ans.— B. **Section of femoral vessels during boning.**

139. Ans.— D. **Hydrogen ions**

## 1(D)—ANEURYSMS, VARICOSE VEINS, THROMBOEMBOLISM, GANGRENE, LYMPHANGITIS

1. Ans.— E. **All of the following**

2. Ans.— B. **Autologous vein**

3. Ans.— A. **Rest pain**

4. Ans.— C. **Immediate anticoagulation**

5. Ans.— C. **Pancreatic Ca**

   **It is called Trouseu's sign**

6. Ans.— A. **Sapheno femoral junction**

7. Ans.— D. **Tobacco**

8. Ans.— D. **Surgical debridement**

9. Ans.— A. **There is loss of consciousness during convulsions.**

10. Ans.— D. **Doppler examination**

11. Ans.— D. **All of the above**

    **Other causes are loss of bases (diarrhoea, fistulas, U. colitis, prolonged aspiration) or increase in fixed acids (DM, starvation, CRF, shock).**

12. Ans.— B. **Measurement of skin-blood flow by fluorence comparison of amputation site to normal reference site.**

13. Ans.— A. **Abrupt, constant pain due to arterial occlusion.**

14. Ans.— C. **Anaerobic myonecrosis**

15. Ans.— D. **Atherosclerosis**

16. Ans.— D. **Internal at the wrist**

17. Ans.— B. **Arterial insufficiency**

18. Ans.— D. **Anterior and posterior tibial**

    **The majority are true fusiform atherosclerotic aneurysms.**

19. Ans.— A. **Aortic and iliac arteries**

20. Ans.— B. **Congenital lymphedema**

21. Ans.— D. **Penicillin**

22. Ans.— C. **Ecchymosis**

23. Ans.— D. **Can be easily incised and the opening resutured.**

24. Ans.— A. **Fusiform**

25. Ans.— A. Dacron

26. Ans.— D. Smoking

27. Ans.— B. Fluid thrill or pulsatile mass

28. Ans.— B. Profunda femoris and Saphenous vein

29. Ans.— D. Amputation

30. Ans.— A. About 10%

31. Ans.— D. The radial pulse is always absent

32. Ans.— B. Unlike hernia there is no impulse felt on coughing.

33. Ans.— C. May by-pass the lymph nodes immediately proximal to the site of infection.

Ac. lymphangitis occurs when infection commonly by streptococcus pyogenes spread beyond a pt. of infection to the group of lymph nodes.

34. Ans.— A. Exercise

35. Ans.— C. Musculofascial anatomy and physiology of the calf.

36. Ans.— C. Used for carotid artery stenosis

37. Ans.— B. Foot

38. Ans.— D. Division and ligation at the sites of a bad leak from the deep to the superficial venous system.

39. Ans.— A. Supportive bandages and ambulation

40. Ans.— B. Colour change and oedema

41. Ans.— A. Subungual melanoma

42. Ans.— A. Deep vein thrombosis

43. Ans.— B. Saphenous vein

44. Ans.— A. Dry cold

45. Ans.— A. Graduated warming

46. Ans.— B. Chronic osteomyelitis

47. Ans.— D. Recurrent bleeding

48. Ans.— C. Pulmonary infarction

49. Ans. A. Poor collaterals

50. Ans.— C. Absent lymphatics

51. Ans.— D. Liver

52. Ans.— A. 1, 2 and 3

53. Ans.— A. Filariasis

54. Ans.— C. Hypoproteinemia

55. Ans.— A. Vein

56. Ans.— C. Intravenous infusion

57. Ans.— B. Atherosclerosis obliterans

58. Ans.— A. Above 50 years of age group

59. Ans.— A. 7-10 days

60. Ans.— D. Patent ventricular septal defects

61. Ans.— D. Whole blood

62. Ans.— D. Claudication

63. Ans.— B. Popliteal artery

It is a condition characterised by occlusive diseases of small and medium sized arteries (Plantars, tibial, radial etc). Does not occur in woman and non-smokers.

64. Ans.— B. Increased skin temperature

It occurs on the brawny oedematous arm of the post -radical mastectomy patient or in a lower limb following groin dissection.

65. Ans.— C. Saphenous vein

66. Ans.— B. Positive Homan's sign

67. Ans.— B. Deep vein thrombosis

68. Ans.— C. Venogram

Venography provides anatomical information and is new only indicated in absence of good duplex ultrasonography.

69. Ans.— D. Applying direct pressure over the bleeding point.

70. Ans.— A. Claudication

71. Ans. C. Age less than forty years

72. Ans.— D. 35%

73. Ans.— A. Thoraco abdominal vessels

It is common in Budd Chiari syndrome.

74. Ans.— A. Sup. Gluteal nerve

When child stands on affected hip, the contralateral hip drops. Also called an abductor limp. Trendelenberg test is for varicose veins.

75. Ans.— A. Long saphenous

76. Ans.— A. Atherosclerosis

Majority are true fusiform atherosclerotic aneurysms. The other causes are trauma, mycotic, syphilitic, collagen disease (Marfan's syndrome).

77. Ans.— B. Co-polymer of glycolide and lectide

78. Ans.— D. Ileo femoral angioplasty

79. Ans.— C. Pulmonary emboli

80. Ans.— C. Pitting oedema upto knee

81. Ans.— B. Rubor

82. Ans.— B. Emergency surgery complication < 10%.

83. Ans.— C. Embolectomy done in all cases

Thrombosis of axillary vein may occur following excessive exercise. Early treatment with anticoagulants may result in rapid resolution. In severe cases, the use of fibrinolytic therapy streptokinase or tissue plasminogen activator may be considered.

84. Ans.— A. Doppler imaging

85. Ans.— D. 1 and 3

86. Ans.— D. All of the above

87. Ans.— B. Respiratory

88. Ans.— A. Ligate the two ends of external femoral vein.

89. Ans.— B. Proximal compression causes increase in heart rate.

90. Ans.— D. Klippel-Trenuayay syndrome

91. Ans.— C. If it occurs in upper limb it is known as writers spasm.

92. Ans.— A. Splenic-A

93. Ans.— D. Absent popliteal pulsation

The disease affect small and medium sized arteries (plantars, tibials, radial etc.) It does not occur in women and non-smokers.

94. Ans.— A. Division of the superficial femoral vein in the groin and transplantation of its vein in the below the level of the complement profound valve.

It will restore the circulation in the limb.

95. Ans.— D. Ethanolamine oleate

96. Ans.— D. Elevate the limb and apply pressure bandage.

97. Ans.— B. Isolated aneurysm

98. Ans.— C. Turn white

99. Ans.— D. Popliteal artery

(Bacteroids fusiformis). It is characterized by papule pustule and a surrounding zone of inflammation.

100. Ans.— C. Cystic Hygroma

101. Ans.— C. a3 b4 c1 d2

102. Ans.— D That resulting from crush or pressure injury.

103. Ans.— B. Simple mastectomy.

104. Ans.— B. Littre's hernia

## 1. (E)—MISCELLANEOUS

1. Ans.— D. Syphilis

2. Ans.— A. Rectal biopsy

3. Ans.— B. Cuffed endotracheal tube

4. Ans.— B. Staphylococcus

5. Ans.— A. Excruciating Pain

6. Ans.— B. Colon

7. Ans.— C. 4.5

8. Ans.— C. Multiple Z plasty

9. Ans.— C. Self-healing nodular lesion with central ulceration.

10. Ans.— D. Media of Monkeberg degeneration

11. Ans.— B. Femoral Hernia

12. Ans.— C. Chronic infection of a sebaceous cyst

It resembles epithelioma.

13. Ans.— C. Schaumann's

14. Ans.— C. Localised pitting oedema of the scalp with underlying osteomyelitis of part of scalp.

Pott's tumor is osteomyelitis of skull with periosteal swelling. Ac. localised headache, tenderness on local percussion of the skull, and localised pitting edema of the scalp over the affected area, collectively form Pott's puffy tumor.

15. Ans.— A.

| A | B | C | D |
|---|---|---|---|
| 4 | 3 | 2 | 1 |

16. Ans.— D. A type of haemangioma

17. Ans.— A. Muscle

18. Ans.— C. Tight bandage

19. Ans.— A. Mucous material

Ganglia are localized, tense (but often painless) cystic swellings containing clear gelatinous fluid.

20. Ans.— C. A developmental malformation

21. Ans.— NONE

22. Ans.— C. Follows ischaemia of the forearm muscles.

23. Ans.— D. All of the above

24. Ans.— A. Distension

25. Ans.— B. An ischaemic condition of the foot following exposure to damp and cold in tight footwear.

26. Ans.— A. Intussusception

**27. Ans.— B. One year**

**28. Ans.— C. Foreign body reaction**

**29. Ans.— A. Carcinoma of liver**

**30. Ans.— C. Popliteal aneurysm**

**31. Ans.— A. Is a form of haemolytic disease of the new born due to ABO blood group incompatibility.**

**32. Ans.— C. Delays the formation of collagen and callus.**

**33. Ans.— B. 4, 3**

**34. Ans.— A. Absence of middle finger**

**35. Ans.— A. Within first year of life**

**36. Ans.— D. No treatment**

**37. Ans.— D. Little finger**

**38. Ans.— D. Index finger**

**39. Ans.— A. Swelling of the whole hand**

**40. Ans.— B. Abscess of intralobar fissure of lung**

**41. Ans.— D. All of the above**

**42. Ans.— A. Hypotension**

**43. Ans.— B. Complete**

**44. Ans.— A. Fresh and old clot**

**45. Ans.— D. Chest tube insertion on the left side**

**46. Ans.— B. Large bowel**

**47. Ans.— C. Retinitis pigmentosa**

**48. Ans.— B. Local palmar fasciectomy**

**49. Ans.— D. Marjolin ulcer**

**50. Ans.— D. Ring finger**

**51. Ans.— B. Lined by epithelium**

**52. Ans.— B. Victor Horsley's sign**

**53. Ans.— D. Flexor digitorum longus and flexor hallucis longus.**

**54. Ans.— B. FNAC**

**55. Ans.— D. All of the above**

**56. Ans.— C. Palmar fascia**

**57. Ans.— A. Atelectasis**

**58. Ans.— B. Involves the extremities only**

**59. Ans.— A. Scrofuloderma**

**60. Ans.— A. Filariasis**

**It is caused by filaria sanguinis, hominis transmitted by mosquito culex fatigans. Microfilaria can be discovered in nocturnal smear.**

**61. Ans.— B. Tachycardia**

**62. Ans.— D. Left supraclavicular space**

**63. Ans.— A. Polymicrogyria**

**64. Ans.— C. 120**

**65. Ans.— B. Gastroesophageal reflux**

**66. Ans.— B. Strawberry angioma**

**67. Ans.— A. Less size**

**68. Ans.— A. Malignancy**

**69. Ans.— A. Capillary hemangioma**

**70. Ans.— C. Hypervolemia**

**71. Ans.— D. Avulsion injury**

**Degloving injuries are seen when hands or limbs are trapped in a moving machinery such as in rollers. Tissue is avulsed, usually from level of deep fascia.**

**72. Ans.— E. Molluscum horns**

**73. Ans.— B. Lax ascitis**

**74. Ans.— A. Gravity**

**75. Ans.— C. Hand-washing of all staff personnel**

**76. Ans.— B. AV fistula**

**77. Ans.— B. Transversalis fascia**

**78. Ans.— A. Saphenous nerve**

**Saphenous nerve involvement is the usual complication.**

**79. Ans.— A. J. Lister**

**80. Ans.— B. Streptococcal infection**

**81. Ans.— C. Localized anaphylaxis**

**82. Ans.— B. It starts as a fissure at the interphalangeal joint of finger and later fibroses to form a fibrous band.**

**Ainhum is a disease, which usually affects male Negroes who have run barefoot in childhood. It is a disease of unknown etiology. A fissure appears at the level of the interphalangeal joint of a toe (usually 5th); the fissure becomes a fibrous band, which completely encircles the digit causing its necrosis. Treatment is either Z plasty or later on amputation**

**83. Ans.— A. Tylosis**

**84. Ans.— D. Lipoma**

**85. Ans.— C. Sir William Osler**

**86. Ans.— A. Ambulatory patients**

**87. Ans.— D. Excessive infusion of 5% glucose**

88. Ans.— B. Veins

Subfascial endoscopic perforator vein surgery

* The procedure is used for patients with either healed or active ulcers (ceap classifications 5 or 6), caused by chronic venous insufficiency, in whom incompetent calf perforating veins are thought to be an important contributing factor, particularly where conservative management (such as leg elevation, compression therapy and medication) has failed.
* Deep venous occlusion and/or infected ulcers are usually contraindications to SEPS.
* SEPS is a minimally invasive alternative to open subfascial perforator vein surgery.

89. Ans.— A. IV injections

* A variety of things can cause inflammation of a superficial vein.
* Most common cause is due to intravenous (IV) catheters or solutions and medications used in hospitals that pierce the vein wall and cause irritation.

90. Ans.— C. Lat

* Aortic dissection is caused by a circumerential or, less frequently, trnsverse tear of the intima.
* It often occurs along the right lateral wall of the ascending aorta where the hydraulic shear stress is high.
* Another common site is the descending thoracic aorta just below the ligamentum arteriosum.

91. Ans.— A. Serum protein electrophoretic studies

* A doctor will request protein electrophoresis of the blood and urine, which might show the presence of a paraprotein (monoclonal protein, or M protein) band, with or without reduction of the other (normal) immunoglobulins (known as immune paresis).
* Myeloma activity appear as "lytic lesions" (with local disappearance of normal bone due to resorption), and on the skull X-ray as "punched-out lesions" (pepper not skull).
* Bone scans are typically not of any additional value in the workup of myeloma patients.

92. Ans.— A. Saphenous upside down

* Vein Graft—gives the best results—either the vein is reversed or valves destroyed by a valvulotome.
* Immediate postop success rate for vein bypass exceeds 90%, but many cases fail in the first 18 months and at 5 years success is 50-60%.
* With PTFE—5 years success is less than 50%.

93. Ans.— B. Blood for cross-matching + Iv fluids

Initial Management

Penetrating

* Resuscitation of airway, breathing, circulation (initial volume replacement should be with colloid or O-negative blood if necessary
* Coagulopathy

Blunt trauma

* For hemodynamically stable patient, imaging by CT should be performed to evaluate the nature of injury
* Can be treated conservatively and blood should be crossmatched
* Discontinuation of conservation is for—ongoing blood loss/ coagulopathy and peritonitis.

94. Ans.— B. Femoral

* Median nerve at the wrist (carpal tunnel syndrome)
* Ulnar nerve at the elbow (cubital tunnel)
* Deep ulnar nerve compression at the wrist (Guyon canal)
* Radial nerve in the forearm—posterior interosseous nerve syndrome
* Lateral femoral cutneous nerve (meralgia paresthetica)
* Tarsal tunnel syndrome

Compression of the posterior tibial nerve behind the medial malleolus,or tarsal tunnel syndrome (TTS), is an uncommon entrapment, neuropathy.

95. Ans.— B. Nasopharynx

* Cigarette smoking causes 87 percent of lung cancer deaths and is responsible for most esophagus and bladder.

**96. Ans.— C.** Lumbar canal stenosis

* Pseudoclaudication and claudication cause similar symptoms—such as leg pain—but for different reasons.
* Pseudoclaudication is due to narrowing of the lumbar spinal canal (spinal stenosis).
* This puts pressure on (compresses) the spinal root nerves, which control movement and sensation in the legs.
* Claudication, on the other hand, is a circulation problem that results in decreased blood flow to the arteries that supply blood to muscles in the legs.

**97. Ans.— D.** Hemoglobin

Five clinical risk factors :

1. Age 60 years
2. Serum lactate dehydrogenase levels elevated
3. Performance status 2 (ECOG) or 70 (Kamofsky)
4. Ann Arbor stage-III or IV
5. > 1 site of extranodal involvement

Patients are assigned a number for each risk factory they have

Patients are groupe differently based upon the type of lymphoma

For diffuse large B cell lymphoma :

| | |
|---|---|
| 0, 1 factor = low risk: | 35% of cases; 5-year survival, 73% |
| 2 factors = low-intermediate risk: | 27% of cases; 5-year survival, 51% |
| 3 factors = high-Intermediate risk: | 22% of cases; 5-year survival, 43% |
| 4, 5 factors = high risk : | 16% of cases; 5-year survival, 26% |

For diffuse large B cell lymphoma treated with R-CHOP:

| | |
|---|---|
| 0 factor = very good : | 10% of cases; 5-year survival, 94% |
| 1, 2 factors = good: | 45% of cases; 5-year survival, 79% |
| 3, 4, 5 factors = poor : | 45% of cases; 5-year survival, 55% |

**98. Ans.— D.** Anhidrosis

Lumbar sympathectomy continues to be controversial. It is probably a useful procedure for selected patients with :

1. Advanced peripheral arterial occlusive disease.
2. Although it is most appropriate for patients with causalgia or hyperhidrosis.

**99. Ans.— A.** CD 117

**100. Ans.— B.** Vicryl

Silk and Nylon are non-absorbable sutures like linon, surgical steel, polyster, polybutester, polyprophylene whereas chronic catgut is collagen derived from health sheep or cattle (obsorbed in 90 days) and vicryl (trademark for polyglctin 910) is a synthetic obsorbable suture absorbed in 60-90 days). The other absorbable sutures are polyglyglyconate, polyglycolic acid, polydioxanone (PDS) and polyglcaprone (read details from table in Bailey & Love).

**101. Ans.— C.** Moderate alcohol intake

The risk factors include Diabetes, Hypertension, hyperlipidemia, hyperhomocysteinemia and smoking

**102. Ans.— A.** C-reactive protein is not routinely used

# 2

# IMPORTANT TEXT OF BURNS & PLASTIC SURGERY

## BLOOD SUPPLY OF DIFFERENT FLAPS

| | Flaps | | Based on |
|---|---|---|---|
| 1. | Pectoralise major myocutaneous flap | — | Pectoral branch of throaco-acromial artery |
| 2. | Latissimus dorsi myocutaneous flap | — | Thoracodorasal artery |
| 3. | Trapezius muscle myocutaneous flap | — | Transverse cervical artery |
| 4. | Radial forearm flap | — | Radial artery |
| 5. | Groïn flap | — | Deep circumflex iliac artery |
| 6. | Forehead flap | — | Superficial temporal artery |
| 7. | Deltopectoral flap | — | Perforating branches of Internal mammary artery |

## COMPOSITION OF I.V. FLUIDS

| | | *Na* | *K* | *Cl* | $HCO_3$ | *Lactate* |
|---|---|---|---|---|---|---|
| 1. | Plasma | 137-147 | 4-5.5 | 95-105 | 22-25 | — |
| 2. | Saline (0.9) | 153 | — | 153 | — | — |
| 3. | Ringer lactate | 130 | 4 | 110 | — | 28 |
| 4. | Darrows | 124 | 36 | 104 | — | 56 |

**Lawson's conditions for graft survival**

Ist Law : 'That the skin should be applied to a healthy granulating surface'.

2nd Law : 'That skin only should be transplanted, and that special care to taken, that there is no fat adherent to it'.

3rd Law : 'That the portion of skin should be accurately and firmly applied to the granulating surface'.

4th Law : 'That the new skin should be kept in its new position without interruption, and that it should be lightly covered with a layer of lint, and over this is a small compress of cotton wool'.

**SKIN GRAFTS**

* **Split-thickness**—Includes the epidermis and a variable amount of dermis. Depending upon the amount of dermis raised these are thick, medium or thin.
* **Full-thickness**—Includes the entire epidermis and dermis.

## FREE SKIN GRAFTS

| | Eponyms | Divisions | Thickness (inches) |
|---|---|---|---|
| * | Reverdin | Epidermal | 0.008=0.010 |
| * | Thiersch | Thin split | 0.012 |
| * | Thiersch | Medium split | 0.015 |
| * | Ollier | Thick split | 0.025 |
| * | Wolf | Full-thickness | 0.030 |

**Tissue Transplants :**

* *Autograft*—Graft in which donor is also recipient
* *Isograft*—Graft between individuals identical in histocompatibility antigens (e.g. Identical twins).
* *Allograft* (Homograft)—Graft between genetically dissimilar members of same species.
* *Xenograft* (Heterograft)—Graft between species.

## BURNS

**First-degree burn** *(Involves only the epidermis)*

* These I° degree burns are dry and quite painful.
* Blistering seldom occurs and no scarring results.
* Gas explosion.
* Brief contact with hot liquids.

**Secondary-degree burn** (*burn all of the epidermis and much of the corium).* Characterised by blisters and accompanied by subcutaneous edema.

* With infection, deep dermal burns are readily converted to full thickness injury.
* Caused by short periods of exposure to intense flash heat.
* Contact with hot liquids.
* Peripheral zone of a deeper flame burn.

## PROPERTIES OF DIFFERENT SPLIT SKIN GRAFTS

| | Properties | Thiersch's Graft | Intermediate | 3/4 Thickness |
|---|---|---|---|---|
| 1. | Thickness | 0.1-0.2 | 0.2-0.4 | 0.4-0.5 |
| 2. | Colour match | Fair | Good | Very Good |
| 3. | Adequate protection | Fair | Good | Very Good |
| 4. | Regeneration of sensation | Rapid and good | Slow and fair | Slower and not very good |
| 5. | Healing of donor site | Very good | Good | Fair |
| 6. | Success of transplantation | Very good | Good | Fair |

## COMMONLY USED FREE SKIN GRAFTS

| *Type* | *Common donor site* | *Uses* | *Comment* |
|---|---|---|---|
| *Split skin graft* (thin, medium, or thick) | Thighs, abdomen, buttocks, back, and elsewhere | To close defects of integument almost anywhere on body | Donor sites epithelialize |
| *Full-thickness skin graft* (Wolfe or whole skin graft) | Retroauricular area, supraclavicular area, antecubital fossa | To close skin defects of limited size, particularly on face | Superior appearance and function; donor sites must be closed surgically |
| *Dermis graft* (whole graft with a thin graft removed from surface) | Abdomen or elsewhere | To fill out defects in contour or to bolster fascial defects | Buried beneath the skin surface |
| *Dermofat graft* (dermis graft with fat attached) | Abdomen, buttocks, or elsewhere | To fill out larger defects in contour | Loses 1/4 to 1/2 of bulk after implantation |
| *Hair follicle-bearing skin grafts* | Scalp, eyebrow | To repair scalp, eyebrow, or lashes | Usually applied in small patches or strips |
| *Composite skin grafts* (whole skin + cartilage; skin + fibrofat or bone) | Helix, anthelix, lobe of external ear<br>Fingertip (accident) | To repair defects of nose, ear, eyelid<br>To replace finger part | Only small grafts will survive<br>Works best for children |

*Other composite grafts finding occasional use are nipple-areolar grafts and nailbed-nail grafts.*

## CAUSES/SIGNS OF IMPORTANT DISEASES

### BURNS

**1. Depth of burn**

1. Partial thickness—Healing can occur from epithelial remnants.
2. Full thickness—Total destruction of all epithelial remnants.

**2. Local effects of burn**

1. Pain
2. Loss of fluid, electrolytes, protein
3. Heat loss—increased calorie requirement
4. Infection—staphylococcal initially
   —Gram negative especially pseudomonas after 5 days
   —Streptococci can convert partial thickness burns to full thickness
5. Thrombosis
   (i) From heat
   (ii) In electrical burns

**3. Systemic effects of burn**

1. Haemolysis
   (i) Direct effect of heat
   (ii) Increased red cell fragility
2. Generalised increase in capillary permeability. With exudation of fluid into ECF and wound
3. Salt and water loss—50% of plasma volume can be lost within 3 hours in 40% burn
4. Diminished cardiac output
   (i) Direct effect of circulating toxic substances
   (ii) Increased blood viscosity and peripheral resistance

5. Oliguria and renal failure
   (i) Hypovolaemia
   (ii) Haemoglobinuria
   (iii) Proteinuria
6. Curling's ulcer—May be related to disruption of mucosal barrier.
7. Respiratory failure
   (i) Sepsis
   (ii) Fluid overload
   (iii) Inhalation of smoke and carbon monoxide
8. Catabolism
   (i) Heat loss
   (ii) Sepsis
   (iii) Complication e.g. renal/respiratory failure

**4. Prognosis**

If age plus % of burn is more than 100, then mortality approaches 100%, mainly from toxaemia. Children do worse.

## ESTIMATION OF SURFACE AREA (%) BY THE RULES OF NINE AND FIVE

| | *Infants* | | *Children* | | *Adults* | |
|---|---|---|---|---|---|---|
| | *R-9* | *R-5* | *R-9* | *R-5* | *R-9* | *R-5* |
| Head | 19 | 20 | 15 | 15 | 10 | 5 |
| One Upper Arm (x2) | 9.5 | 10 | 9.5 | 10 | 9 | 10 |
| Front | 16 | 20 | 16 | 20 | 18 | 20 |
| Back | 16 | 20 | 16 | 20 | 18 | 20 |
| One lower leg (x2) | 15 | 10 | 17 | 15 | 18 | 20 |
| Total (percent) | 100 | 100 | 100 | 105* | 100 | 95** |

N.B. — R-9 — Wallace's 'Rule of Nine'
R-5 — Lynch and Blocker's (1963) 'Rule of Five'
* — 5% may be substracted from the trunk
** — 5% may be added to anterior or to both test

## TYPES OF SKIN FLAPS

1. Local Flap or Sliding Flap (French Method)
   a) Advancement flap (i) V-Y type (ii) Ordinary type
   b) Rotation flap or swinging advancement flap
   c) Transposition flap (Z-plasty)
   d) Multiple interlocking flap
   e) Interpolation flap
2. Pedicle flap (Single pedicle)
   a) Immediate transfer
   b) Delayed non-tubulised transfer
   c) Tubed flap

(Contd.....)

## TYPES OF SKIN FLAPS (Contd....)

d) Reversed tube flap
e) Cross lapped flap (delayed or non-delayed)
f) Direct transfer flap

3. Flaps transferred by regional juxta position—Delayed or non-delayed e.g. abdomen to hand flap.
4. Flaps transferred by intermediate host e.g. jump flaps to via forearm.
5. Tubed flaps transferred by successive migration e.g. caterpillar method.
6. Lined flaps—(i) graft lined flap (ii) Double flap (iii) Marsupialised flap.
7. Bridge flaps or tunnel flaps—Bipedicular flaps.
8. Artery flaps—non-delayed direct transfer.
9. Compound skin flap—When a skin flap carries some other tissue like bone.

## PROPERTIES OF DIFFERENT SPLIT SKIN GRAFTS

| | *Properties* | *Thiersch's Graft* | *Intermediate* | *3/4 Thickness* |
|---|---|---|---|---|
| 1. | Thickness | 0.1-0.2 | 0.-0.4 | 0.4-0.5 |
| 2. | Colour match | Fair | Good | Very good |
| 3. | Adequate protection | | | |
| 4. | Regeneration of sensation | Rapid and good | Slow and fair | Slower and not very good |
| 5. | Healing of donor site | Very good | Good | Fair |
| 6. | Success of transplantation | Very good | Good | Fair |

## SIGNS OF MALIGNANT CHANGE

1. Increase in size
2. Increase in pigment
3. Areas of depigmentation
4. Ulceration or bleeding
5. Irritation
6. Satellite lesions and spread of pigment from edge of lesion.
7. Regional lymph node enlargement—distant metastasis.

## DIFFERENCE BETWEEN BURNS FROM DRY HEAT, MOIST HEAT AND CHEMICALS

| | | *Dry Heat* | *Moist Heat* | *Chemicals* |
|---|---|---|---|---|
| 1. | Examples | Flame, heated solid body, x-rays temperature | Steam, liquid at boiling | Corrosive chemicals |
| 2. | Site of Contact | At and above | At and below | At and below |
| 3. | Skin | Dry, Shrivelled, may be charred | sudden and bleached | May be destroyed |
| 4. | Splashing | — | + | + |
| 5. | Vesicles | At the circumference of burnt area | Over the burnt area | Very rare |

(Contd.....)

## DIFFERENCE BETWEEN BURNS FROM DRY HEAT, MOIST HEAT AND CHEMICALS (Contd...)

| | | *Dry Heat* | *Moist Heat* | *Chemicals* |
|---|---|---|---|---|
| 6. | Red line | + | + | — |
| 7. | Colour | Black | Bleached | Distinctive |
| 8. | Charring | + | — | — |
| 9. | Singeing | + | — | — |
| 10. | Ulceration | — | — | — |
| 11. | Scar | Thick, contracted | Thin, less contracted | Thick, contracted |
| 12. | Clothes | Burnt | Wet, not burnt | May be burnt; show characteristic stains |

## DIFFERENCE BETWEEN PRIMARY AND SECONDARY CONTRACTION OF SKIN GRAFTS

| | *Primary Contraction* | *Secondary Contraction* |
|---|---|---|
| Onset | Immediately | 10th day onward. |
| Cause | Contraction of Elastic Fibres | Contraction of Fibrous Tissues |
| Thicker Graft | More | Less |
| Rigid Recipient Site | More | Less |

## GLASGOW COMA SCALE

| *Eye opening* | *Score* | *Motor response* | |
|---|---|---|---|
| Spontaneous | 4 | Obeys command | 6 |
| To voice | 3 | Localizes pain | 5 |
| To pain | 2 | Withdraw pain | 4 |
| None | 1 | Flexion pain | 3 |
| *Verbal response* | | Extension (pain) | 2 |
| Oriented | 5 | None | 1 |
| Confused | 4 | *Score* | |
| In appropriate words | 3 | 14-15 | V |
| Incomprehensible words | 2 | 11-13 | IV |
| None | 1 | 8-10 | III |
| | | 5-7 | II |
| | | 3-4 | I |

# MCQ's OF BURNS & PLASTIC SURGERY

## What is important in Burns & Plastic Surgery

Burns (degrees, management), Plastic Surgery

1. **Contracture is the most serious complication of burn healing in : AIIMS 1984, 86**
   A. Neck B. Hand
   C. Axilla D. All of the above
2. **The most commonly used formula for fluid replacement in the first 24 hours in burns is : Karnataka 1998**
   A. 2-4 cc/kg. body weight/percentage of burns.
   B. 6 cc/kg. body weight/percentage of burns.
   C. 8 cc/kg. body weight/percentage of burns.
   D. 10 cc/kg. body weight/percentage of burns.
3. **The following sites are unsuitable for skin graft (as they will not be vascularized) except: PGI 1986**
   A. Cortical bone
   B. Periosteum or Perichodrium
   C. Bare cartilage
   D. Bare tendon
4. **The definitive blood and lymph circulation in a graft is established in: AMU 1987**
   A. 2 days B. 3 days
   C. 5 days D. Few days
5. **Partial thickness graft of the hand is expected to heal (if no infection occurs) in——days. Delhi 1988**
   A. 3 to 5 B. 7 to 10
   C. 10 to 14 D. 21 to 31
6. **Full thickness burns of the hand are covered with in the : Delhi 1988**
   A. First 3 or 4 days B. 2 weeks
   C. 3 weeks D. 4 weeks
7. **Sepsis in burn cases is due to: AP 1989**
   A. B.proteus B. Staphylococci
   C. Pneumococci D. Pseudomonas
8. **A 24 years old male with black skin had to undergo extensive surgery for the treatment of burn. Raised dense lesions slowly developed around the sites of surgical incision. They are likely to be: UPSC 1986**
   A. Malignant melanoma
   B. Basal cell carcinoma
   C. Keloids
   D. Areas of chronic
9. **The most important consideration for 30 percent burns is: AIIMS 1984, 85, 86**
   A. Infection B. Contracture
   C. Skin grafting D. Cardiac status
10. **A split skin graft will not take on a bed consisting of: AIIMS 1986**
    A. Fascia B. Muscle
    C. Periostium D. Cartilage
11. **A full thickness loss of middle one third of the upper lips is best reconstructed by: AIIMS 1987**
    A. Naso labial flap B. Cheek flap
    C. Abbey flap D. Esalander flap
12. **Emergency procedures in deep burns case are all except : AIIMS 1990**
    A. Tarsorrhaphy B. Primary excision
    C. Tracheostomy D. Escharotomy
13. **Modern topical antibiotics have improved the prognosis of burns by all except: AIIMS 1990**
    A. ↑ number of bacteria/gm of burnt tissue
    B. Incidence of subeschar sepsis
    C. Penetration by bacteria
    D. Rapid epithelialization
14. **Rhinoplasty is usually done at—— year of age when the nose is fully grown. Rohtak 1985**
    A. 7 B. 9
    C. 12 D. 16

| Ans. | 1. D | 2. A | 3. B | 4. C | 5. C | 6. A | 7. B | 8. C | 9. A | 10. A |
|---|---|---|---|---|---|---|---|---|---|---|
| | 11. C | 12. B | 13. B | 14. D | | | | | | |

15. **Amnion dressings are to be changed every: AMU 1984**
A. 12 hours B. 24 hours
C. 48 hours D. 72 hours

16. **Failure of burn to heal within ———days suggest that depth of burn is greater than partial thickness. AIIMS 1986**
A. 2-3 B. 3-7
C. 7-10 D. 10-14

17. **Wallace's formula of nine for burn is not applicable to the following except : DNB 1990**
A. Children B. Elderly
C. Pregnant females D. Electrical burns

18. **Free skin graft is rejected on: AIIMS 1990**
A. Muscle B. Fat
C. Deep fascia D Dermis

19. **In a 52 years old woman with a 35 percent body surface burn of the trunk. AIIMS 1985**
A. Mortality is mainly secondory to burn shock.
B. The severity of infection can be less end by topical use of sulfamylon.
C. Systematic antimicrobials are of greater effect than are topical agents.
D. Either lactated Ringers solution or isotonic sodium chloride solution will be effective in combating burn shock.

20. **The ideal indicator of sufficient fluid replacement in burns is : AIIMS 1983, 85, 88, 89**
A. CVP
B. Urine output
C. BP
D. Arterial wedge pressure

21. **In case of Burns, the determinants of prognosis are except : AI 1993**
A. Age of patients B. Sex of the patients
C. Extent of burns D. Depth of burns

22. **For split skin graft the best source is: AI 1993, 96**
A. Autograft B. Homograft
C. Isograft D. Xenograft

23. **In burns heat loss is by/due to: Delhi 1992**
A. Dilatation of veins
B. ↑ glucocorticoids
C. ↑ exposed area of evaporation
D. None of the above

24. **Amnion dressing is sterilized by: BHU 1985**
A. Boiling B. Eusol
C. Silver sulphadiazine D. Sulphamylon

25. **Which of the following topical agent penetrates best in an eschar: AMU 1989**
A. Silver nitrate
B. Silver sulphadiazine
C. Mafenide
D. Cerum nitrate silver sulphadiazine

26. **Which of the following cardiovascular effects are not noted to result from a severe burn: AIIMS 1986**
A. Decrease in cardiac output
B. Increase in peripheral vascular resistance
C. Decrease in stroke volume
D. Diarrhoea
E. None of the above

27. **Painful bruising is seen in ———syndrome. DNB 1992**
A. Gardner-Diamond B. Gasser
C. Goldenher's D. Goltz/s

28. **To prevent renal shutdown in burn patient, all of the following can be utilised to aid to the situation, except : AIIMS 1985**
A. Mannitol administration
B. Maintain urine output between 30-50 c.c.per hour
C. Alkalinization of urine
D. Whole blood transfusion

29. **The fluids loss from a burn by evaporation is primarily: PGI 1985**
A. Isotonic
B. Hypertonic
C. Hypotonic
D. Depends upon the type of burn

30. **Dermatome is a: UPSC 1983; AMC 1985, 88**
A. Segment of skin supplied by a single spinal nerve.
B. Segment of skin supplied multiple spinal nerves.
C. Group of skin segments supplied by single spinal nerve
D. None of the above.

31. **Wolfe graft is: PGI 1986; UPSC 1989, 91**
A. Pedical graft
B. Full thickness skin graft
C. Partial thickness skin graft
D. Split thickness skin graft

32. **In 'distal' flap transfer, each stage takes on an average: AIIMS 1983**
A. 1 week B. 2 weeks
C. 3 weeks D. 6 weeks

33. **Full thickness skin graft can be taken for the following sites except: AIIMS 1983**
A. Elbow B. Back to neck
C. Supraclavicular area D. Upper eyelids

| Ans. | 15. C | 16. D | 17. C | 18. B | 19. D | 20. B | 21. B | 22. A | 23. C | 24. A |
|---|---|---|---|---|---|---|---|---|---|---|
| | 25. C | 26. C | 27. A | 28. D | 29. C | 30. A | 31. B | 32. C | 33. B | |

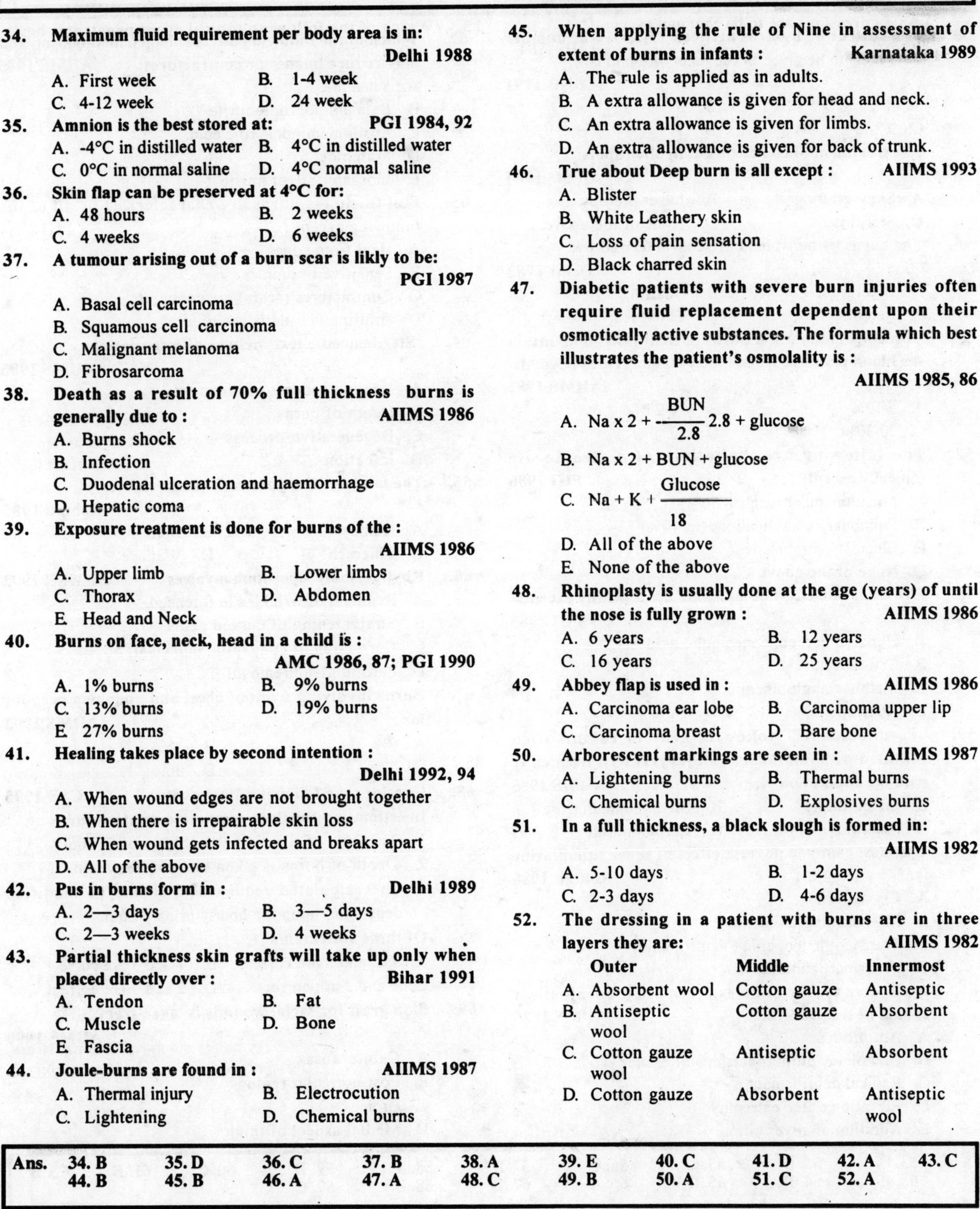

**34. Maximum fluid requirement per body area is in:** **Delhi 1988**

A. First week B. 1-4 week
C. 4-12 week D. 24 week

**35. Amnion is the best stored at:** **PGI 1984, 92**

A. -4°C in distilled water B. 4°C in distilled water
C. 0°C in normal saline D. 4°C normal saline

**36. Skin flap can be preserved at 4°C for:**

A. 48 hours B. 2 weeks
C. 4 weeks D. 6 weeks

**37. A tumour arising out of a burn scar is likly to be:** **PGI 1987**

A. Basal cell carcinoma
B. Squamous cell carcinoma
C. Malignant melanoma
D. Fibrosarcoma

**38. Death as a result of 70% full thickness burns is generally due to :** **AIIMS 1986**

A. Burns shock
B. Infection
C. Duodenal ulceration and haemorrhage
D. Hepatic coma

**39. Exposure treatment is done for burns of the :** **AIIMS 1986**

A. Upper limb B. Lower limbs
C. Thorax D. Abdomen
E. Head and Neck

**40. Burns on face, neck, head in a child is :** **AMC 1986, 87; PGI 1990**

A. 1% burns B. 9% burns
C. 13% burns D. 19% burns
E. 27% burns

**41. Healing takes place by second intention :** **Delhi 1992, 94**

A. When wound edges are not brought together
B. When there is irrepairable skin loss
C. When wound gets infected and breaks apart
D. All of the above

**42. Pus in burns form in :** **Delhi 1989**

A. 2—3 days B. 3—5 days
C. 2—3 weeks D. 4 weeks

**43. Partial thickness skin grafts will take up only when placed directly over :** **Bihar 1991**

A. Tendon B. Fat
C. Muscle D. Bone
E. Fascia

**44. Joule-burns are found in :** **AIIMS 1987**

A. Thermal injury B. Electrocution
C. Lightening D. Chemical burns

**45. When applying the rule of Nine in assessment of extent of burns in infants :** **Karnataka 1989**

A. The rule is applied as in adults.
B. A extra allowance is given for head and neck.
C. An extra allowance is given for limbs.
D. An extra allowance is given for back of trunk.

**46. True about Deep burn is all except :** **AIIMS 1993**

A. Blister
B. White Leathery skin
C. Loss of pain sensation
D. Black charred skin

**47. Diabetic patients with severe burn injuries often require fluid replacement dependent upon their osmotically active substances. The formula which best illustrates the patient's osmolality is :** **AIIMS 1985, 86**

A. $Na \times 2 + \frac{BUN}{2.8} 2.8 + glucose$
B. $Na \times 2 + BUN + glucose$
C. $Na + K + \frac{Glucose}{18}$
D. All of the above
E. None of the above

**48. Rhinoplasty is usually done at the age (years) of until the nose is fully grown :** **AIIMS 1986**

A. 6 years B. 12 years
C. 16 years D. 25 years

**49. Abbey flap is used in :** **AIIMS 1986**

A. Carcinoma ear lobe B. Carcinoma upper lip
C. Carcinoma breast D. Bare bone

**50. Arborescent markings are seen in :** **AIIMS 1987**

A. Lightening burns B. Thermal burns
C. Chemical burns D. Explosives burns

**51. In a full thickness, a black slough is formed in:** **AIIMS 1982**

A. 5-10 days B. 1-2 days
C. 2-3 days D. 4-6 days

**52. The dressing in a patient with burns are in three layers they are:** **AIIMS 1982**

| | Outer | Middle | Innermost |
|---|---|---|---|
| A. | Absorbent wool | Cotton gauze | Antiseptic |
| B. | Antiseptic wool | Cotton gauze | Absorbent |
| C. | Cotton gauze wool | Antiseptic | Absorbent |
| D. | Cotton gauze | Absorbent | Antiseptic wool |

**Ans.** 34. B 35. D 36. C 37. B 38. A 39. E 40. C 41. D 42. A 43. C
44. B 45. B 46. A 47. A 48. C 49. B 50. A 51. C 52. A

**53. In a patient with burns between 25-50% the number of rations to be given in the form of blood is:** **DNB 1991**

A. 4 B. 3
C. 2 D. 1

**54. The treatment of choice for Mongolian spots:** **UPSC 1984**

A. Skin grafting B. Laser therapy
C. Steroids D. None of the above

**55. The burns by moist heat are characterized by:** **Delhi 1982**

A. Ulceration B. Charring
C. Red line D. Thick scar

**56. Vasoconstriction in a burns patient fails to maintain the blood pressure when blood loss increases beyond:** **AIIMS 1982**

A. 5-10% B. 10-20%
C. 20-30% D. 50%

**57. The following are limitations of mafenide use topically except:** **PGI 1986**

A. Maculopapular rash (in 50%)
B. Pulmonary complications (in 40%)
C. Electrolyte imbalance
D. None of the above

**58. The main side effect of mafenide use topically except:** **PGI 1985**

A. Hypercholoraemic metabolic acidosis
B. Crystalluria
C. Methhaemoglobinemia
D. Neutropenia

**59. "Pseudoeschar" (yellowish gray in colour often confused with full thickness injury) is seen frequently with the application of:** **AIIMS 1985**

A. Silver nitrate B. Silver suphadiazine
C. Mafenide D. Cerium nitrate

**60. The most common adverse effect of silver sulfadiazine is:** **Rohtak 1988**

A. Crystalluria
B. Methhaemoglobinemia
C. Transient leucopenia (Neutropenia)
D. Transient jaundice

**61. A circular eschar of an extermity in a burn patient should be treated with :** **AIIMS 1986**

A. Antibiotics
B. Complete spitting incisions of eschar
C. Radical debridement
D. Elevation of the extremity
E. Addition of silver nitrate

**62. Which of the following alters collagen metabolism, and may reduce burn scar contractures:** **AIIMS 1986**

A. Vitamin-C
B. Beta aminopropionitrite
C. Epsilon aminocaproic acid
D. Mafenide
E. Inorganic silver nitrite

**63. Full thickness burns are characterized by all of the following except :** **PGI 1984**

A. Heal from edges
B. Sensitive to pain
C. Contractures (scars) are common
D. Grafting is usually required

**64. 'Sterile needle test' help in differentiating:** **AIIMS 1986**

A. Healing process of burns
B. Depth of burns
C. Degenerative process
D. Infection

**65. The famous 'Rule of nine' was given by:** **Rohtak 1985**

A. Humby B. Muir
C. Thiersch D. Wallace

**66. Rhytidectomy operation involves :** **JIPMER 1992**

A. Removal of wrinkles in forehead
B. Straightening of curved penis
C. Correction of congenital defects of nose
D. Parotid gland removal

**67. Burns involving front of chest and abdomen account for :** **AIIMS 1992**

A. 9% B. 18%
C. 27% D. 36%

**68. Consider the following statements :** **CSE 1995**
**In estimating the fluid requirements after burns :**

1. The Rule of Nine is a valuable guide in adults.
2. Depth of burns is taken into consideration.
3. The calculated requirement should be modified depending upon the hourly urinary output.

**Of these statements**

A. 1, 2 and 3 are correct B. 1 and 3 are correct
C. 1 and 2 are correct D. 2 and 3 are correct

**69. Skin graft for facial wounds is taken from:** **AIIMS 1990**

A. Cubital fossa
B. Post-auricular region
C. Groin
D. Medial aspect of thigh

| Ans. | 53. C | 54. D | 55. C | 56. C | 57. D | 58. A | 59. B | 60. C | 61. B | 62. B |
|---|---|---|---|---|---|---|---|---|---|---|
| | 63. B | 64. B | 65. D | 66. A | 67. B | 68. B | 69. C | | | |

**70. An isograft indicates transfer of tissues between: JIPMER 1993; UPSC 2003**

A. Related donors B. Monozygotic twins
C. Part of some individual D. Unrelated donors

**71. Generalised diffuse pertoinitis has been compared to second and third degree burns of: AIIMS 1984, 86**

A. 13% B. 30%
C. 45% D. 60%

**72. Which one of the following applies best to burn depth of: Orissa 1999**

A. Cannot be estimated clinically.
B. Can be approximated by sensitivity to pin prick.
C. Can be estimated by length of time for slough to occur.
D. Can be estimated by degree of pain.

**73. Leg injury with 10x10 cm bone exposed, ideal graft is : AIIMS 1999**

A. Full thickness B. Amniotic membrane
C. Pedicle D. Split

**74. Head & neck involvement in burns in infant is : PGI 2000**

A. 9% B. 18%
C. 27% D. 32%

**75. Graft survival in Ist 48 hrs. depends on : AIIMS 1999**

A. Plasma imbibation
B. Connection B/W donor & receipient capillaries
C. Ingrowth of capillaries into donors tissue
D. Amount of saline in graft

**76. Which one of the following definitions is false : Kerala 2000**

A. Graft-Transfer of cells or tissue.
B. Autograft-from one part to another part of an individual
C. Syngeneic graft—graft from one individual to a genetically identical individual.
D. Homograft—Graft from one species to another species.
E. Allograft—From one individual to a genetically different individual of the same species.

**77. In chest wall reconstruction the preferred flap is : UPSC 2001**

A. Local random pattern skin flap
B. Pedicled muscle base flap
C. Axial pattern flap
D. Split skin graft

**78. In random pattern flap, safe length to breath ratio is : Delhi 2001**

A. 2:1 B. 3:1
C. 1:2 D. 1:1

**79. True regarding deep burn is all of the following except : SGPGI 2002**

A. Loss of pain
B. Charred appearance
C. Loss of skin reaction
D. Presence of blisters

**80. In a skin graft transfer the word 'take' of graft refers to : SGPGI 2002**

A. Healing of graft
B. Vascularization of graft
C. Dense attachment of graft to surrounding tissue
D. Epithelial ingrowth in the margins

**81. The subdermal plexus forms the vascular basis for : JIPMER 2002**

A. Randomised flaps B. Axial flaps
C. Mucocutaneous flaps D. Fasciocutaneous flaps

**82. A 14 years old girl sustains a steam burn measuring 6 by 7 inches over the ulnar aspect of her right forearm. Blisters develop over the entire area of the burn wound, and by the time the patient is seen after 6 hour the injury. Some of the blisters have ruptured spontaneously. In addition to debridement of the necrotic epithelium, all the following therapeutic regimens might be considered appropriate for this patient, except: AI 2002**

A. Application of silver sulfadiazine and daily washes but no dressing.
B. Application of Polyvinylpyrrolidone foam, daily washes and light occlusive dressing changed daily.
C. Application of mafenide acetate cream, but no daily washes or dressing
D. Heterograft application with sutures to secure in place and daily washes, but no washes.

**83. True about Hickman tube : CMC 2001**

A. Is a silicon tube
B. Indwelling IV transthoracic device
C. Usually needed for T.P.N.
D. All

**84. An isograft is one that is transferred : UPSC 2003**

A. In the same individual.
B. Between monozygotic twins.
C. From 1 belonging to blood group-A and other to blood group B
D. From animal to human when the organ involved is identical.

**85. The ideal temperature of water to cool the burnt surface is : UPSC 2002**

A. 15°C B. 10°C
C. 8°C D. 6°C

| Ans. | 70. B | 71. C | 72. A | 73. C | 74. B | 75. C | 76. D | 77. B | 78. A | 79. D |
|---|---|---|---|---|---|---|---|---|---|---|
| | 80. B | 81. A | 82. D | 83. D | 84. B | 85. A | | | | |

**86. The best cosmetic results for large capillary (port wine) haemangiomas are achieved by : UPSC 2005**

A. Excision and split-thickness skin grafting
B. Laser ablation
C. Cryosurgery
D. Tattooing

**87. The best guide to adequate tissue perfusion in the fluid management of a patient with burns, is to ensure a minimum hourly urine output of : Karnataka 2004**

A. 10-30 ml. B. 30-50 ml.
B. 50-70 ml. D. 70-100 ml.

**88. Sun-burns are : Karnataka 2005**

A. First Degree Burns
B. Second Degree Burns
C. Third Degree Burns
D. Could be any of the above

**89. A full thickness graft can be obtained from al! of the following sites except :**

A. Axilla
B. Elbow
C. Groin
D. Supraclavicular

Ans. 86. C 87. B 88. D 89. D

# EXPLANATIONS OF BURNS & PLASTIC SURGERY

1. Ans.— D. All of the above
2. Ans.— A. 2-4 cc/kg. body weight/percentage of burns.
3. Ans.— B. Periosteum or Perichodrium
4. Ans.— C. 5 days
5. Ans.— C. 10 to 14
6. Ans.— A. First 3 or 4 days
7. Ans.— B. Staphylococci

   Staph aureus is commonest. Streptococcus is a treatment pathogen and pseudomonas pyocyaneus grows on raw surface.
8. Ans.— C. Keloids
9. Ans.— A. Infection
10. Ans.— A. Fascia
11. Ans.— C. Abbey flap
12. Ans.— B. Primary excision
13. Ans.— B. Incidence of subeschar sepsis
14. Ans.— D. 16
15. Ans.— C. 48 hours
16. Ans.— D. 10-14
17. Ans.— C. Pregnant females
18. Ans.— B. Fat
19. Ans.— D. Either lactated Ringers solution or isotonic sodium chloride solution will be effective in combating burn shock.
20. Ans.— B. Urine output

    Pulse, BP and hourly urine volumes are used.
21. Ans.— B. Sex of the patients

    Partial thickness burns heal because remnants of epidermis in hair follicles and sweat glands spread over the wound surface.
22. Ans.— A. Autograft

    It is graft from one part of body to another.
23. Ans.— C. ↑ exposed area of evaporation
24. Ans.— A. Boiling
25. Ans.— C. Mafenide
26. Ans.— C. Decrease in stroke volume
27. Ans.— A. Gardner-Diamond
28. Ans.— D. Whole blood transfusion
29. Ans.— C. Hypotonic
30. Ans.— A. Segment of skin supplied by a single spinal nerve.
31. Ans.— B. Full thickness skin graft
32. Ans.— C. 3 weeks
33. Ans.— B. Back to neck
34. Ans.— B. 1-4 week
35. Ans.— D. 4°C normal saline
36. Ans.— C. 4 weeks
37. Ans.— B. Squamous cell carcinoma
38. Ans.— A. Burns shock
39. Ans.— E Head and Neck

    Majority of facial burns heal spontaneously and should be treated openly with daily application of cream.
40. Ans.— C. 13% burns

    In a child aged one year, the head and neck area is 18% and in a child aged 5, it is 13% of total body area.
41. Ans.— D. All of the above
42. Ans.— A. 2—3 days
43. Ans.— C. Muscle
44. Ans.— B. Electrocution
45. Ans.— B. A extra allowance is given for head and neck.
46. Ans.— A. Blister
47. Ans.— A. $Na \times 2 + \frac{BUN}{2.8} + glucose$ 2.8

**48. Ans.— C. 16 years**

**49. Ans.— B. Carcinoma upper lip**

**50. Ans.— A. LightEning burns**

**51. Ans.— C. 2-3 days**

**52. Ans.— A. Absorbent wool Cotton gauze Antiseptic**

**53. Ans.— C. 2**

**54. Ans.— D. None of the above**

**55. Ans.— C. Red line**

**56. Ans.— C. 20-30%**

**57. Ans.— D. None of the above**

**58. Ans.— A. Hypercholoraemic metabolic acidosis**

**59. Ans.— B. Silver suphadiazine**

**60. Ans.— C. Transient leucopenia (Neutropenia)**

**This is self-limiting.**

**61. Ans.— B. Complete spitting incisions of eschar**

**62. Ans.— B. Beta aminopropionitrite**

**63. Ans.— B. Sensitive to pain**

**64. Ans.— B. Depth of burns**

**65. Ans.— D. Wallace**

**This is used in adults. This rule does not apply to infants and children.**

**66. Ans.— A. Removal of wrinkles in forehead**

**67. Ans.— B. 18%**

**68. Ans.— B. 1 and 3 are correct**

**69. Ans.— C. Groin**

**70. Ans.— B. Monozygotic twins**

**71. Ans.— C. 45%**

**72. Ans.— A. Cannot be estimated clinically**

**73. Ans.— C. Pedicle**

**74. Ans.— B. 18%**

**75. Ans.— C. Ingrowth of capillaries into donors tissue.**

**76. Ans.— D. Homograft-Graft from one species to another species.**

**77. Ans.— B. Pedicled muscle base flap**

**78. Ans.— A. 2 : 1**

**79. Ans.— D. Presence of blisters**

**80. Ans.— B. Vascularization of graft**

**81. Ans.— A. Randomised flaps**

**82. Ans.— D. Heterograft application with sutures to secure in place and daily washes, but no washes.**

**Heterograft application is not indicated at this stage.**

**83. Ans.— D. All**

**84. Ans.— B. Between monozygotic twins**

**Classification of skin graft according to species :**

- **Autograft is graft from one place to another on the same individual.**
- **Isograft is tissue transferred between two genetically idential individuals (identical twins).**
- **Allograft (homograft) is graft from one individual to another of the same species.**
- **Xenograft (heterograft) is graft from one species to a recipient of another species.**

**85. Ans.— A. 15°C**

**86. Ans.— C. Cryosurgery**

**87. Ans.— B. 30-50 ml.**

**88. Ans.— D. Could be any of the above**

# 3

# IMPORTANT TEXT OF NEUROSURGERY

## INTRACRANIAL TUMORS

| | | |
|---|---|---|
| A) | Secondaries (esp. lung) | Commonest |
| B) | Primary | |
| | (i) Glioma | 43% |
| | (ii) Meningioma | 18% |
| | (iii) Pituitary Adenoma | 12% |
| | (iv) Schawannoma | 8% |
| | (v) Chronic pharyngioma | 5% |
| | (vi) Blood vessel Tumor | 2% |
| | (vii) Others | 12% |

## INDICATIONS FOR SKULL X-RAY IN HEAD INJURY

(i) Loss of consciousness/Amnesia
(ii) Focal neurological deficit
(iii) Suspected penetrating injury
(iv) Scalp bruise/Swelling
(v) Alcohol intoxication
(vi) Difficulty in assessing patient

## PRIMARY INTRACRANIAL NEOPLASMS*

*Neuroepithelial*

- Astrocytoma, grades I, II, III, and IV
- Ependymomas
- Oligodendrogliomas
- Medulloblastoma
- Pinealoma
- Papilloma of choroid plexus
- Paraphyseal (colloid) cyst
- Neurilemmoma

*Mesodermal*

- Meningiomas
- Hemangioblastoma
- Chordoma

*Ectodermal*

- Craniopharyngioma
- Pituitary adenomas

*Congenital*

- Epidermoid
- Dermoid

* Neoplasms occurring with extreme rarity have been omitted from this classification, those tumors listed in the plueral term occur with varying histological types and grades of differentiation.

# MCQ's OF NEUROSURGERY

## What is important in Neurosurgery

Head injury (Glasgow coma scale, Management), Haematoma (Subdural, Extradural, Lucid interval), Brain Tumours (Secondaries, Primaries, Calcification, Effects) Aneurysms, Abscesses, Hydrocephalus, Spine (Tumours, Injuries), Nerves (Regeneration, Suturing)

1. **Pseudopapilloedema differs from papilloedema by the absence of the following except : PGI 1986**
   A. Haemorrhage
   B. Engorgement of retinal vessels
   C. Decreased visual acquity
   D. All of the above
2. **By increase in intracranial pressure the fluids pressure is primarly increased in : AMU 1985**
   A. Subdural sheath around optic nerve
   B. Subarachnoid space around optic nerve
   C. Optic nerve itself
   D. All of the above
3. **By increase in intracranial pressure, papilloedema is due to: AIIMS 1986**
   A. Compression of retinal vein
   B. Compression of retinal artery
   C. Dilatation of retinal vein
   D. Not known
4. **Vomiting is prominent in : AMU 1985**
   A. Frontal lobe meningioma
   B. Parietal lobe glioma
   C. Frontal lobe atrophy
   D. Focal lesion in IV ventricle
5. **Patients with thymoma and myasthenia gravis should receive anticholinesterase upto ——before surgery. AMU 1987**
   A. 3-4 hrs B. 6-8 hrs
   C. 12-24 hrs D. 24-48 hrs
   E. 48-72 hrs
6. **Which of the following is the commonest bacterial cause of brain abscess after trauma involving multiple fractures of skull: AMC 1987**
   A. Staphylococcus B. Streptococcus
   C. H.influenzae D. Esch coli
7. **Find the wrong match: AIIMS 1984**

| | Age group | Cause of meningitis |
|---|---|---|
| A. | Infant | Esch.coli |
| B. | Below 4 years | H.influenzae |
| C. | Adults | Meningococcus |
| D. | None of the above | |

8. **The bacteria most often associated with meningitis secondary to ear infection : AIIMS 1985**
   A. Meningococcus B. Pneumococcus
   C. Esch. coli D. Staphylococcus
9. **The commonest cause of secondaries in brain is tumours of: UPSC 1988**
   A. Lung B. Breast
   C. Larynx D. Liver
10. **The following intracranial secondaries may cause bony changes except : Rohtak 1988**
    A. Hodgkin's lymphoma B. Carcinoma stomach
    C. Secondaries D. Multiple myeloma
11. **The following bone tumour may cause dural deposited without causing bony changes : AIIMS 1986**
    A. Hodgkin's lymphoma B. Multiple myeloma
    C. Secondaries D. Fibrous dysplasia
12. **Sturge-Weber syndrome is characterized by all of the following except : AIIMS 1988**
    A. Mental retardation
    B. Visual disturbances
    C. Angiomas of choroid and pia mater
    D. Renal anomalies
13. **A dome shaped skull with a high forehead in the infant with slight hydrocephalus (olympian brow) is seen in: AIIMS 1984**
    A. Marasmus B. Congenital syphilis
    C. Rickets D. Arnold Chiari syndrome

**Ans.** 1. D 2. B 3. A 4. D 5. B 6. A 7. D 8. B 9. A 10. A 11. A 12. D 13. B

**14. In acute head injury, immediate operation is indicated by : UPSC 1985**
A. Bloody spinal fluid on lumbar tap
B. Unilateral fixed dilated pupil
C. Rapidly changing neurological
D. Generalised convulsive seizures

**15. Patient with a history of fall, present a week later with headache and progressive neurological deterioration. The diagnosis is: AI 1989**
A. Acute subdural haemorrhage
B. Extradural haemorrhage
C. Chronic subdural haemorrhage
D. Fracture skull

**16. In a patient with a moderately severe head injury, the development of the following sign suggests an acute increase in the intracranial tension : MAHE 1994**
A. A deterioration in the level of consciousness.
B. A decrease in the arterial blood pressure.
C. An increase in the heart rate.
D. An increase in the rate of respiration.

**17. True about blood picture in Eosinophilic granuloma is: Delhi 1986**
A. ↑ Eosinophilis
B. ↓ Eosinophilis
C. Normal
D. Variable or normal eosinophils and not important for diagnosis

**18. Wrist drop is seen in palsy of : Delhi 1986**
A. Ulnar nerve B. Radial nerve
C. Median nerve D A + B

**19. Feature of extradural haemorrhage include all except : AP 1987**
A. Severe hypotension
B. Deteriorating consciousness
C. Fixed dilated pupil on the same side
D. Fracture line crossing the temporal bone

**20. The involvement of cortical lesions cause the following type of speech defect : AIIMS 1987**
A. Dysphasia B. Dysarthria
C. Dysphonia D. Disarticulation

**21. A patient has meningomyelocele with paraplegia, true is: AIIMS 1988**
A. Can be improved by surgery
B. Can not be improved by surgery
C. Will improve as he gain age
D. None of the above

**22. Vomiting following head injury is: Delhi 1983**
A. A sign of recovery from cerebral contusion.
B. A sign of recovery from cerebral concussion.
C. A sign of recovery from cerebral laceration.
D. A sign of Omen.

**23. Commonest calcified brain mass in children in suprasellar region is: Delhi 1987**
A. Craniopharyngioma B. Meningioma
C. Tuberculoma D. Medulloblastoma

**24. Commonest primary brain tumour is: PGI 1983, 86; Delhi 1986; AIIMS 1986**
A. Astrocytoma B. Glioblastoma
C. Ependymoma D. Meningioma

**25. Commonest intramedullary spinal tumour is: Delhi 1986**
A. Chordoma B. Meningioma
C. Ependymoma D. Oligodendroglioma

**26. Bloody C.S.F. is seen in: Delhi 1992**
A. Sub-arachnoid haemorrhage
B. Sub-dural haemorrhage
C. Extra Dural hematoma
D. Cavernous sinus thrombosis

**27. Seizures in a patient of age 50 years is suggestive of: Delhi 1992**
A. Trauma B. Tumour
C. Hysterical D. CVA

**28. Subdural effusion is caused by : AIIMS 1986, 92; Delhi 1992; AI 1993**
A. Haemophilus influenzae
B. Pneumococcus
C. Str.virdans
D. Staph. aureus

**29. Lumbar puncture is dangerous in : Delhi 1984, 94**
A. Spinal cord tumour
B. Renal failure
C. Metabolic alkalosis
D. All of the above

**30. Complete functional loss in a peripheral nerve without anatomic disruption and sudden complete return of the function in 60-90 days is called : UPSC 1984**
A. Neuropraxis B. Neurolysis
C. Chronaxie D. Demyelinization

**31. For cystic lesions in brain, investigation of choice is: DNB 1990**
A. Angiography B. Ultrasound
C. CT scan D. MRI

**Ans.** 14. C 15. C 16. A 17. C 18. B 19. A 20. A 21. A 22. D 23. A
24. A 25. C 26. A 27. D 28. A 29. A 30. A 31. D

32. **Operative control of bleeding from wounds of the scalp is best achieved by: Rohtak 1986**
A. Diathermy to bleeding vessels
B. Eversion of galea aponeurotica
C. Applying several forceps to the bleeding points
D. Direct pressure applied to the skin

33. **Subarachnoid haemorrhage is commonly due to: UPSC 1987; JIPMER 1992; WB 1995**
A. Hypertension B. Rupture of aneurysm
C. Trauma D. Stroke

34. **The most common site of chondroma in vertebral column is: JIPMER 1992**
A. Sacro-coccygeal B. Cervico-Thoracic
C. Thoracic D. Thoraco lumber

35. **Management of extradural haemorrhage is: AIIMS 1992**
A. Immediate evacuation
B. Evacuation after 24 hours
C. Antibiotics
D. Observation

36. **The first step in the management of head injury is: Rajasthan 1991, 94; AIIMS 1992**
A. Secure airway B. I.V mannitol
C. I.V Dexamethasone D. Blood transfusion

37. **Most common site of meningomyelocele is: AIIMS 1992**
A. Cervical spine B. Lumbo sacral spine
C. Thoracic spine D. Skull

38. **Most common tumour of posterior cranial fossa : PGI 1993**
A. Meningioma B. Glioma
C. Medulloblastoma D. Oligodendroglioma

39. **Glasgow coma scale includes all of the following except : DNB 1991**
A. Eye opening B. Verbal performance
C. Motor activity D. Motor tone

40. **Disorders of limbic system primarily affects: AIIMS 1984**
A. Recall of past memory
B. Recognition of past memory
C. Registration of new memory
D. All of the above

41. **The commonest cause of focal temporal lobe epilepsy is: AIIMS 1984**
A. Tumour B. Idiopathic
C. Abscess D. Tuberculoma

42. **The following are the blood gas changes associated with raised intracranial pressure: AIIMS 1984, 86**

| | Paco2 | Pao2 |
|---|---|---|
| A. | Increase | Increase |
| B. | Increase | Decrease |
| C. | Decrease | Increase |
| D. | Decrease | Decrease |

43. **The organism most often associated with subdural abscess: Delhi 1984**
A. Staphylococcus B. Streptococcus
C. Pneumococcus D. Meningococcus

44. **First symptom of papilloedema is : Delhi 1985**
A. Increased blind spot B. Seeing moving objects
C. Gastric upset D. Lacrimation

45. **Commonest site of meningocele: AI 1989**
A. Lumbosacral B. Occipital
C. Frontal D. Thoracic

46. **In chronic subdural haematoma, not seen is : PGI 1980; AMC 1985**
A. Always preceded with history of unconsciousness
B. Stroke
C. Headache
D. Paraplegia or altered sensorium

47. **Spinal shock due to contusion usually recovers in : AIIMS 1983**
A. 1-2 days B. 5-7days
C. 7-14 days D. 14-21 days

48. **Angular vein infection commonly causes thrombosis of ——sinus. AIIMS 1982**
A. Cavernous B. Sphenoidal
C. Petrosal D. Sigmoid

49. **Infants and children irradiated for the treatment of an enlargement of the thymus are at an increased risk of : MAHE 1995**
A. Carcinoma of the thyroid
B. Leukaemia
C. Malignant thymoma
D. Mediastinal germinoma

50. **The rate of growth in nerves after peripheral nerve suturing is: JIPMER 1986; AIIMS 1986, 87**
A. 1 mm/day B. 1.5 mm/ day
C. 2 mm/day D. 3 mm/day

51. **Most persisting symptom of head injury is: DNB 1990**
A. Amnesia B. Fits
C. Anosmia D. Headache

| Ans. | 32. B | 33. B | 34. C | 35. A | 36. A | 37. B | 38. C | 39. D | 40. C | 41. B |
|---|---|---|---|---|---|---|---|---|---|---|
| | 42. B | 43. B | 44. A | 45. A | 46. A | 47. A | 48. A | 49. A | 50. A | 51. D |

**52. Cauda equina lesion may produce : PGI 1983**

A. Brown Sequard lesion B. Quadriplegia
C. Any of the above D. None of the above

**53. In children, intracranial tumours are more common in: PGI 1984, 85**

A. Anterior fossa
B. Middle fossa
C. Posterior fossa
D. Equal incidences in all fossa

**54. Musculo skeletal abnormality in neurofibromatosis: AMC 1983; PGI 1988**

A. Hypertrophy of limb B. Scoliosis
C. Cafe au lait spots D. Pseudoarthrosis
E. All of the above

**55. The main and the common symptom of vertebro-basilar insufficiency is: AMC 1986, 87**

A. Vertigo B. Diplopia
C. Fainting D. Nausea

**56. Locked-in-syndrome is usually seen in lesions of the following except : AMU 1989**

A. Thalamus B. Pons
C. Tegmentum D. Medulla

**57. Which of the following is not an early feature of extramedullary spinal tumour : AIIMS 1986; AMC 1986**

A. Bladder involvement
B. Touch fibres on the side of lesion
C. Proprioceptive fibres involved on the side of lesion
D. Muscle weakness below lesion

**58. In Infants, papilloedema may be seen in : PGI 1984**

A. Frontal lobe tumors
B. Temporal lobe tumours
C. Medulloblastoma
D. Sagittal sinus thrombosis

**59. Brain space occupying lesion causes death by: UPSC 1982; PGI 1983, 87; Delhi 1984, 86,**

A. Acute Hypertension B. Brain herniation
C. Cushing's syndrome D. Hypotension

**60. The commonest of triad of brain SOL are all except: PGI 1984**

A. Headache B. Vomiting
C. Diplopia D. Papilloedema

**61. Disease which is congenital is: AMU 1985**

A. Glioblastoma B. Medulloblastoma
C. Multiple sclerosis D. Neurofibroma

**62. Tibulant ataxia is typically seen in: AIIMS 1985**

A. Medulloblastoma B. Grave's disease
C. Multiple sclerosis D. Aortic regurgitation

**63. In children below 10 years, commonest cause of Pineal calcification is: AIIMS 1985**

A. Tumour B. Cysticercosis
C. Toxoplasmosis D. Normal

**64. Pineal calcification is usually ——shaped. AIIMS 1985**

A. Spherical B. Oval
C. Comma D. Diamond

**65. Below the level of the lesion in spinal concussion (produced by long axis stretch on the cord accompanying flexion) there is (with one exception): AIIMS 1986**

A. A flaccid paralysis
B. Retention of urine
C. Loss of joint sense
D. Loss of pain and temperature sensation

**66. In the immediate management of patient who may possibly have cervical spinal injury. Which of the following statement is incorrect: UPSC 1985**

A. Cervical injuries should be transported with the head lifted on to a pillow.
B. The patient should be left lying on the stretcher until examination is completed.
C. If a cord lesion is present the best immediate examination is testing the sensory level to pink prick on the trunk.
D. A lateral X-ray should be taken without disturbing the patient.

**67. Ideal treatment to relieve pain after nerve suture is: Delhi 1992**

A. Exercise B. Analgesics
C. Narcotic analgesics D. Sedatives
E. Steroids

**68. Which is not a sign of increased intracranial pressure: AMU 1986**

A. Bitemporal hemianopia
B. Headache
C. Bradycardia
D. Convulsions

**69. The subclavian steal syndrome (giddiness associated with upper limb exercise) can be caused by: DNB 1990**

A. Stenosis of the origin of the vertebral artery.
B. Stenosis of the origin of the internal carotid artery.
C. Stenosis of the origin of the subclavian artery.
D. Stenosis of the subclavian artery where it crosses first rib.

| Ans. | | | | | | | | | |
|---|---|---|---|---|---|---|---|---|---|
| 52. C | 53. C | 54. E | 55. A | 56. A | 57. A | 58. D | 59. B | 60. C | 61. C |
| 62. C | 63. A | 64. C | 65. C | 66. A | 67. A | 68. A | 69. C | | |

**70. Characteristics of the congenital hydrocephalus include each of the following except: AP 1989**

A. Convulsion B. Sun set sign
C. Crack-pot sign D. Transillumination

**71. Witzelsucht syndrome (i.e "Pathological Joking") is seen in : Rohtak 1986**

A. Frontal lobe tumours
B. Parietal lobe tumours
C. Temporal lobe tumours
D. IV ventricular tumour

**72. Empty sella syndrome is often characterized by: AMU 1986**

A. Pituitary tumour B. Cretinism
C. Acromegaly D. None of the above

**73. Protrusion of the lips occurring due tapping the skin at angle of the mouth (Escherich's sign) is seen in: AIIMS 1986**

A. Frontal lobe damage B. Tuberous sclerosis
C. Tetany D. Hyperparathyroidism

**74. The incidence of thymoma development in patient with myasthenia gravis is: AIIMS 1986**

A. 30-45% B. 20-30%
C. 15-20% D. 5-15%

**75. Which of the following lesions of the thymus is most commonly associated with myasthenia gravis : PGI 1987**

A. Lymphoepthelioma
B. Teratoma
C. Granulomatous thymoma
D. None of the above

**76. After an open injury, the optimum time for nerve suture is: PGI 1985**

A. Immediately B. Within one month
C. 1-2 months D. 2-4 months
E. When wound is free from infection

**77. The following are true about the characteristics of sacrococcygeal teratoma except : CMC 1986**

A. One of the most common large tumours seen during first three months of life.
B. Males are more often affected than females.
C. Tumours arise between sacrum and rectum.
D. Prone to become malignant.

**78. All of the following are indications for ventilatory support in patients with head injury except : CSE 1995**

A. $PaO_2$ less than 70 mm Hg
B. $PaCO_2$ more than 45 mm Hg
C. $PaO_2$ saturation less than 90%
D. $PaCO_2$ less than 35 mm Hg

**79. Absolute 3rd nerve palsy occurs in : TN 1998**

A. Aneurysm of middle cerebral-A
B. Aneurysm of anterior cerebral-A
C. Aneurysm of posterior communicating-A
D. Aneurysm of inferior cerebellar-A

**80. Brain abscess may be due to following : AMC 1985**

A. Chronic S.O.M. B. Chronic lung abscess
C. Trauma D. Any of the above

**81. The treatment of cerebral oedema includes : AMC 1985**

A. Restriction of fluid intake
B. Diuretics
C. Glucocorticoids
D. Maintenance of airway
E. All of the above

**82. Non metastatic neurological manifestation in bronchogenic carcinoma includes all of the following, except : CMC 1987**

A. Cerebellar degeneration
B. Hoarseness of voice
C. Myopathy
D. Peripheral neuropathy

**83. The neurosurgical procedure used in Parkinson's disease ,electrocoagulation of a localized area within the brain presumably blocks the output. Which is the form of an excessive feedback, originates in the: UPSC 1985**

A. Basal ganglia
B. Motor cortex
C. Precentral cortex
D. Medullary portion of the reticular formation

**84. Treatment of choice for subgaleal hematoma: UPSC 1987**

A. Incision and evacuation
B. Needle aspiration
C. Antibiotics and then drain
D. Conservative

**85. Facial nerve palsy is seen in the following fracture: PGI 1984**

A. Anterior cranial fossa B. Posterior cranial fossa
C. Middle cranial fossa D. Cranial vault

**86. Consider the following sites of obstruction : CSE 1996**

1. Foramina of Munro
2. Outside the ventricular system
3. At the exist of the fourth system

**Hydrocephalus is described as non-communicating when the obstruction is at : CSE 1996**

A. 1, 2 and 3 B. 1 and 2
C. 2 and 3 D. 1 and 3

| Ans. | | | | | | | | | | |
|---|---|---|---|---|---|---|---|---|---|---|
| | 70. A | 71. A | 72. D | 73. C | 74. A | 75. A | 76. E | 77. B | 78. D | 79. C |
| | 80. D | 81. E | 82. B | 83. A | 84. D | 85. C | 86. A | | | |

**87. Subdural haemorrhage is commonly because of rupture of: UPSC 1983, 84, 86; AIIMS 1984, 85, 87; UPSC 1984, 86; AI 1989**
A. Middle cerebral artery
B. Anterior cerebral artery
C. Posterior cerebral artery
D. Dural sinuses

**88. The cause of slowly progressive paraplegia, root pain and patchy sensory loss is: AIIMS 1984, 85**
A. Motor neurone disease
B. Fluorosis
C. Leprosy
D. Cysticercosis

**89. Which of the following is not a feature of midbrain lesion: AIIMS 1984, 85,88**
A. Upper gaze palsy B. Pupillary dilatation
C. Crossed hemiplegia D. Extension of arm

**90. Head injury with fracture of base of skull may develop: AIIMS 1984, 85**
A. Kernig's sign B. Homan's sign
C. Papilloedema D. CSF Rhinorrhoca

**91. Most useful investigation in head injury is: AIIMS 1984, 85**
A. X-ray lateral view B. Angiogram
C. Ventriculography D. CT scan

**92. A patient 45 years old had suboccipital headache, vomiting, confusion, death in 2 hours. Most common cause is: AIIMS 1985, 86**
A. Glioblastoma degeneration
B. Berry aneurysm rupture
C. Meningitis
D. Hydrocephalus

**93. Following are used to decrease intra-cranial tension except : Rajasthan 1994**
A. Lasix B. Glycerol
C. IV barbiturates D. $PCO_2 > 45$ mmHg

**94. The commonest supratentorial tumour in adults is: UPSC 1984; AMC 1985; AIIMS 1985 , 86, 87 Delhi 1985, 86**
A. Meningioma B. Glioma
C. Medulloblastoma D. Craniopharyngioma

**95. Which of the following does not drain into cavernous sinus: AIIMS 1985, 86**
A. Superficial middle cerebral vein
B. Ophthalmic vein
C. Sphenoparietal sinus
D. Great vein of Galen

**96. A patient with 3rd nerve palsy had no pupillary abnormality. He has: AIIMS 1988**
A. Trauma
B. Diabetes millitus
C. Anterior cerebral artery aneurysm
D. Pituitary tumour

**97. Features of posterior inferior cerebellar artery thrombosis includes all of the following, except : AMU 1990**
A. Sudden onset of severe vertigo.
B. Acute cerebellar S/S with nystagmus to the side of lesion.
C. The involvement of 10,11,12 nerves.
D. Horner's syndrome.

**98. The most commonly affected lower limbs muscle in poliomyelitis is: AIIMS 1986, 87**
A. Quardriceps femoris B. Tibialis anterior
C. Tibialis posterior D. Peroneus longus

**99. Following may be useful management of CSF rhinorrhoea except : AIIMS 1986, 88**
A. Nasal packing
B. Repeated lumbar puncture
C. Antibiotics
D. Craniotomy and dural repair

**100. Acute extradural hematoma may have following features, except : AIIMS 1986**
A. Hematoma under temporalis muscle
B. Presence of lucid interval
C. Tear of superior cerebral vein
D. Fracture squamous temporal bone

**101. All are seen in ulnar nerve palsy except : AIIMS 1986**
A. Loss of sensation over medial aspect of palm
B. Loss of sensation over anatomical snuff box
C. Paralysis of interossei
D. Postive Froment sign

**102. Artery commonly involved in cirsoid Aneurysm is : UPSC 1985; Rajasthan 1994**
A. Superficial temporal artery
B. Carotid artery
C. Femoral artery
D. Tibial artery

**103. Best management of infected subaponeurotic hematoma is: AIIMS 1986**
A. Repeated needle aspiration
B. I and D (Incision and Drainage)
C. Antibiotics alone
D. Open repair

| Ans. | | | | | | | | | |
|---|---|---|---|---|---|---|---|---|---|
| 87. D | 88. B | 89. D | 90. D | 91. D | 92. B | 93. C | 94. B | 95. D | 96. B |
| 97. C | 98. A | 99. A | 100. C | 101. B | 102. A | 103. B | | | |

**104. Hemiplegia is most often caused by thrombosis of : AIIMS 1986, 89**

A. Anterior cerebral artery
B. Posterior cerebral artery
C. Middle cerebral artery
D. Basilar artery

**105. Thalamectomy in Parkinsonism relieves : NIMHANS 1997**

A. Tremor B. Rigidity
C. Ataxia D. Akinesia

**106. Most common extra medullary tumour of spinal cord is: AIIMS 1986, 87; AMC 1987**

A. Neurofibroma B. Meningioma
C. Ependymoma D. Metastatic tumour

**107. In meningioma not seen is: Delhi 1990**

A. Lameller calcification
B. ↑ Diploid space
C. Bone spicule in inner table
D. Decalcification in inner table

**108. Regarding cephalohaematoma: AIIMS 1990**

A. Is due to periosteal injury
B. Focal swelling under periosteum
C. Always associated with jaundice
D. Many lead to cerebral palsy

**109. Central area of face is called Dangerous area because : AIIMS 1990**

A. Infection in this area causes cavernous sinus thrombosis
B. This area is liable to tumour
C. Fatal haemorrhage may occur
D. Connected directly with middle ear

**110. Footdrop results because of injury to: UPSC 1983; PGI 1986; Delhi 1989**

A. Superficial peroneal nerve
B. Deep peroneal nerve
C. Posterior tibial nerve
D. Anterior tibial nerve

**111. Foot drop occurs due to lesion of all, except : PGI 1987**

A. Sciatic nerve
B. Common peroneal nerve
C. $L_5$ root
D. $S_1$ root

**112. Operative indications for paraplegia is: PGI 1987**

A. Progressive motor loss inspite of conservative management.
B. Loss of consciousness.
C. No improvement in sensory loss within 1 week.
D. Incontinence of urine.

**113. Which of the following is a cystic cranial tumour : Kerala 1998**

A. Craniopharyngioma B. Astrocytoma
C. Medulloblastoma D. Ependynoma

**114. Bruising over mastoid process appearing a day or two after head injury indicating fracture of middle cranial fossa is: DNB 1993**

A. Guerin's sign B. Coleman's sign
C. Battle's sign D. Babinski's sign

**115. A patient presents with burning type of severe headache O/E scalp tenderness is severe. Most probable diagnosis is : JIPMER 1997**

A. Migraine B. Temporal arteritis
C. Tension headache D. Hypertension

**116. Bilateral pyramidal signs develop early in: AMC 1986; PGI 1989**

A. Cerebral haemorrhage
B. Subarachnoid haemorrhage
C. Pontine haemorrhage
D. Hemotomyelis

**117. True about meningioma is all except : PGI 1989**

A. 19% of brain tumour
B. Parasagittal meningioma common
C. Reactive hyperostosis
D. Flat
E. Arises from meninges

**118. An elderly patient presents in the casualty with a head injury. Immediate step to be taken is : Bihar 1998**

A. Send for scanning
B. Establish IV access
C. Endotracheal intubation
D. Send blood for cross matching

**119. Raised intracranial pressure is suspected if there is: UPSC 1986; PGI 1990**

A. Unilateral headache B. Ptosis
C. Neck rigidity D. Dilated pupil

**120. Transient syndrome of vertigo, diplopiaslurred speech and paresthesia is : AMC 1984, 86**

A. Anterior communicating artery aneurysm.
B. Basilar artery insufficiency.
C. Middle cerebral artery thrombosis.
D. Posterior communicating artery aneurysm.

**Ans.** 104. C 105. A 106. A 107. D 108. B 109. A 110. C 111. B 112. A 113. A
114. C 115. B 116. D 117. D 118. C 119. D 120. B

**121. A 22-years old male is admitted with fracture of the left femur. Two days later, he becomes mildly confused, has a respiratory rate of 40/min and scattered petechial rash on his upper torso. Chest X-ray shows patchy alveolar opacities bilaterally. His arterial blood gas analysis is abnormal. The most likely diagnosis is : CSE 1998**
A. Cerebral oedema with early neurogenic pulmonary oedema
B. Pulmonary thrombo-embolism
C. Chest contussion
D. Fat embolism

**122. Most common type of spina bifida is: JIPMER 1984, 87**
A. Meningocele B. Meningo myelocele
C. Myelocele D. Spinal bifida occulta

**123. A scooter is hit from behind. The rider is thrown off and he lands with his head hitting the kerb. He does not move, complains of severe pain in the neck and is unable to turn his head. Well-meaning onlookers rush up to him and try to make him sit-up. What would be the best course of action in this situation: UPSC 1997**
A. He should be propped-up and given some water to drink.
B. He should not be propped-up but turned on his face rushed to the hospital.
C. He should be turned on his back and a support should be placed behind his neck and transported to the nearest hospital.
D. He should not be moved at all but carried to the nearest hospital in same position in which he has been since his fall.

**124. After complete division of a nerve, retrograde degeneration occurs as high as——node of Ranvier. DNB 1991**
A. 1st B. 2nd
C. 3rd D. 4th
E. 5th

**125. Meralgia parasethetica is an entrapment neuropathy of the: Delhi 1986; AIIMS 1986**
A. Musculocutaneous nerve
B. Ilio inguinal nerve
C. External cutaneous nerve
D. Lateral popliteal nerve

**126. Consider the following procedures : CSE 1998**
1. Ventriculoperitoneal shunt
2. Ventriculocisternal shunt
3. Ventriculopleural shunt

**Surgical procedures prescribed for the treatment of hydrocephalus would include :**
A. 1 and 3 B. 1 and 2
C. 2 and 3 D. 1, 2 and 3

**127. A child presents with ataxia and incoordination. Nystagmus is observed on lateral gaze towards the right side. Areflexia and hypotonia are also present. The head is titled towards right side and the child walks with a broad base. The site of the lesion is : UPSC 1997**
A. Cerebellum on the right side
B. Cerebellum on the left side
C. Brain stem on the left side
D. None of the above

**128. Malignant astrocytoma is most common in: DNB 1989**
A. Frontal lobe B. Temporal lobe
C. Parietal lobe D. Cerebellum

**129. Patient presents with high fever, signs of raised ICT and a past history of chronic otitis media. Likely diagnosis : AIIMS 1981, 84**
A. Brain abscess
B. Pyogenic meningitis
C. Acute subarachnoid haemorrhage
D. Acute osteomyelitis of skull bone

**130. Dumbell tumour is seen in: AMC 1985**
A. Meningioma B. Neurofibroma
C. Epidendymoma D. Thymoma

**131. A-10 years old child presents with midline cerebellar tumour. Most likely diagnosis is : AI 1994**
A. Medulloblastoma B. Astrocytoma
C. Glioblastoma D. Hemangioblastoma

**132. The most malignant brain tumour is: Karnataka 1987**
A. Glioblastoma multiforme
B. Spongioblastoma
C. Ependymoma
D. Oligodendroglioma

**133. All are true about Glasgow coma scale except : AIIMS 1994**
A. Consists of eye opening, motor and verbal response.
B. Score between 3-15.
C. ↑ Score indicates poor prognosis.
D. Obeying motor command is given maximum score.

**134. Cerebral embolism is common in—— position: AIIMS 1994**
A. Supine B. Trendelenburg's
C. Prone D. Lateral

**Ans.** 121. D 122. D 123. D 124. A 125. C 126. B 127. B 128. A 129. B 130. B
131. A 132. A 133. C 134. A

**135. Arnold Chiari malformation is: UPSC 1994**
A. Agenesis of cerebellum.
B. Herniation of hind brain and cerebellum into cervical canal.
C. Arteriovenous malformation of cerebellum.
D. Healing usually occurs without skin grafting.

**136. In sacral meningomyelocele, false is: AI 1995**
A. Spasticity is a feature of lower limbs
B. Hydrocephalus is often seen
C. Bladder incontinence is present
D. Lax anal sphincter is present

**137. A brain tumour which has CSF metastasis and is radiosensitive: AI 1995, 96**
A. Ependymoma B. Medulloblastoma
C. Pinealoblastoma D. Astrocytoma

**138. Metastasis outside the brain occurs in brain tumour: Kerala 1995**
A. Craniopharyngioma B. Glioblastoma
C. Medulloblastoma D. Hemangioblastoma

**139. In person with rupture of intracranial aneurysm, deterioration in neurological condition after 24 hours may occur due to: PGI 1994**
A. Rerupture
B. Spasm
C. Increased intracranial tension
D. Hydrocephalus

**140. Posteroinferior part of the internal capsule is supplied with : JIPMER 1997**
A. Charcot artery
B. Huyhman's artery
C. Anterior bowel of the posterior choroid artery
D. Inferior choroidal artery

**141. Neuroglia responsible for phagocytosis: AIIMS 1994**
A. Fibrous astrocytes B. Protoplasmic astrocytes
C. Oligodendrocytes D. Microglia

**142. Dysphasia is prominent in disorders of : AIIMS 1984**
A. Dominant parietal lobe
B. Non-parietal lobe
C. Dominant temporal lobe
D. Non-dominant temporal lobe

**143. Which one of the folowing is diagnostic of complete transection of spinal cord after an injury of three weeks duration: UPSC 1995**
A. The rectum of voluntary motor power below the level of the lesion.
B. The rectum of sensations below the levels of the lesion.
C. The rectum of reflex activity with full recovery of sensations below the lesion.
D. The rectum of reflex activity with partial recovery of sensations below the lesion.

**144. A one month old female child has a swelling over the back in the sacral region. There is no cough impulse or erosion of the coccyx. The most likely clinical diagnosis would be: UPSC 1985**
A. Meningocele
B. Lipoma
C. Sacro-coccygeal teratoma
D. Neurofibroma

**145. The most common tumour of pineal gland is: AP 1993**
A. Lipoma B. Astrocytoma
C. Haemangioma D. Germinoma

**146. Plexiform neurofibromatosis most commonly affects: Delhi 1993; MP 1993**
A. Facial nerve
B. Trigeminal nerve
C. Peripheral nerve
D. Glassopharyngeal nerve

**147. Suture separation with proptosis is seen in : PGI 1995**
A. Wilm's tumor B. Neuroblastoma
C. Multiple myeloma D. Phaeochromocytoma

**148. Commonest presentation of spinal cord tumor is : PGI 1996**
A. Pain
B. Bruit over vertebral column
C. Gait deformity
D. All of the above

**149. Most common endocrine tumor of pituitary is : PGI 1996**
A. GH tumor B. ACTH tumor
C. Prolactinoma D. TSH secreting tumor

**150. A lady presents with galactorrhoea and visual defects, investigation of choice is : AI 1997**
A. Prolactin B. GH
C. FSH D. LH

**151. Aneurysm is commonly seen in following except : AI 1997**
A. Ant. cerebral artery
B. Basilar artery
C. Vertebral artery
D. Post. communication artery

**Ans.** 135. B 136. D 137. B 138. C 139. B 140. D 141. D 142. C 143. C 144. C
145. D 146. B 147. B 148. C 149. C 150. A 151. C

**152. Among following, CNS tumor with best prognosis is : AIIMS 1994; AI 1994, 97**

A. Cerebral astrocytoma B. Cerebellar astrocytoma
C. Medulloblastoma D. Glioblastoma

**153. Froment test is used for —— nerve : Delhi 1996**

A. Ulnar B. Radial
C. Median D. Axillary

**154. Aneurysm-8cm, commonest complication is : Delhi 1996**

A. Thromboembolism B. Seizures
C. Hypertension D. Hemiparesis

**155. Pituitary tumor produces : Delhi 1996**

A. Bitemporal hemianopia
B. Binasal hemianopia
C. Unilateral quadrantanopia
D. Increase in blind spot only

**156. The pterion corresponds to the following except : Karnataka 1996**

A. Anterior pole of insula
B. Middle cerebral artery
C. Transverse sinus
D. Lateral cerebral sulcus

**157. Level of lesion in akinetic mutism is in : Delhi 1996**

A. Pons B. Midbrain
C. Cerebellum D. IIIrd ventricle

**158. Nerve most commonly affected in intracranial subclinoid anterior aneurysm is : AI 1996**

A. II B. III
C. VI D. VII

**159. Non-neoplastic compressive lesions of spinal cord are all except : Kerala 1996**

A. Inter-vertebral disc prolapse
B. Aneurysm of special vessels
C. A-V malformation of the spinal vessels
D. Arachnoiditis
E. None of the above

**160. Cranial accessory nerve injury causes paralysis of : AI 1996**

A. Sternocleidomastoid B. Stylopharyngeus
C. Pharyngeal muscles D. Levator scapulae

**161. Craniotomy is indicated in all, except : AI 1996**

A. Depressed fracture
B. Recurrent CSF rhinorrhoea
C. Growing fracture
D. Compound fracture

**162. Spinal cord compression is due to all, except : AI 1996**

A. Lymphoma B. Neurofibroma
C. Ependymoma D. Glioma

**163. Which of the following is not a cause of angiogenic cerebral oedema : Kerala 1998**

A. Normal pressure hydrocephalus
B. Tumors
C. Meningitis
D. None

**164. The most common physical sign of cerebral metastasis is : Karnataka 1998**

A. Epilepsy
B. Focal neurological deficit
C. Papilledema
D. Visual defects

**165. Blood brain barrier is not present in following except : Rajasthan 1998**

A. Neurohypophysis B. Area postrema
C. Subfornical organ D. IVth ventricle

**166. Match List-I (Glasgow coma scale) with List-II (Systolic blood pressure) and select the correct answer using the codes given below the Lists : CSE 1998**

| List-I | List-II |
|---|---|
| A. 13 to 15 | 1. 76 to 89 |
| B. 9 to 12 | 2. 50 to 75 |
| C. 6 to 8 | 3. 1 to 49 |
| D. 4 to 5 | 4. > 89 |

**Codes :**

| | A | B | C | D |
|---|---|---|---|---|
| A. | 4 | 1 | 2 | 3 |
| B. | 1 | 2 | 3 | 4 |
| C. | 4 | 3 | 2 | 1 |
| D. | 3 | 2 | 1 | 4 |

**167. Following an incised wound in the front of the wrist, the patient is unable to oppose the tips of the little finger and the thumb. The nerve involved is : Orissa 1998**

A. Median nerve
B. Ulnar nerve
C. Median and ulnar nerve
D. Radial and ulnar nerve

**168. Revised trauma score includes all of the following, except : CSE 1999**

A. Respiratory rate
B. Urinary output
C. Systolic blood pressure
D. Glasgow coma scale

| Ans. | 152. C | 153. A | 154. A | 155. C | 156. C | 157. D | 158. B | 159. D | 160. C | 161. A |
|---|---|---|---|---|---|---|---|---|---|---|
| | 162. A | 163. A | 164. B | 165. D | 166. A | 167. A | 168. B | | | |

**169. The correct order of priorities in the initial management of head injury is : CSE 1999**

A. Airway, Breathing, Circulation, Treatment of extracranial injuries.

B. Treatment of extracranial injuries, Airway, Breathing, Circulation.

C. Circulation, Airway, Breathing, Treatment of extracranial injuries.

D. Airway, Circulation, Breathing, Treatment of extracranial injuries.

**170. All of the following are the features of congenital hydrocephalus except : CSE 1999**

A. Enlarged tense fontanelles

B. Downward displacement of eyeballs

C. Papilloedema

D. Squint and nystagmus

**171. A non-contrast CT scan in a person brought with hostory of head trauma showed a bi-convex lens shaped lesion. What is the diagnosis : AIIMS 1999**

A. Sub-archnoid haematoma

B. Sub-dural haematoma

C. Extradural haematoma

D. Brain edema

**172. MC causative of infection in spinal epidural space is : Kerala 1999**

A. Proteus B. Pseudomonas

C. Klebsiella D. Staph. aureus

**173. In patient of head injuries with rapidly increasing intracranial tension without haematoma, the drug of choice for initial management would be : UPSC 2000**

A. Lasix B. Steroids

C. 20% Mannitol D. Glycine

**174. Patient having hyperprolactinaemia (20 ng/ml serum) with inappropriate lactation should be investigated by: TNPSC 1998**

A. X-ray of sella turcica

B. CAT scanning of brain

C. Ophthalmoscopic examination

D. All of the above

**175. A comatose patient with head injury at a P.H.C. before transferring to a higher centre, should have the following attended to : TNPSC 2000**

I. Clearing mouth & throat and ensuring that tongue does not fall back.

II. Catheterising the urinary bladder aseptically.

III. Instituting anti-shock measures like I.V. fluids etc.

IV. Sedation using narcotics.

**Of these :**

A. All are correct B. I & III are correct

C. Only III is correct D. I, II & III are correct

**176. True about Berry-aneurysm is following except : PGI 2000**

A. Associated with familial syndrome.

B. Most common site of rupture apex which causes SAH.

C. Wall contains S. muscle fibroblasts.

D. 90% occur in ant. part of circulation at branching points.

**177. A patient has an accident with resultant transection of the pituitary. What will not occur : AI 2001**

A. Diabetes mellitus B. Diabetes insipidus

C. Hyperprolactinemia D. Hypothyroidism

**178. Patient of head injury, has no relatives, requires urgent cranial decompression. Doctor should : AI 2001**

A. Operate without formal consent

B. Take police consent

C. Wait for relatives

D. Should not perform surgery

**179. Consider the following statements : UPSC 2001**
**Cerebral protection in head injury is provided through**

1. Hypothermia at 35°C
2. Hyperventilation
3. Administration of barbiturates
4. Administration of phencyclidine

Which of the above statements are correct :

A. 1, 2, 3 and 4 B. 1, 2 and 3

C. 2, 3 and 4 D. 1 and 4

**180. Which one of the following cranial nerves is most often injured in patients with fracture of the middle cranial fossa : UPSC 2001**

A. Sixth cranial nerve B. Eighth cranial nerve

C. Tenth cranial nerve D. Eleventh cranial nerve

**181. A patient is brought with head injury, head on collision and BP 90/60. Tachycardia present; diagnosis is : AI 2001**

A. Extradural hematoma

B. Subdural hematoma

C. Intracranial haemorrhage

D. Intraabdominal bleed

**182. Characteristic finding in CT Scan of a TB case : AI 2001**

A. Exudates seen in basal cistern

B. Hydrocephalus is commonly seen

C. Tuberculomas are often calcified

D. CT is diagnostic of TBM

| Ans. | | | | | | | | | |
|---|---|---|---|---|---|---|---|---|---|
| 169. A | 170. C | 171. C | 172. D | 173. C | 174. D | 175. B | 176. C | 177. A | 178. A |
| 179. B | 180. B | 181. D | 182. A | | | | | | |

**183. Stereolactic radiosurgery is done for : JIPMER 2002**

A. Glioblastoma multiforme
B. Medullo blastoma spinal cord
C. Epidendymoma
D. AV malformation of brain

**184. Which of the following requires emergency operation in setting without tertiary care facilities : SGPGI 2002**

A. Extradural haemorrhage
B. Subdural haemorrhage
C. Subarachnoid haemorrhage
D. Intacerebral haemorrhage

**185. Which of the following tumors is common in extramedullary intradural location : SGPGI 2002**

A. Ependymoma B. Metastasis
C. Astrocytoma D. Neurofibroma

**186. Post-traumatic increase in ICT, the following drug is not used : JIPMER 2002**

A. Mannitol B. Frusemide
C. Dexamethasone D. Glycerol

**187. All of the following are correct about radiologic evaluation of a patient with Cushing's syndrome except : AI 2002**

A. Adrenal CT scan distinguishes adrenal cortical hyperplasia from an adrenal tumor.
B. CT of sella tursica is diagnostic when a pituitary tumor is present.
C. MRI of the adrenals may distinguish adrenal adenoma from carcinoma.
D. Petrosal sinus sampling is the best way to distinguish tumor from an ectopic ACTH producing tumor.

**188. A 24 years old man falls to the found when he is struck in the right temple by a base ball. While being driven to the hospital he lapses into coma. He is unresponsive with a dilated right pupil when he reaches the emergency department. The most appropriate step in initial management is : AI 2002**

A. CT scan of the head
B. Craniotomy
C. Doppler ultrasound examination of the neck
D. X-rays of the skull and cervical spine.

**189. The following are the clinical features of raised intracranial tension except : UPSC 2002**

A. Headache B. Insomnia
C. Bradycardia D. Papilloedema

**190. A 10 years old child presented with headache, vomiting, gait instability and diplopia. On examination he had papilloedema and gait ataxia. The most probable diagnosis is : AIIMS 2002**

A. Hydrocephalus
B. Brain stem tumour
C. Suprasellar tumour
D. Midline posterior fossa tumour

**191. Which of the following would distinguish hydrocephalus due to aqueductal stenosis when compared to that due to Dandy-Walker malformation : AIIMS 2002**

A. Third ventricle size
B. Posterior fossa volume
C. Lateral ventricular size
D. Head circumference

**192. The lumbar puncture was done in a patient with raised intracranial tension. The patient [illegible]d suddenly on the table. The cause of death is most likely to be : UPSC 2003**

A. Middle cerebral artery haemorrhage
B. Tentorial herniation
C. Rupture of an aneurysm
D. Loss of CSF

**193. Patient sustains head-injury; and develops quadriplegia and respiratory distress. He is suffering from : UPSC 2003**

A. Cervical vertebral fracture dislocation
B. Brainstem haemorrhage
C. Cerebral laceration
D. Cerebral contussion

**194. Which of the following is classic CT appearance of an acute subdural hematoma: AI 2004**

A. Lentiform shaped hyperdense lesion
B. Cresent shaped hypodense lesion
C. Cresent shaped hyperdense lesion
D. Lentiform shaped hypodense lesion

**195. Bleeding from external Auditory Meatus in a case of head injury is suggestive of : UPSC 2005**

A. Anterior cranial fossa fracture
B. Middle cranial fossa fracture
C. Fracture of occipital bone
D. Posterior cranial fossa fracture

**196. The most appropriate route for administration of nutrition to a patient who is comatose for a long period after an automobile accident is : UPSC 2005**

A. Nasogastric tube feeding
B. Gastrotomy tube feeding
C. Jejunostomy feeding
D. Central venous hyperalimentation

**Ans.** 183. A 184. A 185. D 186. C 187. B 188. B 189. B 190. D 191. B 192. B
193. B 194. C 195. B 196. C

**197. Type III category of basal fractures of skull are: Karnataka 2004**

A Those that run in the coronal plane from lateral end of one petrous ridge through sella turcica to lateral end of contralateral petrous ridge.

B Run from side-to-side in the coronal plane but do not pass through the sella turcica.

C Run from front to the contralateral back passing through the sella turcica.

D Run from front-to-back involving all cranial fossae and sella turcica.

**198. The immediate treatment of CSF rhinorrhoea is : Karnataka 2005**

A. Plugging the affected nostril with sterile petrolatum gauze.

B. Frequent blowing and cleaning of the nose.

C. Immediate craniotomy.

D. Wait and watch for 7-10 days, give antibiotics.

**199. The most common neurologic abnormality that occurs with head injury is : Karnataka 2005**

A. Hemiplegia B. Occular nerve palsy

C. Altered consciousness D. Convulsions

**200. In patient of head injuries with rapidly increasing intracranial tension without haematoma, the drug of choice for initial management would be : Delhi 2009**

A. Lasix B. Steroids

C. 20% mannitol D. Glycine

Ans. 197. C 198. D 199. C 200. C

# EXPLANATIONS OF NEUROSURGERY

1. Ans.— D. **All of the above**
2. Ans.— B. **Subarachnoid space around optic nerve.**
3. Ans.— A. **Compression of retinal vein**
4. Ans.— D. **Focal lesion in IVth ventricle**

   **This is because of raised ICT.**
5. Ans.— B. **6-8 hours**
6. Ans.— A. **Staphylococcus**
7. Ans.— D. **None of the above**
8. Ans.— B. **Pneumococcus**
9. Ans.— A. **Lung**

   **Carcinoma bronchus is commonest cause.**
10. Ans.— A. **Hodgkin's lymphoma**
11. Ans.— A. **Hodgkin's lymphoma**

    **Leukemia can also be cause.**
12. Ans.— D. **Renal anomalies**
13. Ans.— B. **Congenital syphilis**
14. Ans.— C. **Rapidly changing neurological**
15. Ans.— C. **Chronic subdural haemorrhage**
16. Ans.— A. **A deterioration in the level of consciousness.**
17. Ans.— C. **Normal**

    **Eosinophils are increased in Tropical eosinophilia and decreased in steroid therapy.**
18. Ans.— B. **Radial nerve**
19. Ans.— A. **Severe hypotension**
20. Ans.— A. **Dysphasia**
21. Ans.— A. **Can be improved by surgery**
22. Ans.— D. **A sign of Omen**
23. Ans.— A. **Craniopharyngioma**
24. Ans.— A. **Astrocytoma**
25. Ans.— C. **Ependymoma**
26. Ans.— A. **Sub-arachnoid haemorrhage**
27. Ans.— D. **C V A**
28. Ans.— A. **Haemophilus influenzae**
29. Ans.— A. **Spinal cord tumour**

    **There is risk of coning and sudden death may occur due to compression of vital medullary centres.**
30. Ans.— A. **Neuropraxis**
31. Ans.— D. **MRI**
32. Ans.— B. **Eversion of galea aponeurotica**
33. Ans.— B. **Rupture of aneurysm**
34. Ans.— C. **Thoracic**
35. Ans.— A. **Immediate evacuation**
36. Ans.— A. **Secure airway**
37. Ans.— B. **Lumbo sacral spine**

    **In spina fibida cystica, meningocele or meningomyelocele are seen. In spina bifida aperta, there is no covering layers and in spina bifida occulta, there is no swelling.**
38. Ans.— C. **Medulloblastoma**
39. Ans.— D. **Motor tone**
40. Ans.— C. **Registration of new memory**
41. Ans.— B. **Idiopathic**
42. Ans.— B. **Increase Decrease**
43. Ans.— B. **Streptococcus**

    **Extradural abscess is associated with history of trauma or disease of middle ear or frontal sinuses. Subdural abscess or empyema is a extremely grave condition associated with paranasal sinus infection.**
44. Ans.— A. **Increased blind spot**
45. Ans.— A. **Lumbosacral**

46. Ans.— A. Always preceded with history of unconsciousness.

Chronic subdural haematoma is produced by rupture of veins passing from cerebral hemisphere to venous sinuses as a result of displacement of brain inside the skull. Superior cerebral veins are usually ruptured. This is produced by blows of small magnum over ant. or post. aspect of skull.

47. Ans.— A. 1-2 days
48. Ans.— A. Cavernous
49. Ans.— A. Carcinoma of the thyroid
50. Ans.— A. 1 mm/day
51. Ans.— D. Headache
52. Ans.— C. Any of the above
53. Ans.— C. Posterior fossa
54. Ans.— E. All of the above
55. Ans.— A. Vertigo
56. Ans.— A. Thalamus
57. Ans.— A. Bladder involvement
58. Ans.— D. Sagittal sinus thrombosis
59. Ans.— B. Brain herniation
60. Ans.— C. Diplopia
61. Ans.— C. Multiple sclerosis

It is a slowly progressive disorder, which results in patchy demyelination of CNS.

62. Ans.— C. Multiple sclerosis
63. Ans.— A. Tumour
64. Ans.— C. Comma
65. Ans.— C. Loss of joint sense
66. Ans.— A. Cervical injuries should be transported with the head lifted on to a pillow.
67. Ans.— A. Exercise
68. Ans.— A. Bitemporal hemianopia

Sixth nerve palsy or lateral rectus palsy can result.

69. Ans.— C. Stenosis of the origin of the subclavian artery.
70. Ans.— A. Convulsion
71. Ans.— A. Frontal lobe tumours
72. Ans.— D. None of the above
73. Ans.— C. Tetany
74. Ans.— A. 30-45%
75. Ans.— A. Lymphoepthelioma

Thymoma is most common mediastinal tumour (25% of total) which is associated with myaesthenia gravis.

76. Ans.— E. When wound is free from infection
77. Ans.— B. Males are more often affected than females.
78. Ans.— D. $PaCO_2$ less than 35 mm Hg
79. Ans.— C. Aneurysm of posterior communicating-A
80. Ans.— D. Any of the above
81. Ans.— E. All of the above
82. Ans.— B. Hoarseness of voice
83. Ans.— A. Basal ganglia
84. Ans.— D. Conservative
85. Ans.— C. Middle cranial fossa
86. Ans.— A. 1, 2 and 3
87. Ans.— D. Dural sinuses

Subdural hematoma more commonly occurs following high velocity injuries and is frequently associated with a cortical contusion. It appears concave hyperdense as compared to convex extradural hematoma.

88. Ans.— B. Fluorosis
89. Ans.— D. Extension of arm
90. Ans.— D. CSF Rhinorrhoea
91. Ans.— D. CT scan
92. Ans.— B. Berry aneurysm rupture
93. Ans.— C. IV barbiturates
94. Ans.— B. Glioma
95. Ans.— D. Great vein of Galen
96. Ans.— B. Diabetes mellitus
97. Ans.— C. The involvement of 10, 11, 12, nerves
98. Ans.— A. Quadriceps femoris
99. Ans.— A. Nasal packing
100. Ans.— C. Tear of superior cerebral vein
101. Ans.— B. Loss of sensation over anatomical snuff box.
102. Ans.— A. Superficial temporal artery

**103. Ans.— B. I and D (Incision and Drainage)**

**104. Ans.— C. Middle cerebral artery**

**105. Ans.— A. Tremor**

**106. Ans.— A. Neurofibroma**

**107. Ans.— D. Decalcification in inner table**

**108. Ans.— B. Focal swelling under periosteum**

**109. Ans.— A. Infection in this area causes cavernous sinus thrombosis.**

**110. Ans.— C. Posterior tibial nerve**

**111. Ans.— B. Common peroneal nerve**

**112. Ans.— A. Progressive motor loss inspite of conservative management.**

**113. Ans.— A. Craniopharyngioma**

**114. Ans.— C. Battle's sign**

**115. Ans.— B. Temporal arteritis**

**116. Ans.— D. Hemotomyelis**

**117. Ans.— D. Flat**

**Meningioma account for 21% of total intra-cranial neoplasms. They originate from arachnoidal cells and most commonly over convexity or at skull base.**

**118. Ans.— C. Endotracheal intubation**

**119. Ans.— D. Dilated pupil**

**120. Ans.— B. Basilar artery insufficiency**

**121. Ans.— D. Fat embolism**

**122. Ans.— D. Spinal bifida occulta**

**123. Ans.— D. He should not be moved at all but carried to the nearest hospital in same position in which he has been since his fall.**

**124. Ans.— A. 1st**

**125. Ans.— C. External cutaneous nerve**

**126. Ans.— B. 1 and 2**

**127. Ans.— B. Cerebellum on the left side**

**128. Ans.— A. Frontal lobe**

**129. Ans.— B. Pyogenic meningitis**

**130. Ans.— B. Neurofibroma**

**131. Ans.— A. Medulloblastoma**

**It is common in vermis in cerebellum.**

**132. Ans.— A. Glioblastoma multiforme**

**It is commonest primary brain tumor, otherwise secondaries are more common.**

**133. Ans.— C. ↑ Score indicates poor prognosis**

**134. Ans.— A. Supine**

**135. Ans.— B. Herniation of hind brain and cerebellum into cervical canal.**

**136. Ans.— D. Lax anal sphincter is present**

**Amniocentesis is a useful test to pickup upto 80% of cases by detecting alphafetoproteins which peak in 16 to 18th weeks of gestation.**

**137. Ans.— B. Medulloblastoma**

**138. Ans.— C. Medulloblastoma**

**139. Ans.— B. Spasm**

**140. Ans.— D. Inferior choroidal artery**

**141. Ans.— D. Microglia**

**142. Ans.— C. Dominant temporal lobe**

**143. Ans.— C. The rectum of reflex activity with full recovery of sensations below the lesion.**

**144. Ans.— C. Sacro-coccygeal teratoma**

**145. Ans.— D. Germinoma**

**146. Ans.— B. Trigeminal nerve**

**147. Ans.— B. Neuroblastoma**

**148. Ans.— C. Gait deformity**

**149. Ans.— C. Prolactinoma**

**150. Ans.— A. Prolactin**

**Normal Prolactin levels are 1-25 ng/mL (0.4-10 nmol/L).**

**151. Ans.— C. Vertebral artery**

**152. Ans.— C. Medulloblastoma**

**153. Ans.— A. Ulnar**

**154. Ans.— A. Thromboembolism**

**155. Ans.— C. Unilateral quadrantanopia**

**156. Ans.— C. Transverse sinus**

**157. Ans.— D. IIIrd ventricle**

**158. Ans.— B. III**

**Headache, epilepsy or focal neurological signs or subarachnoid haemorrhage are symptoms.**

**159. Ans.— D. Arachnoiditis**

**160. Ans.— C. Pharyngeal muscles**

**161. Ans.— A. Depressed fracture**

**162. Ans.— A. Lymphoma**

Lymphoma may cause vertebral bone collapse.

**163. Ans.— A. Normal pressure hydrocephalus**

**164. Ans.— B. Focal neurological deficit**

**165. Ans.— D. IVth ventricle**

**166. Ans.— A. 4 1 2 3**

**167. Ans.— A. Median nerve**

**168. Ans.— B. Urinary output**

**169. Ans.— A. Airway, Breathing, Circulation, Treatment of extracranial injuries.**

**170. Ans.— C. Papilloedema**

**171. Ans.— C. Extradural haematoma**

**172. Ans.— D. Staph. aureus**

Staph. aureus is normally present in skin.

**173. Ans.— C. 20% Mannitol**

**174. Ans.— D. All of the above**

**175. Ans.— B. I & III are correct**

**176. Ans.— C. Wall contains S. muscle fibroblasts**

**177. Ans.— A. Diabetes mellitus**

**178. Ans.— A. Operate without formal consent**

The patient's condition is given priority and the urgency of operation can be certified by at least doctors.

**179. Ans.— B. 1, 2 and 3**

**180. Ans.— B. Eighth cranial nerve**

**181. Ans.— D. Intraabdominal bleed**

**182. Ans.— A. Exudates seen in basal cistern**

Exudates in basal cistern are early and characteristic findings.

**183. Ans.— A. Glioblastoma multiforme**

**184. Ans.— A. Extradural haemorrhage**

**185. Ans.— D. Neurofibroma**

**186. Ans.— C. Dexamethasone**

**187. Ans.— B. CT of sella tursica is diagnostic when a pituitary tumor is present.**

Diagnosis of Cushing's disease is made by radio immunoassay of ACTH in peripheral blood and petrosal venous sinus sampling.

**188. Ans.— B. Craniotomy**

It is important to evacuate haematoma by craniotomy.

**189. Ans.— B. Insomnia**

**190. Ans.— D. Midline posterior fossa tumour**

**191. Ans.— B. Posterior fossa volume**

**192. Ans.— B. Tentorial herniation**

**193. Ans.— B. Brainstem haemorrhage**

In pontine haemorrhages, deep coma with quadriplegia usually occurs over a few minutes. There is prominent decerebrate rigidity and "pin-point" pupils that react to light. There is impairment of reflex horizontal eye movements evoked by head turning (doll's-head or oculocephalic manoeuver). Hyperpnea, severe hypertension, and hyperhidrosis are common. Death usually occurs within a few hours, but there are exceptional survivors.

**194. Ans.— C. Cresent shaped hyperdense lesion**

**195. Ans.— B. Middle cranial fossa fracture**

**196. Ans.— C. Jejunostomy feeding**

**197. Ans.— C Run from front to the contralateral back passing through the sella turcica.**

**198. Ans.— D. Wait and watch for 7-10 days, give antibiotics.**

**199. Ans.— C. Altered consciousness**

**200. Ans.— C. 20% mannitol**

It is used as 0.5-1.0 gm/kg. It must be used with caution in patients with large areas of blood-brain-barrier breakdown, because it can cause mass effect.

# 4

# IMPORTANT TEXT OF MAXILLOFACIAL SURGERY

## EXAMPLES OF WOUNDS AND RECONSTRUCTIONS

| Wounds | Reconstruction |
|---|---|
| ***Congenital*** | |
| Cleft lip | Local flaps |
| Syndactyly | Local flaps with or without skin graft |
| Hypospadias | Local flaps with or without skin graft |
| Giant naevus | Tissue expansion + local flaps |
| ***Developmental*** | |
| Breast asymmetry | Tissue expansion |
| Bell's palsy | Free tissue transfer |
| ***Infection*** | |
| Fournier's gangrene | Skin graft |
| ***Trauma*** | |
| Burns | Skin graft |
| Scar revision | Tissue expansion plus flaps |
| Nasal loss | Local or distant flaps |
| Open tibial fracture | Fascioutaneous flap, muscle flap, free flap |
| Hand or digit amputation | Microvascular replantation |
| Pressure sores | Local flaps, VAC therapy |
| **Neoplasia** | |
| Skin cancer | Local skin flap |
| Oral cancer | Free tissue transfer |
| Breast cancer | Free or distant (pedicled) flaps tissue transfer |

## RADIOLOGICAL VIEWS FOR SPECIFIC FRACTURES

| Site of fracture | Radiographs |
|---|---|
| Mandible : body and ramus | OPT, lateral obliques, lower occlusal, PA mandible |
| Mandible : condyles | OPT, RA mandible with mouth open, Toller transpharyngeal views |
| Maxilla | OM 15 and 30, laterla facial bones |
| Zygomotic complex | OM 15 and 30, submentovertex |
| Orbitl blow-outs | OM 15 and 30 and tomograms |
| Nasal bons | Lateral nasal bones, occipitofrontal |
| Frontal bones | Lateral skull, occipitofrontal |

OPT, orthopantomogram, PA, posteranterior, OM, posteranterior occipitomental

# MCQ's OF MAXILLOFACIAL SURGERY

## What is important in Maxillofacial Surgery

Cleft lip and Palate, Lefort classification of injuries, Jaw swelling (classification, dentigerous cyst), Tongue (Carcinoma), Salivary glands (Ducts, Swelling)

1. **'Prolabium' is seen in : AIIMS 1983**
   A. Unilateral cleft lip B. Bilateral cleft lip
   C. Alveolar cleft D. Median cleft
2. **In unilateral clefts are most common on : AIIMS 1985**
   A. Left side B. Right side
   C. Median D. None of the above
3. **Treacher Collins' syndrome (autosomal dominant) is characterized by all of the following, except : PGI 1986, 92**
   A. Outward slanting of the eyes
   B. Notching of the lower eyelids (coloboma)
   C. High arched or cleft palate
   D. Protrusion of mandible
4. **Vincent's angina affects : AMC 1985; TN 1989**
   A. Pharynx B. Heart
   C. Gums D. Larynx
5. **The most common malignant lesion of parotid gland is : Delhi 1982; Rajasthan 1998**
   A. Mucoepidermoid carcinoma
   B. Adenocystic carcinoma
   C. Acinar cell adenocarcinoma
   D. Anaplastic adenocarcinoma
   E. Squamous cell carcinoma
6. **Parotid tumour which spreads perineurally is : AIIMS 1984**
   A. Mucoepidermoid carcinoma
   B. Epidermoid carcinoma
   C. Carcinoma in pleomorphic adenoma
   D. Adenoid cystic carcinoma
7. **Regarding aphthous stomatitis which of the following is incorrect : AMU 1988**
   A. It is confined to infant
   B. It can be due to a virus
   C. It can caused by Monilia
   D. It can be caused by Candida
8. **A ranula is a : UPSC 1985, 92, 94**
   A. Cystic swelling on the floor of the mouth
   B. Forked uvula
   C. Sublingual thyroid
   D. Thyroglossal cyst
9. **Leukoplakia of the tongue is not associated with : AMC 1985**
   A. A jagged tooth B. Smoking
   C. Dyskeratosis D. Aspergillus niger
10. **Hot spot on Tc Scan in parotid is : PGI 1990, 91, 95**
    A. Adenolymphoma B. Mixed parotid tumour
    C. Calculus D. Mumps
    E. Sjogren's disease
11. **Oral hairy leukoplakia is one of the clinical manifestation seen in : Karnataka 1994**
    A. Mucocutaneous candidiasis
    B. Tertiary syphilis
    C. HIV infection
    D. Leucoderma
12. **Warthin's tumour of the parotid gland is : AMC 1986**
    A. Benign tumour B. Potentially malignant
    C. Malignant D. Highly malignant
13. **Carcinoma of Maxillary antrum may produce : AIIMS 1983**
    A. Epistaxis B. Proptosis
    C. Epiphora D. All of the above
14. **Most common salivary gland tumor in a child is : Rajasthan 1998**
    A. Mucoepidermoid
    B. Adeendymphoma
    C. Acinic cell
    D. A denoid cystic carcinoma

| Ans. | 1. B | 2. A | 3. D | 4. C | 5. A | 6. D | 7. A | 8. A | 9. D | 10. A |
|---|---|---|---|---|---|---|---|---|---|---|
| | 11. C | 12. A | 13. D | 14. A | | | | | | |

**15. Most common tumour of minor salivary glands is : Kerala 1995**

A. Epidermoid carcinoma
B. Mixed tumour
C. Squamous cell carcinoma
D. Epilethioma

**16. Membranous oral lesion are seen in : PGI 1993**

A. Vincent' angina B. Acute glossitis
C. Ludwig's angina D. Papilloma of tongue

**17. Which is most common malignancy on face : PGI 1994**

A. Squamous cell carcinoma
B. Basal cell carcinoma
C. Lymphoma
D. Angiosarcoma

**18. Facial vein injury can lead to thrombosis of : PGI 1994, 96**

A. Cavernous sinus B. Rosenthal sinus
C. Vein of Galen D. Transverse sinus

**19. Which is least Malignant of the following parotid malignancies : PGI 1994**

A. Pleomorphic adenocarcinoma
B. Mucoepidermoid carcinoma
C. Adeno cystic carcinoma
D. Adenocarcinoma

**20. Progressive trismus may result from : AIIMS 1994**

A. Leukoplakia B. Submucous fibrosis
C. Lichen planus D. Congenital syphilis

**21. Common site of malignancy in Plummer Vinson syndrome is at : Delhi 1993**

A. Larynx B. Post. cricoid
C. Tongue D. Oesophagus

**22. Stones are most common in ——— gland. Delhi 1993**

A. Submandibular B. Parotid
C. Submaxillary D. None

**23. Inflammatory enlargement of deep lobe of parotid gland is seen in : Delhi 1992**

A. Post pharyngeal wall B. Supratonsillar area
C. Anterior tonsillar pillar D. Tonsillar fossa/bed

**24. Complication of excision of ranula is : Delhi 1992**

A. Injury to sub-mandibular duct
B. Injury to parotid duct
C. Injury to lingual artery
D. Injury to lingual nerve

**25. Cleft lip is due to non-fusion of : AIIMS 1990, 92**

A. Maxillary process with mandibular process
B. Maxillary with lateral nasal process
C. Maxillary process with medial nasal process
D. All of the above

**26. Most common site of minor salivary gland tumour is : AIIMS 1987, 92**

A. Cheek B. Palate
C. Tonsil D. Tongue

**27. Which is not true of Ca tongue : AIIMS 1992**

A. Commonly adenocarcinoma
B. Lateral border is involved
C. Cervical lymphnode involvement
D. Tabacco chewing is a common risk factor

**28. In submandibular gland surgery, nerve least likely to be injured is: JIPMER 1993**

A. Mandibular branch of facial
B. Lingual
C. Hypoglossal
D. Inferior alveolar

**29. Commonest parotid tumour is: TN 1993**

A. Pleomorphic adenoma B. Warthin's tumour
C. Adenoid cystic ca. D. Secondaries

**30. Most common cause of post-operative parotitis is : AI 1994**

A. Streptococcus B. Staphylococcus
C. Klebsiella D. Pneumococcus

**31. Regarding Ca. lip not true is: AI 1993**

A. Lower lip commonly involved.
B. Early cases surgery and radiotherapy curative.
C. Early metastasis to lymph nodes.
D. Kiss cancer type.

**32. Commonest site for carcinoma tongue is : TN 1990; Delhi 1992**

A. Lateral margin of ant. 2/3
B. Tip of the tongue
C. Dorsum posteriorly
D. Ventral

**33. The operation for short columella is usually done at the age (years) of : AIIMS 1984**

A. 1 to 3 B. 6 to 9
C. 10 to 16 D. 18 to 25

**34. Hynes pharyngoplasty is used to improve a child's : AIIMS 1984**

A. Appearance B. Teething
C. Speech D. Feeding

| Ans. | | | | | | | | | |
|---|---|---|---|---|---|---|---|---|---|
| 15. A | 16. A | 17. A | 18. A | 19. A | 20. B | 21. B | 22. A | 23. D | 24. D |
| 25. C | 26. B | 27. A | 28. D | 29. A | 30. B | 31. C | 32. A | 33. C | 34. C |

35. **The most important factor in operation for cleft lip is : DNB 1989**
A. Age
B. Weight
C. Before speech is developed
D. Hemoglobin

36. **In cleft lip operation, all the stitches are removed on : AIIMS 1986**
A. 2nd day B. 4th day
C. 10th day D. 14th day

37. **The first feed after cleft lip operation should preferably be : AMU 1986; Delhi 1993**
A. Honey B. Warm water
C. Half strength milk D. Full-strength milk

38. **The following are the methods for operating cleft lip except : BHU 1985**
A. Le Mesurier's method B. Tennison's method
C. Millard's method D. Wardill's method

39. **The following are the criteria for operation of cleft lip for achieving the optimum result except : AIIMS 1985**
A. Age 3 to 6 months.
B. Weight more than 4.5 kg (10 lb).
C. Haemoglobin more than 10 gm%.
D. Respiratory swab does not contain any pathogen except streptococcus.

40. **Pierre Robbin syndrome is : AIIMS 1984, 85**
A. Cleft palate with syndactyly
B. Cleft palate with mandibular hypoplasia and respiratory obstruction
C. Cleft lip with mandibular hypoplasia
D. Cleft-up

41. **A patient with cheek cancer has a tumour of 2.5 cm located close to and involving the lower alveolus. A single mobile homolateral lymphnode measured 6 cm is palpable. The TNM stage is : AIIMS 1985, 86, 87**
A. T1, N1, M0 B. T2, N2, M0
C. T2, N1, M0 D. T4, N2, M0

42. **In the reconstruct following excision of previously irradiated cheek cancer, the flap will be : AIIMS 1984, 85**
A. Local tongue
B. Cervical
C. Forehead
D. Pectoralis major myocutaneous

43. **In the treatment of cancer cheek using a single drug, the best results are obtained with : AIIMS 1985, 86**
A. Cisplatinum B. Methotrexate
C. Bleomycin D. Endoxon

44. **Secretomotor fibres to the parotid is via : AIIMS 1983**
A. Auriculo-temporal nerve
B. Facial nerve
C. Trigeminal nerve
D. Maxillary nerve

45. **Dental cyst is cyst in association with chronically infected : AMC 1987; UPSC 1988**
A. Wisdom tooth (unerupted)
B. Normal erupted teeth
C. Carcinoma mandible
D. Carcinoma tongue

46. **In parotid surgery for mixed parotid tumour, there is : Delhi 1988, 89**
A. Facial nerve injury B. Salivary fistula
C. Recurrence D. All of the above

47. **Mixed parotid tumour arises from : Delhi 1987, 88**
A. Epithelium
B. Epithelium + Mesenchyme
C. Mesenchyme
D. None of the above

48. **Regarding carcinoma of tongue which is incorrect : DNB 1989**
A. Starts as painless ulcer
B. May present as a fissure
C. Common site is posterior one third of tongue
D. In late cases, pain may radiate

49. **Which is the muscle flap used over bone : AIIMS 1996**
A. Pedicle B. Full thickness
C. Split thickness D. Distant

50. **Tumours of the palate include the following except : AMU 1989**
A. Ectopic salivary tumour
B. A carcinoma of the maxillary antrum
C. An alveolar abscess of the incisors
D. A transitional-cell carcinoma

51. **Countryman's lip is : UPSC 1987**
A. Swelling due to sensitivity to the sun
B. An early lesion of foot and mouth disease
C. A squamous-cell carcinoma
D. A mucous cyst of the lip

52. **Ca buccal mucosa metastasized to : AI 1997**
A. Submandibular nodes
B. Jugulodiagastric nodes
C. Jugulo omohyoid nodes
D. Brain

| Ans. | | | | | | | | | |
|---|---|---|---|---|---|---|---|---|---|
| 35. C | 36. B | 37. B | 38. D | 39. D | 40. B | 41. C | 42. D | 43. A | 44. A |
| 45. B | 46. D | 47. B | 48. C | 49. A | 50. D | 51. C | 52. B | | |

**53. Axial flap is :** **AI 1997**
A. Flap with artery running along its axis
B. Advanced along an angle to its axis
C. Random pattern flap
D. Transferred to new sites

**54. Lymphatic drainage of pyriform fossa space is to :** **Delhi 1996**
A. Submandibular LN B. Sublingual LN
C. Deep cervical LN D. Post. occipital LN

**55. A Warthin's tumour is :** **AIIMS 1990**
A. An adenolymphoma of the parotid gland
B. A pleomorphic adenoma of the parotidgland
C. A cylindroma
D. A carcinoma of the parotid

**56. The treatment of submandibular calculus lying within the duct is to :** **UPSC 1988**
A. Dilate the duct
B. Remove the stone by making an opening in the duct
C. Site open the duct at the papilla
D. Remove the gland

**57. Which carcinoma does not belong to oral cancer :** **AI 1993**
A. Posterior 1/3 of tongue B. Hard palate
C. Cheek D. Tongue anterior 1/3

**58. In maxillofacial injury where injury to spine cannot be ruled out, the first measure is :** **AI 1993**
A. Airway maintaining B. Check of spinal lying
C. Start an I/V line D. Check the pupils

**59. What traverses the parotid gland :** **AI 1993**
A. Facial nerve B. Axillary nerve
C. Internal carotid artery D. Mandibular nerve

**60. Painless ulcer of the tongue is due to :** **UPSC 1987**
A. Dyspepsia B. Syphilis
C. Tuberculosis D. None of the above

**61. Warthin's tumor is best treated by :** **AI 1996**
A. Superficial parotidectomy
B. Enucleation
C. Radiotherapy
D. Chemotherapy

**62. In carcinoma of tip of tongue, lymph nodes not involved are :** **PGI 1983; AIIMS 1984**
A. Juglodiagastric B. Retropharyngeal
C. Submandibular D. None of the above

**63. Epidermoid carcinoma of following has best prognosis :** **AIIMS 1986**
A. Lip B. Buccal mucosa
C. Palate D. Tongue

**64. Commonest oral cancer is :** **UPSC 1986; AIIMS 1989; Delhi 1990; PGI 1990**
A. Squamous cell carcinoma (Epidermoid carcinoma)
B. Adenocarcinoma
C. Transitional cell carcinoma
D. Columnar cell carcinoma

**65. Orodental fistula of the following predisposes to carcinoma lung :** **Delhi 1985, 90**
A. 2nd incisor B. 1st premolar
C. 2nd premolar D. 1st molar

**66. Operation on inferior part of tongue may injur nerve :** **Delhi 1990**
A. IX B. XI
C. XII D. Lingual

**67. Most effective and safest treatment for pleomorphic adenoma parotid :** **AIIMS 1995**
A. Enucleation
B. Superficial parotidectomy
C. Deep parotidectomy
D. Radiotherapy

**68. A 28 years old male with recurrent oral ulcer with erythema. Diagnosis is :** **AI 1996**
A. Aphthous ulcer B. Pemphigus
C. Herpes genitalis D. Malignancy

**69. Trismus in parapharyngeal abscess is due to spasm of :** **PGI 1998**
A. Masseter B. Medial pterygoid
C. Lateral pterygoid D. Temporalis

**70. After mandibulectomy, muscle preventing falling back of tongue is :** **PGI 1998**
A. Genioglossus B. Hyoglossus
C. Palatoglossus D. All of the above

**71. Treatment of submandibular salivary gland duct calculi is :** **AMC 1988**
A. Excision of submandibular gland.
B. Opening the duct at the frenulum.
C. Opening the duct and removal of calculus.
D. Excision of gland and duct.

**72. Reparative granuloma of jaw is treated by :** **AIIMS 1990**
A. Antibiotics
B. Wedge resection
C. Resection and bone grafting
D. Curettage

| Ans. | 53. A | 54. C | 55. A | 56. B | 57. B | 58. A | 59. A | 60. B | 61. A | 62. B |
|---|---|---|---|---|---|---|---|---|---|---|
| | 63. A | 64. A | 65. D | 66. D | 67. B | 68. A | 69. C | 70. C | 71. C | 72. D |

**73. Dentigerous cyst arises from : AI 1988; JIPMER 1987**

A. An unerupted tooth
B. Apex of an infected tooth
C. Nasopalatine cysts
D. Solitary bone cyst
E. Multi locular keratocytes

**74. The most common site of the internal opening of a branchial fistula is at the : UPSC 1995**

A. Lateral nasopharyngeal wall
B. Fossa of Rosenmuller
C. Gingivo-labial sulcus
D. Tonsilar fossa

**75. Pleomorphic adenoma (mixed tumour) of the parotid gland : AIIMS 1985**

A. Is best treated by superficial lobectomy.
B. Frequently requires removal of the facial nerve for adequate treatment.
C. Has tendency to locally recur following removal.
D. Frequently metastasize to cervical lymph nodes.

**76. Warthin's tumour is : AI 1988**

A. Malignant
B. Rapidly
C. Gives a hot pertechnetate scan
D. Cold pertenchnetate scan

**77. The most common cyst of the jaw is : AMC 1984**

A. Odontogenic cyst B. Dentigerous cyst
C. Radicular cyst D. Follicular cyst

**78. A patient with a fistula and chronic pus discharge from lower face and mandible is most commonly suffering from : UPSC 1984**

A. Dental cyst B. Vincent's angina
C. Ludwig's angina D. Actinomycosis

**79. A persistent or recurring abscess of anterior part of the cheek is most likely due to : PGI 1982**

A. Aberrant Stenson's duct
B. Branchial cleft cyst
C. Alveolar abscess
D. Thyroglossal duct
E. None of the above

**80. Patient has tumor of the lower jaw, involvement of the alveolar area and is edentulous. Rx is choice : AI 2001**

A. Hemimandibulectomy
B. Commando operation
C. Segmental mandibulectomy
D. Marginal mandibulectomy

**81. Medial mental sinus is due to : Karnataka 1989**

A. Persistence of thyroglossal tract
B. Failure of the branchial pouch to disappear
C. Caries of lower molar teeth
D. Apical abscess of lower incisors

**82. Salivary gland calculi are : Karnataka 1989**

A. Most common in the parotid gland
B. Diagnosed by probing and palpating with a lacrimal duct probe
C. Easily palpable with the fingers
D. Associated with renal calculi

**83. Orodynia is seen in all except : AIIMS 1994**

A. Candida infection B. Barret's Esophagus
C. Cardiospasm D. Gumma

**84. Incision for sublingual dermoid : AP 1993, 94**

A. Submandibular
B. Submental
C. Vertical incision from the tip of the tongue
D. Transverse incision from the tip of the floor of the mouth

**85. Cancer tongue may have all the following features except : Delhi 1992, 94**

A. Pain in the ear B. Pain in swallowing
C. Ankyloglossis D. Nasal regurgitation

**86. A 60-years old female presents with a non-healing ulcer with raised edges on the face four years duration, without any significant lymph node enlargement. The most likely diagnosis is : UPSC 1996**

A. Basal cell carcinoma B. Epidermoid carcinoma
C. Malignant melanoma D. Mycosis fungoides

**87. In Plummer Vinson syndrome which is true : PGI 1996**

A. Glossitis
B. Slough in pyriform fossa
C. Sympathetic overactivity
D. Parasympathetic overactivity

**88. 2.5 cm involvement of oral cavity carcinoma with contralateral mobile lymph node, staging is : PGI 1996**

A. T2N2 B. T2N3
C. T1N1 D. T2

**89. In radical neck dissection, which nerve is sometimes sacrificed : PGI 1996**

A. 9 B. 10
C. 11 D. 12

**90. Superficial part of parotid overlies : AIIMS 1996**

A. Ramus of mandible B. Palatine tonsil
C. Pharyngeal tonsil D. Soft palate

| Ans. | 73. A | 74. A | 75. A,C | 76. C | 77. C | 78. D | 79. C | 80. C | 81. D | 82. C |
|---|---|---|---|---|---|---|---|---|---|---|
| | 83. D | 84. C | 85. D | 86. A | 87. A | 88. A | 89. C | 90. A | | |

**91. Bilateral enlargement of parotid is seen in all except : AIIMS 1996**

A. Sjogren's syndrome B. SLE
C. Chronic pancreatitis D. Sarcoidosis

**92. A bacterial pyogenic parotitis is found most commonly in which of the following : Orissa 1999**

A. Mumps
B. Debilitation after major surgery
C. Drug reaction (iodide mumps)
D. Uveoparotid fever

**93. Compressible swelling at root of nose in 2 years old boy : AIIMS 1999**

A. Meningoencephalocoele
B. Supraorbital artery aneurysm
C. Cystic hygroma
D. Lacrimal cyst

**94. Cusp of Carabelli is seen in : TN 1999**

A. Ist molar upper B. IInd molar lower
C. IIIrd molar upper D. IIIrd molar lower

**95. A T2 oral cancer adjacent to the mandible with 1 cm ulcer is treated by: JIPMER 2000**

A. Surgery B. Radiotherapy
C. Chemotherapy D. Laser therapy

**96. Regarding submandibular salivary gland, the following are true except : Kerala 2000**

A. Superficial lobe lies in the submandibular triangle and deep lobe in the floor of the mouth.
B. Calculi are more common.
C. Pleomorphic adenomas are less common than in parotid
D. Damage to Lingual nerve during surgery will cause loss of sensation in the post one third of the tongue.
E. Hypoglosal nerve loops under the submandibular duct.

**97. Most common cause of post-operative parotitis is : AI 1994**

A. Streptococcus B. Staphylococcus
C. Klebsiella D. Pneumococcus

**98. Brawing swelling 'of submandibular region with inflammatory oedema is a feature of : JIPMER 2001**

A. Vincent's disease B. Ludwig's angina
C. Plunging ranula D. Diphtheria

**99. Carcinoma of lip is histologically : PGI 1994; Kerala 2001**

A. Squamous cell ca. B. Adeno ca.
C. Basal cell ca. D. None

**100. Referred pain in ear in Ca base of tongue is through : Rohtak 2001**

A. Facial N. B. Glossopharyngeal
C. Hypoglossal D. V Lingual nerve

**101. The most common tumor in the mandible is : AIIMS 2001**

A. Osteoblastoma
B. Ameloblastoma
C. Squamous cell carcinoma
D. Lymphoma

**102. The most common location of ameloblastoma is near the : AIIMS 2001**

A. Alveolar margin in the midline
B. Molar region in the mandible
C. Symphysis menti
D. Any of the above

**103. A child presents with hypoplasia of mandible, absent condyle and ramus of mandible with deformities of pinna & bearing defects. The probable : JIPMER 2002**

A. Treaches Collin syndrome
B. Crouzon's syndrome
C. Hemifacial microsomia
D. Pierre robbin syndrome

**104. A 55 years old man presents with 1x2 cm ulcer in the right lateral border of tongue. Biopsy from the lesion revealed well-differentiated squamous cell carcinoma. The most appropriate management is : AIIMS 2002**

A. Interstitial brachytherapy
B. External beam irradiation + immunotherapy
C. Laser ablation
D. Chemotherapy

**105. An edentulous patient has carcinoma of the oral cavity infiltrating into the alveolar margin. Which of the following would not be indicated in managing the case : AI 2002**

A. Segmental mandibulectomy.
B. Marginal mandibulectomy with removal of the outer table.
C. Marginal mandibulectomy with removal of upper-half mandible.
D. Radiotherapy.

**106. Nerve damaged in radical mastoidectomy is : Maharashtra 2000**

A. Facial B. Cochlear
C. Vestibular D. All

**107. Persistent bucconasal membrane results in : Maharashtra 2002**

A. Cleft lip B. Choanal atresia
C. Cleft palate D. T-O fistula

**108. Which one of the following odontomas is locally invasive malignant tumor : UPSC 2002**

A. Odontogenic myxoma
B. Fibromatous epulis
C. Dentigerous cyst
D. Ameloblastoma

| Ans. | | | | | | | | | |
|---|---|---|---|---|---|---|---|---|---|
| 91. C | 92. B | 93. A | 94. A | 95. B | 96. A | 97. B | 98. B | 99. A | 100. D |
| 101. C | 102. B | 103. C | 104. A | 105. B | 106. A | 107. B | 108. D | | |

**109. A man presents to a STD clinic with urethritis and urethral discharge. Gram stain shows numerous pus cells but no microorganism. The culture is negative on the routine laboratory media. The most likely agent is : AIIMS 2002**

A. Chlamydia trachomatis
B. Haemophilus ducreyi
C. Treponema pallidum
D. Neisseria gonorrhoae

**110. A 24 years old male presents to a STD clinic with a single painless ulcer on external genitalia. The choice of laboratory test to look for the etiological agent would be: AIIMS 2002**

A Scrappings from ulcer for culture on chocolate agar with antibiotic supplement.
B Serology for detection of specific IgM antibodies.
C Scrappings from ulcer for dark field microscopy.
D Scrappings from ulcer for tissue culture.

**111. Tooth is fixed in its socket by the : COMEDEK-2005**

A. Cementocytes
B. Peridontal membrane
C. Cement
D. Dentine

Ans. 109. A 110. C 111. B

# EXPLANATIONS OF MAXILLOFACIAL SURGERY

1. Ans.— B. **Bilateral cleft lip**
2. Ans.— A. **Left side**
3. Ans.— D. **Protrusion of mandible**
4. Ans.— C. **Gums**

   Borrelia vincenti and fusiformis are the cause.
5. Ans.— A. **Mucoepidermoid carcinoma**
6. Ans.— D. **Adenoid cystic carcinoma**
7. Ans.— A. **It is confined to infant**
8. Ans.— A. **Cystic swelling on the floor of the mouth.**
9. Ans.— D. **Aspergillus niger**
10. Ans.— A. **Adenolymphoma**
11. Ans.— C. **HIV infection**
12. Ans.— A. **Benign tumour**

    It is adenolymphoma of parotid gland.
13. Ans.— D. **All of the above**
14. Ans.— A. **Mucoepidermoid**
15. Ans.— A. **Epidermoid carcinoma**
16. Ans.— A. **Vincent' angina**
17. Ans.— A. **Squamous cell carcinoma**
18. Ans.— A. **Cavernous sinus**
19. Ans.— A. **Pleomorphic adenocarcinoma**
20. Ans.— B. **Submucous fibrosis**
21. Ans.— B. **Post. cricoid**
22. Ans.— A. **Submandibular**
23. Ans.— D. **Tonsillar fossa/bed**
24. Ans.— D. **Injury to lingual nerve**
25. Ans.— C. **Maxillary process with medial nasal process.**
26. Ans.— B. **Palate**
27. Ans.— A. **Commonly adeno carcinoma**
28. Ans.— D. **Inferior alveolar**
29. Ans.— A. **Pleomorphic adenoma**

    It accounts for 70% of parotid tumours and 50% of all salivary tumors. It is common in women and in fifth decade Malignant transformation is uncommon.
30. Ans.— B. **Staphylococcus**

    It is infection of parotid gland, limited entirely to elderly, debilitates, malnourished patients with poor oral hygiene. It is common in second post-operative week and is associated with nasogastric intubation. First symptom is pain or tenderness at angle of Jaw.
31. Ans.— C. **Early metastasis to lymph nodes**
32. Ans.— A. **Lateral margin of ant. 2/3**
33. Ans.— C. **10 to 16**
34. Ans.— C. **Speech**
35. Ans.— C. **Before speech is developed**
36. Ans.— B. **4th day**

    The optimal time for operation of cleft lip can be described as the accepted "rule of ten". This includes body weight of 10lb (4.5 kg) or more and a hemoglobin of 10 g/dL or more. This is usually at sometime after the 10th week of life. Manchester repair is used.
37. Ans.— B. **Warm water**
38. Ans.— D. **Wardill's method**
39. Ans.— D. **Respiratory swab does not contain any pathogen except streptococcus.**
40. Ans.— B. **Cleft palate with mandibular hypoplasia and respiratory obstruction.**
41. Ans.— C. **T2, N1, M0**
42. Ans.— D. **Pectoralis major myocutaneous**
43. Ans.— A. **Cisplatinum**
44. Ans.— A. **Auriculo-temporal nerve**
45. Ans.— B. **Normal erupted teeth**
46. Ans.— D. **All of the above**

47. Ans.— B. Epithelium + Mesenchyme

48. Ans.— C. Common site is posterior one third of tongue.

49. Ans.— A. Pedicle

50. Ans.— D. A transitional-cell carcinoma

51. Ans.— C. A squamous-cell carcinoma

52. Ans.— B. Jugulodiagastric nodes

The carcinoma is well differentiated and locally infiltrating. It metastasises (50% to regional LN—submaxillary, parotid and periglandular LN and the deep Jugular and submental LN).

53. Ans.— A. Flap with artery running along its axis.

It is a single—pedicle flap. They are deltopectoral, forehead, grain, cervico-humeral and transverse back flaps.

54. Ans.— C. Deep cervical LN

55. Ans.— A. An adenolymphoma of the parotid gland

56. Ans.— B. Remove the stone by making an opening in the duct.

57. Ans.— B. Hard palate

Carcinoma of oral cavity is commonest malignancy among Indian males.

58. Ans.— A. Airway maintaining

Airway may obstruct due to aspiration of blood, clot formation etc.

59. Ans.— A. Facial nerve

It is likely to be paralysed in its surgery.

60. Ans.— B. Syphilis

Ulcers can be produced by spices, sharp tooth, squamous all carcinoma in addition to syphilis.

61. Ans.— A. Superficial parotidectomy

Also called Adeno lymphoma, a benign tumor markedly eosinophilic whose inner cells are columnar. Forms 10% of parotid tumor, rare in submandibular & minor glands. Unlike all other, 'hot' spot on 99Tc "pertechnetate scan so that a firm diagnosis is possible without biopsy."

62. Ans.— B. Retropharyngeal

63. Ans.— A. Lip

64. Ans.— A. Squamous cell carcinoma (Epidermoid carcinoma).

65. Ans.— D. 1st molar

66. Ans.— D. Lingual

67. Ans.— B. Superficial parotidectomy

68. Ans.— A. Aphthous ulcer

It is of 3 types —minor, major and herpetiform.

69. Ans.— C. Lateral pterygoid

70. Ans.— C. Palatoglossus

71. Ans.— C. Opening the duct and removal of calculus.

72. Ans.— D. Curettage

73. Ans.— A. An unerupted tooth

Dentigerous cyst arises as a result of separation of the reduced enamel epithelium from the surface of the crown of an unexpected tooth and accumulation of fluid in the internal unerupted upper third molars seen in a radiograph displaced upto the orbital floor are usually involved in dentigerous cyst. Most frequent is lower third molar.

74. Ans.— A. Lateral nasopharyngeal wall

75. Ans.— A. Is best treated by superficial lobectomy

76. Ans.— C. Gives a hot pertechnetate scan

77. Ans.— C. Radicular cyst

78. Ans.— D. Actinomycosis

79. Ans.— C. Alveolar abscess

80. Ans.— C. Segmental mandibulectomy

Once the cancellous bone is substantially involved, segmental resection is necessary for large tumors, combined radiotherapy and surgery are used. Surgery alone is used for recurrence after radiotherapy and radiotherapy for small tumors.

81. Ans.— D. Apical abscess of lower incisors

82. Ans.— C. Easily palpable with the fingers

83. Ans.— D. Gumma

84. Ans.— C. Vertical incision from the tip of the tongue.

85. Ans.— D. Nasal regurgitation

The ca. tongue is most common in lateral margin 47%, other sites are Post. 1/3rd 20%, ventral surface & frenulum - 9%, dorsum 6.5%, faucio lingual 6%.

**86. Ans.— A. Basal cell carcinoma**

**87. Ans.— A. Glossitis**

**88. Ans.— A. T2N2**

**89. Ans.— C. 11**

**90. Ans.— A. Ramus of mandible**

**91. Ans.— C. Chronic pancreatitis**

**92. Ans.— B. Debilitation after major surgery**

**93. Ans.— A. Meningoencephalocele**

**94. Ans.— A. Ist molar upper**

**95. Ans.— B. Radiotherapy**

**96. Ans.— A. Superficial lobe lies in the submandibular triangle and deep lobe in the floor of the mouth.**

**97. Ans.— B. Staphylococcus**

**It is infection of parotid gland, limited entirely to elderly, debilitates, malnourished patients with poor oral hygiene. It is common in second post-operative week and is associated with nasogastric intubation. First symptom is pain or tenderness at angle of Jaw.**

**98. Ans.— B. Ludwig's angina**

**99. Ans.— A. Squamous cell ca.**

**100. Ans.— D. V Lingual nerve**

**101. Ans.— C. Squamous cell carcinoma**

**102. Ans.— B. Molar region in the mandible**

**103. Ans.— C. Hemifacial microsomia**

**104. Ans.— A. Interstitial brachytherapy**

**105. Ans.— B. Marginal mandibulectomy with removal of the outer table.**

**Mandibulectomy is the treatment of choice.**

**106. Ans.— A. Facial**

**107. Ans.— B. Choanal atresia**

**108. Ans.— D. Ameloblastoma**

**109. Ans.— A. Chlamydia trachomatis**

**110. Ans.— C Scrappings from ulcer for dark field microscopy.**

**111. Ans.— B. Peridontal membrane**

# 5

# IMPORTANT TEXT OF NECK

## DIFFERENTIAL DIAGNOSIS OF LUMP INSIDE OF THE NECK

1. Sebaceous cyst
2. Lipoma
3. Lymph node
4. Thyroid/parathyroid tumour
5. Cystic hygroma
6. Carotid artery aneurysm/carotid body tumour
7. Submandibular pouch
8. Branchial cyst

## RESULTS OF THYROID FUNCTION TESTS IN NORMAL AND PATHOLOGICAL STATES

| Thyroid functional state | TSH (0.3-3.3 mU $l^{-1}$) | Free T4 (10-30 nmol $l^{-1}$) | Free T3 (3.5-7.5 μmol $l^{-1}$) |
|---|---|---|---|
| Euthyroid | Normal | Normal | Normal |
| Thyrotoxic | Undetectable | High | High |
| Myxoedema | High | Low | Low |
| Suppressive $T_4$ therapy | Undetectable | High | High |
| $T_3$ toxicity | Low/undetectable | Normal | High |

## CLASSIFICATION OF THYROID SWELLINGS

***Simple goitre (euthyroid)***
Diffuse hyperplastic
- Physiological
- Pubertal
- Pregnancy

Multinodular goitre

***Toxic***
Diffuse
- Graves' disease

Multinodular
Toxic adenoma

***Neoplastic***
Benign
Malignant

***Inflammatory***
Autoimmune
- Chronic lymphocytic thyroiditis
- Hashimoto's disease

Granulomatous
- De Quervain's thyroidits

Fibrosing
- Riedel's thyroiditis

Infective
- Acute (bacterial thyroiditis, viral thyroiditis, subacute thyroiditis)

Chronic (tuberculous, syphilitic)
Other
- Amyloid

# MCQ's OF NECK

## What is important in Neck

Branchial cyst, Cystic hygroma, Carotid body tumour, Block dissection (Crile's) Thyroid Function tests, Swellings, Tumours, Wayne's index, Post-operative Complications, Thyroglossal cysts

1. **Congenital toticollis is due to : Rohtak 1986**
   A. Infarction of the sternomastoid at birth
   B. A hemi-cervical vertebra
   C. Failure of the clavicle to develop
   D. A rhabadomyoma of the sternomastoid

2. **By far most frequent sign of hyper-parathyroidism is : AMU 1986**
   A. Bone cyst
   B. Pancreatitis
   C. Renal stones
   D. Right superior vena cava
   E. None of the above

3. **Retrosternal goitre usually develops from : TN 1996**
   A. Upper pole B. Lower pole
   C. Isthmus D. Ectopic thyroid tissue

4. **A soft swelling at the lower end of sternucleiomastoid which moves on deglutination is : AIIMS 1986**
   A. Branchial cyst B. Thyroglossal cyst
   C. Carcinoma thyroid D. Hodgkin's lymphoma

5. **Thymus gland abscess seen in congenital syphilis is called : AIIMS 1986**
   A. Fouchier's abscess B. Politzeri abscess
   C. Douglas abscess D. Dobois abscess

6. **Signs & symptoms of hyperthyroidism may include following, except : AMU 1989**
   A. Sleeping tachycardia B. Atrial fibrillation
   C. Exophthalmos D. Decreased sweating
   E. Pretibial myxoedema

7. **Most common type of parathyroid adenoma is : AIIMS 1986**
   A. Clear cell adenoma B. Chief cell adenoma
   C. Oxyphil cell adenoma D. A + B
   E. B + C

8. **Feature of Hashimoto's disease include following, except : BHU 1987**
   A. Soft diffuse enlargement of thyroid.
   B. Increased levels of circulating thyroid antibodies.
   C. May be associated with pernicious anaemia.
   D. Initial hyperthyroidism followed by hypothyroidism.
   E. Hyperthyroidism occurs usually in middle aged females.

9. **The only reason for operating in case of thyroiditis is : AIIMS 1984**
   A. To prevent cancerous degeneration.
   B. For relief of pain in neck and ear.
   C. To overcome pressure on trachea or oesophagus.
   D. To cure the toxic reaction.
   E. If there is autoimmune reaction.

10. **Medullary carcinoma of thyroid associated with each of the following except : AIIMS 1983**
    A. Prostaglandins
    B. Serotonin
    C. Calcitonin
    D. Multiple endocrine adenomatosis
    E. Better prognosis than papillary carcinoma

11. **The most common complication after subtotal thyroidectomy is : AMU 1987; UPSC 1988, 93**
    A. Tetany
    B. Hypothyroidism
    C. Recurrent laryngeal curve injury
    D. Hypoparathyroidism

12. **Cervical sympathectomy is most effective in the management of : CSE 1997**
    A. Raynaud's disease
    B. Buerger's disease
    C. Atherosclerotic vascular disease
    D. Hyperthirosis

| Ans. | 1. A | 2. C | 3. B | 4. B | 5. D | 6. D | 7. B | 8. A | 9. C | 10. E |
|---|---|---|---|---|---|---|---|---|---|---|
| | 11. B | 12. A | | | | | | | | |

**13. Symptoms of endemic goitre are following, except : BHU 1985, 87**

A. Cold intolerance B. Hoarseness
C. Dysphagia D. Heat intolerance

**14. Treatment of Hashimoto's disease is : AMC 1985**

A. Carbimazole
B. Thyroxine
C. Radio iodine
D. Subtotal thyroidectomy

**15. Parathyroid gland develop from —— bronchial pouches. AMC 1988**

A. 1st and 2nd B. 2nd and 3rd
C. 3rd and 4th D. 5th and 6th

**16. In hypothyroidism, following are seen, except : AMC 1993**

A. Large thick tongue B. Umbilical hernia
C. Constipation D. Brachycephalic head

**17. Cystic compressible, translucent swelling in the posterior triangle of neck : AIIMS 1984; AI 1991**

A. Cystic hygroma B. Branchial cyst
C. Thyroglossal cyst D. Dermoid cyst

**18. Lymphnode metastasis commonest in —— carcinoma thyroid. DNB 1990**

A. Follicular B. Papillary
C. Anaplastic D. Medullary

**19. Cystic hygroma is a kind of : PGI 1980; AMC 1985**

A. Lymphoma B. Lymphangioma
C. Hemangioma D. Capillary angioma

**20. FNAC is not of much in use in which thyroid pathology: AI 1995; TN 1996**

A. Papillary carcinoma B. Follicular carcinoma
C. Medullary carcinoma D. Thyroiditis

**21. All except —— are true about Riedel's thyroiditis. DNB 1989**

A. Auto-immune disease
B. Collagen disorder
C. May cause obstructive symptoms
D. May be associated with retroperitoneal fibrosis

**22. Which is a never cause of thyroglossal fistula : PGI 1982; AIIMS 1985**

A. Infection of thyroglossal cyst
B. Inadequate removal of thyroglossal cyst
C. Congenital
D. None of the above

**23. The commonest and least common sites of thyroglossal cyst are respectively : AIIMS 1987, 90; PGI 1980, 89, 92; DNB 1990**

A. Beneath the foramen caecum
B. At the level of cricoid cartilage
C. In the floor of mouth
D. Beneath hyoid
E. On the thyroid cartilage

**24. Median ectopic thyroid is a : DNB 1990**

A. Thyroglossal cyst B. Normal thyroid tissue
C. Carcinoma metastasis D. Strauma ovari

**25. Which of the following is incorrect regarding the thyroid : AMU 1986**

A. The gland develops from the third pharyngeal pouch.
B. The C-cells are developed from the ultimobranchial body.
C. The normal gland weight is 20-25 gms.
D. The resting follicle contains colloid in which iodine is stored.

**26. Long-acting thyroid stimulator is : UPSC 1987; Delhi 1989**

A. A glycoprotein
B. Di-iodothyronine
C. An IgM immunoglobulin
D. An IgG immunoglobulin

**27. Thyroid carcinoma with best prognosis is : AI 1996**

A. Papillary carcinoma B. Follicular carcinoma
C. Anaplastic type D. Medullary type

**28. The disadvantage of using radio-iodine to treat thyrotoxicosis is following except : PGI 1982**

A. Drug therapy is prolonged.
B. An indefinite follow-up is essential.
C. There is a progressive incidence of thyroid insufficiency.
D. It should be avoided under the age of 45.

**29. The term lateral aberrant thyroid implies : AIIMS 1986**

A. Congenital aberrant thyroid tissue lateral to the thyroid.
B. A metastasis in a cervical lymph node from an occult thyroid carcinoma.
C. A metastasis from carcinoma of the larynx.
D. A type of branchial cyst.

**30. Movement of thyroid during deglutition is due to : AIIMS 1986**

A. Its attachment with trachea
B. Its development with tongue together
C. Its attachment with hyoid
D. Sheathed with the same fascia
E. None of the above

**Ans.** 13. D 14. B 15. C 16. D 17. A 18. B 19. B 20. B 21. A 22. C
23. D,E 24. B 25. A 26. D 27. A 28. A 29. B 30. C

**31. Osteitis fibrosa cystica is associated with :** **AI 1995**
A. Hyperparathyroidism
B. Congenital bone disease
C. Hypoparathyroidism
D. Hyperthyroidism

**32. Parathyroid adenoma is associated with following, except :** **AMU 1987**
A. Low serum alkaline phosphatase
B. Low serum phosphorus
C. Increased serum calcium
D. Pathological fracture

**33. A 21-year old woman has a 3 cm node in the lower deep cervical chain on the left. The biopsy is interpreted as revealing normal thyroid tissue in a lymph node. The most likely diagnosis is :** **UPSC 1995**
A. Subacute thyroiditis
B. Metastatic carcinoma thyroid
C. Hashimoto's disease
D. Lateral aberrent thyroid

**34. All of the following are used in effectively treating recurrent thyroid cancer except :** **MAHE 1994**
A. Chemotherapy
B. Further surgery
C. High doses of $I^{131}$
D. High doses of thyroxine

**35. Characteristic feature of primary hyperparathyroidism is :** **AIIMS 1992**
A. Diffuse osteopenia
B. Swelling lamina dura
C. Sub-peritoneal resorption of terminal phalanges
D. Salt & pepper appearance of skull

**36. All are the complications of total Thyroidectomy except :** **AIIMS 1992**
A. Airway obstruction
B. Haemorrhage
C. Hypercalcemia
D. Recurrent laryngeal nerve palsy

**37. Hypocalcemia in immediate post-operative period following excision of parathyroid adenoma is due to:** **AIIMS 1992**
A. Increased calcitonin
B. Stress
C. Hypercalciuria
D. Increased uptake by bone

**38. Multiple cold nodules in a thyroid scan is a feature of :** **AIIMS 1992**
A. Multi-nodular goitre
B. Multicentric papillary Ca.
C. Grave's disease
D. Hashimoto's thyroiditis

**39. Secondaries in the neck with no obvious primary malignancy is most often due to :** **JIPMER 1993; AIIMS 2002**
A. Ca. Larynx B. Ca. Nasopharyx
C. Ca. Thyroid D. Ca. Stomach

**40. Treatment of choice for cold nodule in thyroid is :** **JIPMER 1993**
A. $I^{131}$
B. Hemithyroidectomy
C. Subtotal thyroidectomy
D. Wait and watch

**41. The type of Thyroid Ca. which produces high level of serum calcitonin is :** **JIPMER 1993**
A. Follicular B. Papillary
C. Anaplastic D. Medullary

**42. Medullary carcinoma of thyroid arises from :** **Delhi 1993**
A. Follicular cell lining
B. Interfollicular C-cells
C. Parathyroid cells in thyroid
D. Parathyroid gland

**43. Hyoid bone is removed to prevent the recurrence of :** **Delhi 1993**
A. Thyroid nodule B. Thyroglossal cyst
C. Ectopic thyroid D. Papillary carcinoma

**44. Calcitonin is a marker in serum for :** **AI 1995**
A. Anaplastic carcinoma B. Medullary carcinoma
C. Papillary carcinoma D. Follicular carcinoma

**45. $I^{131}$ scan of thyroid is useful to :** **TN 1989**
A. Estimate function B. Detect cold nodules
C. Diagnose carcinoma D. All of the above

**46. Retrotracheal extension of thyroid mass can be recognised by :** **AP 1989**
A. X-ray neck B. C.T. scan
C. Barium swallow D. Ultrasound

**47. Occult carcinoma of the thyroid is seen in :** **DNB 1991**
A. Papillary carcinoma B. Medullary
C. Anaplastic D. Hurthle-cell carcinoma

**48. A cold nodule of the thyroid may be due to the following except :** **TN 1988**
A. Cyst of the thyroid
B. Degeneration in a nodule
C. Carcinoma
D. Parenchymatous goitre

| Ans. | 31. A | 32. A | 33. D | 34. A | 35. D | 36. C | 37. D | 38. A | 39. B | 40. B |
|---|---|---|---|---|---|---|---|---|---|---|
| | 41. D | 42. B | 43. B | 44. B | 45. B | 46. B | 47. A | 48. D | | |

**49. In non-endemic zones, solitary nodule of the thyroid is result of: PGI 1985**

A. Thyroditis B. Adenoma
C. Follicular carcinoma D. Colloid goitre

**50. Following are true about thyroid tumor except : JIPMER 1997**

A. Malignant tumors are solid in USS.
B. 40-50% malignant nodules are cold in isotopes scanning.
C. FNAC biopsy is not diagnostic.
D. Calcitonin is a tumor marker for medullary Ca. thyroid.

**51. Which of the following is not an histological type of carcinoma of the thyroid : AIIMS 1991**

A. Transitional B. Papillary
C. Anaplastic D. Medullary

**52. Multinodular goitre least commonly leads to : AMC 1993, 94**

A. Hypothyrodism B. Hyperthyroidism
C. Carcinoma D. All of the above

**53. After operation for hyperparathyroidism which of the following does not take place : AMU 1986, 89**

A. Renal stones disappear
B. Bones recalcify
C. Psychiatric patients improve
D. Hyperparathyroidism recurs in a small minority of patients

**54. Regarding the clinically solitary nodule of the thyroid, which statement is incorrect : UPSC 1987**

A. The solitary toxic nodule is almost never malignant.
B. The solitary toxic nodule may be treated by radio cobalt.
C. The cold nodule is suspect (may be malignant).
D. The cold nodule should be excised.

**55. About branchial cyst, incorrect is : Karnataka 1987; DNB 1990**

A. Arises from the second branchial cleft.
B. Usually appears between the ages of 20-25 years.
C. Protrudes beneath the anterior border of the sternomastoid.
D. Is always lined by squamous epithelium.

**56. Which of the following is inappropriate to cystic hygroma : DNB 1990**

A. It is a type of cavernous haemangioma
B. It can be the earliest swelling of the neck to appear in life
C. It can obstruct labour
D. It is brilliantly translucent

**57. The 'Potato's tumour of the neck is a : DNB 1990**

A. Sternomastoid tumour B. Carotid body tumour
C. Thyroid tumour D. Parotid tumour

**58. Which of the following is used in the treatment of thyrotoxic crisis: DNB 1991**

A. Propranolol
B. Metoclopramide
C. Tetraiodophenolphthalein
D. Radio-iodine

**59. Tertiary hyperparathyroidism is due to : AIIMS 1996**

A. Autonomy in functioning
B. CRF
C. Adenoma
D. Malabsorption syndrome

**60. Sternomastoid tumour appears : UPSC 1984**

A. Congenitally
B. Soon after birth
C. In first week of life
D. At the age of 2—6 weeks

**61. Regarding carotid body tumour, which of the following is not true : AMU 1987**

A. It increases gradually.
B. It responds very well to radiotherapy.
C. It is usually unilateral.
D. Vertical movements are not possible whereas it can be moved horizontally.
E. None of the above.

**62. The blood supply and venous drainage of thyroid composes of : AMC 1987, 92**

A. Superior thyroid artery and vein
B. Middle thyroid vein
C. Inferior thyroid artery and vein
D. All of the above

**63. Indication of operation in cases of thyroiditis is : UPSC 1988**

A. To achieve relief from pain
B. To prevent malignant change
C. To remove pressure on trachea and oesophagus
D. None of the above

**64. Following are true about branchial cyst, except : AI 1997**

A. Transilluminate
B. Common in mediastinum
C. Toothpaste like content
D. Remnant of IInd branchial arch

**65. With which of the following medullary carcinoma of thyroid is associated : PGI 1985; Delhi 1985**

A. Cushing's syndrome B. Carcinoid syndrome
C. Phaeochromocytoma D. Hyperparathyroidism
E. All of the above

**Ans.** **49. B** **50. B** **51. A** **52. C** **53. A** **54. B** **55. D** **56. A** **57. B** **58. A**
**59. A** **60. B** **61. B** **62. D** **63. C** **64. B** **65. E**

**66. Sistrunk's operation is used in : PGI 1982**
A. Parotid tumour B. Thyroglossal fistula
C. Thyroglossal cyst D. Branchial fistula

**67. In thyrotoxicosis which of the following is seen : UPSC 1985**
A. Pretibial myxedema
B. Glycosuria
C. Unilateral exophthalmos
D. All of the above

**68. The treatment of hypercalcemia in hyperparathyroidism includes following, except : PGI 1981, 88**
A. Hydration B. Mithramycin
C. Steroids D. Inj. Vitamin-C

**69. Inferior thyroid artery ligation in subtotal thyroidectomy is done : PGI 1987, 88**
A. As close to the thyroid as possible
B. As far as possible
C. At its origin
D. Anywhere

**70. Treatment of cystic hygroma is : JIPMER 1986, 88**
A. Surgical excision B. Injection of sclerosants
C. Irradiation D. Majesty inactivity

**71. Carotid sheath contains following except : AIIMS 1983**
A. Carotid artery B. Internal jugular vein
C. Vagus nerve D. Phrenic nerves

**72. Treatment of tuberculous cervical lymph node is : AMC 1993**
A. Incision + dependent drainage
B. Incision + nondependent drainage
C. Dependent aspiration
D. Non-dependent aspiration

**73. Radical dissection of neck includes following, except : Delhi 1989; DNB 1993; PGI 1994**
A. Cervical lymph nodes
B. Strenocleidomastoid
C. Phrenic nerves
D. Internal jugular vein

**74. Commonest cause of the hypoparathyroidism is : Delhi 1988**
A. Idiopathic B. Surgery in neck area
C. Familial D. Di George's syndrome

**75. Diagnostic of thyrotoxic thyroid adenoma is : Delhi 1984, 88**
A. ↑ T3, ↑ T4, ↑ TSH
B. Normal T3, ↑ T4, ↑ TSH
C. ↑ T3, Normal T4 and TSH
D. Normal T3 and T4, ↑ TSH

**76. In 26 years old lady with prominent eyes, anxious - T3/T4, tachycardia and tremors has, except : AIIMS 1998**
A. Diffuse goitre B. Adenomatous goitre
C. Riedel's struma D. Hashimoto's disease

**77. Best treatment of anaplastic carcinoma of thyroid is : Delhi 1986**
A. Chemotherapy
B. Subtotal thyroidectomy
C. Total thyroidectomy
D. External radiation

**78. The special danger of a carotid body tumour is that : AIIMS 1986, 87**
A. It recurs after excision
B. It is blended with the carotid artery
C. It is blended with the external jugular vein
D. It is radioresistant

**79. Regarding retrosternal goitre, which is false : TN 1989**
A. Produces a scabbard trachea
B. Mediastinal syndrome occurs
C. Can be plunging goitre
D. Can be treated by antithyroid drugs

**80. Patients with severe hypocalcemia may exhibit spontaneous tetany. Tying the blood pressure cuff in the upper arm and inflating above the systolic pressure for over 3 minutes may result in a carpal spasm in cases of mild hypocalcaemia This is ______. Bihar 1989**
A. Trousseau B. Chvostek
C. Babinski D. Romberg

**81. Endemic goitre usually presents with : AI 1996**
A. Diffuse goitre B. Hypothyroidism
C. Hyperthyroidism D. Solitary nodule

**82. Supraclavicular lymph node can be involved in following except : AP 1993; Kerala 1993**
A. Hepatoma B. Carcinoma of breast
C. Carcinoma of stomach D. Testicular tumour

**83. Patient having hypothyroidism shows psuedohypertrophy of calf muscles. He is having : UP 1995**
A. Farber Albright syndrome
B. Laron's syndrome
C. Gouerot-Nulock Houwe syndrome
D. Kocher-Debre Semelaigne syndrome

**84. Wayne's clinical diagnostic index is based on : DNB 1990**
A. Symptoms alone B. Signs alone
C. ECG changes D. A & B
E. A, B, C

| Ans. | | | | | | | | | |
|---|---|---|---|---|---|---|---|---|---|
| 66. B | 67. D | 68. D | 69. B | 70. A | 71. D | 72. D | 73. C | 74. B | 75. C |
| 76. A | 77. D | 78. B | 79. D | 80. A | 81. A | 82. A | 83. D | 84. D | |

**85. Thyroid storm is due to excessive secretion of : AIIMS 1985, 90**

A. TSH B. Thyroxine
C. Catecholamines D. Steroids

**86. A solitary nodule in thyroid in a middle aged lady is : AIIMS 1985, 94**

A. Carcinoma B. Multinodular goitre
C. Adenoma D. Physiological goitre

**87. Most common indication for surgery in multinodular intrathoracic goitre is : AIIMS 1985, 86**

A. Dyspnea
B. Dysphagia
C. Risk of carcinoma
D. Pressure on great vessels

**88. Thyroid storm after operation is due to : Delhi 1992, 93**

A. Inadequate Preoperative treatment
B. Massive bleeding
C. Recurrent laryngeal nerve injury
D. Rough handling during surgery

**89. A multiloculated translucent swelling in posterior triangle of neck of a child : AIIMS 1987; Delhi 2001**

A. Cystic hygroma B. Thyroglossal cyst
C. Hemangiomas D. Branchial cyst

**90. Treatment of metastasis by $I^{131}$ is for which type of carcinoma thyroid : Kerala 1996**

A. Follicular B. Papillary
C. Anaplastic D. Medullary

**91. Regarding branchial fistula : AIIMS 1990**

A. Opens internally near tonsil
B. Situated in midline of neck
C. Remnant of 3rd branchial arch
D. Excised by single transverse incision

**92. Killian's area is commonly complicated by : PGI 1986**

A. Carcinoma B. Diverticulum
C. Polyp D. Diphtheria

**93. Pharyngeal pouch originates from : PGI 1987**

A. Killian's dehiscence
B. Anterosuperior part
C. Posterosuperior part
D. Upper part of inferior constrictor muscle

**94. Metastatic calcium deposits are seen in : JIPMER 1997**

A. Thyroid neoplasm B. Parathyroid neoplasm
C. Thyrotoxicosis D. Thymoma

**95. A lymphnode like swelling in the neck of a child is most likely due to : PGI 1993, 94**

A. Cervical Cyst B. Branchial Cyst
C. Carotid body tumor D. Hygroma

**96. Vascular symptoms occur only when a cervical rib is : TN 1996**

A. Complete
B. Expand into a large bony mass
C. Ending in a tapering point
D. Like a fibrous band

**97. Example of radiation induced Ca is : Kerala 1996**

A. Papillary carcinoma thyroid
B. Follicular carcinoma thyroid
C. Lymphoma
D. Hepatoma
E. Seminoma

**98. Treatment of choice in well-differentiated thyroid carcinoma : PGI 1982, 85; Kerala 1996; AIIMS 2001**

A. Radio iodine
B. Near total thyroidectomy
C. Subtotal thyroidectomy
D. Radiation
E. Total thyroparathyroidectomy

**99. Commonest site of branchial cyst is : PGI 1989, 90, 94**

A. Thyroid.
B. Junction of upper and middle third of sternocleido-mastoid.
C. Junction of middle and lower third of sternocleido-mastoid.
D. Apical lobe of lungs.
E. Superior mediastinum.

**100. Carotid blowout is due to : AIIMS 1998**

A. Hemimandibulectomy B. Radical neck resection
C. Thyroid surgery D. Sistrunk operation

**101. Therapy of choice for diffuse toxic goitre in a patient over 45 years : Delhi 1984**

A. Surgery
B. Antithyroid drug
C. Radio iodine
D. Antithyroid drugs first followed by surgery

**102. Among following most common cause of solitary thyroid nodule is : AIIMS 1994**

A. Adenomatous goitre B. Follicular adenoma
C. Papillary adenoma D. Papillary carcinoma

| Ans. | | | | | | | | | | |
|---|---|---|---|---|---|---|---|---|---|---|
| 85. B | 86. C | 87. D | 88. A | 89. A | 90. A | 91. D | 92. B | 93. A | 94. B |
| 95. B | 96. A | 97. A | 98. B | 99. B | 100. B | 101. C | 102. B | | |

**103. Hypothyroidism with increased TSH levels is seen in following except : PGI 1989, 90**

A. Sheehan's syndrome
B. Lithium carbonate therapy
C. Post radio iodine ablation
D. Endemic goitre

**104. All of the following regarding papillary carcinoma thyroid is true except : AI 1990**

A. Multicentric origin
B. Secondaries to lymph nodes
C. Slowly growing
D. Bony metastasis in early stage

**105. Protein bound iodine measures secretory function of thyroid in all of the following circumstances except: AI 1990**

A. Nephrotic syndrome
B. Following hemithyroidectomy
C. During ampicillin therapy
D. Asthmatics on ephedrine

**106. In the fresh surgically removed specimen, adenomatous goitre is recognised by : Karnataka 1987**

A. Diffuse fleshy appearance of the gland.
B. Large honeycombed colloid filled areas.
C. Variable sized nodules of variegated appearance.
D. Multiple solid white nodules.

**107. Collar stud abscess occurs in : Karnataka 1987**

A. Tuberculous infection of deep cervical lymph nodes
B. Terminal pulp space infection
C. Deep palmar abscess
D. All of the above

**108. 'Brown Tumors' are seen in : Karnataka 1989**

A. Secondaries of bones B. Hyperparathyroidism
C. Hypothyroidism D. Adrenal tumors

**109. A patient presents with sore throat followed by mid line tender swelling with pain, diagnosis is : AIIMS 1993**

A. Subacute Thyroiditis B. Acute Thyroiditis
C. Thyroglossal cyst D. Toxic Thyroid Nodule

**110. Of the following methods which one is the most sensitive for detecting parathyroid adenomas : Karnataka 1993**

A. Barium cine esophagography
B. Selenomethionine scanning
C. Thallium-Technitium Substraction Scanning
D. Inferior thyroid arteriography

**111. All of the following are causes of goitrous hypothyroidism except : Karnataka 1993**

A. Hashimoto's thyroiditis
B. Prolonged Iodine intake
C. Iodine deficiency
D. Secondary hypothroidism

**112. Papillary Carcinoma of thyroid is associated with following except : Karnataka 1993**

A. Psammoma Bodies
B. Papillary processes
C. Follicular pattern with papillary processes
D. Amyloid stroma

**113. Medullary carcinoma of thyroid is characterized by following except : AIIMS 1994**

A. Secretes calcitonin
B. Hereditary in nature
C. Amyloid stroma is seen
D. Hormone dependent

**114. In radical neck dissection on right side, the common complication is : AIIMS 1994**

A. Laryngeal oedema B. Flap necrosis
C. Thoracic duct injury D. Parotid salivary fistula

**115. A 20-years old male presents with enlarged lymph nodes on the right side of the neck. The glands are discrete, mobile, non-tender and vary from 1 to 3 cm diameter. Most are moderately firm in consistency, but some of the larger ones are soft and cystic. There is a hard one centimeter nodule in the isthmus of the thyroid gland. What is the most likely diagnosis : UPSC 1994**

A. Carcinoma of the thyroid gland
B. Tuberculous lymphadenitis
C. Hodgkins disease
D. Lymphosarcoma

**116. Untrue about ectodermal cleft is : AIIMS 1995**

A. Dorsal part of first cleft forms lining of ext. ear.
B. Cervical sinus is found between 2nd to 6th arches.
C. Ventral part of cleft is obliterated.
D. None of the above.

**117. Thyroid carcinoma with pulsating vescular skeletal metastasis is : AI 1995**

A. Papillary B. Anaplastic
C. Follicular D. Medullary

**118. Which is the least common in thyroid scan in case of follicular carcinoma : AI 1995**

A. Hot B. Warm
C. Cold D. Isothermic

**119. Medullary carcinoma thyroid is associated with : Kerala 1996**

A. Pheochromocytoma B. Pituitary carcinoma
C. Carcinoid syndrome D. Testicular tumour
E. Neuroblastoma

| Ans. | 103. A | 104. D | 105. A | 106. B | 107. A | 108. B | 109. B | 110. C | 111. B | 112. D |
|---|---|---|---|---|---|---|---|---|---|---|
| | 113. D | 114. C | 115. A | 116. D | 117. C | 118. D | 119. A | | | |

**120. Hurthle cells are seen in : AI 1995**
A. Hashimoto's thyroiditis
B. Hyperthyroidism
C. Medullary carcinoma of thyroid
D. Acute thyroiditis

**121. Following are true about actinomycosis except : AI 1995**
A. Cervicofacial is commonest form
B. Sulphur granules present
C. Can be caused by higher fungi and bacteria
D. Chronic infection and may require surgery

**122. Which is not true regarding carotid body tumour : PGI 1994**
A. Is radio resistant
B. Is a non-chromafin paraganglioma
C. May have massive bleeding
D. Surgical removal is treatment of choice

**123. Diagnostic feature of branchial cyst is : TN 1996**
A. Relation to sternomastoid
B. Brilliantly transilluminant
C. Cholesterol crystals in the aspirated fluid
D. Clear fluid aspirated

**124. Treatment of choice for de Quervain's thyroiditis is : Rohtak 1995, 96**
A. Corticosteroids B. Aspirin
C. TSH D. ACTH
E. T3, T4

**125. A patient with thyroid surgery in the morning develops hematoma in the operated side, most dangerous immediate complication is : AIIMS 1999**
A. Respiratory Obstruction
B. Recurrent Laryngeal Nerve injury
C. Dysphagia
D. Shock

**126. Thyrotoxicosis is due to : TN 1999**
A. Total thyroxin B. Free T3, T4
C. Total T3 D. Total T4

**127. Sudden pain in thyroid nodule indicates : UP 1999**
A. Necrosis B. Infarction
C. Haemorrhage D. Malignant change

**128. Respiratory distress after thyroid surgery can be due to following, except : Delhi 1992; AIIMS 2000**
A. Hematoma at local site
B. Laryngomalacia
C. Bilateral recurrent laryngeal nerve injury
D. Hypocalcemia

**129. The following are true regarding solitary nodule of Thyroid except one : Kerala 2000**
A. 20% are malignant.
B. More than 50% of cold nodules are malignant.
C. FNAC has become established as the investigation of choice.
D. More common in women.
E. The only indication for isotope scanning is combination of toxicity and nodularity.

**130. Kalloo, 45 years, presents with a swelling in the thyroid gland and a lymphnode in the neck. Aspiration of the node shows amyloid material. What is the management of choice for this patient : AIIMS 2000**
A. Hemithyroidectomy with neck dissection.
B. Total thyroidectomy, with neck dissection.
C. Total thyroidectomy with neck irradiation.
D. Hemithyroidectomy.

**131. Long standing case of multinodular goitre develops hoarseness and increase in size. Likely diagnosis is : AI 2001**
A. Follicular ca. B. Papillary ca.
C. Medullary ca. D. Anaplastic ca.

**132. A patient with B/L proptosis, heat intolerance and tolerance, unlikely diagnosis is : AI 2001**
A. Hashimoto's thyroiditis
B. Thyroid adenoma
C. Diffuse thyroid goitre
D. Reidel's thyroiditis

**133. Risk factors for thyroid carcinoma are following except : NIMHANS 2000**
A. Family H/o papillary Ca.
B. Family H/o medullary Ca.
C. Low dose irradiation
D. None of the above

**134. Occult thyroid malignancies are usually : DNB 2001**
A. Follicular B. Medullary
C. Papillary D. Anaplastic

**135. Which one of the following statements regarding medullary carcinoma of thyroid is correct : UPSC 2001**
A. Total thyroidectomy is curative.
B. It is TSH dependent.
C. Radioactive iodine is useful in the treatment.
D. Chemotherapy and total thyroidectomy are curative.

**136. After thyroidectomy, patient feels prostration, lethargy, tingling and tetany. Immediate relief is by : AI 2000**
A. Calcium gluconate B. PTH
C. Calcitonin D. Vit. D.

| Ans. | | | | | | | | | |
|---|---|---|---|---|---|---|---|---|---|
| 120. A | 121. C | 122. D | 123. C | 124. A | 125. A | 126. B | 127. C | 128. C | 129. B |
| 130. B | 131. A | 132. D | 133. A | 134. C | 135. A | 136. A | | | |

**137. Patient on same evening after thyroidectomy has swelling and difficulty in breathing. Next management is : AI 2001**

A. Open immediately B. Intubate orotracheally
C. Wait and watch D. Oxygen by mask

**138. Swelling of deep parotid gland presents as swelling in : DNB 2001**

A. The neck B. Floor of mouth
C. Temporal region D. None

**139. In a 50 years old male presenting with mobile hard non- tender nodule in thyroid, diagnosis can be established by : Delhi 2001**

A. Radioisotope scan B. X-ray soft tisue neck
C. FNAC D. Serum T3 and T4 levels

**140. Which malignancy would occur in prolonged multinodular goiter : AIIMS 2001**

A. Papillary carcinoma B. Follicular carcinoma
C. Anaplastic carcinoma D. Medullary carcinoma

**141. A patient with carcinoma of the tongue was found to have lymph nodes in the lower neck. The treatment of choice for the lymph nodes is : AIIMS 2001**

A. Radical neck dissection
B. Chemotherapy
C. Tele radiotherapy
D. Local excision

**142. Thyroidectomy was done for a patient. 2 hours post-operative, the patient developed difficulty in breathing and stridor. All the following are possible causes except: AIIMS 2001**

A. Tracheomalacia
B. Recurrent laryngeal nerve palsy
C. Hypocalcemia
D. Wound hematoma

**W.143. In a patient with parathyroid hyperplasia, surgery is planned. The amount of parathyroid to be removed is : AIIMS 2001**

A. All four glands
B. Enlarged gland to be removed
C. 4.5 parathyroids to be removed
D. Radical parathyroidectomy

**144. A 6 years old child complains of difficulty in swallowing and on examination there is a sublingual swelling, which is suspected to be Lingual thyroid. The Ist step in the management of this child would be : SGPGI 2002**

A. Tracheostomy and airway maintenance
B. Thyroid scan
C. Intubation
D. Explain to child that it require immediate surgery

**145. A 45 yearsold man presents with pisodic headache, palpitation and flushing. His sister died of a thyroid cancer. The most appropriate investigation is : AIIMS 2002**

A. 24 hours urine catecholamines
B. 24 hours urine 5-HIAA
C. Thyroid scan
D. Serum calcium, phosphorus and alkaline phosphatase.

**146. Parathyroid adenoma most commonly involves : AIIMS 2002**

A. Inferior glands
B. Superior glands
C. Substance of thyroid
D. Arises from ectopic parathyroid in mediastinum

**147. A patient presents with solid submandibular node, hard inconsistency. Clinical examination was not fruitful. The next appropriate investigation is : AIIMS 2002**

A. X-ray chest
B. Triple endoscopy
C. Oral staining with acetic acid
D. CT scan

**148. Thyroid storm is seen in all except : AI 2002**

A. Thyrotoxicosis
B. Surgery for thyroiditis
C. Surgery on normal thyroid
D. $I^{131}$ therapy in thyrotoxicosis

**149. A 75 years old woman underwent neck exploration for hyperthyroidism 5 years ago, and a parathyroid adenoma was excised. At the present time, she is recovering from a myocardial infarction 6 weeks ago, and she is in mild congestive heart failure. Her electrocardiogram shows a slow atrial fibrillation. Measurement of her serum calcium shows a level of 13.0 mg/dl and urine calcium is 300 mg/24 th. Studies suggest a small mass in the orotracheal position behind the right clavicle : AI 2002**

Appropriate management at this time is :

A. Observation and repeat calcium levels in two months.
B. Repeat neck exploration.
C. Treatment with technetium-99.
D. Ultrsound guided alcohol injection of the mass.

**150. In hyperthyroidism during pregnancy, which of the following is absolutely contraindicated : AI 2002**

A. Surgery B. Radioiodine ($I^{131}$)
C. Antithyroid drugs D. Iodine

| Ans. | | | | | | | | | |
|---|---|---|---|---|---|---|---|---|---|
| 137. A | 138. C | 139. C | 140. B | 141. A | 142. A | 143. A,C | 144. B | 145. B | 146. A |
| 147. B | 148. D | 149. D | 150. B | | | | | | |

**151. A 26 years woman presents with a palpable thyroid nodule, and needle biopsy demonstrates amyloid in the stroma of the lesion. A cervical lymph node is palpable on the same side as the lesion. The preferred treatment should be : AI 2002**

A. Removal of the involved node, the isthmus, and the enlarged lymph node.
B. Removal of the involved lobe, the isthmus, a portion of the opposite lobe, and the enlarged lymph node.
C. Total thyroidectomy and modified neck dissection on the side of the enlarged lymph node.
D. Total thyroidectomy and irradiation of the cervical lymph nodes.

**152. Main problem associated with carotid body tumor operation is : Maharashtra 2000**

A. The tumor blends with bifurcation of carotid artery
B. The tumor blends with jugular vein
C. Recurrence
D. Shock

**153. Ca++ levels are normal in : CMC 2001**

A. 1° (primary) hyperparathyroidism
B. 2° (secondary) hyperparathyroidism
C. Tertiary hyperparathyroidism
D. None

**154. Common position of thyroglossal cyst is : CMC 2001**

A. Suprahyoid B. Subhyoid
C. Sublingual D. Lower neck

**155. Podophyllum resin is indicated in the treatment of : CMC 2001, 2003**

A. Psoriasis
B. Pemphigus
C. Condyloma acuminata
D. Condylomata lata

**156. What is the most appropriate operation for a solitary nodule in one lobe of the thyroid : AI 2003**

A. Lobectomy
B. Hemithyroidectomy
C. Nodule removal
D. Partial lobectomy with 1 cm margin around the nodule

**157. The most suitable isotope of iodine for treating hyperthyroidism is : AI 2003**

A. 1-123 B. 1-125
C. 1-131 D. 1-132

**158. In a patient with thyroid surgery the block to be given is at the : MAHE 2003**

A. Stellate ganglion
B. Upper cervical ganglion
C. Dorsal sympathetic ganglia
D. Any of the above

**159. Thoracic extension of cervical goitre is usually approached through: AI 2004**

A. Neck
B. Chest
C. Combined cervico-thoracic route
D. Thoracoscopic

**160. In which of the following is medullary thyroid cancer in most aggresive form : Karnataka 2005**

A MEN Type-I B. MEN Type-II a
C. MEN Type-II b D. Sporadic cases

**161. On USG of thyroid which is not sign of malignancy : AI 2009**

A. Hypoechogenicity B. Hyperechogenicity
C. Microcalcification D. Colloids

**162. Thoracic outlet syndrome is diagnosed by : AI 2009**

A. Clicical examinations
B. X-ray
C. Electromyography
D. CT scan

**163. Differance between follicular adenoma and carcinome : AI 2009**

A. Hurthle cell B. Increased mitosis
C. Vascular invasion D. None

**164. A 21 years old woman has 3 cm node in the lower deep cervical chain on the left. The biopsy is interpreted as revealing normal thyroid tissues in a lymph node. The most likely diagnosis is : Delhi 2009**

A. Subacute thyroids B. Metastatic carcinoma
C. Hashimato's disease D. Lateral aberrant thyroid

| Ans. | | | | | | | | | |
|---|---|---|---|---|---|---|---|---|---|
| 151. C | 152. A | 153. B | 154. B | 155. C | 156. A | 157. C | 158. B | 159. A | 160. C |
| 161. A | 162. C | 163. C | 164. B | | | | | | |

# EXPLANATIONS OF NECK

1. Ans.— A. Infarction of the sternomastoid at birth.
2. Ans.— C. Renal stones
3. Ans.— B. Lower pole

   Deviation of trachea on X-ray is an important sign.
4. Ans.— B. Thyroglossal cyst
5. Ans.— D. Dobois abscess
6. Ans.— D. Decreased sweating
7. Ans.— B. Chief cell adenoma
8. Ans.— A. Soft diffuse enlargement of thyroid
9. Ans.— C. To overcome pressure on trachea or oesophagus.
10. Ans.— E. Better prognosis than papillary carcinoma.
11. Ans.— B. Hypothyroidism

    Thyroxine hormone therapy is given life long.
12. Ans.— A. Raynaud's disease
13. Ans.— D. Heat intolerance
14. Ans.— B. Thyroxine
15. Ans.— C. 3rd and 4th
16. Ans.— D. Brachycephalic head
17. Ans.— A. Cystic hygroma

    The gland develops from the third pharyngeal pouch.
26. Ans.— D. An IgG immunoglobulin
27. Ans.— A. Papillary carcinoma

    Papillary Ca.Thyroid gives best prognosis since their spread to lymph nodes is very rare.
28. Ans.— A. Drug therapy is prolonged
29. Ans.— B. A metastasis in a cervical lymph node from an occult thyroid carcinoma.
30. Ans.— C. Its attachment with hyoid
31. Ans.— A. Hyperparathyroidism

    Hyperparathyroidism affects the skeletons, marked osteoclastic activities are seen and resorbed bone is replaced with fibrous tissue called as Brown tumor.
32. Ans.— A. Low serum alkaline phosphatase
33. Ans.— D. Lateral aberrent thyroid
34. Ans.— A. Chemotherapy
35. Ans.— D. Salt & pepper appearance of skull
36. Ans.— C. Hypercalcemia
37. Ans.— D. Increased uptake by bone

    Persistent post-operative hypocalcemia may occur in upto 10% patients and recurrent laryngeal nerve is seen in about 6%.
38. Ans.— A. Multi-nodular goitre
39. Ans.— B. Ca. Nasopharyx
40. Ans.— B. Hemithyroidectomy
41. Ans.— D. Medullary
42. Ans.— B. Interfollicular C-cells
43. Ans.— B. Thyroglossal cyst
44. Ans.— B. Medullary carcinoma

    These are tumors of parafollicular (C-cells) derived from neural cyst. Calcitonin is a valuable tumor marker; associated with pheochromocytoma and hyper-parathyroidism (MEN IIa).
45. Ans.— B. Detect cold nodules
46. Ans.— B. C.T. scan
47. Ans.— A. Papillary carcinoma
48. Ans.— D. Parenchymatous goitre
49. Ans.— B. Adenoma
50. Ans.— B. 40-50% malignant nodules are cold in isotopes scanning.
51. Ans.— A. Transitional
52. Ans.— C. Carcinoma
53. Ans.— A. Renal stones disappear
54. Ans.— B. The solitary toxic nodule may be treated

by radio cobalt.

55. Ans.— D. Is always lined by squamous epithelium.

56. Ans.— A. It is a type of cavernous haemangioma.

It is a capillary haemangioma. It manifests in infancy and childhood.

57. Ans.— B. Carotid body tumour

58. Ans.— A. Propranolol

59. Ans.— A. Autonomy in functioning

60. Ans.— B. Soon after birth

61. Ans.— B. It responds very well to radiotherapy.

62. Ans.— D. All of the above

63. Ans.— C. To remove pressure on trachea and oesophagus.

64. Ans.— B. Common in mediastinum

It protrudes from beneath the anterior border of upper third of the sternomastoid as a fluctuant swelling which may transilluminate. It develops from vestigeal remnants of second branchial cleft, lined by squamous epithelium, contents are either clear fluid or like tooth paste.

65. Ans.— E. All of the above

66. Ans.— B. Thyroglossal fistula

67. Ans.— D. All of the above

68. Ans.— D. Inj. Vitamin-C

69. Ans.— B. As far as possible

70. Ans.— A. Surgical excision

71. Ans.— D. Phrenic nerves

72. Ans.— D. Non-dependent aspiration

73. Ans.— C. Phrenic nerves

74. Ans.— B. Surgery in neck area

75. Ans.— C. ↑ T3, Normal T4 and TSH

76. Ans.— A. Diffuse goitre

77. Ans.— D. External radiation

78. Ans.— B. It is blended with the carotid artery

It is also called chemodectomy or 'Potato' tumor. It is situated at bifurcation of carotid artery, is most important moiety of the chemoreceptor system. It is sensitives to changes in blood pH and temperature. It is unilateral in middle life and arteriography is useful. Special dangers of excision are haemorrhage and the way it is blended with carotid bifurcation.

79. Ans.— D. Can be treated by antithyroid drugs

80. Ans.— A. Trousseau

81. Ans.— A. Diffuse goitre

82. Ans.— A. Hepatoma

83. Ans.— D. Kocher-Debre Semelaigne syndrome

84. Ans.— D. A & B

85. Ans.— B. Thyroxine

Antithyroid drugs or radioactive iodine should be given before surgery.

86. Ans.— C. Adenoma

87. Ans.— D. Pressure on great vessels

88. Ans.— A. Inadequate Preoperative treatment

89. Ans.— A. Cystic hygroma

90. Ans.— A. Follicular

91. Ans.— D. Excised by single transverse incision

92. Ans.— B. Diverticulum

93. Ans.— A. Killian's dehiscence

94. Ans.— B. Parathyroid neoplasm

They are seen in Kidney, Pancreas, salivary glands and prostate.

95. Ans.— B. Branchial Cyst

96. Ans.— A. Complete

97. Ans.— A. Papillary carcinoma thyroid

98. Ans.— B. Near total thyroidectomy

99. Ans.— B. Junction of upper and middle third of sternocleido mastoid.

100. Ans.— B. Radical neck resection

101. Ans.— C. Radio iodine

102. Ans.— B. Follicular adenoma

103. Ans.— A. Sheehan's syndrome

104. Ans.— D. Bony metastasis in early stage

Spread of papillary Ca thyroid to lymph nodes is common. But blood born metastasis are rare unless the tumors are extrathyroidal.

105. Ans.— A. Nephrotic syndrome

106. Ans.— B. Large honeyeombed colloid filled areas

107. Ans.— A. Tuberculous infection of deep cervical lymph nodes.

108. Ans.— B. Hyperparathyroidism

109. Ans.— B. Acute Thyroiditis

110. Ans.— C. Thallium-Technitium Substraction Scanning.

111. Ans.— B. Prolonged Iodine intake

112. Ans.— D. Amyloid stroma

113. Ans.— D. Hormone dependent

114. Ans.— C. Thoracic duct injury

115. Ans.— A. Carcinoma of the thyroid gland

116. Ans. D. None of the above

117. Ans.— C. Follicular

It is also most common. Thyroidectomy with resection of extrathyroid tumors done.

118. Ans.— D. Isothermic

A hot nodule takes up isotop whereas cold nodule does not.

119. Ans.— A. Pheochromocytoma

120. Ans.— A. Hashimoto's thyroiditis

121. Ans.— C. Can be caused by higher fungi and bacteria.

Penicillin is treatment of choice.

122. Ans.— D. Surgical removal is treatment of choice

123. Ans.— C. Cholesterol crystals in the aspirated fluid.

124. Ans.— A. Corticosteroids

125. Ans.— A. Respiratory Obstruction

126. Ans.— B. Free T3, T4

127. Ans.— C. Haemorrhage

128. Ans.— C. Bilateral recurrent laryngeal nerve injury.

129. Ans.— B. More than 50% of cold nodules are malignant.

130. Ans.— B. Total thyroidectomy, with neck dissection

131. Ans.— A. Follicular ca.

Blood borne metastasis are almost twice common than papillary cycle. Recurrent laryngeal nerve palsy can cause hoarseness.

132. Ans.— D. Reidel's thyroiditis

It is very rare accounting for 0.5% of goiter thyroid tissue is replaced by cellular fibrous tissue diagnosed by biopsy.

133. Ans.— A. Family H/o papillary Ca.

134. Ans.— C. Papillary

135. Ans.— A. Total thyroidectomy is curative.

136. Ans.— A. Calcium gluconate

Tetany due to parathyroid removal is a complication occurring in 0.5% and 2-5 days after operation.

137. Ans.— A. Open immediately

The wound is open immediately to relieve the tension before taking the patient to theatre to evacuate the haematoma.

138. Ans.— C. Temporal region

139. Ans.— C. FNAC

140. Ans.— B. Follicular carcinoma

141. Ans.— A. Radical neck dissection

142. Ans.— A. Tracheomalacia

W143. Ans.— A. All four glands

C. 4.5 parathyroids to be removed

144. Ans.— B. Thyroid scan

145. Ans.— B. 24 hours urine 5-HIAA

146. Ans.— A. Inferior glands

147. Ans.— B. Triple endoscopy

148. Ans.— D. $I^{131}$ therapy in thyrotoxicosis

Pre-operative codine betablockers and carbimazole are used for preoperative preparation.

149. Ans.— D. Ultrsound guided alcohol injection of the mass.

Parathyroid adenoma (single gland disease) constitutes 90% of cases of primary hyperparathyroidism.

150. Ans.— B. Radioiodine ($I^{131}$)

Radioiodine is teratogenic.

151. Ans.— C. Total thyroidectomy and modified neck dissection on the side of the enlarged lymph node.

The findings are suggestive of medullary Ca thyroid. High levels of serum calcitonin (>0.08 ng/ml) are also seen.

152. Ans.— A. The tumor blends with bifurcation of carotid artery.

153. Ans.— B. 2° (secondary) hyperparathyroidism

**154. Ans.— B. Subhyoid**

**155. Ans.— C. Condyloma acuminata.**

**156. Ans.— A. Lobectomy**

**Solitary Thyroid nodule :**

* **MC cause-Adenoma thyroid**
* **Investigation - First - FNAC, Best - Trucut biopsy**

| **Condition** | **Surgery of choice** |
|---|---|
| **Thyrotoxicosis** | **Sub total thyroidectomy** |
| **Solitary thyroid swelling** | **Lobectomy, Hemithyroidectomy** |
| **Diffuse carcinoma** | **Near total/total thyroidectomy** |

* **"Thyroid lobectomy is usually recommended for solitary Thyroid nodule".**

**157. Ans.— C. 1-131**

**Most appropriate management of Hyper-Thyroidism -**

* **Iodine 131 for 8-12 weeks (I/C are Age > 40, Recurrent hyperthyroidism, Poor risk patients.**
* **Than surgical management is done by Sub-total thyroidectomy, (leaving 4-8 grams of tissue on each side).**

**158. Ans.— B. Upper cervical ganglion**

**159. Ans.— A. Neck**

**Substernal (Retrosternal) Goiter**

- **It is an unusual presentation of intra-thoracic component of an enlarged thyroid, usually as a result of multi-nodular goiter.**
- **Mostly are labelled secondary because they are extensions of multinodular goiters.**
- **Most substernal goiters can be approached through a cervical incision (neck incision).**

**160. Ans.— C. MEN Type-II b**

**161. Ans.— D. Colloids**

**Echogenicity : The incidence of malignancy is 4% when a solid thyroid nodule is hyperechoic. If the lesion is hypoechoic, the incidence of malignancy rises to 26%.**

***Margins :*** **A malignant thyroid nodule tends to have ill-defined margins on ultrasound.**

***Calcification :*** **Fine punctate calcification due to calcified psammoma bodies within the nodule is seen in pappillary carcinoma in 25-40% of cases. If used as the sole predictive sign of malignancy.**

***Comet tail sign :*** **The presence of a cornet tail sign in a thyroid nodule indicates the presence of *colloid* within a benign colloid nodule and is strong predictor of benignity.**

***Colour flow patterns :*** **In general there are three patterns of vascular distribution within a thyroid nodule :**

* **Type I - Complete absence of flow signal within the nodule**
* **Type II - Exclusive perinodular flow signals**
* **Type III : Intranodular flow with multiple vascular poles chaotically arranged, with or without significant perinodular vessels.**

**162. Ans.— A. Clinical examination**

***Diagnosis***

* **There are not specific diagnostic tests for thoracic outlet syndromes.**
* **The diagnosis is made by rulling out other diseases and by observing the patient.**
* **Two nonspecific tests that can suggest the presence of thoracic outlet syndrome are the Adson test and the Allen test.**

**163. Ans.— C. Vascular invasion**

**FNAC—Investigation of choice in discrete thyroid swellings. It cannot distinguish between a follicular adenoma and carcinoma (capsular and vascular invasion)**

**164. Ans.— B. Metastatic carcinoma**

**Normal thyroid tissue found laterally separate from thyroid tissue must be considered and treated as a metastasis in a cervical LN from an ocult papillary thyroid carcinoma.**

# 6

# IMPORTANT TEXT OF BREAST

## DIFFERENTIAL DIAGNOSIS OF LUMP IN BREAST

1. Carcinoma
2. Fibroadenosis 95%
3. Fibroadenoma

**Less commonly**

1. Fat necrosis
2. Cysts (chronic abscess—retention cyst)
3. Lipoma
4. Cystic Hygroma

**Differential diagnosis of discharge**

1. Blood stained
   (i) Intraductal papilloma/carcinoma
   (ii) Duct ectasia
   (iii) Fibroadenosis with cysts
2. Serous
   Pregnancy
3. Brown-green
   Fibroadenosis
4. Milky
   (i) Following lactation
   (ii) Galactocele
5. Purulent
   Abscess

**Differential diagnosis of pain in breast**

1. Abscess
2. Fibroadenosis
3. Carcinoma
4. Chondritis

## SYMPTOMS & SIGN OF BREAST DISEASE

**Nipple discharge :**

* *Milky*
  * Pregnancy
  * Hyperprolactenaemia
* *Clear*
  * Physiological
* *Clear serous*
  * Duct papilloma (+ontest for occult blood)
  * Mammary dysplasia
* *Green*
  * Perimenopausal
  * Duct ectasia
* *Blood-stained*
  * Intraduct papiloma (common)
  * Carcinoma
  * Duct ectasia
* *Varying with menstrual cycle*
  * Premenstrual
  * Fibroadenosis
* *Independent of menstrual cycle*
  * Carcinoma
  * Fibroadenosis
  * Infection

**Lump in the Breast**

*Hard lump :*

* Discrete lump with a smooth surface and solid—*Fibroadenoma.*
* Discrete lump with a smooth surface and fluctuant—*Fibroadenotic cyst.*

# MCQ's OF BREAST

## What is important in Breast

Lymphatic drainage, Secretions (D/D), Abscess, Benign tumor, Carcinoma breast, Types of Mastectomy

1. **In breast cancer, stage T.N.M. indicates : AIIMS 1984**
   A. Tumour more than 2 cm diameter with axillary nodes.
   B. Tumour <2 cm, no nodes, no metastasis.
   C. Tumour fixed to chest wall, no axillary nodes, no metastasis.
   D. Fixed to pectoralis, no axillary nodes.
2. **Danazol is useful in the treatment of : UPSC 1984**
   A. Fibroadenoma B. Fibroadenosis
   C. Plasma-cell mastitis D. Paget's disease
3. **Mastitis of infants stops secretion by ——— weeks. AMU 1988**
   A. First B. Second
   C. Third D. Never unless treated
4. **Amazia (congenital absence of breast) may sometimes be associated with the absence of a portion of : AMU 1990**
   A. Pectoralis major B. Pectoralis minor
   C. Teres major D. Latissimus dorsi
5. **The most frequent site of accessory breasts is : AMU 1987; PGI 1995**
   A. Groin B. Thigh
   C. Axilla D. Buttock
6. **Prognosis in cancer of the breast is most favourable in : AIIMS 1986**
   A. Upper-outer quadrant B. Lower-outer quadrant
   C. Upper-inner quadrant D. Lower-inner quadrant
7. **In Paget's disease nipple secretions is mainly : AMC 1983**
   A. Mucous material B. Water
   C. Blood D. All of the above
8. **Paget's disease of nipple is treated by : AI 1995**
   A. Radiotherapy
   B. Biopsy and simple mastectomy
   C. Radical mastectomy
   D. Chemotherapy
9. **Most common regime used in Ca. breast : PGI 1996**
   A. CMF B. CAV
   C. CHOP D. PEB
10. **Non-malignant conditions of the breast include following except : PGI 1984**
    A. Cystosarcoma phylloides
    B. Duct ectasia
    C. Giant fibroadenoma
    D. Paget's disease of the nipple
11. **Detection of lipoma like swelling in breast is indicative of : AIIMS 1985**
    A. Presence of true lipoma
    B. Fibroadenosis
    C. Underlying cancer
    D. A benign condition
    E. None of the above
12. **Lymphnode which is first to be involved in carcinoma breast : AIIMS 1989, 93, 95; AI 1998**
    A. Pectoral group B. Internal mammary
    C. Apical D. Central
    E. Supra-clavicular
13. **Massive swellings of the breast include the following, except : Kerala 1988, 94**
    A. Cystosarcoma phylloides
    B. Atrophic scirrhous carcinoma
    C. Diffuse hypertrophy
    D. Giant fibroadenoma
14. **The following are clinical signs supporting an early diagnosis of carcinoma of the breast : Kerala 1989**
    A. A prickling sensation in a breast lump
    B. Peau d' Orange
    C. Brawny arm
    D. Cancer en Cruisse

| Ans. | 1. B | 2. B | 3. C | 4. A | 5. C | 6. A | 7. B | 8. B | 9. A | 10. D |
|---|---|---|---|---|---|---|---|---|---|---|
| | 11. D | 12. A | 13. B | 14. A | | | | | | |

**15. Regarding follow-up of patients with carcinoma of the breast, except : DNB 1989**

A. It is unnecessary for a surgeon to follow-up his patients. with carcinoma of the breast after operation. It is done by other specialist.
B. A rectal examination may be necessary.
C. The liver should be examined
D. X-ray of the chest is a routine follow-up examination.

**16. In TNM classification, stage-II carcinoma breast is : AIIMS 1984, 85**

A. T2N2M0 B. T2N1M0
C. T3N1M0 D. T1N0M0

**17. Breast development during intrauterine life begins at : AIIMS 1984, 85**

A. 6 weeks B. 8 weeks
C. 10 weeks D. 12 weeks

**18. Best position for self-palpation of breast is : AIIMS 1987**

A. Lying down pillow under shoulder
B. Standing with Arms raised
C. 45° reclining
D. Any of the above

**19. Carcinoma breast is common in : AIIMS 1986, 90; Delhi 1996**

A. Cystic disease B. Duct ectasia
C. Epithelial hyperplasia D. Sclerosing adenosis

**20. In radical mastectomy, the structure to be ligated is : PGI 1986; AIIMS 1986**

A. Axillary vein B. Axillary artery
C. Innominate vein D. Phrenic nerve

**21. "Breast mouse" is found in cases of : UPSC 1987**

A. Bite by a mouse B. Hard fibroadenoma
C. Soft fibroadenoma D. Papillary cystadenoma
E. Fibroadenosis

**22. The early sign suggestive of carcinoma breast is : AMC 1984**

A. Peau d'orange
B. Brawny arm
C. Breast lump with pricking sensation
D. Hyperpyrexia

**23. Breast abscess should always be treated by : UPSC 1989**

A. Antibiotics B. Incision and drainage
C. Excision D. Aspiration

**24. A milk fistula : AIIMS 1983**

A. Occurs in lactating woman
B. Is related to recurrent abscesses of areolar region
C. Is related to carcinoma breast
D. Is a milk born disease

**25. Which of the following are indicative of inoperability in patients with breast cancer except : PGI 1986**

A. Inflammatory cancer
B. Satellite skin nodules
C. Parasternal nodules
D. Involved axillary lymphnodes

**26. Duct ectasia of the breast : AIIMS 1983**

A. Occurs in young multipara
B. Presents with a worm like swelling extending radially from the nipple
C. Is a precursor of carcinoma breast
D. None of the above

**27. Which of the following represents Mondor's disease : UPSC 1984**

A. Chronic mastitis
B. Fibro-adenoma breast
C. Fat necrosis
D. Thrombophlebitis of breast veins

**28. Radical mastectomy is contraindicated in : AIIMS 1986; BHU 1986**

A. Peau d'orange
B. Breast lesion with appearance of shotty axillary lymphnodes
C. Blood stained nipple discharge
D. Acute inflammatory reaction

**29. Which of the following is least frequent site for breast metastasis: DNB 1986**

A. Lung B. Liver
C. Bone D. Contralateral breast

**30. A cracked nipple is : UPSC 1984**

A. A retention cyst
B. Paget's disease of breast
C. Caused by syphilis
D. Precursor of breast abscess

**31. A 50-years old female presents with a fungating carcinoma of the breast, 8 cm in diameter. Mobile 1 cm diameter nodes are palpable in the ipsilateral axilla. Chest X-ray and bone scan are normal. The treatment of choice for her would be : CSE 1995**

A. Simple mastectomy with axillary clearance and post-operative chemotherapy.
B. Simple mastectomy with axillary node sampling and post-operative radiotherapy; chemotherapy if nodes are positive.
C. Radiotherapy to breast and chemotherapy.
D. Radical mastectomy and chemotherapy.

**Ans.** 15. A 16. B 17. D 18. C 19. C 20. B 21. B 22. C 23. B 24. B
25. D 26. B 27. D 28. D 29. D 30. D 31. B

32. **Of the operations listed, the interests of a patient with a stage-III carcinoma of the breast are best served by : AMU 1986**
A. A radical mastectomy
B. A super-radical mastectomy
C. Simple mastectomy
D. Lumpectomy

33. **A 50-years old woman was operated for left radical mastectomy. During physical examination she was asked to face a wall and push hard against it with both hands outstretched. It was noticed that inferior angle and medial border of the left Scapula projected medially. Which nerve was injured during the left mastectomy : CSE 1996**
A. Nerve to deltoid
B. Nerve to serratus anterior
C. Nerve to trapezius
D. Nerve to lattismus dorsi

34. **A 40-years old female presents with a 9-months history of a swelling in the outer quadrant of the breast. It is 3 cm diameter and is not attached to the skin or deep fascia. Lymph nodes are enlarged and mobile in the axilla. There are no supraclavicular lymph nodes. Chest X-ray is normal. Biopsy showed scirrhous carcinoma. The correct course of treatment in this case would be : CSE 1997**
A. Simple mastectomy and radiotherapy
B. Radical mastectomy
C. Radical mastectomy and radiotherapy
D. Radiotherapy

35. **The diagnosis of breast carcinoma is established by local excision of the palpable lump, and residual or multicentric cancer may be demonstrated in —— of mastectomy specimens. AMC 1987**
A. 10% B. 20%
C. 30% D. 60%

36. **A 40-years old lady underwent radical mastectomy for a 2 cm carcinoma of the breast. Histopathology of axillary nodes removed did not show any secondaries. The most appropriate future line of management would be : UPSC 1996**
A. Periodic follow-up for any recurrence and treatment thereof
B. Radiotherapy
C. Chemotherapy
D. Hormone therapy

37. **Secondary deposits from carcinoma breast are commonest in : AIIMS 1986; AI 1989**
A. Lung B. Liver
C. Brain D. Bone

38. **Risk factor for carcinoma breast is : AI 1989**
A. Fibroadenoma on the side
B. Sister dead from cancer breast
C. Jewish origin
D. All of the above

39. **Fibroadenosis is a : AIIMS 1983; AMC 1985, 87; Delhi 1987**
A. Benign condition
B. Premalignant
C. Sarcoma
D. Spontaneously remitting lesion

40. **Greenish discharge from the nipple is suggestive of : UPSC 1985; AIIMS 1998**
A. Carcinoma B. Duct papilloma
C. Duct carcinoma D. Fibroadenosis

41. **Treatment of choice in duct papilloma is : AI 1996**
A. Radiotherapy B. Microdochectomy
C. Chemotherapy D. No treatment

42. **Most common type of carcinoma breast is : PGI 1984, 85; AIIMS 1993**
A. Paget's B. Lobular
C. Comedo D. Ductal

43. **Paget's disease of the breast has all of the following, except : Karnataka 1989**
A. Nipple scaling
B. Sanguinous nipple discharge
C. Constitutes 10% of all breast carcinomas
D. Arises from the ductal tissue above the nipple

44. **Reconstruction of the breast following total mastectomy for cancer is done ideally by using : AIIMS 1984, 86**
A. Distant tube pedicle
B. Opposite breast
C. Trapezius myocutaneous flap
D. Latissmus dorsi myocutaneous flap

45. **True about Gynaecomastia is following except : AIIMS 1993**
A. Usually unilateral in young males.
B. Bilateral cases are due to manifestation of endocrinopathy.
C. Arises from duct with fibrosis, Acini not involved.
D. May be seen in Addison's disease.

**Ans.** 32. B 33. B 34. A 35. D 36. A 37. D 38. B 39. A 40. D 41. B
42. D 43. C 44. D 45. A

**46. Adrenelectomy in carcinoma breast is indicated when the following is involved : Delhi 1989**
A. Liver B. Lung
C. Bone D. Lymphnode

**47. In Axillary tail carcinoma, treatment is : Delhi 1989**
A. Simple mastectomy B. Radical mastectomy
C. Extended mastectomy D. Chemotherapy

**48. In carcinoma breast with axillary lymph node involvement and partial mastectomy done in the past, next treatment is : Delhi 1987, 88**
A. Radiotherapy B. Chemotherapy
C. Oophrectomy D. Hypophysectomy

**49. Commonest site of carcinoma breast is : Delhi 1987**
A. Upper and outer quadrant
B. Upper and medial quadrant
C. Lower and medial quadrant
D. Lower and lateral quadrant

**50. Breast abscess occurs in patients with : JIPMER 1997**
A. Cracked fissured nipple
B. Duct obstruction
C. Mammary duct ectasia
D. Nipple retraction

**51. Paget's disease of the breast is : UPSC 1994**
i. A premalignant condition
ii. A disease primarily involving the nipple
iii. Treated by simple mastectomy
**Of these statements :**
A. (i), (ii) and (iii) are correct
B. (i) and (ii) are correct
C. (ii) and (iii) are correct
D. (i) and (iii) are correct

**52. Chemotherapy in carcinoma breast is particularly useful in one of the following : AMU 1988**
A. Local lesion (Primary)
B. Bony secondaries
C. Lymph node involvement
D. Visceral spread

**53. One of these has a greater prognostic value in carcinoma breast : AMU 1988; AIIMS 1996**
A. Size of the tumour
B. Age of the patient
C. Presence of the pain
D. Involvement of lymph nodes

**54. Blood stained discharge from the nipple is typical of : AI 1988; AMU 1990, 94**
A. Paget's disease of the nipple
B. Intra-ductal papilloma
C. Fibroadenosis
D. Filarial mastitits

**55. Skin retraction over the breast is least likely in : AP 1989**
A. Fat necrosis B. Paget's disease
C. Carcinoma D. Fibroadenosis

**56. Retromammary abscess is due to : Kerala 1988**
A. Tuberculosis of rib B. Empyema necesitatis
C. Infected haematoma D. All of the above

**57. The treatment of fibroadenoma of the breast is : AIIMS 1984**
A. Simple mastectomy B. Local excision
C. Observation D. Radiotherapy

**58. Which is the incorrect statement about the lymphatic system draining the breast : AIIMS 1985**
A. There is free communication between the subclavicular and supraclavicular lymph nodes.
B. The lymph nodes along the internal mammary chain are involved in about half the cases in which the axillary nodes are implicated by carcinoma.
C. The thoracic chain of lymph nodes along the internal mammary vessels.
D. Some lymph nodes lie between the greater and lesser pectoral muscles.

**59. A breast lump is safe to leave alone after aspiration if : AMU 1987**
A. It is a cyst which does not subsequently refill.
B. It is solid and not cystic.
C. There is minimal blood stain in the aspirate.
D. Cytology reveals cells with hyperchromatic nuclei.

**60. Which of the following rule out radical mastectomy for breast cancer : UPSC 1984**
A. Enlarged and fixed axillary nodes
B. Fixation of lesion to chest wall
C. Proven distant metastasis
D. Skin ulceration
E. All of the above

**61. Nipples may be constructed by using skin from : Rohtak 1986**
A. Labia minora B. Groin or medial thigh
C. Buttock D. Any of the above

| Ans. | | | | | | | | | |
|---|---|---|---|---|---|---|---|---|---|
| 46. C | 47. B | 48. A | 49. A | 50. B | 51. C | 52. D | 53. D | 54. B | 55. D |
| 56. D | 57. B | 58. C | 59. A | 60. E | 61. D | | | | |

**62. The reconstruction of breast should not be carried out earlier than —— months after the mastectomy (to permit scars and tissue to soften). PGI 1984**

A. 1 to 3 B. 3 to 6
C. 6 to 12 D. 12 to 18

**63. Acute mastitis most commonly occurs early in : AMU 1985; AIIMS 1985; UPSC 1986; JIPMER 1988**

A. Pregnancy B. Menopause
C. Puberty D. Lactation

**64. Which of the following are indications for breast biopsy following aspiration of cyst : AIIMS 1984**

A. Aspiration of solid tumour.
B. Presence of a residual mass after aspiration.
C. Aspiration of serosanguinous or grossly bloody fluid.
D. Abnormal cytologic finding in fluid.
E. All of the above

**65. The least effective palliative treatment for advanced carcinoma of the male breast is : AIIMS 1985**

A. Orchiectomy B. Hormone therapy
C. Adrenalectomy D. Hypophysectomy
E. Cytotoxic agents

**66. Tumours of aberrant breast tissue are rare, in which of the following may be an aberrant carcinoma present most frequently : UPSC 1986**

A. Axilla B. Infraclavicular region
C. Sternal area D. Epigastrium
E. Close to xiphistrium

**67. Prognosis in male breast Ca depends on : AIIMS 1995**

A. Duration of disease B. Ulceration of nipple
C. Nipple discharge D. L.N. Status

**68. A false negative rate of 11% exists for mammography which of the following causes is most frequently listed : AMU 1986**

A. Dense breasts B. Small lesions
C. Faulty technique D. Recent aspiration

**69. Which of the following may not be considered "minimal" breast cancer : AIIMS 1986**

A. Duct cancer less 1 cm in outer quadrants
B. Lobular carcinoma in situ
C. Duct carcinoma less than 1 cm in inner quadrants
D. Colloid carcinoma
E. Early "Paget's disease"

**70. Which of the following is true of cystosarcoma phylloides : UPSC 1988; JIPMER 1992**

A. Small tumour B. Locally invasive
C. Highly malignant D. Early metastasis

**71. Peau d'orange in carcinoma breast is due to : AI 1988; DNB 1989; JIPMER 1992**

A. Lymphatic blockage
B. Invasion of ligament of Cooper
C. Sweat gland blockage
D. Lactiferous duct invasion

**72. Carcinoma breast which is most often bilateral is : AIIMS 1986, 92, 96, 97; AI 1989**

A. Medullary carcinoma
B. Lobular carcinoma
C. Ductal adenocarcinoma
D. Paget's disease

**73. In the treatment of breast cancer, Tamoxifen is used in : AIIMS 1992; PGI 1996**

A. Pre-menopausal woman
B. Estrogen receptor positive tumor
C. Presence of lymph nodes
D. Presence of bone metastasis

**74. Treatment of choice in cystosarcoma phylloides is : PGI 1993**

A. Simple mastectomy
B. Modified Radical Mastectomy
C. Radical mastectomy
D. Lumpectomy

**75. Hypercalcemia in breast cancer is most often due to : JIPMER 1993**

A. Tumor necrosis B. Ectopic parathormone
C. Bone Secondaries D. Chest wall invasion

**76. The most common organism found in breast abscess is : DNB 1990**

A. Streptococcus
B. Bacteriodes
C. Staphylococcus aureus
D. No growth i.e. sterile abscess

**77. Commonest cause of bleeding from nipple is : Delhi 1993; Kerala 1996**

A. Scirrhous carcinoma B. Fibrocystic disease
C. Duct papilloma D. Paget's disease

**78. Which carcinoma breast is not invasive : Delhi 1993**

A. Comedo carcinoma B. Scirrhous carcinoma
C. Lobular carcinoma D. Paget's disease

**79. The most favourable prognosis in breast carcinoma is associated with : Rohtak 1986, 89**

A. Medullary carcinoma
B. Scirrhous carcinoma
C. Atrophic scirrhous carcinoma
D. Duct carcinoma
E. Invasive lobular carcinoma

**Ans.** 62. C 63. D 64. E 65. B 66. A 67. A 68. A 69. C 70. B 71. A
72. B 73. B 74. A 75. C 76. C 77. C 78. A 79. A

**80. Cystosarcoma phylloides is : PGI 1994**

A. A type of carcinoma
B. A type of sarcoma
C. Fibroadenoma of breast
D. None of the above

**81. Patey's modification of radical mastectomy involves removal of following except : PGI 1994**

A. Pectoralis minor muscle and its covering fascia.
B. Axillary vein.
C. The skin surrounding the carcinomatous zone.
D. Pectoralis major muscle with fascia.

**82. Fibrocystic disease is characterized by following except : PGI 1983**

A. Precancerous
B. Bilateral
C. Treatment is complete exision
D. Incidence increases after menopause
E. Benign

**83. A 50-years old post-menopausal woman has undergone modified radical mastectomy for a 4 cm sized T2 cancer breast. Examination of the axillary lymphnodes by the pathologist does not show any metastatic disease. Post-operative management of this patient would be : CSE 1998**

A. Radiotherapy
B. Chemotherapy
C. Tamoxifen
D. Close monitoring and follow-up

**84. In inflammatory Ca. breast with metastasis to axilla, treatment of choice is : PGI 1996**

A. Radical mastectomy + chemotherapy
B. Radical mastectomy + radiotherapy
C. Simple mastectomy + radiotherapy
D. Chemotherapy + radiotherapy

**85. McGovern nipple is : DNB 1994**

A. Secondaries in breast
B. Spread of Ca. breast to opposite side
C. Radical mastectomy but nipple preserved
D. Used for choanal atresia

**86. Most malignant type of carcinoma breast is : PGI 1984, 91**

A. Paget's disease
B. Anaplastic carcinoma
C. Scirrhous's carcinoma
D. Atrophic Scirrhous's carcinoma
E. Mastitis carcinomatosa

**87. Of the following pathological findings in the breast, which is least likely to be precancerous : PGI 1984**

A. Fibroadenoma  B. Intraductal papilloma
C. Sclerosing adenosis  D. Lobular hyperplasia
E. Cancer of the breast

**88. The recurrence of carcinoma breast is indicated by enlargement of : AIIMS 1982, 88**

A. Axillary lymphnodes  B. Cervical lymph nodes
C. Dysphagia  D. Dyspnoea

**89. A solitary breast mass is malignant if following are present, except : PGI 1982, 88; AMC 1987**

A. Serous discharge  B. Gritty sensation
C. Oedema of arm  D. Skin involvement

**90. Carcinoma of the breast 4 cm. in size fixed to the pectoralis muscle would qualify as : JIPMER 1986, 87; Kerala 1987**

A. Stage-I  B. Stage-II
C. Stage-III  D. Stage-IV

**91. A distressing complication of radical mastectomy is: Orissa 1999**

A. Paralysis of the fifth finger of the hand.
B. Oedema of the arm.
C. Loss of sensation of the medial side of the arm.
D. Frequent skin infections of the hand on the affected side.

**92. Match List-I with List-II and select the correct answer using the codes given below the lists : CSE 1999**

| List-I | List-II |
|---|---|
| A. Inflammatory carcinoma | 1. Bilateral |
| B. Lobular | 2. Malignant infiltration of lactiferous ducts |
| C. Retraction of nipple | 3. Cuts like an unripe pear |
| D. Peau d'orange | 4. Highly aggressive cancer |
| | 5. Cutaneous lymphatic edema |

Codes :

| | A | B | C | D |
|---|---|---|---|---|
| A. | 4 | 3 | 2 | 5 |
| B. | 2 | 1 | 5 | 4 |
| C. | 4 | 1 | 2 | 5 |
| D. | 1 | 2 | 4 | 3 |

**Ans.** 80. C 81. D 82. B 83. D 84. B 85. D 86. E 87. A 88. A 89. A
90. C 91. B 92. C

**93. A painless, hard swelling of breast in old woman is generally due to : Karnataka 1999**

A. Cancer
B. Calcified haematoma
C. Fat necrosis
D. Fibroadenoma

**94. Match List-I (Clinical stage of breast cancer) with List-II (Therapeutic option) and select the correct answer by using the codes given below the Lists: UPSC 2000**

| List-I | List-II |
|---|---|
| A. T1N0M0 | 1. Modified radical mastectomy + adjuvant chemotherapy |
| B. T2N1M0 | 2. Quadrantectomy + radiotherapy |
| C. T4N2M0 | 3. Palliative chemotherapy/Hormone therapy |
| D. T4N2M1 | 4. Primary chemotherapy + adjuvant surgery |

**Codes:**

| | a | b | c | d |
|---|---|---|---|---|
| A. | 2 | 1 | 3 | 4 |
| B. | 1 | 2 | 4 | 3 |
| C. | 1 | 2 | 3 | 4 |
| D. | 2 | 1 | 4 | 3 |

**95. Breast mass of 6 x 3 cm size with hard mobile ipsilateral axillary lymph node and ipsilateral supraclavicular lymph node, the staging is : AIIMS 2000**

A. $T_4N_2M_0$
B. $T_3N_2M_0$
C. $T_3N_1M_1$
D. $T_4N_1M_1$

**96. Regarding moderately increased risk for Invasive Breast carcinoma which of the following conditions is true : Kerala 2000**

A. Sclerosing adenoma
B. Apocrine metaplasia
C. Duct Ectasia
D. Atypical ductal hyperplasia
E. Fibroadenoma

**97. The breast reconstruction which of the following is not used : AIIMS 2000**

A. Transverse rectus abdominus myocutaneous flap.
B. Transverse rectus abdominus free flap.
C. Pectoralis major myocutaneous flap.
D. Lattismus dorsi myocutaneous flap.

**98. 4 cm breast nodule with ipsilatral mobile LN in axilla staging : PGI 2000**

A. $T_2N_1M_0$
B. $T_2N_2M_0$
C. $T_1N_1M_0$
D. $T_3N_2M_1$

**99. In which one of the following types of carcinoma of the breast, is a biopsy of the opposite breast advised : UPSC 2001**

A. Inflammatory carcinoma
B. Medullary carcinoma
C. Lobular carcinoma
D. Scirrhous carcinoma

**100. Mondor's disease is : AI 1996**

A. Superficial thrombophlebitis of breast veins
B. Carcinoma breast
C. Filariasis of breast
D. Premalignant breast lesion

**101. A 45 years old woman presents with hard and mobile lump in breast confirmatory investigation is : Delhi 1992; AI 2001**

A. FNAC
B. USG
C. Mammography
D. Excision biopsy

**102. The following drugs are used in Rx of cyclical mastalgia, except : JIPMER 2002**

A. Danazol
B. Tamoxifen
C. Evening primrose oil
D. Estrogen

**103. In a mammogram all of the following are features of Ca. breast except : UPSC 2002**

A. Solid lesion with illdefined edge or stellate configuration
B. True microcalcification
C. Areas of microcalcification
D. Increased skin thickness

**104. A 45 years old male has multiple grouped vesicular lesions present on the T10 segment dermatome associated with pain. The most likely diagnosis is : AIIMS 2002**

A. Herpes zoster
B. Dermatitis herpetiformis
C. Herpes simplex
D. Scabies

**105. A 56 years old man has painful rashes over his right upper eyelid and forehead for the last 48 hours. He underwent chemotherapy for Non-Hodgkin's lymphoma one year ago. His temperature is 98°F, blood pressure 138/76 mm Hg and pulse is 80/minute. Examination shows no other abnormalities. Which of the following is the most likely diagnosis : AIIMS 2002**

A. Impetigo
B. Herpes zoster
C. Pyoderma gangrenosum
D. Erysipelas

**Ans.** 93. B 94. D 95. C 96. D 97. C 98. A 99. C 100. A 101. D 102. D 103. C 104. A 105. B

**106. Which layer of epidermis is underdeveloped in the VLBW infants in the initial 7 days : AIIMS 2002**

A. Stratum germinativum B. Stratum granulosum
C. Stratum lucidum D. Stratum corneum

**107. A 28 years old patient has multiple grouped papulo-vesicular lesions on both elbows, knees, buttocks and upper back associated with severe itching. The most likely diagnosis is : AIIMS 2002**

A. Pemphigus vulgaris
B. Bullous pemphigoid
C. Dermatitis Herpetiformis
D. Herpes zoster

**108. An 8 years old child presented with itchy, exudative lesions on the face, palms and soles. The siblings also have similar complaints. The treatment of choice in such a patient is : AI 2003**

A. Systemic ampicillin
B. Topical betamethasone
C. Systemic prednisolone
D. Topical permethrin

**109. A 24 years old female has flaccid bullae in the skin and oral erosions. Histopathology shows intraepidermal acantholytic blister. The most likely diagnosis is : AI 2003**

A. Pemphigoid
B. Erythema multiforme
C. Pemphigus vulgaris
D. Dermatitis herpetiformis

**110. Most suggestive of malignancy on a breast mammogram is : CUPGME 2003**

A. True microcalcification
B. Stellate
C. Irregular opacities
D. All of the above

**111. In a female patient of Breast Cancer with lung metastasis, the most common presenting symptoms is : Burdwan 2003**

A. Chronic cough B. Hemoptysis
C. No specific complaint D. Dyspnoea

**112. Worst prognosis in breast carcinoma is seen in : JIPMER 2003**

A. Colloid B. Lobular
C. Inflammatory D. Papillary

**113. After radical mastectomy there was injury to the long thoracic nerve. The integrity of the nerve can be tested at the bedside by asking the patient to: AI 2004**

A. Shrug the shoulders
B. Raise the arm above the head on the affected side
C. Touch the opposite shoulder
D. Lift a heavy object from the ground

**114. All of the following are hormonal agents used against breast cancer, except : AI 2004**

A. Letrazole B. Exemestrane
C. Taxol D. Tamoxifen

**115. Which of the following microscopic features is typical of Paget's disease : Karnataka 2005**

A. Presence of large vaculated cells
B. Epidermal hypertrophy
C. Subdermal round cell infiltration
D. All of the above

**116. Triple assessment for Ca breast is : AI 2009**

A. History, clinical examination and mammogram
B. History , clinical examination and FNAC
C. History and mammogram and FNAC
D. Clinical examination, mammogram and FNAC/ biopsy

**Ans.** 106. C 107. C 108. D 109. C 110. A 111. C 112. C 113. B 114. C 115. D 116. D

# EXPLANATIONS OF BREAST

**1. Ans.— B. Tumour <2 cm, no nodes, no metastases**

**2. Ans.— B. Fibroadenosis**

**3. Ans.— C. Third**

**4. Ans.— A. Pectoralis major**

**5. Ans.— C. Axilla**

**6. Ans.— A. Upper- outer quadrant**

**Adenocystic variety has the best prognosis.**

**7. Ans.— B. Water**

**8. Ans.— B. Biopsy and simple mastectomy**

**Paget's disease is a superficial manifestation of an underlying breast carcinoma and presents as an eczema like condition of nipple and areola.**

**9. Ans.— A. CMF**

**10. Ans.— D. Paget's disease of the nipple**

**11. Ans.— D. A benign condition**

**12. Ans.— A. Pectoral group**

**Lymphnode status is best prognostic factor. It indicates extent of spread.**

**13. Ans.— B. Atrophic scirrhous carcinoma**

**14. Ans.— A. A prickling sensation in a breast lump**

**15. Ans.— A. It is unnecessary for a surgeon to follow up his patients with carcinoma of the breast after operation. It is done by other specialist**

**16. Ans.— B. T2N1M0**

**17. Ans.— D. 12 weeks**

**18. Ans.— C. 45° reclining**

**19. Ans.— C. Epithelial hyperplasia**

**20. Ans.— B. Axillary artery**

**21. Ans.— B. Hard fibroadenoma**

**22. Ans.— C. Breast lump with pricking sensation**

**23. Ans.— B. Incision and drainage**

**24. Ans.— B. Is related to recurrent abscesses of areolar region.**

**25. Ans.— D. Involved axillary lymphnodes**

**26. Ans.— B. Presents with a worm like swelling extending radially from the nipple.**

**27. Ans.— D. Thrombophlebitis of breast veins**

**28. Ans.— D. Acute inflammatory reaction**

**Radical surgery should not be done in presence of acute inflammatory reaction.**

**29. Ans.— D. Contralateral breast**

**30. Ans.— D. Precursor of breast abscess**

**Cracked nipple may occur during lactation and forerunner of acute infective mastitis. It should be rested for 24 to 45 hours.**

**31. Ans.— B. Simple mastectomy with axillary node sampling and post-operative radiotherapy; chemotherapy if nodes are positive**

**32. Ans.— B. A super-radical mastectomy**

**33. Ans.— B. Nerve to serratus anterior**

**34. Ans.— A. Simple mastectomy and radiotherapy**

**35. Ans.— D. 60%**

**36. Ans.— A. Periodic follow-up for any recurrence and treatment thereof.**

**37. Ans.— D. Bone**

**Carcinoma Breast spreads by local, lymphatic & Blood stream. By local spread it goes to skin & peritoneal muscle & chest wall. By lymphatic spread Permeation occurs to lymphatic channels. By blood stream it goes to lumbar vertebra & femur, cause vertebral osteolysis. In most of the cases it by this way the metastasis occurs in liver, lung fields and brain.**

**38. Ans.— B. Sister dead from cancer breast**

**39. Ans.— A. Benign condition**

**40. Ans.— D. Fibroadenosis**

**41. Ans.— B. Microdochectomy**

**Majority of these tumors are single and seen in between 35-50 years. Dark blood stained discharge from nipple is the only symptom in majority.**

**42. Ans.— D. Ductal**

**43. Ans.— C. Constitutes 10% of all breast carcinomas.**

**44. Ans.— D. Latissmus dorsi myocutaneous flap**

**45. Ans.— A. Usually unilateral in young males**

**46. Ans.— C. Bone**

**47. Ans.— B. Radical mastectomy**

**48. Ans.— A. Radiotherapy**

**49. Ans.— A. Upper and outer quadrant**

**50. Ans.— B. Duct obstruction**

**51. Ans.— C. (ii) and (iii) are correct**

**52. Ans.— D. Visceral spread**

**53. Ans.— D. Involvement of lymph nodes**

**54. Ans.— B. Intra-ductal papilloma**

**Commonest cause of Blood discharge from nipple is duct papilloma. Chronic cystic mastitis & cystosarcoma phylloides is not a cause of Blood stained discharge from nipple.**

**55. Ans.— D. Fibroadenosis**

**56. Ans.— D. All of the above**

**57. Ans.— B. Local excision**

**58. Ans.— C. The thoracic chain of lymph nodes along the internal mammary vessels.**

**59. Ans.— A. It is a cyst which does not subsequently refill**

**60. Ans.— E. All of the above**

**61. Ans.— D. Any of the above**

**62. Ans.— C. 6 to 12**

**63. Ans.— D. Lactation**

**64. Ans.— E. All of the above**

**65. Ans.— B. Hormone therapy**

**66. Ans.— A. Axilla**

**67. Ans.— A. Duration of disease**

**68. Ans.— A. Dense breasts**

**69. Ans.— C. Duct carcinoma less than 1 cm in inner quadrants.**

**70. Ans.— B. Locally invasive**

**71. Ans.— A. Lymphatic blockage**

**Peaud'orange is due to cutaneous lymphatic oedema It is a sign of advanced. ca. But some time it is seen in chronic abscess also.**

**72. Ans.— B. Lobular carcinoma**

**Bilateraly it is common in lobular type and in those below 50 years of age.**

**73. Ans.— B. Estrogen receptor positive tumor**

**74. Ans.— A. Simple mastectomy**

**75. Ans.— C. Bone Secondaries**

**76. Ans.— C. Staphylococcus aureus**

**77. Ans.— C. Duct papilloma**

**78. Ans.— A. Comedo carcinoma**

**79. Ans.— A. Medullary carcinoma**

**Medullary carcinoma have solid sheets of large cells often associated with a marked lymphocytic reaction.**

**80. Ans.— C. Fibroadenoma of breast**

**81. Ans.— D. Pectoralis major muscle with fascia**

**82. Ans.— B. Bilateral**

**83. Ans.— D. Close monitoring and follow-up**

**84. Ans.— B. Radical mastectomy + radiotherapy**

**85. Ans.— D. Used for choanal atresia**

**86. Ans.— E. Mastitis carcinomatosa**

**87. Ans.— A. Fibroadenoma**

**88. Ans.— A. Axillary-lymph nodes**

**They are usually removed in modified radical mastectomy.**

**89. Ans.— A. Serous discharge**

**90. Ans.— C. Stage III**

**91. Ans.— B. Oedema of the arm**

**92. Ans.— C.**

| A | B | C | D |
|---|---|---|---|
| 4 | 1 | 2 | 5 |

**93. Ans.— B. Calcified haematoma**

**Calcified haematoma is very hard.**

**94. Ans.— D. 2 1 4 3**

**95. Ans.— C. $T_3N_1M_1$**

**96. Ans.— D. Atypical ductal hyperplasia**

**97. Ans.— C. Pectoralis major myocutaneous flap**

**98. Ans.— A. $T_2N_1M_0$**

**99. Ans.— C. Lobular carcinoma**

**100. Ans.— A. Superficial thrombophlebitis of breast veins.**

**It may be seen in arm. The treatment is restricted arm movements and the condition subsides spontaneously.**

**101. Ans.— D. Excision biopsy**

**102. Ans.— D. Estrogen**

**103. Ans.— C. Areas of microcalcification**

**104. Ans.— A. Herpes zoster**

**105. Ans.— B. Herpes zoster**

**106. Ans.— C. Stratum lucidum**

**107. Ans.— C. Dermatitis Herpetiformis**

**108. Ans.— D. Topical permethrin**

- **Two siblings showing itchy lessions**
- **The diagnosis is surely scabies**
- **Causative organisms - itch mite (life cycle of 21 days).**
- **C/s feature burrows in Horny layer of skin.**
- **Treatment-Benzyl Benzoate/Superior ointment/ Permethrins/GBHC.**

**109. Ans.— C. Pemphigus vulgaris**

**110. Ans.— A. True microcalcification**

**111. Ans.— C. No specific complaint**

**112. Ans.— C. Inflammatory**

**113. Ans.— B. Raise the arm above the head on the affected side.**

**114. Ans.— C. Taxol**

**All of the above are used in Ca breast but Taxol (paclitaxel) is cytotoxic agent not hormonal agents.**

**Hormonal Therapy in Ca. Breast**

- **The potent antiestrogen tamoxifen, is the endocrine treatment of choice in the premenopausal patients and is the initial therapy of choice for post-menopausal women with metastatic breast cancer.**

- **Hormonal agents used in Ca breast are —**

| | |
|---|---|
| **1. Antiestrogen** | **— Tamoxifen, Raloxifen, Toremifen** |
| **2. Estrogen** | **— Diethylstilbestrol** |
| **3. Progestin** | **— Megestrol acetate** |
| **4. Aromatase inhibitor** | **— Aminoglutethimide, Letrazol<br>— Anastrazole, Exemestane** |

- **Aromatase inhibitors (e.g. anastrazole, letrazole) and inactivators (exemestane) block the peripheral conversion of adrenal androgens into estrogens and have been shown to be at least as effective as or more effective than tamoxifen as first-line therapy for metastatic hormone receptors-expressing breast cancer.**
- **Aromatase inhibitors are effective only in postmenopausal women.**
- **A new pure antiestrogen. Fulvestrant, has now been FDA-approved as second-line therapy for metastatic hormone receptor-positive breast cancer.**

**115. Ans.— D. All of the above**

**116. Ans.— D. Clinical examination, mammogram and FNAC/biopsy**

- **Triple assessment :**
- **Combination of clinical assessment, radiological imaging and cyto/histo-logical diagnosis. PPV is 99.9% (Positive Predictive Value).**

# 7

# IMPORTANT TEXT OF CARDIOTHORACIC SURGERY

## DISTRIBUTION OF TUMOURS AND OTHER MASSES IN MEDIASTINUM

*All parts of Mediastinum*
- Lymph node lesions
- Bronchogenic cysts

*Anterior Mediastinum*
- Teratoma
- Lymphangioma
- Angiomas
- Pericardial cysts
- Esphageal lesions

*Middle Mediastinum*
- Teratoma
- Thymona
- Parathyroid adenoma
- Aneurysm
- Lipoma
- Myxoma
- Goitre

*Posterior Mediastinum*
- Neurogenic tumours
- Pheochromocytoma
- Aneurysms
- Enterogenous cysts
- Spinal lesions
- Hiatus hernia

## TYPES OF BRONCHIAL ADENOMA

| | *Carcinoid* | *Cylindroma* |
|---|---|---|
| Location | Proximal bronchus | Primary bronchi and trachea |
| Comparative incidence | 85% | 15% |
| Histologic features | Squamous metaplasia, small uniform cell with acidophilic neoplasm; mitosis and argentaffin granules rare | Cells less uniform, smaller. occasionally oncocytic |
| Lymph node metastasis | Uncommon | Twice as common (30%), also distant metastasis more common |
| Bronchoscopic appearance | Smooth, rounded protrusion into lumen, mucosa intact, bleeds freely | Extends along the bronchus wall; paler and firmer |
| Invasiveness | Local *iceberg effect* common : small intraluminal component with rather large endobronchial component | Recurrence rate 7 times that of carcinoid |
| Symptoms | Obstruction, infection, bleeding, wheezing | Same |

## WHO CLASSIFICATION OF PRIMARY NEOPLASMS OF LUNG

A. Epithelial tumors
   1. Epidermoid carcinomas (with keratinization).
   2. Small cell anaplastic (oat cell) carcinoma.
   3. Adenocarcinoma (with formation of glands or papillarity, may or may not have mucus)
   4. Large cell undifferentiated carcinoma (may or may not have mucus, no glands or keratinization, includes giant cell variant).
   5. Combined epidermoid and adenocarcinoma.
   6. Bronchoalveolar cell carcinoma (localized and disseminated forms).
   7. Carcinoid tumors.
   8. Tumors of mucus glands (adenocystic carcinoma, mucoepidermoid tumors and others).
   9. Squamous papillomas of surface epithelium (with or without goblet cells).

B. Sarcoma

C. Combined tumors of epithelial and mesodermal cells (carcinosarcomas, blastomas)

D. Mesotheliomas (localized and diffuse)

E. Unclassified tumors

## CARCINOMA BREAST : VARIOUS METHODS OF MANAGEMENT OPERABLE BREAST CANCER

**Local only :**

**Stage-I :** $T_1$, $N_0$ or $N_1a$, $M_0$

**Stage-II:** $T_1$, $N_1b$, M0; or $T_2$, $N_0$, $M_0$

T2, $N_1a$, $M_0$; or $T_2$, $N_1b$, $M_0$

*Irradiation to breast & Draining nodes + Either Adrenalectomy + Oophorectomy or Hypophysectomy*

***Stage-III*** **:** $T_1 N_2 M_0$ or $T_2 N_2 M_0$ or $T_3 N_{1 \text{ or } 2}$ $M_0$

**Stage-IV :** Any T, any N with M1

**Systemic only**

Oophorectomy

Adrenalectomy, oophorectomy + 5 Fluorouracil

Hypophysectomy

* *Single and Multiple*

Chemotherapy

* *Estogen, Androgen, Corticosteroid*

Hormone therapy

Immunotherapy

Radiotherapy

## STAGING OF BREAST CANCER

Clinical—TNM Classification

T— Primary Tumour
- T1 — tumour diameter 2 cm or less—not fixed. Includes Paget's
- T2 — tumour diameter 2-5 cm-not fixed
- T3 — tumour diameter more than 5 cm
- T4 — skin or chest wall involvement (skin tethering/nipple retraction not include)

N— Regional Lymph Node
- N0 — no palpable homolateral nodes
- N1 — mobile homolateral axillary lymph node
- N2 — homolateral supra/infraclavicular lymph nodes or oedema of arm

M— Distant Metastases
- M0 — no distant metastases
- M1 — distant metastases

N.B. Enlarged lymph nodes may represent reactive hyperplasia.

Clinical error of 20% in assessing lymph node involvement. Clinical staging should be supplemented by investigation: e.g., Bone scan, liver function tests etc.

*Higher risk woman*

1. Positive family history
2. Prior breast cancer (8%)
3. Gross cystic disease
4. Prior history of intraductal papilloma
5. Prior history of endometrial carcinoma
6. Childless woman and those conceiving after the age of 30

## SURGICAL ANATOMY

**Calot's triangle**

* Above by liver
* Medially by common hepatic duct
* Below by cystic duct

**Sherren's triangle :**

* Umbilicus
* Anterior superior iliac spine
* Symphisis pubis

**White bile**

— Opalescent secretion (not white) by bile duct with distal obstruction contains mucus, cholesterol and traces of none of bite salts (formed partly of mucous secretion & partly of transudate from the duct wall).

**Limey bile**

— A condition in which there is as much calcium in the bile that the gall bladder shows upon plain X-ray and is due to gradual obstruction of CBD and is seen in chronic pancreatitis and carcinoma panceas.

## SUSPECT A TESTICULAR TUMOR WITH

1. Painless lump - not necessarily
2. Lymphadenopathy
3. Abdominal mass
4. Secondary hydrocoele
5. Gynaecomastia
6. History of undescended testicle
7. Any young patient with scrotal swelling

## FEATURES OF ACOUSTIC NEUROMA

1. VIII nerve palsy - deafness tinnitus, vertigo
2. VII nerve palsy - facial weakness, unilateral taste loss
3. V nerve palsy - facial numbness, loss of corneal reflex
4. IX, X, nerve palsy - dysphagia, hoarseness
5. Cerebellar syndrome
6. Raised intracranial pressure

# MCQ's OF CARDIOTHORACIC SURGERY

## What is Important in Cardiothoracic Surgery

Thorax (injuries, effusions, haemorrhage, management), Bypass Surgery, Surgery, Surgery for valvular lesions

1. **A Taussig-Bing malformation is best treated by : AIIMS 1984**
   A. Diversion of V.S.D. simultaneously with Mustard operation.
   B. Diversion of the septal defect.
   C. Reattachment and reversal of aorta and pulmonary arteries.
   D. No corrective procedure for this anomaly.
   E. Methods similar to double outlet right ventricle.
2. **The organism most frequently related to the cause of mediastinal fibrosis is : PGI 1985**
   A. Actinomycosis  B. Histoplasma
   C. Hansen bacillus  D. Staphylococcus
   E. Koch bacillus
3. **The most important consideration in determining whether or not to treat an atrial septal defect is : AMC 1985**
   A. Paradoxical embolus
   B. Magnitude of the shunt
   C. Location of the defect
   D. Possibly of local infection
   E. Conduction changes
4. **The most common anatomic variation of coronary artery fistula connects : AIIMS 1986**
   A. Left coronary to right ventricle
   B. Left coronary to left ventricle
   C. Right coronary with right ventricle
   D. Right coronary to right atrium
   E. Right coronary and great cardiac vein
5. **The most common cause of death, after palliative operations for tetralogy of fallot is : BHU 1986**
   A. Haemorrhage
   B. Hypoxia
   C. Respiratory failure
   D. Acute pulmonary oedema
   E. Congestive failure
6. **A 50-years-old male, a known hypertensive, suddenly experiences excruciating pain in his back between the shoulder blades. The pain does not radiate to the neck or arm. A physical examination reveals a systolic murmur over the aortic area, radiating to the major vessels and a 40 mmHg-difference in the arterial blood pressure between the two arms. The probable diagnosis is : MAHE 1993**
   A. Angina pectoris
   B. Aortic stenosis
   C. Coarctation of the aorta
   D. Dissecting aneurysm of the aorta
7. **The most useful initial diagnostic procedure in the patient described is : MAHE 1993**
   A. Oesophagogram (barium swallow)
   B. Resting electrocardiogram
   C. Stress test
   D. X-ray of the chest
8. **Which of the following is not a mediastinal cyst : DNB 1989**
   A. Spring water cyst
   B. Foregut cyst
   C. Pleuropericardial cyst
   D. 'Water lily' cyst
   E. All of the above
9. **Which of the following histological types of lung cancer is associated with the myasthenic (Eaton-Lambert) syndrome: MAHE 1996**
   A. Adenocarcinoma
   B. Epidermoid carcinoma
   C. Large cell carcinoma
   D. Small cell carcinoma

**Ans.** 1. A  2. B  3. B  4. C  5. E  6. D  7. A  8. D  9. D

**10. Bronchiectasis associated with tuberculosis : UPSC 1989**

A. Is almost always the direct result of the tuberculous infection.
B. In the upper lobes, often represents healed tuberculous cavities.
C. Has a different distribution than non-tuberculous bronchiectasis.
D. Is characterized by the presence of stratified squamous epithelium.

**11. 'Shock lung' is usually seen : UPSC 1986**

A. With head injuries
B. With haemorrhagic shock
C. After prolonged cardiopulmonary bypass
D. With multiple trauma
E. All of the above

**12. The symptoms of recurrent infection, intractable cough, sputum production, and frequent hemoptysis refractory to medical therapy are indicative of : UPSC 1985**

A. Oat cell carcinoma of the lung
B. Bronchiectasis
C. Coccidioidomycosis
D. Pulmonary sequestration
E. Empyema

**13. The most favourable pulmonary metastatic lesions include all except : PGI 1986**

A. Breast B. Kidney
C. Testis D. Uterus
E. Melanoma

**14. A patient presents with injury to the lower chest, which among the followings is not a correct step in the management : Kerala 1998**

A. Arrange USS abdomen
B. Intercostal drainage through the second space
C. Caring of # ribs
D. X-ray chest

**15. The stage of myasthenia gravis that best responds to thymectomy is : PGI 1986**

A. Stage 1 : active
B. Stage 2 : inactive
C. Stage 3 : burned out
D. Those with thymoma present
E. None of the above

**16. The central venous pressure (CVP) is maintained at : AIIMS 1986**

A. 50-100 mm water B. 10-15 mm water
C. 100-150 mm water D. 10-15 mm Hg

**17. The classic signs of cardiac temponade include except : Rohtak 1986**

A. Muffled heart sounds
B. Diminished pulse pressure
C. Hypotension
D. Increase of cardiac size, by X-ray
E. Increased venous pressure

**18. The oxygen consumption in the arrested, asystolic heart is : AMU 1984**

A. 10 ml/min/100 gm B. 100 ml/min/100 gm
C. 2 ml/min/100 gm D. 30 ml/min/100 gm
E. None of the above

**19. Pulmonary neoplasm associated with smoking : AIIMS 1986**

A. Oat cell carcinoma
B. Squamous cell carcinoma
C. Adenocarcinoma
D. None of the above

**20. There is a clear-cut indication for exploratory laparotomy in blunt abdominal trauma if the peritoneal lavage fluid shows : CSE 1995**

A. 10 to 50 RBC/microlitre
B. 10 to 50,000 RBC/microlitre
C. 50,000 to 1,00,000 RBC/microlitre
D. Above 1,00,000 RBC/microlitre

**21. Aspiration pneumonia most commonly occurs in : UPSC 1990; PGI 1993; Rohtak 1995**

A. Right anterior lobe B. Left posterior basal lobe
C. Right upper lobe D. Right lower lobe

**22. Surgical intervention in tuberculosis is required for : AI 1993**

A. Hemoptysis B. Miliary tuberculosis
C. Tuberculous empyema D. Tuberculoma

**23. Superior vena caval syndrome is most commonly caused by : PGI 1981, 89; UPSC 1985; AIIMS 1987, 90; Delhi 1993, 98**

A. Secondaries B. Bronchiectasis
C. Consolidation D. Lung tumor

**24. Which of the following is the commonest cause of calcified pulmonary metastasis : Delhi 1993**

A. Adenocarcinoma kidney
B. Squamous cell carcinoma
C. Seminoma
D. Carcinoma thyroid

**25. Which of the following is the commonest tumor of anterior mediastinum : Delhi 1993**

A. Thymoma B. Neurofibroma
C. Ectopic thyroid D. Lymphoma

**Ans.** 10. B 11. E 12. B 13. E 14. B 15. A 16. C 17. D 18. C 19. B
20. B 21. D 22. C 23. D 24. D 25. A

**26. The effects of supporting the heart with intra-aortic balloon counterpulsation include all of the following except : MAHE 1993**

A. Increase in diastolic coronary perfusion.
B. Increase in myocardial oxygen demand.
C. No change in the preload.
D. Reduction in the afterload.

**27. Bilateral phrenic nerve palsy is caused by : Delhi 1993**

A. Carcinoma bronchus
B. Polio
C. Medullary carcinoma thyroid
D. Paget's disease

**28. A case presented with Multisystem trauma with variable blood loss with irregular breathing. The diagnosis is : Delhi 1992**

A. Extradural hematoma B. Rupture lung
C. Spleen rupture D. None of the above

**29. A soft tissue tumour causing rib erosion is : PGI 1986; Delhi 1992**

A. Mesothelioma B. Fibrosarcoma
C. Thymoma D. Neurofibroma

**30. Hamman's sign is most characteristic of : UPSC 1988; WB 1996**

A. Subcutaneous emphysema
B. Pneumothorax
C. Pneumopericardium
D. Pneumomediastinum

**31. Which of the following is true about adenocarcinoma of the bronchus: AMU 1987**

A. Is closely associated with pipe smoking.
B. Has often spread into the pulmonary veins by the time of diagnosis.
C. Equally common in both sexes.
D. Account for 25% of bronchogenic carcinomas.

**32. Myocardial oxygen consumption in a breathing heart is : AIIMS 1985**

A. 10 ml/min/gram
B. 14 ml/sec/gram
C. 10 ml/minute/100 gram
D. 100 ml/minute/100 gram
E. None of the above

**33. A patient with aorta-pulmonary fistula characteristically shows all of the following, except : AMU 1986**

A. Wide pulse pressure
B. Mild cyanosis
C. Cardiomegaly
D. Failure to gain weight
E. Frequent respiratory infections

**34. The most common cause of lung abscess is : AIIMS 1987; Rohtak 1988; Delhi 1997**

A. Failure to use porphylactic antibiotics
B. Chronic atelectasis
C. Aspiration of foreign material
D. Tuberculosis

**35. Goals of IPPR are the following except : DNB 1990**

A. To maintain $PaO_2$ between 60-80 mm Hg.
B. Avoid hypoxia ($PaO_2$ below to 50 mmHg) or hyperoxia (above $PaO_2$ 100 mmHg).
C. Maintain $PaCO_2$ between 35-45 mmHg.
D. None of the above.

**36. Mediastinal bronchogenic cysts are commonest in : AMU 1985**

A. Anterior B. Middle
C. Posterior D. Any where

**37. Apnea is defined as cessation of breathing for —— sec or longer but associated with bradycardia, cyanosis or pallor. DNB 1989**

A. 5 B. 10
C. 15 D. 20

**38. Cyanosis in which $PaO_2$ are normal often result due to : UPSC 1984**

A. Congenital heart disease
B. Respiratory disease
C. Valvular lesion
D. Abnormal hemoglobin

**39. In trauma to the heart, the area most often injured is : UPSC 1986**

A. Left atrium B. Left ventricle
C. Right atrium D. Right ventricle

**40. The presence of a post-operative bronchopleural fistula is characterized by all, except : PGI 1983**

A. Secondary empyema
B. Pink frothy sputum
C. Increased coughing in the upright position
D. Symptoms appearing on the 5th or 6th day
E. Spontaneous closure

**41. Haemorrhagic pleural effusion with a mass adherent to the chest wall most likely is : AMU 1984**

A. Tuberculosis
B. Bronchogenic carcinoma
C. Pulmonary infarction
D. Mesothelioma
E. Histoplasmosis

| Ans. | 26. D | 27. B | 28. B | 29. D | 30. D | 31. B | 32. C | 33. B | 34. C | 35. D |
|---|---|---|---|---|---|---|---|---|---|---|
| | 36. A | 37. D | 38. D | 39. D | 40. C | 41. D | | | | |

**42. In a patient of mesothelioma, one often finds : AIIMS 1984**
A. Hypoglycaemia
B. An association with asbestosis
C. Haemorrhagic pleural effusion
D. Clubbing of fingers
E. All of the above

**43. Bronchiectasis may develop from all of the following, except : PGI 1985**
A. Congenital malformation
B. Chronic pulmonary infection
C. Retained bronchial foreign body
D. Tuberculous
E. Chronic pleural effusion

**44. Congenital lobar emphysema is usually treated by : AMU 1985**
A. Lobectomy
B. Pneumonectomy
C. Tube drainage
D. Bronchoscopy and aspiration
E. None of the above

**45. Thin-walled intra-pulmonary cavities are most frequently associated with : AIIMS 1986**
A. Isoniazid therapy
B. Corticosteroid therapy
C. Coccidiodomycosis
D. Acute miliary tuberculosis
E. All of the above

**46. Pleural fluid with the appearance of anchovy sauce is characteristic of : UPSC 1985**
A. E. coli B. Entamoeba histolytica
C. Staphylococcus aureus D. Echinococcus
E. None of the above

**47. The primary treatment of empyema which results from tuberculosis is : UPSC 1985**
A. Open tube drainage
B. Systemic antibiotic therapy
C. Closed tube drainage
D. Thoracoplasty
E. Thoracocentesis

**48. Failure to establish adequate drainage in an empyema with a bronchopleural fistula is indicated by : AMC 1985**
A. Drainage less than 100 c.c. per day.
B. Haemorrhagic drainage less than 100 c.c per day.
C. The development of haemoptysis.
D. Continued productive cough with purulent material.
E. All of the above.

**49. Tension Pneumothorax results in : CSE 1998**
A. Alkalosis
B. Increased cardiac output
C. Decreased Venous return
D. All of the above

**50. The most common fungal disease confused with tuberculosis is : Delhi 1984**
A. Nocardiosis B. Coccidiodomycosis
C. Histoplasmosis D. Actinomycosis
E. Blastomycosis

**51. The most common cause of mediastinitis is : AIIMS 1986, 91**
A. Cervical cellulitis
B. Osteomyelitis of vertebrae
C. Pleural empyema
D. Rupture of oesophagus
E. Pericarditis

**52. Contraindications to surgery in patients with an atrial septal defects are : AIIMS 1986**
A. Patients over 50 years of age.
B. Pulmonary hypertension without increased pulmonary vascular resistance.
C. Pulmonary hypertension with increased pulmonary vascular resistance.
D. Pulmonary blood flow one-to-two times greater than systemic flow.
E. All of the above.

**53. The most frequently causes of haemoptysis : AIIMS 1985, 89, 92; UPSC 1985, 87, 91**
A. Bronchogenic carcinoma
B. Pulmonary tuberculosis
C. Mitral stenosis
D. Pulmonary embolism
E. Bronchiectasis

**54. Development of which of the following is the most ominous sign in aortic stenosis : PGI 1986, 91, 96**
A. Angina pectori
B. Left ventricular hypertrophy
C. Left ventricular failure
D. Syncope

**55. The use of serum creatine phosphokinase (CPK) to support a clinical impression of acute myocardial damage is of little use until which day post-operative: AMU 1986, 87**
A. Ist B. 3rd
C. 12th D. 15th
E. 42nd

| Ans. | 42. E | 43. E | 44. A | 45. C | 46. B | 47. B | 48. D | 49. C | 50. C | 51. D |
|---|---|---|---|---|---|---|---|---|---|---|
| | 52. C | 53. B | 54. C | 55. B | | | | | | |

56. **Most common source for thrombus in Pulmonary Embolism is : AIIMS 1992**
A. Posterior tibial vein B. Ilio femoral vein
C. Popliteal vein D. Soleal vein

57. **In Pneumothorax due to blunt injury, treatment of choice is : AIIMS 1992**
A. Intercostal drainage B. Observation
C. Thoractomy D. Pneumonectomy

58. **Blalock-Tausig shunt is used in the correction of : AIIMS 1992**
A. PDA B. VSD
C. Tetralogy of Fallot D. TAPVC

59. **Ganglioneuroma is most common in : Delhi 1983**
A. Ant. mediastinum
B. Middle mediastinum
C. Post. mediastinum
D. Retroperitoneum region

60. **Which nerve is easily injured in PDA ligation : UPSC 1984**
A. Phrenic B. Sympathetic trunk
C. Cardiac nerves D. Recurrent laryngeal

61. **Most common congenital defect associated with pulmonary stenosis is : UPSC 1986**
A. ASD B. VSD
C. Patent foramen ovale D. PDA

62. **Development of the heart takes place during —— week. JIPMER 1985**
A. 2nd and 8th B. 3rd and 5th
C. 1st and 3rd D. 22nd-24th

63. **Highest frequency of coarctation of aorta is seen in : UPSC 1988**
A. Klinefelter's syndrome
B. Down's syndrome
C. Rubella's syndrome
D. Turner's syndrome

64. **Chest tubes must not be inserted posterior to : PGI 1985, 86**
A. Midaxillary line B. Posterior axillary line
C. Anterior axillary line D. Mid-clavicular line

65. **Bronchogenic carcinoma commonly metastatise to which endocrine organ : AIIMS 1985**
A. Ovaries B. Testes
C. Thyroid D. Adrenals

66. **Pleura usually heals in : AMU 1987**
A. 1—3 days B. 3—5 days
C. 5—7 days D. 21—28 days

67. **All of the following are anterior mediastinal tumours except : UPSC 1984, 85, 87; AIIMS 1985; Delhi 1986, 89, 93; AI 1995**
A. Thymoma B. Teratoma
C. Neurofibroma D. Retrosternal goitre

68. **The contraindication for surgery in PDA includes : PGI 1982**
A. Cardiomegaly B. Left-to-right shunt
C. Polycythemia D. Reversal of shunt

69. **The contraindication for operation in mitral value disease is : PGI 1983**
A. Recurrent pulmonary oedema
B. Opening snap
C. Recurrent stensosis after surgery
D. Gross cardiomegaly

70. **All of the following statements are true regarding secundum defect, except : Delhi 1984**
A. Commonest among atrial septal defects.
B. Pulmonary systolic murmurs are present.
C. ECG shows bundle branch block and left ventricular hypertrophy.
D. Direct suture closure is often possible.

71. **The length from incisior teeth to cricopharyngeal constriction is : AIIMS 1983**
A. 10 cms B. 12.5 cms
C. 2.5 cms D. 3.5 cms
E. 4.5 cms

72. **Complications of external cardiac message are all except : PGI 1983, 86**
A. Liver rupture B. Stomach rupture
C. Rib fracture D. Kidney rupture

73. **A solitary nodule in a chest X-ray is indicative of malignancy if following are present except : PGI 1985, 86**
A. The patient is over 45 years
B. Egg shell calcification
C. Indistinct margins
D. Doubling time of 2 weeks

74. **Foreign body commonly lodges in : AIIMS 1981, 83; ESI 1985; PGI 1986**
A. Right lower bronchus
B. Right upper bronchus
C. Left upper bronchus
D. Left lower bronchus

| Ans. | | | | | | | | | | |
|---|---|---|---|---|---|---|---|---|---|---|
| | 56. B | 57. C | 58. C | 59. D | 60. D | 61. A | 62. A | 63. D | 64. B | 65. D |
| | 66. C | 67. C | 68. D | 69. D | 70. C | 71. C | 72. D | 73. B | 74. B | |

**75. Which one of the following is the most important diagnostic physical sign of pneumothorax: CSE 1995**

A. Resonant note on percussion with absent or decreased breath sounds.
B. Decreased vocal fremitus.
C. Making of heart sounds.
D. Decreased respiratory movement of chest on the affected side.

**76. A coin shaped lesion in apical lobes with erosion of ribs and thoracic vertebra is : Delhi 1982, 87; AIIMS 1984, 86; UPSC 1984**

A. Coarctation of aorta B. Pancoast tumour
C. Bronchiectasis D. Any of the above

**77. The following pneumoconiosis has increased risk of developing pleural malignancies : PGI 1980**

A. Anthracosis B. Silicosis
C. Asbestosis D. Bagassosis

**78. All are causes of bilateral common laryngeal nerve palsy except : Delhi 1989**

A. Thyroid surgery
B. Thyroid malignancy
C. Carcinoma bronchus
D. Carcinoma oesophagus (upper part)

**79. Right bronchus is : DNB 1989**

A. Short and thin B. Short and broad
C. Long and broad D. Long and thin

**80. "Frozen chest" usually follows : PGI 1985**

A. Emphyema thoracic
B. Pneumothorax
C. Pulmonary tuberculosis
D. Carcinoma transversalis
E. Pleural effusion

**81. Injury to recurrent laryngeal nerve produces : AMU 1988**

A. Pitch is altered B. Permanent hoarseness
C. Temporary hoarseness D. Stridor

**82. Nasogastric suction should be done post-operatively until —— is there. PGI 1987**

A. Patient develops sore throat
B. Flatus passed
C. Pulse rate becomes normal
D. No more gastric secretions

**83. Post-operative atelectasis from obstruction of a major airway may require intrabronchial suction through : PGI 1988**

A. Nasotracheal suction B. Direct laryngoscopy
C. Mediastinoscopy D. Endoscopy

**84. The mediastinum is shifted to the affected side in : UPSC 1988**

A. Atelectasis B. Pleural effusion
C. Pneumothorax D. Chronic bronchitis

**85. Surgery in cases of pulmonary tuberculosis is indicated in all except : AMC 1986, 87**

A. Tuberculosis bronchiectasis.
B. Miliary tuberculosis.
C. Tuberculoma of destroyed region.
D. Frank destructive lesion not responding to medical treatment.

**86. The initial treatment of a bacterial lung abscess is: AMC 1986**

A. Antibiotic agents, bronchoscopy and postural drainage
B. Lobectomy
C. Open thoracotomy drainage
D. Antibiotic agents followed by resection

**87. The ideal way to relieve increasing spontaneous pneumothorax : PGI 1989**

A. Suprasternal decompression
B. Thoracotomy
C. Subxiphoid decompression
D. None of the above

**88. Which of the following tumours occur commonly in the posterior mediastinum : Delhi 1986; AI 1995**

A. Thymoma B. Neurofibroma
C. Teratoma D. Pericardial cyst

**89. In which of the following ways a patient of chronic empyema of chest can present : AMU 1987**

A. Localised empyema
B. Bronchopleural fistula
C. Discharging sinus at the chest wall
D. All of the above

**90. Which one of the following pairs regarding staging of bronchogenic carcinoma is not correctly matched: CSE 1996**

A. Occult carcinoma TX, NO, MO
B. Stage-I T2, NO, MO
C. Stage-II T3, N1, MO
D. Stage-III T2, N1, M1

**91. An elderly man has abdominal pain, found to have fusiform dilated descending aorta. Likely cause is : AI 2001**

A. Dissected aneurysm
B. Atherosclerosis
C. Right ventricular failure
D. Syphilis aortitis

**Ans.** 75. A 76. B 77. C 78. D 79. B 80. A 81. B 82. B 83. D 84. A
85. B 86. A 87. D 88. B 89. D 90. D 91. B

**92. Regarding development of diaphragm : AIIMS 1983**

A. It develops during 8th week of foetal life.
B. Left dome closes later than right.
C. It grows partly from pleuroperitoneal fold.
D. All of the above are true.
E. None of the above.

**93. How long does a part of lung remain uninflated (atelectatic) in a new born : AIIMS 1984**

A. Two minutes B. Two hours
C. Two days D. Two weeks
E. Two years

**94. Which of the following is true regarding Carcinoma bronchus : Rohtak 1987**

A. Usually presents as haemoptysis.
B. Resolves on administration of a course of antibiotics.
C. Does not occur in non smokers.
D. Should be suspected if a consolidation lungs does not. result with all possible treatment for chest infection.

**95. Which of the following is a contraindication for bronchoscopy : PGI 1984**

A. Emphysema B. Bronchiectasis
C. Tuberculosis lungs D. Aortic aneurysm

**96. Which of the following is not a contraindication for bronchoscopy ? Delhi 1983; AIIMS 1984**

A. Lesions of cervical spine
B. Cardiac failure
C. Active bleeding
D. Trismus

**97. The most common mediastinal tumour is : AIIMS 1985**

A. Neurogenic tumour
B. Bronchogenic carcinoma
C. Plasma cell myelomas
D. Pericardial cysts

**98. Which of the following provides the earliest suggestion of post-operative ventilatory failure : Delhi 1983**

A. Abdominal chest X-ray
B. Rash on the chest wall
C. Restlessness
D. Hyperthermia

**99. Which of the following is the most common inifial symptom of primary cancer of the hilum of the lung : DNB 1990**

A. Cough B. Haemoptysis
C. Wheeze D. Dyspnoea

**100. A 25-years old male is admitted with blunt injury chest. On examination, patient is found to have significant flail chest. The choice of immediate treatment is : UPSC 2001**

A. Intercostal drainage
B. Tracheal intubation and positive pressure ventilation
C. Aspiration
D. Strapping of chest wall

**101. Post-operative pulmonary embolism can be prevented by all except : DNB 1989**

A. Leg exercises B. Early ambulation
C. Pillows under the calf D. Compression stockings

**102. Following cardiac arrest, brain injury is likely to follow within : DNB 1990**

A. 2 minutes B. 3-4 minutes
C. 8 minutes D. 10 minutes

**103. The sequence of symptoms in pulmonary embolism is : DNB 1990**

A. Fever, pain, dyspnoea
B. Fever, dyspnoea, pain
C. Dyspnoea, pain, haemoptysis
D. Dyspnoea, cough, purulent sputum

**104. Which one of the following consequences of chest trauma represents the greatest immediate threat to life : JIPMER 1993; CSE 1996**

A. Sub-cutaneous emphysema of neck
B. Sucking pneumothorax
C. Tension pneumothorax
D. Haemothorax

**105. Diagnosis of cardiac arrest is based on all of the following except : PGI 1982**

A. Absent carotid pulse
B. Absent or gasping respiration
C. Dilated pupils
D. Dilated and fixed pupils

**106. The commonest cause for not being able to tap out pus in a case of chronic empyema is : AP 1989**

A. Selection of wrong site
B. Use of narrow needle
C. Employment of inefficient syringe
D. Presence of excessive fibrin in pus
E. Clotted pus

**107. The most common cardiac malformation at birth is: AIIMS 1986**

A. Atrial septal defect
B. Ventricular septal defect
C. Aortic stenosis
D. Tetralogy of fallot

**Ans.** 92. D 93. D 94. D 95. D 96. C 97. B 98. C 99. A 100. B 101. C 102. B 103. C 104. B 105. D 106. A 107. B

**108. Blood supply to a portion of lung via anomalous systemic artery defines the congenital anomaly as : AIIMS 1987**

A. Pulmonary atresia
B. Pulmonary sequestration
C. Pulmonary agenesis
D. Congenital lobar pneumonia

**109. The major advantage of homograft or heterograft valve prosthesis over a mechanical one is : AIIMS 1984**

A. Ready availability
B. Long-term durability
C. Hemodynamic superiority
D. The low incidence of thromboembolism

**110. Which of the following may not be seen in Tetralogy of Fallot if occurring in children : AIIMS 1984**

A. Ventricular septal defect
B. Patient ductus arteriorus
C. Overriding of the aorta
D. Right ventricular hypertrophy

**111. True position of the intersegmental plane in lungs is indicated by : AIIMS 1984**

A. Pulmonary arteries B. Pulmonary veins
C. Bronchial arteries D. None of the above

**112. All generations of bronchus are fully presented by ——— week of intrauterine life. AMU 1987**

A. 6th B. 10th
C. 16th D. 24th

**113. Intralobar sequestration of lung is commonest in the : UPSC 1989**

A. Apical segment of upper lobe
B. Medial segment of middle lobe
C. Lateral basal segment of lower lobe
D. Posterior basal segment of lower lobe

**114. The following valves are commonly used for mitral valve replacement except : AIIMS 1985**

A. Starr Ball valve
B. Bjork Disc valve
C. Porcine aortic valve heterograft
D. None of the above

**115. Myxoma is most common in : UPSC 1988**

A. Left atrium B. Right atrium
C. Left ventricle D. Right ventricle

**116. The only true indication of a aortocoronary bypass surgery is : AMU 1986**

A. Deterioration in left ventricular function
B. Repeated Cerebral embolism
C. Angina controlled with drugs
D. Angina uncontrolled with medical means

**117. Colt's umbrella and Blakemore's wire are used for the treatment of : AMU 1986**

A. Coronary thrombosis B. Pulmonary embolism
C. Cardiac tumours D. Aortic aneurysm

**118. Blalock's operation in Fallot's tetralogy consists of an anastomosis between : AIIMS 1986**

A. Left subclavian artery and left pulmonary artery.
B. Right subclavian artery and left pulmonary artery.
C. Right subclavian artery and right pulmonary artery.
D. Left subclavian artery and left pulmonary artery.

**119. The most important complication of patent ductus arteriosus in a child is : AMU 1989**

A. Bacterial endocarditis
B. Brain abscess
C. Cardiac failure
D. Ventricular fibrillation

**120. The treatment of choice for patent ductus arteriosus in a child is : AP 1988**

A. Digoxin B. Anticoagulants
C. Diuretics D. Surgical correction

**121. Which of the following sign of coarctation of aorta is rare in children : TN 1988**

A. Differential cyanosis
B. Left ventricular failure
C. Prominent ascending aorta on X-ray
D. Notching of the ribs

**122. In an adult, operative treatment for coarctation of aorta relieves all of the following except : DNB 1990**

A. Hypertension
B. Cyanosis
C. Risks of serious complications
D. Intermittent claudication

**123. Congenital valvular lesions are commonest in : DNB 1990**

A. Aortic and Tricuspid valves
B. Aortic and pulmonary valves
C. Mitral and Tricuspid valves
D. Mitral and Aortic valves

**124. The diagnosis of haemothorax can be confirmed by: AMU 1987**

A. X-ray chest B. Tomography
C. Thoracoscopy D. Bronchography
E. None of the above

**125. Extralobar bronchogenic cysts may communicate with the following except : AP 1989**

A. Oesophagus B. Stomach
C. Bronchus D. None of the above

| Ans. | | | | | | | | | |
|---|---|---|---|---|---|---|---|---|---|
| 108. B | 109. D | 110. D | 111. A | 112. C | 113. D | 114. D | 115. A | 116. D | 117. B |
| 118. A | 119. C | 120. D | 121. D | 122. A | 123. D | 124. E | 125. C | | |

**126. Consider the following statements regarding the involvement of mediastinal lymph nodes in lung cancer : CSE 1997**
1. It is detected by CT scan of chest.
2. Its enlargement is diagnosed by CT scan of chest.
3. Non-homogenous enhancement of glands is characteristic.

**Of these statements**
A. 1 and 3 are correct B. 2 and 3 are correct
C. 1 and 2 are correct D. 1, 2 and 3 are correct

**127. The immediate treatment for cardiac tamponade is: AMC 1991**
A. Vasopressors B. Blood transfusion
C. Beta blockers D. Pericardiocentesis

**128. Commonest cause of spontaneous pneumothorax is : UPSC 1989**
A. Malignancy B. Lung abscess
C. Bronchiectasis D. Rupture of Bulla

**129. Most important measure in all serious cases of crush injuries to chest is : AIIMS 1986**
A. Relief of pain B. Oxygen
C. Tracheostomy D. Antibiotics

**130. The minor degrees of stove-in-chest usually require: AMC 1984**
A. Little specific treatment
B. Tracheostomy
C. Surgical correction
D. Positive pressure ventilation

**131. The immediate treatment of choice in most cases of flail chest is : AMC 1986; AIIMS 1992, 93**
A. Analgesics
B. Intermittent positive pressure ventilation
C. Tracheostomy
D. Breathing exercises

**132. Daily aspirations in mild traumatic haemothorax are usually started after an initial interval of 24 hours as this is the time : AMC 1985**
A. When bleeding is not much
B. Blood may not be liquified
C. To allow bleeding vessel to seal
D. None of the above

**133. The commonest site of fracture of bronchus is : PGI 1986**
A. Upper most part
B. Junction of mediastinal and hilar bronchus
C. Hilar bronchus
D. None of the above

**134. "Pump lung" is a term used for : DNB 1990**
A. Shock lung resulting due to microthrombo-embolism.
B. Shock lung following extensive intravascular coagulation.
C. Stiff lung due to markedly decreased lung compliance.
D. Shock lung following heart lung bypass.

**135. Tietz's disease is most common in ——— costal cartilages. PGI 1987**
A. 1st, 2nd B. 2nd, 3rd
C. 3rd, 4th D. 4th, 5th

**136. The commonest cause of cold abscess of chest wall is: AMC 1987**
A. Tuberculous intercostal lymphadenitis
B. Pott's spine
C. TB of ribs
D. TB of sternum

**137. Cold abscess in chest most commonly presents in the : AMC 1988**
A. Anterior axillary line B. Midaxillary line
C. Posterior axillary line D. Spine

**138. The most important sign of cardiac arrest is : AMC 1986**
A. Dilated pupils B. Absent carotid pulse
C. Gasping respiration D. Cold body

**139. In deep hypothermia, the heart fibrillates at about : AMU 1988**
A. 35°C B. 30°C
C. 25°C D. 5°C

**140. In patent ductus arteriosus, the ductus connects : AIIMS 1987**
A. Left pulmonary artery with aorta just proximal to the origin of the left subclavian artery.
B. Left pulmonary artery with aorta just distal to the origin of left subclavian artery.
C. Right pulmonary artery with aorta just distal to the origin of left subclavian artery.
D. Right pulmonary artery with aorta just distal to the origin of left subclavian artery.

**141. For pleurodesis, the following may be used except : Delhi 1989**
A. Silver nitrate (5%)
B. Iodised talc
C. Comphor in oil (0.5%)
D. Ethyl alcohol (20%)

**142. Fluid in pleural effusion first collects at : AIIMS 1984**
A. Anterior costophrenic angle
B. Posterior costophrenic angle
C. Parasternal area
D. Any of the above

| Ans. | | | | | | | | | |
|---|---|---|---|---|---|---|---|---|---|
| 126. A | 127. D | 128. D | 129. C | 130. A | 131. B | 132. C | 133. B | 134. D | 135. B |
| 136. A | 137. A | 138. B | 139. C | 140. B | 141. D | 142. B | | | |

**143. Normal amount of pleural fluid is approximately : AIIMS 1984**
A. 5 ml B. 15 ml
C. 50 ml D. 100 ml

**144. A majority of surgically produced chylous effusions require the following measures except : PGI 1987**
A. Low fat diet
B. Chest aspiration
C. Thoracotomy and suturing
D. None of the above

**145. The following may arise anywhere in the mediastinum except : DNB 1990**
A. Tuberculous adenitis B. Secondaries
C. Sarcoids D. Teratoma

**146. Which is the commonest congenital anomaly of diaphragm : USPC 1984**
A. Eventration
B. Oesophageal hiatus hernia
C. Hernia through forament of Morgagni
D. Hernia through foramen of Bochdalek

**147. Biot's respiration is seen in : DNB 1990**
A. Hypnosedative poisoning
B. Appendicitis
C. Cholecystitis
D. Bulbar poliomyelitis

**148. The one which does not require cardiopulmonary bypass is : DNB 1991**
A. M S with M R B. VSD
C. Fallot's tetralogy D. PDA

**149. Rashkind's balloon septostomy is done in : DNB 1990**
A. Coarctation of aorta
B. Patent ductus arteriosus
C. Transposition of great vessels
D. Fallot's tetralogy

**150. Which is the commonest rheumatic cardiac valvulitis : UPSC 1987, 92; AI 1989, 92**
A. Mitral regurgitation B. Mitral stenosis
C. Tricuspid stenosis D. Aortic regurgitation

**151. Active rheumatic carditis is ——— contraindication to surgical therapy. DNB 1989**
A. Relative and temporary
B. Relative and permanent
C. Absolute and temporary
D. Absolute and permanent

**152. The ideal age of surgical correction in mitral stenosis is : DNB 1990**
A. 0-5 years B. 5-12 years
C. 12-20 years D. 20-50 years

**153. The following are the indications of surgery in mitral stenosis except : AIIMS 1987**
A. Associated valvular lesions e.g. aortic regurgitation
B. Thromboembolism
C. Symptoms aggravated by pregnancy
D. Persistent congestive cardiac failure

**154. The majority of emboli occur in mitral valvotomy : AIIMS 1986**
A. At the time of operation
B. 1-2 weeks after operation
C. 2-4 weeks after operation
D. 6-12 weeks after operation

**155. Which of the following is an indication of underdigitalization in a patient undergoing mitral valvotomy: PGI 1984**
A. Tachycardia B. Ventricular ectopics
C. Systemic embolism D. Atrial fibrilation

**156. Following are the irreducible hazards of operation for mitral valvotomy except : AIIMS 1983**
A. Cerebral embolism B. Cardiac arrest
C. Auricular tears D. Suppurative bronchitis

**157. Glasgow's sign (a systolic murmur over the brachial artery) is seen in : AIIMS 1986, 90**
A. Aortic regurgitation
B. Tracheo oesophageal fistula
C. Mitral stenosis
D. Aortic aneurysm

**158. All of the following may produce the thoracic outlet syndrome except : MAHE 1993**
A. Cervical rib
B. Costoclavicular compression
C. Raynaud's disease
D. Scalenus anticus syndrome

**159. Closed tracheal injury due to trauma most often involves the trachea or bronchi near the : UPSC 1987**
A. Cricoid B. Mid-trachea
C. Carina D. Secondary bronchi

**160. The best treatment of hemothorax with 500 cc or more of blood in the pleural space is : UPSC 1987**
A. Closed thoracostomy and tube drainage
B. Needle aspiration
C. Thoracotomy
D. Wait and watch

**W161. All are the manifestations of superior vena caval syndrome except : AIIMS 1987**
A. Increased venous pressure
B. Edema of the head and neck
C. Cyanosis
D. Dyspnea

| Ans. | | | | | | | | | |
|---|---|---|---|---|---|---|---|---|---|
| 143. A | 144. C | 145. D | 146. B | 147. B | 148. D | 149. C | 150. A | 151. C | 152. D |
| 153. D | 154. A | 155. A | 156. D | 157. D | 158. C | 159. C | 160. A | 161. NONE | |

**162. A 20-yearS-old man falls from the roof of a two-storey building, landing on a heap of rubble. The initial evaluation reveals a flail chest to be the only obvious injury. The patient is in severe respiratory distress with tachypnoea (rate = 40/minute). The percussion note is bilaterally symmetrical and the breath sounds on the right side are slightly decreased. Arterial blood gases on facemask oxygen are : PaOz, 45 mmHg; $PaCO_2$ mmHg and pH 7.47. Which component of his injury is most likely to have caused these abnormal blood gases ? MAHE 1993**

A. Chest wall instability B. Hypovolaemia
C. Pain D. Pulmonary contussion

**163. Fluoroscopically guided transthoracic needle biopsy of lung is least useful in : AIIMS 1986**

A. Central lesions less than 2 cm in size
B. Peripheral lesions less than 1 cm in size
C. Cavitating lesions in all position
D. All of the above are equal

**164. The incidence of neoplastic degeneration is greater in : AMC 1987**

A. Infant pulmonary hamartomas
B. Adult pulmonary hamartomas
C. Both of the above all equal
D. Neither of the above malignant tendencies

**165. Amoebic lung abscess is commonly due to : AIIMS 1994; AI 1997**

A. Direct extension B. Haematogenous spread
C. Lymphatic spread D. From liver

**66. Post operative pneumonia is most commonly due to: AI 1996**

A. Gram negative bacilli B. Streptococcus
C. Staphylococcus D. Mycoplasma

**167. The commonest cause of aortic aneurysm is : Rohtak 1988**

A. Trauma
B. Syphilis
C. Rheumatic heart disease
D. Atherosclerosis
E. Congenital

**168. The procedure to be adopted in emergency operation for tetralogy of fallot's is : TN 1988**

A. Direct aortic-pulmonary anastomosis
B. Open heart definitive reconstruction
C. Pott's type anastomosis
D. Pulmonary artery bending

**169. Ca lung mainly metastasize to : AI 1996**

A. Liver B. Brain
C. Bone D. Skin

**170. The following may be useful in children undergoing mitral valvotomy except : AIIMS 1986**

A. Digoxin B. Oral anticoagulants
C. Antibiotics D. Vigorous exercises

**171. In patients who underwent upper abdominal surgery, post-operative pulmonary atelectasis occurs in : AMU 1990**

A. 100% B. 50%
C. 25% D. 10%

**172. Lung carcinoma and non-smoking indicates : AI 1996**

A. Multifactorial etiology
B. Unifactorial etiology
C. Unpredictable association
D. No association

**173. Pancoast tumor produces : AI 1996**

A. Marked Erythema B. Horner's syndrome
C. Monoplegia D. Hemiparesis

**174. Left atrial enlargement causes injuries to : AI 1996**

A. Right recurrent laryngeal nerve
B. Left recurrent laryngeal nerve
C. Bilateral recurrent laryngeal nerve
D. Any of the above

**175. The most common type of bronchogenic carcinoma is : DNB 1989; UP 1995; AI 1996**

A. Epidermoid B. Anaplastic
C. Alveolar D. Bronchiolar

**176. Contraindications to PEEP include all, except : UPSC 1987**

A. Pulmonary oedema B. Emphysema
C. Cardiogenic shock D. Pneumonia

**177. Treatment of flail chest include all, except : UPSC 1988**

A. Tracheostomy to reduce dead space.
B. Positive pressure respiration.
C. Traction on the broken fragments of ribs.
D. Internal fixation of fragments by wire.

**178. Treatment of 10% spontaneous pneumothorax is : AIIMS 1986**

A. Observation
B. Immediate thoracotomy
C. Tube thoracostomy
D. Endotracheal intubation

| Ans. | | | | | | | | | |
|---|---|---|---|---|---|---|---|---|---|
| **162. A** | **163. A** | **164. D** | **165. A** | **166. A** | **167. D** | **168. A** | **169. A** | **170. D** | **171. B** |
| **172. A** | **173. B** | **174. B** | **175. A** | **176. A** | **177. C** | **178. A** | | | |

**179. Prolonged post-operative respiratory support is better provided by : UPSC 1987**

A. Volume cycled respirators
B. Pressure cycled respirators
C. Both of the above are equal
D. Neither of the above

**180. Paradoxical respiration is seen in : UPSC 1996**

A. Flail chest
B. Tension pneumothorax
C. Empyema necessitans
D. Mediastinal emphysema

**181. Dyspnea, chest pain, hypoglycemia, hypertrophic pulmonary osteoarthropathy and a haemorrhagic pleural effusion is most likely in : AMU 1986**

A. Pulmonary tuberculosis
B. Alveolar cell carcinoma
C. Metastatic thymoma
D. Mesothelioma

**182. All are true with bronchial adenoma, except : Delhi 1987**

A. Uncommon benign tumours of the bronchus.
B. 10% of them are malignant.
C. 80% of them arise from a major bronchus.
D. They produce localized emphysema.

**183. Empyema necessitans is defined as a pleural empyema which : UPSC 1996**

A. Is under pressure
B. Has ruptured into the bronchus
C. Has ruptured into the pericardium
D. Is showing extension to the subcutaneous tissue

**184. The greatest incidence of bronchopleural fistula is following : Delhi 1988**

A. Segmental resection B. Lobectomies
C. Pneumonectomies D. Thoracotomy

**185. The most useful investigation in the diagnosis of bronchiectasis is : Delhi 1984**

A. Pulmonary angiography
B. Bronchography
C. Arterial blood gases
D. Lung scan

**186. Brochiogenic lung cysts are due to : AIIMS 1985**

A. Metastatic carcinoma
B. Klebsilla infection
C. Abnormal budding of the bronchial buds
D. Chest trauma

**187. Indications for coronary bypass operations include all of the following except : AIIMS 1983**

A. Severe angina not responding to medical therapy.
B. Occlusive disease of the left main coronary artery.
C. Triple vessel disease.
D. Previous infarction and congestive cardiac failure.

**188. Horner's syndrome associated with pain shoulder and arm is suggestive of : Delhi 1987**

A. Aortic aneurysm
B. Myocardial infarction
C. Cervical Spondylosis
D. Pancoast's tumour
E. Shoulder girdle syndrome

**189. Common cause of microabscesses in lungs includes : TN 1996**

A. Streptococcus B. Staphylococcus
C. Pneumococcus D. Klebsiella

**190. Hoarseness of voice when present alongwith a suspected abnormal mediastinal mass shadow is probably due to : AIIMS 1984**

A. Mediastinal lymphadenitis
B. An abscess in mediastinum
C. Aortic aneurysm
D. Carcinoma oesophagus

**191. Which of the following is not associated with pulmonary arterio-venous aneurysm : AIIMS 1984**

A. Haemoptysis B. Continous murmur
C. Skin pigmentation D. Polycythemia

**192. Which of the following often metastasizes to opposite lung: AIIMS 1985; Rohtak 1989**

A. Epidermoid carcinoma
B. Alveolar cell carcinoma
C. Adenocarcinoma
D. Carcinoid

**193. Muscle not cut in posterolateral thoracotomy is : PGI 1998**

A. Serratus ant. B. Latissimus dorsi
C. Rhomboid major D. Serratus posterior sup.

**194. All are features of Cardiac temponade, except : AMC 1985**

A. Week heart sounds
B. Paradoxical pulse
C. Low J.V.P
D. Increased cardiac dullness

**195. Chest tubes must not be inserted posterior to : PGI 1984**

A. Mid-axillary line B. Posterior axillary line
C. Anterior axillary line D. Mid clavicular line

| Ans. | | | | | | | | | |
|---|---|---|---|---|---|---|---|---|---|
| 179. A | 180. A | 181. D | 182. A | 183. D | 184. C | 185. D | 186. C | 187. D | 188. D |
| 189. B | 190. C | 191. C | 192. C | 193. C | 194. C | 195. B | | | |

**196. Intrabronchial foreign bodies may require which of the following : AIIMS 1984**

A. Bronchoscopy B. Bronchotomy
C. Lung resection D. All of the above

**197. The chemotherapy is most useful for : AIIMS 1984, 86**

A. Squamous cell carcinoma
B. Oat cell carcinoma
C. Adenocarcinoma
D. Neuroblastoma

**198. Best treatment for thoracic duct rupture is : AIIMS 1984**

A. Operative correction B. Fat emulsion
C. Observation D. Antibiotics

**199. Thoracotomy is best indicated in : AIIMS 1984, 85**

A. Cardiac temponade
B. Multiple fracture of ribs
C. Multiple fracture of ribs with hemothorax
D. Spontaneous pneumothorax

**200. Which of the following primaries do not produce a smooth secondary in lungs : PGI 1985; AIIMS 1985**

A. Seminoma B. Carcinoma lymph node
C. Carcinoma thyroid D. Carcinoma lung

**201. Multiple interstitial nodules are not seen in : AIIMS 1985, 86**

A. Miliary tuberculosis B. Tropical eosinophilia
C. Lobar pneumonia D. Asbestosis

**202. The following are recognised late complications of cardiac valve prosthesis replacement, except : AIIMS 1986**

A. Haemolytic anemia
B. Paravalvular leak
C. Bacterial endocarditis
D. Thromboembolic episodes

**203. Three most common symptoms of bronchogenic carcinoma are the following except : DNB 1991**

A. Cough with sputum for more than 2-3 weeks
B. Pain chest
C. Haemoptysis
D. Dyspnoea

**204. Addison's manoeuver is employed to detect : AIIMS 1986**

A. Thoracic outlet obstruction
B. Incompetent saphenofemoral junction
C. Site of AV malformation
D. Deep vein thrombus site

**205. Commonest cause of hydropneumothorax in our country is : AIIMS 1987**

A. Broncheogenic carcinoma
B. Sarcoidosis
C. Emphysematous bulla
D. Pulmonary tuberculosis

**206. Commonest indication for surgery in pectus excavatum is : AIIMS 1987**

A. Recurrent respiratory infections
B. Respiratory deficiency
C. Cosmetic reasons
D. Presses great vessels

**207. Mustard operation is often done for : AIIMS 1989**

A. PDA B. COA
C. TOF D. TGA

**208. Treatment of choice in severe flail chest is : UPSC 1984, 94; AIIMS 1985, 87, 93**

A. Inter costal block
B. Strapping + analgesics
C. Fixation of fractured ribs with wire
D. Intermittent positive pressure ventilation

**209. An infant achieves adult levels of Pulmonary vascular resistance and pulmonary artery pressure by the age of : DNB 1990**

A. Birth B. 1-3
C. 3-6 D. 6-12

**210. The cause of massive haemoptysis is : AMC 1985**

A. Tuberculosis
B. Viral pneumonia
C. Bronchiectasis
D. Bronchogenic carcinoma

**211. In thoracic outlet syndrome, following are true except : AIIMS 1998**

A. Neurological symptoms are common.
B. Radial nerve most commonly involved.
C. Posturing and physiotherapy relieves the symptoms.
D. Resection of 1st rib relieves symptoms.

**212. Most common cause of death in blunt trauma chest is : AIIMS 1998, 2000**

A. Tracheobronchial injury
B. Aspiration
C. Esophageal rupture
D. Pericardial effusion

**213. Most common type of diaphragmatic hernia is : JIPMER 1985, 87**

A. Bochdalek's hernia
B. Morgagni's hernia
C. Hernia through the dome
D. Hiatus hernia

| Ans. | 196. D | 197. B | 198. C | 199. C | 200. B | 201. C | 202. B | 203. B | 204. A | 205. C |
|---|---|---|---|---|---|---|---|---|---|---|
| | 206. C | 207. D | 208. D | 209. D | 210. C | 211. B | 212. A | 213. D | | |

**214. In pulmonary embolism, treatment is started when there is : AIIMS 1981; AMC 1984, 87**

A. Definite evidence of disease
B. Clinical suspicion of disease
C. Pain in the legs
D. None of the above

**215. Best treatment of tension pneumothorax is : PGI 1984**

A. Immediate letting out of air
B. Wait and watch
C. Rib resection
D. Underwater drainage

**216. Ectopic ACTH secretion by carcinoma bronchus is differentiated from Cushing's disease by : AIIMS 1986, 89**

A. Purple striae
B. Glucose intolerance
C. Centripetal obesity
D. Hypokalemia and calf pain

**217. Cavity formation in bronchogenic carcinoma occurs in : AIIMS 1985, 89**

A. Oat cell carcinoma
B. Squamous cell carcinoma
C. Adenocarcinoma
D. Bronchoalveolar carcinoma

**218. A 8 years old underdeveloped boy is seen because of signs of heart failure. He also has hypertension in the arm, but not in the legs and prominent notching of the lower rib margins. The most likely diagnosis is : AIIMS 1988**

A. Patent ductus arteriosus
B. Tetralogy of Fallot
C. Pulmonary stenosis
D. Coarctation of the aorta

**219. Open drainage of empyema is indicated only : PGI 1983, 92, 2002**

A. In streptococcal infections
B. When the pus is thick
C. When the mediastinum is fixed
D. In bilateral disease
E. When thoracostomy tube drainage is ineffective

**220. In an unconscious patient following multiple injuries resulting due to an accident after taking alcohol, the following is preferred : AMC 1983, 84, 87**

A. Endotracheal tube (uncuffed)
B. Endotracheal tube (cuffed)
C. Tracheostomy
D. Oropharyngeal tube

**221. Blood stained sputum may be the only symptom in : AI 1990**

A. Bronchiectasis
B. Carcinoma bronchus
C. Adenoma bronchus
D. Pulmonary TB

**222. Investigation of choice in pulmonary embolism is : AI 1990**

A. Chest X-ray
B. Ultrasound
C. CT Scan
D. Ventilation-perfusion scan

**223. Left ventricular failure is indicated if pulmonary artery wedge pressure exceeds : AIIMS 1984, 86**

A. 5 mmHg
B. 10 mmHg
C. 15 mmHg
D. 20 mmHg

**224. Bronchogenic carcinoma which produce paraneoplastic syndrome : Kerala 1987; AI 1988**

A. Squamous cell carcinoma
B. Oat cell carcinoma
C. Adenocarcinoma
D. Large cell carcinoma

**225. Treatment of recurrent pulmonary embolism in adults includes all except : PGI 1989**

A. Mobin Udin umbrella
B. Kimray Greenfield filter
C. Plication of IVC
D. Femoral thromboembolectomy

**226. Treatment of uncomplicated hydatid cyst in lung is : PGI 1989**

A. Marsupialisation
B. Lobectomy
C. Enucleation
D. Extended tube drainage

**227. Spontaneous rupture of a major bronchus would cause all except : AI 1994**

A. Massive pneumothorax
B. Haemothorax
C. Subcutaneous emphysema
D. Mediastinal emphysema

**228. In patient suspected to have suffered a pulmonary embolism, immediate primary treatment consists of : Karnataka 1987**

A. Pulmonary embolectomy
B. Infusion of streptokinase
C. Anticoagulant drugs
D. Inferior vena caval clipping

**Ans.** 214. B 215. A 216. D 217. B 218. D 219. C 220. B 221. C 222. D 223. D
224. B 225. C 226. C 227. B 228. B

**229. The clinical features of thoracic outlet syndrome include all of the following except : Karnataka 1987**
A. Paresthesia along the ulnar border
B. Ischaemic gangrene of the digits
C. Atrophy and wasting of the thenar eminence
D. Bruit in the neck

**230. Following an operation a pt. developed pulmonary rupture. Sign is : West Bengal 1994**
A. Dyspnoeic with slow pulse
B. Tachycardia
C. Haemoptysis
D. Asymptomatic

**231. Most common cause of acute mediastinitis is : AI 1997**
A. Oesophageal rupture
B. Tracheal rupture
C. Inflammation of thoracic vertebra
D. Fracture of ribs

**232. Quantitative estimation of Air embolism is by : AIIMS 1993**
A. Doppler
B. Pulmonary wedge pressure
C. End tidal $CO_2$ estimation
D. ECG

**233. Young male with accident - massive left sided haemothorax. Immediate treatment is : AIIMS 1993**
A. Tube thoracostomy
B. Strapping
C. Endotracheal intubation, IPPV and pleural aspiration
D. Observation

**234. All of the following are cavitating lesions of lung except : AIIMS 1994**
A. Sq. cell carcinoma
B. Caplan's syndrome
C. Hamartoma
D. Wegner's granulomatosis

**235. Commonest tumor to metastasise to heart is : AI 1995, 96**
A. Malignant melanoma
B. Bronchogenic carcinoma
C. Ca breast
D. Leomyosarcoma

**236. Common cause of SVC obstruction is : AI 1995**
A. Thrombosis
B. Extrinsic compression
C. Congenital web
D. Neoplastic encroachment

**237. Least likely cause of lung secondaries is : Kerala 1994; Rohtak 2001**
A. Ca breast B. Ca testis
C. Ca ovary D. Ca prostate

**238. Which is true regarding adenocarcinoma of lung : AIIMS 1994**
A. Cause 50% of lung cancers
B. More common in females
C. Associated with subcutaneous angio-myolipomas
D. Peripheral location

**239. Majority of lung cysts occur : AIIMS 1994**
A. Near the carina B. In Mediastinum
C. Peribronchial tissue D. Base

**240. Rastelli operation is often done for : DNB 1994**
A. TOF B. ASD
C. TGA D. MS
E. VSD

**241. Most common sign of aspiration pneumonitis : AIIMS 1994**
A. Tachypnea B. Bronchospasm
C. Cyanosis D. Crepitations

**242. Intralobar sequestration of lung gets its blood supply from : AIIMS 1994**
A. Descending aorta
B. Pulmonary artery
C. Internal mammary artery
D. None of the above

**243. B/L diphragmatic paralysis which is not true : AIIMS 1994**
A. Causes normocapnic failure
B. Shift test is positive in fluoroscopy
C. Diaphragmatic pacing may be helpful
D. None of the above

**244. Commonest complication of blunt injury thorax : AIIMS 1995**
A. Aortic rupture B. Pneumothorax
C. Haemopneumothorax D. # rib

**245. Rx of choice of post-operative lung collapse : AIIMS 1995**
A. Endoscopic suction B. Pulmonary resection
C. Corticosteroids D. Needle drainage

**246. C.V.P. (central venous pressure) and pulmonary wedge pressure give an accurate assessment of all of the following except : UPSC 1995**
A. Tissue perfusion B. Volume depletion
C. Volume overload D. Myocardial function

| Ans. | 229. C | 230. A | 231. C | 232. B | 233. C | 234. B | 235. A | 236. D | 237. D | 238. D |
|---|---|---|---|---|---|---|---|---|---|---|
| | 239. A | 240. C | 241. A | 242. A | 243. A | 244. D | 245. A | 246. A | | |

**247. A young female patient has been admitted following a road accident with complaints of pain in the right side of the chest. On examination she is found to have rapid and shallow breathing, a fast pulse rate and hyper-rosonant chest with absent breath sound on the right side. The most appropriate immediate course of action would be to : UPSC 1995**

A. Perform a diagnostic chest aspiration on right side and put in a chest tube.
B. Order for urgent chest X-ray and start oxygen.
C. Put the patient on positive pressure ventilation.
D. Send for the cardiothoracic surgeon for exploration of chest.

**248. Eventration of diaphragm does not occur in : AP 1993**

A. Vagotomy B. Post-lobectomy
C. Phrenic nerve palsy D. Mediastinal mass

**249. Commonest symptom associated with thoracic outlet syndrome is : AP 1993; AIIMS 1996**

A. Intermittent claudication
B. Pain in radial nerve distribution
C. Pain in ulnar nerve distribution
D. Gangrene

**250. Elective surgery after Myocardial infarction is done after : Delhi 1992; DNB 1993**

A. 2 months B. 3 months
C. 5 months D. 6 months

**251. The following are the indications for the tube thoracostomy of parapneumonic effusion, except : Orissa 1998**

A. Pleural fluid glucose level less than 50mg/dl.
B. Presence of gross amount of pus in the pleural space.
C. Organism visible on gram stain of pleural fluid.
D. Pleural fluid protein is more than 3gm/dl.

**252. A patient aspirated a foreign body in the standing position. Where is it likely to lodge : AIIMS 1999**

A. Right anterobasal B. Right medial basal
C. Right posterobasal D. Right lateral basal

**253. Commonest cause of Hypotension in fracture ribs (T10-T12) : AIIMS 1999**

A. Intercostal artery damage
B. Pulmonary confusion
C. Abdominal solid visceral organ injury
D. Damage to aorta

**254. In hiatus hernia with haematemesis, the cause is likely to be : AP 1999**

A. Reflux esophagitis B. Chr. duodenal ulcer
C. Variceal blood D. Chr. gastritis

**255. The commonest tumor associated with acquired pure red cell aplasia is : UPSC 2000**

A. Bronchogenic carcinoma
B. Hepatic carcinoma
C. Hodgkin's lymphoma
D. Thymoma

**256. A patient presents with respiratory distress, hypotension and dilated bulging neck veins after chest trauma. Most likely cause is : AIIMS 2000**

A. Hemothorax
B. Tension Pneumothorax
C. Flail chest
D. None of the above

**257. All of the following regarding Bochdalech hernia is true, except : AIIMS 2000**

A. Early respiratory distress leading to early diagnosis and treatment are good prognostic sign.
B. Common on left posterior side.
C. Stomach and transverse colon are commonest content to herniate.
D. Diagnosed prenatally by ultrasound.

**258. A patient having fever, heaviness in chest and difficulty in breathing was found to have pleural effusion, chest drain has to be put in. Most common site of drainage is : AIIMS 2000**

A. 2nd intercostal space midclavicular line.
B. 5th intercostal space just lateral to vertebral column.
C. 7th intercostal midaxillary line.
D. 5th intercostal space midclavicular line.

**259. After thyroid surgery, patient developed sudden respiratory distress, dressing was removed and it was found to be slightly blood stained and wound was bulging. First thing to do is : AIIMS 2000**

A. Remove the stitch and take the patient to O.T.
B. Laryngoscopy and intubation
C. Tracheostomy
D. Cricothyroidotomy

**260. Which of the following features denote a contraindication for surgical resection in a case of carcinoma lung : AIIMS 2000**

A. Malignant pleural effusion
B. Involvement of visceral pleura
C. Hilar lymphadenopathy
D. Consolidation of one lobe

| Ans. | | | | | | | | | |
|---|---|---|---|---|---|---|---|---|---|
| 247. A | 248. D | 249. C | 250. D | 251. D | 252. A | 253. A | 254. A | 255. D | 256. B |
| 257. A | 258. C | 259. A | 260. A | | | | | | |

**261. Lalloo, a 55 years old chronic smoker, presents with complaints of hoarseness of voice. On examination there is a single enlarged painless lymphnode in the left supraclavicular area. What is the next step to be done : AIIMS 2000**

A. Excision biopsy of the node
B. Laryngoscopy and chest X-ray
C. CT scan of chest
D. Sputum for AFB

**262. Minimum diameter required for bypass surgery is: MAHE 2001**

A. 3.5 mm B. 5 mm
C. 7 mm D. 1 cm

**263. True statement about thoracic outlet syndrome is : Delhi 2001**

A. Results from compression of brachial artery and brachial plexus.
B. Neurological symptoms are seen in distribution of C5 and C6.
C. Occurs due to compression of neurovascular bundle between insertion of anterior and middle scalenus muscle.
D. None of the above.

**264. 60 years old man with suspected bronchogenic Ca. TB has been ruled out in this patient. What investigation would be chosen : AI 2001**

A. CT guided FNAC
B. Bronchoscopy and biopsy
C. X-ray
D. Sputum examination

**265. Investigation of choice in a solitary pulmonary nodule is: AIIMS 2002**

A. High resolution CT scan
B. MRI
C. Contrast enhanced CT scan
D. Image guided FNAC

**266. Epithelium in Barret's mucosa is : AI 2002**

A. Ciliated columnar B. Columnar
C. Stratified squamous D. Squamous

**267. True adenocarcinoma of esophagus is most likely to be due to : AI 2002**

A. Achalasia
B. Barret's esophagus
C. Patterson Brown syndrome
D. Scleroderma

**268. The treatment modality of achalasia which has the maximum probability of causing a recurrence is : AI 2002**

A. Pneumatic dilatation B. Laparoscopic myotomy
C. Botulinum toxin D. Open surgical myotomy

**269. Clotted haemothorax is treated by : A.P. 2002**

A. Rib resection
B. Tube drainage
C. Injection of streptokinase
D. Surgery

**270. Consider the following statements : UPSC 2002**

1. Pharyngeal diverticulum is a protrusion of pouch through the neck defect called Killian's dehiscence.
2. It is initiated by imperfect relaxation of strap muscles.
3 It is common in mated & usually presents as a left sided neck swelling.
4. Cricopharyngeal myotomy is an essential compovent of its surgical procedure.

**Which of these statements are correct for pharyngeal diverticulum :**

A. 1, 2 & 4 B. 1, 3 & 4
C. 1, 2 & 3 D. 3 & 4

**271. The following are true about bronchogenic carcinoma, except : UPSC 2002**

A. It is the commonest malignant tumour in men.
B. One-Lung-Anaesthesia has improved results of surgery.
C. Most lung cancers are unresectable at presentation.
D. Small cell carcinoma carries better survival rate.

**272. A post-operative cardiac surgical patient developed sudden hypotension, raised central venous pressure, pulsus paradoxus at the 4th post-operative hour. The most probable diagnosis is : AI 2003**

A. Excessive mediastinal bleeding
B. Ventricular dysfunction
C. Congestive cardiac failure
D. Cardiac tamponade

**273. The classical triad of post-traumatic cardiac tamponade consists of : UPSC 2003**

A. Low BP low CVP, distant heart sounds.
B. High BP, high CVP, distant heart sounds.
C. Low BP, high CVP, distant heart sounds.
D. High BP, low CVP, distant heart sounds.

**274. 'Popcorn' calcification in a lung nodule is pathognomonic of : UPSC 2003**

A. Hamartomas B. Histoplasmosis
C. Tuberculosis D. Benign nodule

**Ans.** 261. B 262. A 263. C 264. B 265. A 266. B 267. B 268. C 269. D 270. B 271. D 272. D 273. C 274. A

**275. A 60 years old male was diagnosed as carcinoma right lung. On CECT chest there was a tumor of 5´ 5 cm in upper lobe and another 2 ´2 cms size tumor nodule in middle lobe. The primary modality of treatment is: AI 2004**

A. Radiotherapy B. Chemotherapy
C. Surgery D. Supportive treatment

**276. In which of the following conditions is Paradoxical respiration observed : UPSC 2004**

A. Stove-in-chest B. Flail chest
C. Pneumothorax D. Haemopneumothorax

**277. Poorest prognosis in lung cancer is associated with : COMEDK 2005**

A. Small cell carcinoma
B. Squamous cell carcinoma
C. Columnar cell carcinoma
D. Adenosquamous cell carcinoma

278. All are true regarding FLAIL Chest except :

A. Fracture of at least three ribs bilaterally
B. Paradoxical breathing is not seen in consicous patient
C. Patient should be intubated if PO2 is less than 40 % with 60 % oxygen
D. If overlapping is seen then it should be treated with open reducation

**Ans. 275. C 276. B 277. A 278. B**

# EXPLANATIONS OF CARDIOTHORACIC SURGERY

1. Ans.— A. Diversion of V.S.D. simultaneously with Mustard operation.
2. Ans.— B. Histoplasma
3. Ans.— B. Magnitude of the shunt
4. Ans.— C. Right coronary with right ventricle
5. Ans.— E. Congestive failure
6. Ans.— D. Dissecting aneurysm of the aorta
7. Ans.— A. Oesophagogram (barium swallow)
8. Ans.— D. 'Water lily' cyst
9. Ans.— D. Small cell carcinoma
10. Ans.— B. In the upper lobes, often represents healed tuberculous cavities.
11. Ans.— E. All of the above
12. Ans.— B. Bronchiectasis
13. Ans.— E. Melanoma

    Malignant melanoma spreads by lymphatic (to regional LN) and blood (to lungs, liver, brain, skin, and rarely bones, SI, heart, breast).
14. Ans.— B. Intercostal drainage through the second space.
15. Ans.— A. Stage 1 : active
16. Ans.— C. 100-150 mm water
17. Ans.— D. Increase of cardiac size, by X-ray
18. Ans.— C. 2 ml/min/100 gm
19. Ans.— B. Squamous cell carcinoma
20. Ans.— B. 10 to 50,000 RBC/microlitre
21. Ans.— D. Right lower lobe
22. Ans.— C. Tuberculous empyema

    Indications for surgery are :

    * Suspicious lesion on chest X-ray in which neoplasia can not be ruled out.
    * Chronic tubercular abscess, resistant to chemotherapy.
    * Aspergilloma in tuberculous cavity.
    * Life threatening hemoptysis.
23. Ans.— D. Lung tumor

    Radiotherapy is often indicated.
24. Ans.— D. Carcinoma thyroid
25. Ans.— A. Thymoma
26. Ans.— D. Reduction in the afterload
27. Ans.— B. Polio
28. Ans.— B. Rupture lung
29. Ans.— D. Neurofibroma
30. Ans.— D. Pneumomediastinum
31. Ans.— B. Has often spread into the pulmonary veins by the time of diagnosis.
32. Ans.— C. 10 ml/minute/100 gram
33. Ans.— B. Mild cyanosis
34. Ans.— C. Aspiration of foreign material

    In post-operative period, aspiration of saliva and gastric secretions is common.
35. Ans.— D. None of the above
36. Ans.— A. Anterior
37. Ans.— D. 20
38. Ans.— D. Abnormal hemoglobin
39. Ans.— D. Right ventricle
40. Ans.— C. Increased coughing in the upright position.
41. Ans.— D. Mesothelioma

    Asbestosis is a predisposing factor.
42. Ans.— E. All of the above
43. Ans.— E. Chronic pleural effusion
44. Ans.— A. Lobectomy
45. Ans.— C. Coccidiodomycosis
46. Ans.— B. Entamoeba histolytica
47. Ans.— B. Systemic antibiotic therapy

    It also requires surgery.
48. Ans.— D. Continued productive cough with purulent material.

49. Ans.— C. **Decreased Venous return**

50. Ans.— C. **Histoplasmosis**

51. Ans.— D. **Rupture of oesophagus**

52. Ans.— C. **Pulmonary hypertension with increased pulmonary vascular resistance.**

53. Ans.— B. **Pulmonary tuberculosis**

In developing countries, it is the most common cause.

54. Ans.— C. **Left ventricular failure**

55. Ans.— B. **3rd**

56. Ans.— B. **Ilio femoral vein**

57. Ans.— C. **Thoractomy**

58. Ans.— C. **Tetralogy of Fallot**

Subclavian artery is anastamosed to pulmonary artery.

59. Ans.— D. **Retroperitoneum region**

60. Ans.— D. **Recurrent laryngeal**

61. Ans.— A. **ASD**

62. Ans.— A. **2nd and 8th**

63. Ans.— D. **Turner's syndrome**

64. Ans.— B. **Posterior axillary line**

65. Ans.— D. **Adrenals**

66. Ans.— C. **5—7 days**

67. Ans.— C. **Neurofibroma**

Thymoma is most common mediastinal tumor (25%). It is commonest in Anterior mediastinum. Lymphoma is commonest in superior and cystic (Branchial cyst) in middle and neurogenic in posterior mediastinum.

68. Ans.— D. **Reversal of shunt**

69. Ans.— D. **Gross cardiomegaly**

70. Ans.— C. **ECG shows bundle branch block and left ventricular hypertrophy.**

71. Ans.— C. **2.5 cms**

72. Ans.— D. **Kidney rupture**

73. Ans.— B. **Egg shell calcification**

74. Ans.— B. **Right upper bronchus**

75. Ans.— A. **Resonant note on percussion with absent or decreased breath sounds.**

76. Ans.— B. **Pancoast tumour**

77. Ans.— C. **Asbestosis**

78. Ans.— D. **Carcinoma oesophagus (upper part)**

79. Ans.— B. **Short and broad**

80. Ans.— A. **Emphyema thoracic**

81. Ans.— B. **Permanent hoarseness**

82. Ans.— B. **Flatus passed**

83. Ans.— D. **Endoscopy**

84. Ans.— A. **Atelectasis**

85. Ans.— B. **Miliary tuberculosis**

86. Ans.— A. **Antibiotic agents, bronchoscopy and postural drainage.**

87. Ans.— D. **None of the above**

88. Ans.— B. **Neurofibroma**

89. Ans.— D. **All of the above**

90. Ans.— D. **Stage III — T2, N1, M1**

91. Ans.— B. **Atherosclerosis**

Atherosclerosis is the cause in 95% cases and 95% occur below the renal artery.

92. Ans.— D. **All of the above are true**

93. Ans.— D. **Two weeks**

94. Ans.— D. **Should be suspected if a consolidation lungs does not result with all possible treatment for chest infection.**

95. Ans.— D. **Aortic aneurysm**

96. Ans.— C. **Active bleeding**

97. Ans.— B. **Bronchogenic carcinoma**

98. Ans.— C. **Restlessness**

99. Ans.— A. **Cough**

100. Ans.— B. **Tracheal intubation and positive pressure ventilation.**

101. Ans.— C. **Pillows under the calf**

102. Ans.— B. **3-4 minutes**

103. Ans.— C. **Dyspnoea, pain, haemoptysis**

104. Ans.— B. **Sucking pneumothorax**

105. Ans.— D. **Dilated and fixed pupils**

106. Ans.— A. **Selection of wrong site**

107. Ans.— B. **Ventricular septal defect**

It is the commonest congenital cardiac abnormality and causes acyanotic disease whereas tetralogy of fallot is commonest cyanotic heart disease.

108. Ans.— B. **Pulmonary sequestration**

109. Ans.— D. **The low incidence of thromboembolism.**

110. Ans.— D. Right ventricular hypertrophy

111. Ans.— A. Pulmonary arteries

112. Ans.— C. 16th

113. Ans.— D. Posterior basal segment of lower lobe

114. Ans.— D. None of the above

115. Ans.— A. Left atrium

116. Ans.— D. Angina uncontrolled with medical means

117. Ans.— B. Pulmonary embolism

118. Ans.— A. Left subclavian artery and left pulmonary artery.

119. Ans.— C. Cardiac failure

120. Ans.— D. Surgical correction
CHF is most important complication.

121. Ans.— D. Notching of the ribs

122. Ans.— A. Hypertension

123. Ans.— D. Mitral and Aortic valves

124. Ans.— E. None of the above

125. Ans.— C. Bronchus

126. Ans.— A. 1 and 3 are correct

127. Ans.— D. Pericardiocentesis

128. Ans.— D. Rupture of Bulla
It is seen in emphysema.

129. Ans.— C. Tracheostomy

130. Ans.— A. Little specific treatment

131. Ans.— B. Intermittent positive pressure ventilation

132. Ans.— C. To allow bleeding vessel to seal

133. Ans.— B. Junction of mediastinal and hilar bronchus.

134. Ans.— D. Shock lung following heart lung bypass.

135. Ans.— B. 2nd, 3rd

136. Ans.— A. Tuberculous intercostal lymphadenitis.

137. Ans.— A. Anterior axillary line

138. Ans.— B. Absent carotid pulse
Myocardial infarction is commonest cause.

139. Ans.— C. 25°C

140. Ans.— B. Left pulmonary artery with aorta just distal to the origin of left subclavian artery.

141. Ans.— D. Ethyl alcohol (20%)

142. Ans.— B. Posterior costophrenic angle

143. Ans.— A. 5 ml

144. Ans.— C. Thoracotomy and suturing

145. Ans.— D. Teratoma

146. Ans.— B. Oesophageal hiatus hernia

147. Ans.— B. Appendicitis

148. Ans.— D. PDA

149. Ans.— C. Transposition of great vessels

150. Ans.— A. Mitral regurgitation

151. Ans.— C. Absolute and temporary

152. Ans.— D. 20-50 years

153. Ans.— D. Persistent congestive cardiac failure

154. Ans.— A. At the time of operation

155. Ans.— A. Tachycardia

156. Ans.— D. Suppurative bronchitis
Suppurative bronchitis can be controlled with drugs.

157. Ans.— D. Aortic aneurysm

158. Ans.— C. Raynaud's disease

159. Ans.— C. Carina

160. Ans.— A. Closed thoracostomy and tube drainage.

161. Ans.— NONE

162. Ans.— A. Chest wall instability

163. Ans.— A. Central lesions less than 2 cm in size

164. Ans.— D. Neither of the above malignant tendencies.

165. Ans.— A. Direct extension
Amoebia spread via inf. mesenteric vein and portal vein. It is common in upper and outer quadrant.

166. Ans.— A. Gram negative bacilli

167. Ans.— D. Atherosclerosis

168. Ans.— A. Direct aortic-pulmonary anastomosis

169. Ans.— A. Liver
Hilar lymph nodes are commonly involved whereas blood born metastases are to brain (85%), adrenals (45%), liver (45%) and bone (35%).

170. Ans.— D. Vigorous exercises

171. Ans.— B. 50%

172. Ans.— A. Multifactorial etiology

173. Ans.— B. Horner's syndrome
Due to involvement of branchial plexus.

174. Ans.— B. Left recurrent laryngeal nerve

It is common in mitral stenosis.

175. Ans.— A. Epidermoid

Three main types of Bronchogenic Ca are seen sq. cell Ca (epidermoid) 50%. Anaplastic (a) Small cell or/oat 15% (b) Large cell 5%.

176. Ans.— A. Pulmonary oedema

177. Ans.— C. Traction on the broken fragments of ribs.

In non-smokers, adenocarcinoma and in smokers, squamous cell carcinoma are common.

178. Ans.— A. Observation

179. Ans.— A. Volume cycled respirators

180. Ans.— A. Flail chest

181. Ans.— D. Mesothelioma

182. Ans.— A. Uncommon benign tumours of the bronchus.

183. Ans.— D. Is showing extension to the subcutaneous tissue.

184. Ans.— C. Pneumonectomies

185. Ans.— D. Lung scan

186. Ans.— C. Abnormal budding of the bronchial buds.

187. Ans.— D. Previous infarction and congestive cardiac failure.

188. Ans.— D. Pancoast's tumour

189. Ans.— B. Staphylococcus

190. Ans.— C. Aortic aneurysm

191. Ans.— C. Skin pigmentation

192. Ans.— C. Adenocarcinoma

193. Ans.— C. Rhomboid major

194. Ans.— C. Low J.V.P

Cardiac temponade may prove fatal if not immediately managed which is done by aspiration. It is done by a short Bevelled needle introduced along side of the xiphoid process in an upward and backward direction with needle at 45° to skin.

195. Ans.— B. Posterior axillary line

196. Ans.— D. All of the above

197. Ans.— B. Oat cell carcinoma

198. Ans.— C. Observation

199. Ans.— C. Multiple fracture of ribs with hemothorax.

200. Ans.— B. Carcinoma lymph node

201. Ans.— C. Lobar pneumonia

202. Ans.— B. Paravalvular leak

203. Ans.— B. Pain chest

204. Ans.— A. Thoracic outlet obstruction

205. Ans.— C. Emphysematous bulla

Commonest cause of pleural effusion is T.B.

206. Ans.— C. Cosmetic reasons

207. Ans.— D. TGA

208. Ans.— D. Intermittent positive pressure ventilation.

The initial treatment for flail chest is IPPV which is followed by fixation of the fractured rib (this can be done with stainless steel wire, Rush nails, judet clips).

209. Ans.— D. 6-12

210. Ans.— C. Bronchiectasis

Massive haemoptysis is seen bronchiectasis.

211. Ans.— B. Radial nerve most commonly involved

212. Ans.— A. Tracheobronchial injury

213. Ans.— D. Hiatus hernia

214. Ans.— B. Clinical suspicion of disease

215. Ans.— A. Immediate letting out of air

216. Ans.— D. Hypokalemia and calf pain

217. Ans.— B. Squamous cell carcinoma

218. Ans.— D. Coarctation of the aorta

219. Ans.— C. When the mediastinum is fixed

220. Ans.— B. Endotracheal tube (cuffed)

221. Ans.— C. Adenoma bronchus

Cough, recurrent haemoptysis are common and it arises peripherally. They are mainly carcinoid (80%).

222. Ans.— D. Ventilation-perfusion scan

223. Ans.— D. 20 mmHg

224. Ans.— B. Oat cell carcinoma

225. Ans.— C. Plication of IVC

226. Ans.— C. Enucleation

227. Ans.— B. Haemothorax

228. Ans.— B. Infusion of streptokinase

229. Ans.— C. Atrophy and wasting of the thenar eminence.

230. Ans.— A. Dyspnoeic with slow pulse

231. Ans.— C. Inflammation of thoracic vertebra

TB of Thoracic spine is a common cause.

232. Ans.— B. Pulmonary wedge pressure

233. Ans.— C. Endotracheal intubation, IPPV and pleural aspiration.

234. Ans.— B. Caplan's syndrome

235. Ans.— A. Malignant melanoma

Melanoma may also rarely spread.

236. Ans.— D. Neoplastic encroachment

237. Ans.— D. Ca prostate

238. Ans.— D. Peripheral location

239. Ans.— A. Near the carina

240. Ans.— C. TGA

241. Ans.— A. Tachypnea

242. Ans.— A. Descending aorta

243. Ans.— A. Causes normocapnic failure

244. Ans.— D. # rib

245. Ans.— A. Endoscopic suction

246. Ans.— A. Tissue perfusion

247. Ans.— B. Perform a diagnostic chest aspiration on right side and put in a chest tube

248. Ans.— D. Mediastinal mass

249. Ans.— C. Pain in ulnar nerve distribution

250. Ans.— D. 6 months

251. Ans.— D. Pleural fluid protein is more than 3gm/dl.

252. Ans.— A. Right anterobasal

253. Ans.— A. Intercostal artery damage

254. Ans.— A. Reflux esophagitis

255. Ans.— D. Thymoma

Thymoma is also associated with myaesthenia gravis.

256. Ans.— B. Tension Pneumothorax

257. Ans.— A. Early respiratory distress leading to early diagnosis and treatment are good prognostic sign.

258. Ans.— C. 7th intercostal midaxillary line

259. Ans.— A. Remove the stitch and take the patient to O.T.

260. Ans.— A. Malignant pleural effusion

261. Ans.— B. Laryngoscopy and chest X-ray

262. Ans.— A. 3.5 mm

263. Ans.— C. Occurs due to compression of neuro-vascular bundle between insertion of anterior and middle scalenus muscle.

264. Ans.— B. Bronchoscopy and biopsy

265. Ans.— A. High resolution CT scan

266. Ans.— B. Columnar

Epithelium in Barret's oesophagus is columnar and cause adenocarcinoma oesophagus.

267. Ans.— B. Barret's esophagus

Squamous cell type is commonest (in upper two thirds) and adenocarcinoma affects lower one third, Barret's oesophagus affects cardia of stomach and is premalignant.

268. Ans.— C. Botulinum toxin

Heller's operation is treatment of choice. Botulinum toxin acts by interfering with cholinergic excitatory neural activity at LOS and its effect waves off.

269. Ans.— D. Surgery

270. Ans.— B. 1, 3 & 4

271. Ans.— D. Small cell carcinoma carries better survival rate.

272. Ans.— D. Cardiac temponade

During Cardiac Surgery or post-operative patients cardiac surgery develops cardiac temponade as a common complication.

*Cardiac Temponade -*

* Low BP, High CVP (because of back pressure), pulsus paradoxus, tachycardia, faint heart-sounds.
* T/t - Emergency-Aspiration (from left side of xiphisternum).
* Then-Surgical Decompression (Median sternotomy midline approach, or Left Thoracotomy approach).

Note - Bullets in pericardial cavity should be removed under "Cardio-pulmonary Bypass."

**273. Ans.— C. Low BP, high CVP, distant heart sounds.**

**The accoumulation of fluid in the pericardium in an amount sufficient to cause serious obstruction to the inflow of blood to the ventricles is known as cardiac tamponade. The most common causes of tamponade are malignant disease idopathic pericarditis, and uremia. The three principles features of tamponade are elevation of intracardiac pressures, limitation of ventricular filling and reduction of cardiac output.**

**274. Ans.— A. Hamartomas**

***Hamartomas* are typically round; smooth, slightly lobulated peripheral masses < 4 cm in size without lobar predominance. Calcification is present in < 5% of cases. The typical pattern of "popcorn" calcification seen in chest X-ray is pathognomonic of hamartoma.**

**275. Ans.— C. Surgery**

**276. Ans.— B. Flail chest**

**277. Ans.— A. Small cell carcinoma**

# 8

# IMPORTANT TEXT OF OESOPHAGUS

## CLASSIFICATION OF OESOPHAGEAL MOTILITY DISORDERS

**Disorder of the pharyngo-oesophageal junction**
Stroke
Myasthenia
Cricopharyngeal 'achalasia'
**Disorders of the body of the oesophagus**
Diffuse oesophageal spasm
Nutracker oesophagus
**Hypoperistalsis**
Systemic sclerosis [CREST]
Reflux-associated
Idiopathic

**Allergic**
Eosinophilic oesophagitis
Non-specific oesophageal dysmotility

**Disorders of the lower oesophageal sphincter**
Achalsia
Hypertensive lower sphincter
Incompetent lower sphincter (i.e. GORD)

CREST : calcinosis, Raynaud syndrome, (o) oesophageal motility disorders, sclerodactyly and telangiectasia

## CARCINOMA OF OESOPHAGUS

* Squamous cell usually affects upper two thirds; adenocarcinoma usually affets lower third
* Common aetiological factors are tobacco and alcohol (squamous cell) and GORD (adenocarcinoma)
* Incidence of adenocarcinoma increasing
* Lymph node involvement, especially coeliac, is a bad prognostic factor
* Dysphagia is the most common presenting symptom, but is a late feature
* Increasing endoscopy rate has increased detection of earlier lesions with better prognosis
* Staging CT is essential; EUS, bronchoscopy and laparoscopy may be useful

## GASTRO-OESOPHAGEAL REFLUX DISEASE (GORD)

* GORD is due to loss of competence of LOS and is extremely common
* May be associated with a hiatus hernia, which may be sliding or less commonly rolling (para-oesophageal)
* Most common symptoms are heartburn and regurgitation, which are worse on stooping and lying
* Dysphagia may occur, but neoplasm must be eliminated
* Diagnosis should include endoscopy/24-h pH is gold standard
* Management is primarily medical but surgery may be required, laparoscopic fundoplication being the most popular technique
* Stricture may develop time

# MCQ's OF OESOPHAGUS

## What is important in Oesophagus

Oesophagus (Achalasia, Congenital Anomalies, Hiatus Hernia, Carcinoma, Rupture)

1. **Best diagnosis of tracheo-oesophageal fistula is by : Delhi 1989**
   A. Barium sulphate B. Conary 240
   C. Dianosil D. Urograffin
2. **All are premalignant conditions of oesophagus except : Rajasthan 1994**
   A. Varices
   B. Barret's oesophagus
   C. Achalasia cardia
   D. Plummer Vinson syndrome
3. **Dysphagia lusoria is due to : UPSC 1987; PGI 2000**
   A. An oesophageal diverticulum
   B. Oesophageal webs
   C. An aneurysm of the aorta
   D. Compression by aberrent great vessels
4. **Mallory-Weiss Syndrome is due to a mucosal tear of: AMC 1984**
   A. Pylorus B. Oesophagus
   C. Colon D. Duodenum
5. **Most common cause of benign strictures in oesophagus is : AMU 1985**
   A. Achalasia cardia
   B. Foreign body in oesophagus
   C. Strictures due to caustics & alkalies
   D. Congenital
6. **Maximum dilatation of oesophagus occurs in : Kerala 1994; Rohtak 2001**
   A. Carcinoma at gastroesophageal junction
   B. Achalasia cardia
   C. Stricture at lower end
   D. CREST syndrome
7. **True about carcinoma esophagus is : Kerala 1994; Rohtak 2001**
   A. Most common site of lower end
   B. Both adeno and squamous cell carcinoma occurs
   C. Commonest histology adenocarcinoma
   D. More common in females
8. **Which is true regarding Barret's oesophagus : AIIMS 1994**
   A. Squamous metaplasia of lower esophagus
   B. Seen mainly in females
   C. Premalignant
   D. Responds to conservative management
9. **Oesophagus and duodenum share : AIIMS 1995**
   A. Mucous cells
   B. Submucosal glands
   C. Pseudostratified columnar epith.
   D. All of the above
10. **True about Ca Esophagus : Delhi 1995**
    A. Multicentric
    B. Commonest in upper one third
    C. Submucosal spread not common
    D. Colon is used for reconstruction
11. **One of the following is true regarding Zenker's diverticulum : AI 1995**
    A. It is asymptomatic
    B. Occurs in the mid oesophagus
    C. Treatment is simple excision
    D. It occurs in young males
12. **In total oesophageal resection, best replacement is : PGI 1995**
    A. Jejunum B. Duodenum
    C. Ileum D. Transverse colon
13. **Pressure of oesophagus is ———. PGI 1995**
    A. 2 mm below the ambient pressure
    B. 7 mm below the ambient pressure
    C. 15 mm below the ambient pressure
    D. 20 mm above the ambient pressure

**Ans.** 1. C 2. A 3. D 4. B 5. C 6. B 7. B 8. C 9. B 10. D 11. C 12. A 13. B

**14. Adenocarcinoma oesophagus, following is true :** **AIIMS 1996**

A. Ba emulsion is used for diagnosis
B. Occurs mostly in lower 1/3rd
C. Upper 1/3rd commonly involved
D. Radiotherapy useful

**15. A 55-years old male has retro-sternal discomfort unrelated to physical exertion. Pain gets worse after lying down; there is partial relief with antacids. The most likely diagnosis is :** **UPSC 1996**

A. Ischaemic heart disease
B. Carcinoma oesophagus
C. Achalasia cardia
D. Hiatus hernia

**16. A neonate presenting with dribbling of saliva, diagnosis is :** **Delhi 1992**

A. Oesophageal atresia
B. Duodenal atresia
C. Tracheo oesophageal fistula
D. Choanal atresia

**17. Schatzki ring is :** **PGI 1998**

A. Mucosal ring at squamocolumnar junction
B. Muscular ring
C. Dysphasia alike for solids and liquids
D. Inflammatory stricture

**18. Esophageal burns are severe with :** **AP 1997**

A. $NaHCO_3$ B. NaOH
C. HCl D. Carbolic acid

**19. Commonest cause of death in Ca. oesophagus anastomosis by Ivor Lewis method is :** **AIIMS 1998**

A. Anastomatic leak
B. Anastomatic necrosis
C. Pulm. atelectasis
D. Myocarditis

**20. A male complains of foul-smelling regurgitation of food taken 2 days earlier. The likely diagnosis is :** **AIIMS 1999**

A. Achalasia cardia
B. Carcinoma esophagus
C. Pharyngeal pouch
D. Tracheoesophageal fistula

**21. True about Ca Esophagus :** **Delhi 1995**

A. Mostly stenotic.
B. Histology of tumour indicates prognosis.
C. Perirectal involvement is treated by local resection.
D. Spread to adjacent tissue affects the final prognosis after surgery.

**22. Esophageal carcinoma most commonly occurs at :** **Delhi 1983; AIIMS 1992**

A. Upper third B. Middle third
C. Lower third D. Post-cricoid region

**23. Gastro-esophageal reflex is best diagnosed by :** **AIIMS 1992; PGI 1994; AIIMS 1995**

A. Endoscopy B. Ultrasound
C. Barium meal D. Barium swallow

**24. Following are true of Achalasia cardia except :** **TN 1993**

A. Mostly occurs in women
B. Heller's operation is Rx of choice
C. Dilated esophagus narrowing inferiorly
D. Not premalignant

**25. In Oesophageal achalasia, which of the following is not true :** **UPSC 1994**

A. Pain on ingestion is rare.
B. Peristalsis in the oesophagus disturbed.
C. Dysphagia is usually the first symptom.
D. Ganglion cell in Auerbach's plexus in the oesophageal wall are absent.

**26. Indications of immediate primary repair of oesophageal atresia are following except :** **AMC 1985**

A. Weight of child above 2-2.5 kg.
B. Gap between distal and proximal oesophagus less than 2 cm.
C. Other congenital malformations.
D. No pulmonary complication.

**W.27. One endoscopy, the transition epithelial zone in the lower part of esophagus is termed as :** **PGI 1993, 94**

A. C-zone B. Z-zone
C. Barrett's zone D. Transition zone

**28. The most common cause of reflux oesophagitis is :** **AIIMS 1984**

A. Sliding hiatus hernia
B. Paraoesophageal hiatus hernia
C. Carcinoma of the oesophagus
D. Ectopic gastric mucosa in the oesophagus
E. Achalasia

**29. Oesophageal web is commonest in which portion :** **AMU 1986**

A. Proximal B. Middle
C. Distal D. Any of the above

**Ans.** **14. B** **15. D** **16. A** **17. A** **18. B** **19. A** **20. A** **21. B** **22. B** **23. A**
**24. D** **25. A** **26. C** **27. B, D** **28. A** **29. A**

30. **The most frequent cause of death in patient with tracheo-oesophageal fistula is : AIIMS 1985**
A. Vomiting
B. Malnutrition
C. Pulmonary complications
D. Other congenital anomalies
E. Diarrhoea

31. **Pulsion diverticulum of the oesophagus : AIIMS 1994**
A. Usually occurs in mid-oesophagus.
B. Has the neck of sac usually in midline.
C. It is true diverticulum with all oesophageal layers.
D. Is caused by pull of extrinsic inflammatory lesion.
E. Is usually small and not clinically significant.

32. **Gott's tetrad in cases of oesophageal rupture shows following, except : PGI 1984**
A. Pain in the lower chest
B. Cheyne stokes breathing
C. Vomiting and haematemesis
D. Respiratory distress and prostration
E. Subcutanous neck emphysema

33. **A 32-years-old man presents with a history of episodic dysphagia for solids. Typically, the episode occurs after swallowing a bolus of meat or bread, relief of the symptoms occurring only when the bolus is vomited. The most likely diagnosis is : MAHE 1996**
A. Achalasia cardia
B. Carcinoma of the cardio-oesophageal junction
C. Schatzki's ring
D. Zenker's diverticulum

34. **The most common site of spontaneous oesophageal perforation (Boerhaave's syndrome) is : AIIMS 1984**
A. Lower third B. Middle third
C. Upper third D. Near the cricothyroid
E. None of the above

35. **The ideal treatment of achalasia of oesophagus is : UPSC 1984**
A. Dilatation B. Oesophagomyotomy
C. Bypass procedure D. Vagotomy
E. Vagotomy and drainage

36. **Commonest cause of esophageal perforation is : PGI 1982**
A. Acid ingestion B. Hyperemesis
C. Instrumentation D. Carcinoma infiltration

37. **Commonest benign tumour of the esophagus is : AMU 1984; PGI 1985, 88**
A. Leiomyoma B. Papilloma
C. Adenoma D. Hemangioma

38. **Features of Achalasia cardia (Cardiospasm) include all of the following except : UPSC 1996**
A. Increasing difficulty in swallowing, more for liquids than for solids.
B. Regurgitant vomiting.
C. Dilated and elongated oesophagus.
D. Filling defect and "rat-tail" deformity on barium study.

39. **In a patient with swelling in neck, dyspnoea, dysphagia and gurgling, diagnosis is : Delhi 1983, 89**
A. Cervical lymphadenopathy
B. Incoordinate peristalis
C. Oesophageal web
D. Achalasia cardia

40. **Cardiospasm is a disease of : UPSC 1983**
A. Heart
B. Peripheral blood vessels
C. Oesophagus
D. Stomach
E. Pancreas

41. **Which is the least common type of congenital atresia of the oesophagus : AIIMS 1986**
A. Lower pouch opening into the trachea.
B. Upper pouches opening into the trachea.
C. Both pouches opening into the trachea.
D. Both pouches ending blindly.

42. **The following are the common causes of stenosis in lower third of oesophagus except : PGI 1984**
A. Congenital B. Oesophagitis
C. Ulceration D. Achalasia

43. **In isolated tracheoesophageal fistula the following are seen except : AMU 1990**
A. Excessive salvation B Choking with feeding
C. Pneumonia D. None of the above

44. **For bleeding varices of the oesophagus the common operation is/are : DNB 1989**
A. Portocaval shunt B. Gastrectomy
C. Splenectomy D. All of the above

45. **Tracheooesophageal fistula (congenital) may have all of the following presentations, except : Delhi 1994; MP 1994**
A. Regurgitation of all feeds
B. Continuous pouring saliva from mouth
C. Attacks of coughing, cyanosis on feeds
D. Bilious vomiting

| Ans. | | | | | | | | | |
|---|---|---|---|---|---|---|---|---|---|
| 30. C | 31. B | 32. B | 33. C | 34. A | 35. B | 36. C | 37. A | 38. C | 39. C |
| 40. C | 41. C | 42. A | 43. A | 44. A | 45. D | | | | |

**46. Regarding oesophageal varices which is not true : UPSC 1985**

A. Confined to oesophagus only
B. Can be diagnosed by splenoportography
C. Can be diagnosed by oesophagoscope
D. Can be treated by injection therapy

**47. Commonest symptom of oesophageal perforation is : AIIMS 1985, 90**

A. Pain B. Dysphagia
C. Respiratory distress D. Haematemesis

**48. The commonest type of presentation of carcinoma oesophagus is : AMC 1984; AIIMS 1985, 86, 87**

A. Stricturous growth B. Cauliflower growth
C. Infilterating growth D. Polypoid growth

**49. Commonest site of corrosive strictures is : AIIMS 1987**

A. Pharynx B. Oesophagus
C. Duodenum D. Stomach

**50. Corkscrew esophagus is characteristic of : AIIMS 1985; Delhi 1989**

A. Hiatus hernia
B. Achalasia cardia
C. Carcinoma oesophagus
D. Diffuse spasm of oesophagus

**51. The commonest congenital abnormality in oesophagus is : UPSC 1986; PGI 1987**

A. Upper end communicates with trachea and lower part ends blindly.
B. Upper pouch ends blindly and lower pouch communicates with trachea.
C. Both pouches communicate with trachea.
D. Opening in trachea and both pouches of oesophagus end blindly.
E. Cord like stricture.

**52. In Achalasia cardia, features are following except : PGI 1985, 90**

A. ↓ L.O.S. pressure
B. ↓ Myenteric neurons
C. Absence of air bubble in stomach
D. Presence of air fluid level in chest X-ray in up-right posture
E. Reflux esophagitis

**53. In majority of patients with oesophageal leaks in thoracic cavity of less than 12 hours duration, the treatment of choice is : UPSC 1997**

A. Primary closure, drainage and antibiotics
B. Early oesophagogastrostomy
C. Exclusion and diversion of continuity
D. Total oesophagectomy and gastric pull upper

**54. In a 32-years-old female, the least likely cause of dysphagia is : AMC 1986**

A. Achalasia cardia
B. Plummer Vinson syndrome
C. Oesophageal malignancy
D. Scleroderma

**55. The Sengstaken tube must maintain a pressure of —— to stop bleeding from varices. JIPMER 1987**

A. 20 mm Hg B. 25 mm Hg
C. 35 mm Hg D. 45 mm Hg

**56. Scleroderma commonly involves : JIPMER 1990; PGI 1995**

A. Stomach B. Duodenum
C. Esophagus D. Colon

**57. Which one of the following statements about neoplasia in the oesophagus is correct : UPSC 1994**

A. Benign tumours are more frequent than carcinomas.
B. Metastatic spread is not an important feature of carcinoma of the oesophagus.
C. Massive haematemesis is a feature of oesophageal carcinoma.
D. Adenocarcinomas of the proximal stomach can invade the lower end of the oesophagus and cause Dysphagia.

**58. A 32-years old woman had been troubled by progressive dysphagia for several years with the necessity to drink water to force food down. There had been no weight loss or loss of appetite but sometimes there was voluminous regurgitation after meals. Recently, there have been several bouts of pneumonia. The most likely diagnosis is : UPSC 1994**

A. Oesophageal hiatal hernia
B. Achalasia cardia
C. Carcinoma of oesophagus
D. Stricture of oesophagus

**59. Perforation of esophagus during instrumentation commonly occurs at the level of : JIPMER 1992**

A. Cricopharyngeal sphincter
B. Bronchial constriction
C. Aortic constriction
D. Diaphragm

**60. True about Achalasia cardia, except : MAHE 1999**

A. Absence of air bubble in stomach
B. Fluid levels seen
C. Cork screw appearance
D. Huge dilatation

**Ans.** 46. A 47. A 48. D 49. B 50. D 51. B 52. A 53. A 54. C 55. C
56. C 57. D 58. B 59. A 60. C

**61. Peptic oesophagitis : UPSC 2000**
A. Is effectively demonstrated by barium swallow.
B. Is always associated with hiatus hernia.
C. Can be readily confirmed by oesophagoscopy.
D. Is associated with the production of higher than normal amounts of gastric acid.

**62. Male aged 60 has foul breath, regurgitates food that is eaten 3 days back : AI 2001**
A. Zenker's diverticulum B. Meckel's diverticulum
C. Scleroderma D. Achalasia cardia

**63. Following are features of oesophageal rupture except : UP 2000**
A. Pain B. Fever
C. Bradycardia D. Low B.P.

**64. Patterson BrownKelly syndrome is characterized by all except : PGI 2000**
A. Lower oesophageal web
B. Iron deficiency anemia
C. Common in adult female
D. Premalignant

**65. In achalasia cardia, true is : PGI 2000**
A. Pressure at distal end ↑ with no peristalsis
B. Low pressure at LES with no peristalsis
C. Pressure > 50 mmHg with peristalsis
D. Pressure falls at distal end

**66. Heller's operation is performed for : AI 1990**
A. Pyloric stenosis
B. Achalasia cardia
C. Peptic ulcer
D. Carcinoma of the oesophagus

**67. Achalasia cardia is : AI 1991**
A. A motor disorder due to failure of relaxation of lower oesophageal sphincter
B. An inborn error of metabolism
C. Infective in origin
D. Related to dietary deficiency of Vit. A

**68. A company executive presents with hemetemesis of about 5 L of bright red blood. His previous history is normal, most likely cause of bleeding is : AI 2000**
A. Duodenal ulcer B. Gastritis
C. Variceal bleeding D. Oesophagitis

**69. Most common site for squamous ca. esophagus : PGI 1994; AI 2001**
A. Upper-third
B. Mid-third
C. Lower-third
D. Cricoesophageal junction

**70. Adenocarcinoma of esophagus is commonest in : AIIMS 2000; AI 2001**
A. Uppe- one-third
B. Children
C. Barrett's esophagus
D. Plummer Vinson syndrome

**71. Not used for acute variceal bleed : Punjab 1997; MAHE 2001**
A. Propranolol B. Vasopressin
C. Somatostatin D. Balloon temponade

**72. A patient came with history of dysphagia with recurrent chest infections and was diagnosed to have an esophageal diverticulum at the level of the cricopharyngeus. The treatment of choice is : AIIMS 2001**
A. Cricopharyngeal myotomy alone
B. Excision of the sac and myotomy
C. Laser vaporization of the sac
D. Marsupialization of the sac

**73. Which is true for scleroderma's effects on esophagus : Kerala 2001**
A. Normal LES & UES, decreased peristalsis.
B. Decreased tone & UES, normal LES, decreased peristalsis.
C. Normal UES, decreased LES, normal peristalsis.
D. Normal UES, decreased LES tone & decreased peristalsis.

**74. True adenocarcinoma of esophagus is most likely to be due to : AI 2002**
A. Achalasia
B. Barrett's esophagus
C. Patterson Brown syndrome
D. Scleroderma

**75. The treatment modality of achalasia which has the maximum probability of causing a recurrence is : AI 2002**
A. Pneumatic dilatation B. Laparoscopic myotomy
C. Botulinum toxin D. Open surgical myotomy

**76. The confirmatory diagnostic feature of congenital atresia of the oesophagus is : UPSC 2005**
A. Regurgitation of feed
B. Continuous pouring of saliva
C. Attacks of coughing and cyanosis
D. Obstruction to passage of a nasogastric tube about 10 cm from the lips

| Ans. | 61. C | 62. A | 63. C | 64. A | 65. A | 66. B | 67. A | 68. C | 69. B | 70. C |
|---|---|---|---|---|---|---|---|---|---|---|
| | 71. A | 72. B | 73. D | 74. B | 75. C | 76. D | | | | |

# EXPLANATIONS OF OESOPHAGUS

1. Ans.— C. Dianosil
2. Ans.— A. Varices
3. Ans.— D. Compression by aberrent great vessels
4. Ans.— B. Oesophagus
5. Ans.— C Strictures due to caustics & alkalies
6. Ans.— B. Achalasia cardia
7. Ans.— B. Both adeno and squamous cell carcinoma occurs.
8. Ans.— C Premalignant
9. Ans.— B. Submucosal glands
10. Ans.— D. Colon is used for reconstruction
11. Ans.— C. Treatment is simple excision
    Cervical pulsion diverticulum is called pharyngeal pouch or Zenker's diverticulum.
12. Ans.— A. Jejunum
13. Ans.— B. 7 mm below the ambient pressure
14. Ans.— B. Occurs mostly in lower 1/3rd
15. Ans.— D. Hiatus hernia
16. Ans.— A. Oesophageal atresia
17. Ans.— A. Mucosal ring at squamocolumnar junction.
    This is thin submucosal web completely encircling the whole of the lumen situated near the middle of lower sphincter.
18. Ans.— B. NaOH
19. Ans.— A. Anastomatic leak
20. Ans.— A. Achalasia cardia
21. Ans.— B. Histology of tumour indicates prognosis
22. Ans.— B. Middle third
    Squamous cell carcinoma is commonest in middle one third and adenocarcinoma is commonest in lower one third (Some books mention commonest site as middle one third (BL-661) and some as lower one third (CSDT-434).
23. Ans.— A. Endoscopy
24. Ans.— D. Not premalignant
25. Ans.— A. Pain on ingestion is rare
26. Ans.— C. Other congenital malformations

W27. Ans.— B. Z-zone
D. Transition zone

28. Ans.— A. Sliding hiatus hernia
    For acute oesophagitis, following burns or scalds, infective or peptic or indwelling stomach tube or chronic - most important cause is reflux of acid gastric juices due to a sliding hiatus hernia. Alkaline juices reflex due to oesophagodudenostomy or oesophagoje junostomy. It is common in pregnancy.
29. Ans.— A. Proximal
30. Ans.— C Pulmonary complications
31. Ans.— B. Has the neck of sac usually in midline
32. Ans.— B. Cheyne-stokes breathing
33. Ans.— C Schatzki's ring
34. Ans.— A. Lower third
    Full thickness rupture is Boerhaave's syndrome, as a result of vomiting with a full stomach. A longitudinal tear in the lower oesophagus leads to mediastinitis and a left pleural effusion. Partial thickness mucosal rupture is seen in Mallory Weiss syndrome.
35. Ans.— B. Oesophagomyotomy
36. Ans.— C. Instrumentation
    Iatrogenic or injuries is commonest cause. Often the perforation goes unrecognized. If cervical oesophagus is required, it is closed in 2 layers and if, mid or lower oesophagus is involved, thoracotomy
37. Ans.— A. Leiomyoma
38. Ans.— C. Dilated and elongated oesophagus
39. Ans.— C. Oesophageal web

40. Ans.— C. Oesophagus

41. Ans.— C. Both pouches opening into the trachea

42. Ans.— A. Congenital

43. Ans.— A. Excessive salvation

44. Ans.— A. Portocaval shunt

45. Ans.— D. Bilious vomiting

46. Ans.— A. Confined to oesophagus only

47. Ans.— A. Pain

48. Ans.— D. Polypoid growth

49. Ans.— B. Oesophagus

50. Ans.— D. Diffuse spasm of oesophagus

51. Ans.— B. Upper pouch ends blindly and lower pouch communicates with trachea.

52. Ans.— A. ↓ L.O.S. pressure

53. Ans.— A. Primary closure, drainage and antibiotics.

54. Ans.— C. Oesophageal malignancy

55. Ans.— C. 35 mm Hg

56. Ans.— C. Esophagus

Scleroderma is a collagen disease usually occurring in females and presenting with skin changes (esp. seen on fingers of hands) and Raynaud's phenomenon. There are smooth muscle changes both in the small arterial walls and in the esophagus and small bowel. Radiologically there is dilatation of oesophagus.

57. Ans.— D. Adenocarcinomas of the proximal stomach can invade the lower end of the oesophagus and cause Dysphagia.

58. Ans.— B. Achalasia cardia

59. Ans.— A. Cricopharyngeal sphincter

60. Ans.— C. Cork screw appearance

61. Ans.— C. Can be readily confirmed by oesophagoscopy.

62. Ans.— A. Zenker's diverticulum

63. Ans.— C. Bradycardia

64. Ans.— A. Lower oesophageal web

65. Ans.— A. Pressure at distal end ↑ with no peristalsis

66. Ans.— B. Achalasia cardia

The essential treatment of achalasia cardia is disruption of constricting fibres of the cardia either from without (by Heller's opn.) or within (by Negus hydrostatic bag).

67. Ans.— A. A motor disorder due to failure of relaxation of lower oesophageal sphincter.

68. Ans.— C. Variceal bleeding

Variceal bleeding (due to alcoholism) is common in the executive with past history normal.

69. Ans.— B. Mid third

Most common site of Sq. cell carcinoma is middle third and the leading symptom is dysphagia.

70. Ans.— C. Barrett's esophagus

The main complications of Barrett's esophagus are high peptic stricture or adenocarcinoma anywhere along the whole length of columnar epithelium. In both the presenting symptom is dysphagia Adenocarcinoma is common in lower-third esophagus.

71. Ans.— A. Propranolol

72. Ans.— B. Excision of the sac and myotomy

73. Ans.— D. Normal UES, decreased LES tone & decreased peristalsis.

Epithelium in Barret's oesophagus is columnar and cause adenocarcinoma oesophagus.

74. Ans.— B. Barrett's esophagus

Squamous cell type is commonest (in upper two-thirds) and adenocarcinoma affects lower one-third. Barrett's oesophagus affects cardia of stomach and is premalignant.

75. Ans.— C. Botulinum toxin

Heller's operation is treatment of choice. Botulinum toxin acts by interfering with cholinergic excitatory neural activity at LOS and its effect wanes off.

76. Ans.— D. Obstruction to passage of a nasogastric tube about 10 cm from the lips.

# 9

# IMPORTANT TEXT OF STOMACH

## COMMON EXAMPLES OF ACUTE ABDOMINAL PAIN

| | *Peptic Ulcer* | *Acute Cholecystitis* | *Acute Pancreatitis* | *Ureteric Colic* |
|---|---|---|---|---|
| *Main site* | Epigastrium | Epigastrium or Rt. hypochond. | Epigastrium | From loin to groin |
| *Radiation* | Sometimes into the back | Beneath R. scapula R. shoulder tip | Into the back May become generalised | Into scrotum or labia |
| *Character* | Gnawing | Constant once | Sudden onset maximal | Constant Constant |
| *Severity* | Mild to moderate | Moderate to severe | Very severe | Very severe |
| *Duration* | 1/2-3 hours | Usually several hours | Days | Usually hours |
| *Frequency & periodicity* | Remissions for weeks or months. | Unpredictable | Unpredictable | — |
| *Special times of occurrence* | Between meals | — | — | — |
| *Aggravating factors* | Irregular meals Smoking | — | After alcohol or heavy meals | Dehydration Previous infection of urine |
| *Relieving factors* | Food, antacids Vomiting | — | May be eased by sitting upright | — |
| *Associated phenomena* | Family history. G.I. haemorrhage Perforation | Restless & vomiting Jaundice | Gallstones Paralytic ileus | Restless & vomiting Haematuria |

## COMPLICATIONS OF GASTRIC SURGERY

*Early*

1. Haemorrhage
2. Paralytic ileus
3. Stomal obstruction
4. Duodenal fistula
5. Acute post. operative pancreatitis
6. Post. gastrectomy syndromes
7. Int. obstruction
8. Pulmonary T.B.
9. Anaemia
10. Carcinoma
11. Gallstones

*Late :*

1. Recurrent ulcer
2. Gastro-jejuno-colic fistula

# MCQ's OF STOMACH

## What is important in Stomach

Stomach (Blood and Lymphatic supply, Investigations, Ulcer, Tumors)

1. **The following are the complications of Ramstedt's operation except : Rohtak 1986**
   A. Pyrexia
   B. Gastroenteritis
   C. Disruption of wound
   D. Renal failure
2. **The peak incidence of onset of symptoms in hypertrophic pyloric stenosis of infants is at the age of : Kerala 1989**
   A. 1-2 weeks B. 2-3 weeks
   C. 3-6 weeks D. 9-12 weeks
3. **The appropriate time for correction of congenital pyloric stenosis of infants is : AP 1989**
   A. Immediately B. At 1 year of age
   C. At 3 months of age D. At 3 years of age
4. **Atropine methylnitrate was introduced in the treatment of congenital pyloric stenosis by —— in 1935. AMU 1988**
   A. Ramstedt B. Hellar
   C. E. Svensgaard D. William E. Ladd
5. **The vomit in congenital atresia of duodenum differs from that in congenital pyloric stenosis of infants. It is : AMU 1989**
   A. Regurgitant B. Projectile
   C. Contains bile D. Not always present
6. **Which of the following is the most essential step in reaching the diagnosis of hypertrophic stenosis of infants : AIIMS 1986**
   A. Constipation
   B. Vomiting
   C. Visible peristalsis
   D. Palpation of hypertrophic pylorous
7. **A 45-years-old man presented with intractable peptic ulcers, gastric hyperacidity and diarrhoea. These symptoms did not respond to aggressive anti-peptic ulcer therapy. Elevated levels of gastrin were demonstrated in the serum. At exploratory laparotomy, a tumour was found. In which of the following anatomical locations was the tumour likely to have been found : MAHE 1995**
   A. Stomach B. Duodenum
   C. Pancreas D. Small intestine
8. **Which of the following statements about acute erosive ulceration of the stomach and/or duodenum is false : MAHE 1996**
   A. It is a recognised sequel of head injury.
   B. It usually presents with upper gastrointestinal haemorrhage.
   C. It can be prevented by giving $H_2$ receptor blockers.
   D. When medical treatment fails, it responds well to surgery.
9. **Which of the following is diagnostic of carcinoma stomach : Delhi 1983**
   A. Bleeding per rectum B. Plain X-ray abdomen
   C. Barium meal D. Gastroscopy
10. **Carcinoma stomach at the pyloric end in a manageable condition should be managed by : Delhi 1986**
    A. Upper radical partial gastrectomy
    B. Lower radical partial gastrectomy
    C. Gastro-jejunostomy
    D. Radiotherapy
11. **Presenting symptom of carcinoma stomach is : AIIMS 1987**
    A. Weight loss B. Perforation
    C. Bleeding D. Obstruction

**Ans.** 1. D 2. C 3. A 4. C 5. C 6. D 7. C 8. D 9. D 10. B 11. A

12. **Of the serious complications that are likely to arise after gastric resection, the most common is : PGI 1982**

A. Thrombophlebitis
B. Blowout of the duodenal stump at 4th day
C. Sepsis and haemorrhage
D. Lung complication

13. **All of the following are true of leimyosarcoma of the stomach except : CSE 1995**

A. Histological diagnosis is easily obtained by endoscopic biopsy.
B. They are asymptomatic until they become very large.
C. They commonly present with pain and occult or massive haemorrhage.
D. They arise more commonly from the proximal stomach.

14. **Krukenberg tumour of ovary arises from : AIIMS 1987**

A. Breast B. Stomach
C. Liver D. Rectum

15. **The treatment of Hodgkin's disease of stomach is : NIMHANS 1986**

A. Gastric resection
B. Gastric resection and chemotherapy
C. Purely medical
D. None of the above

16. **Rx of gastric adenocarcinoma is : PGI 1986; AIIMS 1990**

A. Surgery with Chemotherapy
B. Chemotherapy
C. Radiotherapy/Chemotherapy
D. Preoperative RT with surgery

17. **Which of the following does not need drainage operation : PGI 1986**

A. Truncal vagotomy
B. Highly selective vagotomy
C. Selective vagotomy
D. Partial gastrectomy

18. **Consider the following statements : CSE 1995**
**In carcinoma of the stomach :**

1. A fixed abdominal lump indicates inoperability.
2. Radiotherapy offers a good chance of cure.
3. In advanced disease, paliative resection is better than palliative bypass operation.

A. 1,2 and 3 are correct B. 1 and 2 are correct
C. 2 and 3 are correct D. 1 and 3 are correct

19. **Diarrhoea following truncal vagotomy is due to : Delhi 1998**

A. Increased gastric emptying
B. Increased small bowel activity
C. Decreased absorption of fat
D. Gastric mucosal atrophy

20. **Which of the following is true about Zollinger Ellison syndrome : Delhi 1998**

A. Increased basal acid output and further increase by histamine.
B. Increased basal acid output and no further increase by histamine.
C. Decreased basal acid output and increased by histamine.
D. Decreased basal acid output and is not increased by histamine.

21. **Hour glass deformity of the stomach is seen in : AIIMS 1992**

A. Gastric ulcer B. Gastric carcinoma
C. Gastric lymphoma D. Corrosive strictures

22. **The most common benign tumor of the Stomach is : PGI 1993, 95, 97**

A. Leiomyoma B. Adenoma
C. Hamartoma D. Lipoma

23. **Most common site of Carcinoma stomach is : UPSC 1985; PGI 1987, 93; Delhi 1986, 91, 97**

A. Fundus B. Pylorus
C. Antrum D. Cardia

24. **Erosive gastritis can predispose to Carcinoma stomach at following sites except : JIPMER 1993**

A. Lesser curvature B. Antrum
C. Body D. Fundus

25. **Treatment of Zollinger Ellison syndrome is : TN 1993**

A. Total gastrectomy
B. Partial gastrectomy
C. Excision of tumor alone
D. $H_2$ receptor antagonist

26. **Immediate complication of Truncal vagotomy and gastrojejunostomy is : TN 1993**

A. Loss of motility
B. Diarrhoea
C. Small intestinal muscle hypertrophy
D. Anastomotic leak

27. **Most common cause of weight loss following Gastrojejunostomy is : TN 1993**

A. Poor appetite
B. Afferent loop syndrome
C. Diarrhoea
D. Dumping syndrome

| Ans. | | | | | | | | | |
|---|---|---|---|---|---|---|---|---|---|
| 12. B | 13. A | 14. B | 15. B | 16. A | 17. B | 18. D | 19. B | 20. B | 21. A |
| 22. A | 23. B | 24. D | 25. C | 26. D | 27. A | | | | |

**28. Which of the following is more common in the first born child : TN 1993**

A. Duodenal atresia
B. Congenital pyloric stenosis
C. Congenital megacolon
D. Renal agenesis

**29. Gastric ulcer occurs most commonly in the : TN 1993; AI 2001**

A. Pylorus B. Fundus
C. Antrum D. Cardia

**30. Which of the following gastric tumor is most likely to bleed : Delhi 1993**

A. Fibromyosarcoma B. Gastric lymphoma
C. Carcinoid D. Adenocarcinoma

**31. Gastric cancer : MAHE 1992**

A. Most commonly occurs in the fundus of the stomach.
B. Is most commonly a squamous cell carcinoma.
C. Frequently metastasis via the blood stream.
D. Is most frequently an ulcerating lesion.

**32. Which of the following is not true about uncomplicated benign gastric ulcers : UPSC 1983**

A. Commonly recur after medical treatment.
B. Should receive surgical treatment if healing has not occurred after 4 to 6 weeks of medical treatment.
C. Occur most commonly on the greater curvature.
D. Should initially be treated medically.

**33. Normal pyloric canal is —— mm long and in congenital hypertrophic pyloric stenosis it is usually greater than —— mm. AIIMS 1984**

A. 4, 6 B. 10, 14
C. 14, 17 D. 17, 20

**34. Gastric mucosa normally reverses itself every after —— days. AMU 1987**

A. 10 B. 30
C. 50 D. 70

**35. After closure of a perforated duodenal ulcer, a 50-years old man has been maintained on gastric suction for seven days and has been receiving 5% dextrose in water, normal saline and vitamins as intravenous therapy. The average daily volume of gastric aspirate is 1500 ml/day. The patient has developed adynamic ileus and is extremely weak and lethargic. The most likely abnormality is : UPSC 1998**

A. Metabolic acidosis
B. Low serum magnesium level
C. Low serum sodium level
D. Hypokalaemic alkalosis

**36. Which disease state is not associated with an increase in incidence of peptic ulceration : UPSC 1983**

A. Chronic, pulmonary emphysema
B. Laennec's cirrhosis
C. Crohn's disease
D. Parathyroid hyperplasia
E. Zollinger-Ellison tumour

**37. In pernicious anemia, carcinoma stomach is commonest in : Delhi 1984**

A. Prepylorus B. Fundus
C. Lesser curvature D. Cardiac end

**38. The operation of choice for carcinoma of the distal 2/3rd of the stomach is : UPSC 1984**

A. Antrectomy
B. Subtotal gastrectomy
C. Total gastrectomy
D. Wedge resection of the lesion
E. Any of the above

**39. All of the following are risk factors for cancer stomach except : Delhi 1994**

A. Pernicious Anaemia
B. Hyperacidity
C. Post-gastrectomy stomach
D. Post-truncal vagotomy stomach

**40. Surgery in peptic ulcer is indicated in the following except : AMU 1987**

A. Bleeding ulcer B. Duodenal obstruction
C. Perforation D. Curling's ulcer

**41. The signs of inoperateble gastric cancer are : DNB 1990**

A. Virchow's nodes
B. Liver metastasis
C. Mobile subpyloric nodes
D. All of the above

**42. The following is true of pyloric stenosis except : DNB 1990**

A. It results a healed duodenal ulcer
B. Visible peristalsis of stomach
C. Pyloric mass is felt
D. Vomiting of previous day's food ingested

**43. The best method to estimate gastric acid secretion is: Delhi 1983**

A. F.T.M. B. Night secretion
C. Pentagastrin test D. A.H.T.

**44. Regarding hourglass stomach, untrue is : AIIMS 1984**

A. It mostly occurs in men
B. It is usually silent
C. A Billroth-I gastrectomy is required
D. Weight loss is very great

| Ans. | 28. B | 29. B | 30. A | 31. A | 32. C | 33. C | 34. B | 35. D | 36. C | 37. B |
|---|---|---|---|---|---|---|---|---|---|---|
| | 38. B | 39. B | 40. D | 41. D | 42. A | 43. C | 44. A | | | |

**45. Which of the following is not related clinically or pathologically to carcinoma of the stomach : UP 1991**

A. Blood group-O B. Trousseau's sign
C. Linitis plastica D. Krukenberg tumours

**46. The prognosis following resection of carcinoma of the stomach is determined by : PGI 1985**

A. The extent of stomach removed
B. The margin of apparently healthy stomach removed above the growth
C. A short clinical history
D. The histology of the growth

**47. The post-gastrectomy "dumping" syndrome is due to : AIIMS 1985**

A. Hypoglycaemia
B. Serotonin release
C. Sudden hypovolaemia
D. Small gastric pouch
E. Dumping of hypertonic material into jejunum

**48. Diverticulum of the stomach : UPSC 1986**

A. Pain is the main symptom
B. Usually at cardiac end
C. Usually on posterior surface
D. inversion is the satisfactory treatment
E. All of the above

**49. Which of the following is true about hypertrophic pyloric stenosis : UPSC 1984**

A. The musculature of the pyloric antrum is atrophied.
B. First born female infants are most commonly affected.
C. The cause is unknown.
D. None of the above.

**50. The following are the common presentations of adenomatous polyp in stomach except : AIIMS 1984**

A. Bleeding
B. Abdominal pain
C. Vomiting (bile stained)
D. Achlorhydria

**51. The following is premalignant potential of adenomatous polypus of stomach : PGI 1985**

A. Multiple
B. Associated pernicious anaemia
C. Recurrence
D. All of the above

**52. Post-Vogotomy diarrhoea can be effectively managed by : UPSC 2001**

A. Steroids B. Thyroxin
C. Somatostatin analogue D. Parathormone

**53. In congenital pyloric stenosis, the defect usually less in ——of antrum. PGI 1983**

A. Never fibres
B. Circular muscle fibres
C. Longitudinal muscle fibres
D. Mucosa

**54. The following indicate the premalignant potential of adenomatous polypus of stomach : AIIMS 1982**

A. Multiple
B. Associated Pernicious anaemia
C. Recurrence
D. All of the above

**55. All of the following are indications for gastroduodenoscopy except : UPSC 1986**

A. For differential diagnosis between chronic peptic ulcers and a carcinoma.
B. Diagnosis of shallow gastric ulcer which does not show on radiography.
C. To assess results of medical treatment of peptic ulcer.
D. For taking biopsy from the duodenum.

**56. The following are common presentations of trichobezoar except : AMU 1990**

A. Vomiting B. Lump in epigastrium
C. Loss of weight D. Gall stones

**57. An important predisposing factor in volvulus of the stomach is : AMU 1988**

A. Trauma
B. Eventation of the diaphragm
C. Absence of Auerbach's plexus
D. Prematurity

**58. After Ramstedt's operation for congenital pyloric stenosis, first feed (not more than 5 ml) is given : Rohtak 1986; AIIMS 1986, 87**

A. Immediately B. After one hour
C. After 24 hours D. After 1 week

**59. If the mucosa was accidentally opened at operation (Ramstedt), it is wise not to feed the child orally for : AMU 1990**

A. 12 hours B. 24 hours
C. 48 hours D. 1 week

**60. The commonest aetiological factor in trichobezoar is : AIIMS 1985**

A. Worm infestation
B. Diabetes mellitus
C. Congenital defect in pyloric antrum
D. Psychological disturbances

| Ans. | 45. A | 46. D | 47. E | 48. E | 49. C | 50. C | 51. D | 52. C | 53. B | 54. D |
|---|---|---|---|---|---|---|---|---|---|---|
| | 55. D | 56. D | 57. B | 58. B | 59. C | 60. D | | | | |

**61. The most useful method to diagnose cause of upper GI haemorrhage is : UPSC 1984**

A. Barium study B. Celiac angiography
C. Gastric biopsy D. Endoscopy

**62. Which of the following statement are correct concerning the blind loop sydrome : AMU 1986**

A. Steatorrhea appears to be caused by reduction in micelle concentration of conjugated bile salts.
B. Diarrhoea possible is caused by dehydroxylation of fatty acids by bacteria.
C. Both of the above.
D. Neither of the above.

**63. Adequate margins of resection are essential for gastrectomy for carcinoma. With positive margins, the 5-years survival rate is less than 15. Ideal margins both proximal and distal are at least : AMU 1988**

A. 4 cm B. 6 cm
C. 8 cm D. 10 cm
E. 12 cm

**64. The cause of alternation of serum gastrin and gastric secretion in patients with hyperparathyroidism is : PGI 1982**

A. Parathormone B. Calcium iron
C. $PO_2$- D. Mg+2
E. All of the above

**65. The treatment of choice for a Curling's ulcer is : AMC 1987**

A. Prophylaxis
B. Vagotomy and hemigastrectomy
C. Vagotomy and pyloroplasty
D. Total gastrectomy
E. Suture ligation of ulcer base

**66. Duodenal fistula ('Blow out') is a complication of Polya partial gastrectomy which occurs due to : AIIMS 1986**

A. Anaemia
B. Haemorrhage from anastomatic line
C. Stomal obstruction
D. Avascular stump necrosis

**67. In acute dilatation of stomach, an early sign is : Delhi 1983, 97.**

A. Unexplained restlessness
B. Brown vomitus
C. Shock
D. Hypotension

**68. All of the following are seen in congenital Pyloric stenosis except : AI 1994**

A. Preterm infant
B. Projectile vomiting
C. Weight loss
D. Manifests 2 weeks after birth

**69. A premenopausal female presents with stage-II carcinoma breast which of the following procedures would not be done : Kerala 1998**

A. Lumpectomy B. Quadrancetomy
C. Radical mastectomy D. Radiotherapy

**70. All of the following are common causes of haematemesis except : DNB 1988**

A. Chronic peptic ulcer B. Pernicious anemia
C. Esophageal varices D. Carcinoma of stomach

**71. The best method of treatment for gastrojejunocolic fistula is by : AMU 1990**

A. Superficial colostomy
B. Resection of stomach, jejunum and colon
C. Jejunostomy feeding
D. Conservative

**72. Electrolyte disturbance in chronic pyloric stenosis with vomiting tends to be : AMU 1989; AI 2001**

A. Hyperchloraemic acidosis
B. Hypochloraemic alkalosis
C. Hypochloraemic acidosis
D. Hyperchloraemic alkalosis

**73. The most frequent complication of vagotomy is : AIIMS 1986; AI 2001**

A. Dysphagia B. Diarrhoea
C. Dryness of mouth D. Tachycardia

**74. Which of the following is not a contraindication to curative resection of a gastric carcinoma : TN 1989**

A. Peritoneal dissemination.
B. Pancreatic involvement.
C. Involvement of lymph nodes along the lesser and greater curvatures.
D. Involvement of coeliac lymph nodes.

**75. Treatment of diffuse linitis plastica is : UPSC 1984**

A. Radiotherapy B. Partial gastrectomy
C. Gastroscopic dilation D. Total gastrectomy
E. No treatment is desired

**76. All of the following statements are true regarding night fasting secretion of gastric juice except : AIIMS 1985**

A. It is used for assessment of the inter-digestive or resting secretion of the stomach.
B. Normal volume is 800 ml (12 hours).
C. Free HCl content is an index of vagal activity.
D. Free HCl content is reduced in gastric ulcer.

| Ans. | 61. D | 62. C | 63. B | 64. B | 65. B | 66. D | 67. A | 68. A | 69. C | 70. B |
|---|---|---|---|---|---|---|---|---|---|---|
| | 71. B | 72. B | 73. B | 74. C | 75. D | 76. B | | | | |

**77. All of the following may be features of a silent carcinoma of the body of the stomach except : AMU 1989, 92**

A. Obstructive jaundice B. Ascites
C. Dysphagia D. Krukenberg's tumours

**78. Which is not true of Infantile hypertrophic pyloric stenosis: JIPMER 1992**

A. Hypertrophy of circular muscle fibres
B. Billous vomitus
C. Palpable lump abdomen
D. Profound weight loss

**79. Carcinoma stomach with good prognosis is : AIIMS 1985, 92; AI 1995**

A. Superficial spreading B. Ulcerative
C. Fungating type D. Linitus plastica

**80. A boy of 8 years presents with epigastric lump with non-billious vomiting. Diagnosis likely is : AIIMS 1998**

A. Jejuno-jejunal intussusception
B. Hypertrophic pyloric stenosis
C. Ileal atresia
D. Choledochal cyst

**81. Linitis plastica is not seen in : AIIMS 1998**

A. Ca stomach B. Syphilis
C. Sarcoidosis D. Leiomyosarcoma

**82. After gastric surgery, urinary output of 800 cc per day indicates : AMC 1984, 87**

A. ↑ Fluid intake B. ↓ Fluid intake
C. Normal condition D. None of the above

**83. Burning epigastric pain is due to : AIIMS 1986**

A. Vomiting B. Reflux esophagitis
C. Duodenal ulcer D. Gastric ulcer

**84. A 43 years old man is brought to the emergency room when he fainted after vomiting an undeterminated amount of bright red blood. The history and physical examination were uninformative. Laboratory studies: WBC 9.600, RBC 3,200,000 hemoglobin 9 gm per 100 ml, hematocrit 32 percent. The next diagnostic procedure should be : AIIMS 1988**

A. Selective angiography
B. Upper gastrointestinal roentgenograms
C. Barium enema
D. Endoscopic examination of esophagus, stomach and duodenum
E. None of the above

**85. Barium meal picture of carcinoma stomach shows following : Kerala 1987**

A. Filling defect
B. Loss of rugosity
C. Small capacity of stomach
D. Delayed emptying barium
E. All of the above

**86. H. Pylori causes following except : AI 1999**

A. Duodenal ulcer B. Gastric carcinoma
C. Gastric lymphoma D. Fundal gastritis

**87. All of the following predispose to gastric carcinoma except : AI 1990**

A. Achlorhydria B. 'O' blood group
C. Pernicious anaemia D. Post gastrectomy

**88. A stomach with diffuse thickening with leathery feeling and multiple haemorrhagic spots is diagnostic of : Kerala 1990**

A. $B_{12}$ deficiency
B. Colloid carcinoma stomach
C. Peptic ulcer
D. Squamous cell cancer stomach

**89. Which of the following conditions show marked elevation of serum gastrin level : CSE 1995**

1. Pernicious anaemia
2. Duodenal ulcer
3. Zollinger-Ellison syndrome
4. Massive resection of small intestine

**Select the correct answer :**

A. 1, 2 and 3 B. 1, 3 and 4
C. 1, 2 and 4 D. 2, 3 and 4

**90. Intractable peptic ulceration with renal stones occurs in : JIPMER 1990**

A. Zollinger Ellison syndrome
B. Parathyroid adenoma
C. Milk alkali syndrome
D. MEA-I syndrome

**91. Commonest cause of death in peptic ulcer patients is : AI 1990**

A. Perforation B. Haemorrhage
C. Pyloric stenosis D. Malignancy

**92. Commonest operation done for peptic ulcer with gastric outlet obstruction is : PGI 1983**

A. Truncal vagotomy with gastrojejunostomy .
B. Highly selective vagotomy with pyloroplasty.
C. Truncal vagotomy with gastrojejunostomy.
D. Gastrojejunostomy.

| Ans. | | | | | | | | | |
|---|---|---|---|---|---|---|---|---|---|
| 77. C | 78. B | 79. A | 80. B | 81. D | 82. B | 83. B | 84. D | 85. E | 86. D |
| 87. B | 88. B | 89. A | 90. D | 91. B | 92. C | | | | |

**93. Which of the following signs are present in an advanced case of carcinoma of stomach : CSE 1996**

1. Trousseau's sign
2. Troisier's sign
3. Depostis in the pouch of Douglas
4. Murphy's sign

**Select the correct answer :**

A. 1 and 4 B. 1 and 2
C. 1, 2 and 3 D. 2, 3 and 4

**94. A patient with a perforated ulcer may be treated by : AIIMS 1985**

A. Conservative means
B. Plication of the perforation
C. Subtotal gastrectomy
D. All of the above means
E. None of the above

**95. Commonest site of Leiomyoma in GIT is : AI 1994, 96**

A. Stomach B. Ileum
C. Jejunum D. Rectum

**96. Troiseir's sign is seen in all except : AI 1994**

A. Ca stomach B. Seminoma
C. Medulloblastoma D. Ca Pancreas

**97. Achlorhydria is diagnostic of : Karnataka 1989**

A. Pernicious anaemia
B. Carcinoma stomach
C. Gastric mucosal atrophy
D. None of the above

**98. All of the following are associated with acid peptic disease except : Karnataka 1993**

A. Cirrhosis of liver B. Thyrotoxicosis
C. Hyperparathyroidism D. Chronic lung disease

**99. Consider the following types of growths : CSE 1998**

1. Pyloric growth
2. Carcinoma of body of stomach
3. Growth at cardia

**The correct sequence in Descending order of the degree of accuracy of barium meal examination for the diagnosis of carcinoma stomach in respect of the given types of growths is :**

A. 2, 1, 3 B. 3, 1, 2
C. 1, 2, 3 D. 1, 3, 2

**100. Bilious vomiting is seen in all except : Kerala 1994**

A. Jejunal atresia
B. Volvulus of small intestine
C. Duodenal atresia
D. Pyloric stenosis

**101. Dilatation of stomach does not occur in : Kerala 1994**

A. Pyloric obstruction B. Hypokalaemia
C. Cardiospasm D. Pneumonia

**102. Most valuable provocative test for Zollinger Ellison syndrome is : AI 1999**

A. ACTH infusion test
B Secretin stimulation test
C. Ca2+ infusion test
D. Food stimulation test

**103. Late postcibal syndrome is due to : PGI 1994**

A. Rapid gastric emptying with increased small bowel activity
B. Distension of afferent loop
C. Hypoglycaemia
D. Short band

**104. Lowest recurrence rate in duodenal ulcer treatment is seen with : AIIMS 1994, 95**

A. Truncal vagotomy
B. Highly selective vagotomy
C. Truncal vagotomy + pyloroplasty
D. Truncal vagotomy + antrectomy

**105. Which is not true regarding Mentrier's disease : AIIMS 1994**

A. Exophytic growth
B. Protein loss
C. Hypertrophy of gastric mucosa
D. Predispose commonly to carcinoma

**106. Following are true of Ac. gastric dilatation except : AIIMS 1995**

A. Hypokalemia
B. Tachycardia
C. Profuse vomiting
D. Respiratory embarasment

**107. Early gastric carcinoma is : TN 1996**

A. Mucosa involved without lymph node involvement.
B. Mucosa involved irrespective of lymph node involvement.
C. Submucosa involved irrespective of lymph node involvement.
D. Submucosa involved without lymph node involvement.

**108. False about recurrent peptic ulcer : AI 1995**

A. Periodicity of pain lost
B. Refractory to Cimetidine therapy
C. Barium meal detects almost all ulcers
D. Endoscopy can miss the ulcers

| Ans. | | | | | | | | | | |
|---|---|---|---|---|---|---|---|---|---|---|
| | 93. C | 94. B | 95. A | 96. C | 97. B | 98. B | 99. A | 100. D | 101. C | 102. B |
| | 103. A | 104. D | 105. D | 106. C | 107. C | 108. C | | | | |

**109. All of the following drugs are used for eradication of Helicobacter pylori except : UPSC 1995**

A. Bismuth subcitrate B. Sucralfate
C. Metronidazole D. Amoxycillin

**110. In Holliander's test, significant rise of acid output should be ———meq. UPSC 1995**

A. 5 B. 10
C. 15 D. 20

**111. Treatment of choice for Type-II Zollinger Ellison's syndrome is : UPSC 1995**

A. Total Gastrectomy with removal tumor
B. Paritial Gastrectomy
C. Excision tumor
D. $H_2$ receptor antagonist

**112. Anticholinergic that is used in peptic ulcer is : AI 1997**

A. Omeprazole B. Pirenzepine
C. Cimetidine D. Famotidine

**113. Gastric mucosal hypertrophy occurs in : Kerala 1996**

A. Gastrinoma B. Duodenal ulcer
C. Gastric ulcer D. Gastric cancer
E. APUDOMA

**114. Chronic duodenal ulcer with pyloric stenosis is best treated by : UPSC 1996**

A. Cimetidine and endoscopic dilatation
B. Gastrojejunostomy and vagotomy
C. Highly selective vagotomy
D. Sub-total gastrectomy

**115. Total capacity of the stomach is markedly reduced in : UPSC 1996**

A. Cauliflower growth of stomach
B. Hourglass stomach
C. Pyloric stenosis
D. Linitis plastica

**116. A 50-years old male who had chronic duodenal ulcer for the last six years presents with worsening of symptoms, loss of periodicity of symptoms, pain on rising in the morning, sense of epigastric bloating and post-prandial vomiting. The most likely cause of the worsening of his symptoms is the development of : UPSC 1996**

A. Posterior penetration
B. Gastric outlet obstruction
C. Carcinoma
D. Pancreatitis

**117. Parietal cell vagotomy must be done in association with : Rajasthan 1995**

A. Pyloroplasty
B. Gastrojejunostomy
C. Anterectomy with gastrojejunostomy
D. None of the above

**118. Autoimmune diseases are associated with : Rajasthan 1996**

A. Type-A chronic gastritis
B. Type-B chronic gastritis
C. Both
D. None

**119. Consider the following drugs : UPSC 1997**

1. Ranitidine/$H_2$ receptor β-blockers
2. Somatostatin
3. Pitressin
4. Glucagon

**Drugs used in the treatment of bleeding duodenal ulcer would include :**

A. 1 and 2 B. 1 and 3
C. 2, 3 and 4 D. 1, 2 and 4

**120. Gastrojejunostomy wound is an example of : JIPMER 1998**

A. Clean wound
B. Clean contaminated wound
C. Contaminated wound
D. Dirty wound

**121. Benign chronic gastric ulcer : MAHE 1999**

A. Common in acid secreting region
B. Increased risk of gastric Ca
C. Hour glass stomach
D. Associated with hyperacidity

**122. Consider the following statements : CSE 1999**

In an endoscopic examination for gastric malignancy, mucosa looks quite normal in :

1. Colloid carcinoma
2. Linitis plastica
3. Lymphoma

Which of the above statements are correct :

A. 1, 2 and 3 B. 1 and 2
C. 1 and 3 D. 2 and 3

**123. About Dumping syndrome all are true, except : AI 2000**

A. Surgery is the treatment of choice
B. Due to entry of hypertonic fluid into intestine
C. Abdominal distention is present
D. Can be managed by diet

**Ans.** 109. B 110. D 111. D 112. B 113. A 114. B 115. D 116. B 117. A 118. A
119. B 120. B 121. C 122. B 123. D

**124. Following are sites of Cushings ulcer except : AI 1999**

A. Oesophagus B. Stomach
C. Proximal duodenum D. Distal duodenum

**125. A young patient has been diagnosed to have antral gastric carcinoma with obstruction. His clinical evaluation reveals enlarged left supraclavicular nodes without ascites and metastasis on the liver on palpable mass. In this case, the treatment of choice would be : UPSC 2000**

A. Radical gastrectomy
B. Palliative gastrectomy
C. Gastrojejunostomy
D. Devine's gastric exclusion

**126. Which of the following malignancies is associated with staple diet : JIPMER 2000**

A. Carcinoma colon B. Liver cancer
C. Stomach cancer D. Ca Pancreas

**127. The following are contraindications for the Gastrostomy except : Kerala 2000**

A. Gastric Diseases
B. Thin abdominal wall
C. Significant gastro-oesophageal reflux
D. Delayed gastric emptying
E. Loss of gas reflux

**128. Endoscopy of a patient having peptic ulcer disease showed features of chronic antral gastritis. Which of the following dyes will stain a specimen taken from the stomach : AIIMS 2000**

A. PAS B. Gram stain
C. Warthin starry stain D. Zeil Nielson stain

**129. Which of the following ↓ LES without gastric acid production : NIMHANS 2000**

A. Cimetidine B. Omeprazole
C. Cisapride D. Ranitidine

**130. A gastrojejunostomy without any spillage of contents is a : DNB 2001**

A. Clean wound
B. Clean contaminated wound
C. Dirty wound
D. Contaminated wound

**131. A 45 years old male is operated upon for benign gastric ulcer. A partial gastrectomy has been done. On the early post-operative period the patient is lethargic, drowsy and confused. The most likely diagnosis is: UPSC 2001**

A. Post-operative psychosis
B. Hypokalemia
C. Hyponatremia
D. Hypovolaemic shock

**132. Gastric acid output is influenced by all of the following hormones except : UPSC 2001, 2002**

A. Gastrin B. Glucagon
C. Secretin D. Cholecystokinin

**133. Ulcer recurrence rate is least with : JIPMER 2001**

A. GJ Vagotomy
B. Highly selective vagotomy
C. Vagotomy + antrectomy
D. Vagotomy + pyloroplasty

**134. Treatment of choice of a tumor of 5 cm size present in prepyloric region of stomach is : Delhi 2001**

A. Entrectomy B. Subtotal gastrectomy
C. Total gastrectomy D. Gastrojejunal anastomosis

**135. Which of the following procedures is associated with least complications like dumping syndrome, post-prandial vomiting and diarrhoea : AIIMS 2001**

A. Highly selective vagotomy
B. TV + GJ
C. Antrectomy
D. Truncal vagotomy + pyloroplasty

**136. Acute gastric dilatation is best prevented by : SGPGI 2002**

A. Nasogastric tube
B. Gastrostomy
C. Stopping of oral feeds until improvement in condition
D. Steroids

**137. Gastric malignancy is predisposed with : JIPMER 1993; PGI 2000; AI 2002**

A. Duodenal ulcer
B. Gastric hyperplasia
C. Intestinal metaplasia-III
D. Blood group-O

**138. All the following indicates early gastric cancer except : AI 2002**

A. Involvement of mucosa.
B. Involvement of mucosa and submucosa.
C. Involvement of mucosa, submucosa and muscularis.
D. Involvement of mucosa, submucosa and adjacent lymph nodes.

**139. The least recurrence of gastric hypersecretion following surgery for peptic ulcer is seen with : AI 2002**

A. Vagotomy with gastrojejunostomy
B. Antrectomy with vagotomy
C. Highly selective vagotomy
D. Truncal vagotomy

**Ans.** **124. D** **125. C** **126. C** **127. B** **128. C** **129. C** **130. B** **131. C** **132. D** **133. C** **134. B** **135. A** **136. A** **137. C** **138. C** **139. B**

**140. The tries as originally described by Zollinger and Ellison is : AI 2002**

A. Hypergastrinemia, raised gastric acid output, beta cell tumor.

B. Hypergastrinemia, raised gastric acid output, beta cell. tumor.

C. Hypochlorhydria, raised gastric acid output, beta cell tumor.

D. Tumor of papilla of Vater, hypergastrinemia, raised gastric acid output.

**141. In gastric outlet obstruction in a duodenal ulcer patient, the site of obstruction is most likely to be : AI 2002**

A. Antrum B. Duodenum

C. Pylorus D. Pyloric canal

**142. Consider the following features with reference to Zollinger-Ellison syndrome : UPSC 2002**

1. Intractable peptic ulceration
2. Hypergastrinaemia
3. β-islet-cell tumour of the pancreas

**Which of these features are present in Zollinger-Ellison syndrome :**

A. 1 and 3 B. 2 and 3

C. 1, 2 & 3 D. 1 and 2

**143. All of the following are indications for surgery in gastric lymphomas except : AIIMS 2002**

A. Bleeding

B. Perforation

C. Residual disease following chemotherapy

D. Intractable pain

**144. What is the most characteristic of congenital hypertrophic pyloric stenosis : AI 2003**

A. Affects the first born female child

B. The pyloric tumor is best felt during feeding

C. The patient is commonly marasmic

D. Loss of appetite occurs early

**145. A posteriorly perforating ulcer in the pyloric antrum of the stomach is most likely to produce initial localised peritonitis or abscess formation in the following : AI 2003**

A. Omental bursa (lesser sac)

B. Greater sac

C. Right subphrenic space

D. Hepatorenal space (pouch of Morrison)

**146. A 65 years old woman with known duodenal ulcer being treated by $H_2$ blocker therapy is admitted with upper gastrointestinal bleeding. After blood replacement is begun the next step is her management should be : UPSC 2004**

A. Institute anti H. pylori treatment

B. Repeated gastric lavage

C. Endoscopy and coagulation of bleeding vessel

D. Pyloroduodenotomy and oversewing of the bleeding vessel

| **Ans.** | **140. B** | **141. B** | **142. D** | **143. D** | **144. A** | **145. A** | **146. D** |
|---|---|---|---|---|---|---|---|

# EXPLANATIONS OF STOMACH

1. Ans.— D. Renal failure
2. Ans.— C. 3-6 weeks
3. Ans.— A. Immediately
4. Ans.— C. E. Svensgaard
5. Ans.— C. Contains bile
6. Ans.— D. Palpation of hypertrophic pylorous
7. Ans.— C. Pancreas
8. Ans.— D. When medical treatment fails, it responds well to surgery.
9. Ans.— D. Gastroscopy
10. Ans.— B. Lower radical partial gastrectomy
11. Ans.— A. Weight loss
12. Ans.— B. Blowout of the duodenal stump at 4th day.
13. Ans.— A. Histological diagnosis is easily obtained by endoscopic biopsy.
14. Ans.— B. Stomach
15. Ans.— B. Gastric resection and chemotherapy
16. Ans.— A. Surgery with Chemotherapy
17. Ans.— B. Highly selective vagotomy
18. Ans.— D. 1 and 3 are correct
19. Ans.— B. Increased small bowel activity
20. Ans.— B. Increased basal acid output and no further increase by histamine.

    Normal gastrin levels are below 200 pg/ml but in this they rise above it. Secretion is used for diagnosis (2 units/Kg) preceded by I/V calcium (2 mg over 1 minute as bolus).
21. Ans.— A. Gastric ulcer
22. Ans.— A. Leiomyoma
23. Ans.— B. Pylorus
24. Ans.— D. Fundus
25. Ans.— C. Excision of tumor alone
26. Ans.— D. Anastomotic leak
27. Ans.— A. Poor appetite
28. Ans.— B. Congenital pyloric stenosis
29. Ans.— B. Fundus
30. Ans.— A. Fibromyosarcoma

    Malaena, Mild indigestion and epigastric pain are common (in that order). Haematemesis is, however, the most common symptom.
31. Ans.— A. Most commonly occurs in the fundus of the stomach.
32. Ans.— C. Occur most commonly on the greater curvature.
33. Ans.— C. 14, 17
34. Ans.— B. 30
35. Ans.— D. Hypokalaemic alkalosis
36. Ans.— C. Crohn's disease
37. Ans.— B. Fundus
38. Ans.— B. Subtotal gastrectomy
39. Ans.— B. Hyperacidity
40. Ans.— D. Curling's ulcer
41. Ans.— D. All of the above
42. Ans.— A. It results a healed duodenal ulcer
43. Ans.— C. Pentagastrin test
44. Ans.— A. It mostly occurs in men
45. Ans.— A. Blood group-O
46. Ans.— D. The histology of the growth
47. Ans.— E. Dumping of hypertonic material into jejunum.
48. Ans.— E. All of the above
49. Ans.— C. The cause is unknown
50. Ans.— C. Vomiting (bile stained)
51. Ans.— D. All of the above
52. Ans.— C. Somatostatin analogue
53. Ans.— B. Circular muscle fibres
54. Ans.— D. All of the above
55. Ans.— D. For taking biopsy from the duodenum
56. Ans.— D. Gall stones

    Obstruction, perforation and peritonitis and haematemesis are common.

**57. Ans.— B. Eventation of the diaphragm**

**58. Ans.— B. After one hour**

**59. Ans.— C. 48 hours**

**60. Ans.— D. Psychological disturbances**

**Trichobezoar is also called hair ball of the stomach. In 90% cases it is found in females and most of them are psychiatric.**

**61. Ans.— D. Endoscopy**

**62. Ans.— C. Both of the above**

**63. Ans.— B. 6 cm**

**64. Ans.— B. Calcium iron**

**65. Ans.— B. Vagotomy and hemigastrectomy**

**66. Ans.— D. Avascular stump necrosis**

**67. Ans.— A. Unexplained restlessness**

**68. Ans.— A. Preterm infant**

**Type affected infant is fullterm.**

**69. Ans.— C. Radical mastectomy**

**70. Ans.— B. Pernicious anemia**

**71. Ans.— B. Resection of stomach, jejunum and colon**

**72. Ans.— B. Hypochloraemic alkalosis**

**73. Ans.— B. Diarrhoea**

**74. Ans.— C. Involvement of lymph nodes along the lesser and greater curvatures.**

**75. Ans.— D. Total gastrectomy**

**76. Ans.— B. Normal volume is 800 ml (12 hours)**

**77. Ans.— C. Dysphagia**

**78. Ans.— B. Billous vomitus**

**79. Ans.— A. Superficial spreading**

**Even when metastasis is present, prognosis is better than advanced or deep involving lesions.**

**80. Ans.— B. Hypertrophic pyloric stenosis**

**81. Ans.— D. Leiomyosarcoma**

**Commonest cause is linitis plastica. There is a gerneralised and localised form of leather bottle stomach.**

**82. Ans.— B. ↓ Fluid intake**

**83. Ans.— B. Reflux esophagitis**

**84. Ans.— D. Endoscopic examination of esophagus, stomach and duodenum.**

**85. Ans.— E. All of the above**

**86. Ans.— D. Fundal gastritis**

**Question is wrong, as all the complication may occur.**

**87. Ans.— B. 'O' blood group**

**'A' blood group is important. Blood group 'O' is important in duodenal ulcer.**

**88. Ans.— B. $B_{12}$ deficiency**

**89. Ans.— A. 1, 2 and 3**

**90. Ans.— D. MEA- I syndrome**

**91. Ans.— B. Haemorrhage**

**Of all the complication of Peptic ulcer, Perforation is the most acute and lethal complication.**

**92. Ans.— C. Truncal vagotomy with gastrojejunostomy**

**93. Ans.— C. 1, 2 and 3**

**94. Ans.— B. Plication of the perforation**

**95. Ans.— A. Stomach**

**First symptom is massive haematemesis and/or melaena. The presence of a barium filled sinus extending into the tumor visualized by X-rays is extremely characteristic. Gastric acidity remains unchanged. It should be removed by enucleation or wedge resection.**

**96. Ans.— C. Medulloblastoma**

**97. Ans.— B. Carcinoma stomach**

**98. Ans.— B. Thyrotoxicosis**

**99. Ans.— A. 2, 1, 3**

**100. Ans.— D. Pyloric stenosis**

**101. Ans.— C. Cardiospasm**

**102. Ans.— B Secretin stimulation test**

**103. Ans.— A. Rapid gastric emptying with increased small bowel activity.**

**104. Ans.— D. Truncal vagotomy + antrectomy**

**105. Ans.— D. Predispose commonly to carcinoma**

**106. Ans.— C. Profuse vomiting**

**Unexplained restlessness is commonest symptom.**

**107. Ans.— C. Submucosa involved irrespective of lymph node involvement.**

**108. Ans.— C. Barium meal detects almost all ulcers**

**109. Ans.— B. Sucralfate**

**110. Ans.— D. 20**

**111. Ans.— D. $H_2$ receptor antagonist**

**Treatment of Z-E syndrome : Type-I — partial gastrectomy to remove G cell bearing area. Type- II—Resection of pancreatic tumor and total gastrectomy may**

be advised only if medical therapy fails, If tumor is inoperatable truncal vagotomy be performed.

112. Ans.— B. Pirenzepine

113. Ans.— A. Gastrinoma

114. Ans.— B. Gastrojejunostomy and vagotomy

115. Ans.— D. Linitis plastica

116. Ans.— B. Gastric outlet obstruction

117. Ans.— A. Pyloroplasty

118. Ans.— A. Type-A chronic gastritis

119. Ans.— B. 1 and 3

120. Ans.— B. Clean contaminated wound

121. Ans.— C. Hour glass stomach

122. Ans.— B. 1 and 2

123. Ans.— D. Can be managed by diet

Symptoms fall into 2 categories CVS and GIT. Dietary treatment or surgery is required.

124. Ans.— D. Distal duodenum

Acute ulcers associated with CNS tumor or injuries different from stress ulcers because they are associated with elevated levels of serum gastrin and serum gastric acid secretion and are more prone to perforate. They also similar to ordinary gastroduodenal ulcers.

125. Ans.— C. Gastrojejunostomy

126. Ans.— C. Stomach cancer

127. Ans.— B. Thin abdominal wall

128. Ans.— C. Warthin starry stain

129. Ans.— C. Cisapride

130. Ans.— B. Clean contaminated wound

131. Ans.— C. Hyponatremia

132. Ans.— D. Cholecystokinin

133. Ans.— C. Vagotomy + antrectomy

134. Ans.— B. Subtotal gastrectomy

135. Ans.— A. Highly selective vagotomy

136. Ans.— A. Nasogastric tube

137. Ans.— C. Intestinal metaplasia-III

H. pylori infection, pernicious anemia and gastric atrophy, gastric polyps, Menetuer's disease smoking and genetic factors are other risk factors.

138. Ans.— C. Involvement of mucosa, submucosa and muscularis.

It indicates late stage.

139. Ans.— B. Antrectomy with vagotomy

It controls gastric hypersecretion by decreasing the area and secretion.

140. Ans.— B. Hypergastrinemia, raised gastric acid output, beta cell tumor.

It occurs in duodenum in 'gastrinoma triangle' defined by (a) junction of cystic duct and common bile duct superiorly (b) junction of neck and body of pancreas medially (especially sup. mesenteric artery) duodenum inferiorly. Proton pump inhibitors or gastrectomy is the treatment.

141. Ans.— B. Duodenum

The two common causes of gastric outlet obstruction are gastric cancer and pyloric stenosis secondary to peptic ulceration.

142. Ans.— D. 1 and 2

143. Ans.— D. Intractable pain

144. Ans.— A. Affects the first born female child

145. Ans.— A. Omental bursa (lesser sac)

* MC site of gastric ulcer is lesser curvature (anterior wall).
* May be associated with H. pylori infection.
* Most sensitive investigation in management of suspected peptic ulceration is gastro duodenoscopy.
* Common complication of peptic ulcer are perforation, bleeding & stenosis).
* Most common site of perforation is anterior wall which lead to spill of contents in lesser sac.
* Investigation - X ray-gas under diaphragm confirm by- DPL (diagnostic peritoneal lavage).

146. Ans.— D. Pyloroduodenotomy and oversewing of the bleeding vessel.

# 10

# IMPORTANT TEXT OF HEPATOBILIARY SYSTEM (LIVER, SPLEEN, PANCREAS)

## CHILD'S CRITERION (FOR SHUNT SURGERY IN PORTAL HYPERTENSION)

| | *Observation* | *Suitable* | *Marginal* | *Unsuitable* |
|---|---|---|---|---|
| 1. | Bilirubin (mg%) | Below 2.0 | 2.0-3.0 | Above 3.0 |
| 2. | Albumin (mg%) | Over 3.5 | 3.0-3.5 | Below 3.0 |
| 3. | Ascites | None | Early Controlled | Poorly controlled |
| 4. | Neurological Disorder | None | Minimal | Coma |
| 5. | Nutritional Status | Excellent | Good | Poor |

## LAPAROSCOPIC CHOLESCYSTECTOMY

*Universally agreed contraindications*

Severe cholecystitis
Jaundice
Portal hypertension
Pregnancy

*Universally agreed investigations and Precautions*

Liver function tests
GB ultrasonography
Group and save serum
Prophylactic antibiotics

## INDICATIONS OR CONTRAINDICATIONS FOR LIVER TRANSPLANTATION

| | |
|---|---|
| Should be considered | Primary biliary cirrhosis<br>Cryptogenic cirrhosis<br>Chronic Non-A, Non-B hepatitis<br>Sclerosing cholangitis<br>Reformed alcoholic |
| Contraindications | Schistosomiasis<br>Extrahepatic portal vein<br>Severe cardiac disease<br>Severe pulmonary disease<br>AIDS<br>Uncontrolled sepsis |
| Undecided | Unreformed alcoholic |

## PORTAL HYPERTENSION
(more than 30 cm water)

Classification

*Prehepatic*

Portal vein thrombosis following :

1. Umbilical sepsis/exchange transfusion
2. Pylephlebitis—e.g., from appendicitis/diverticulitis
3. Platelet disorder e.g., myelofibrosis/following splenectomy
4. Pancreatic tumour

*Hepatic*

All forms of cirrhosis

*Posthepatic*

1. Hepatic vein obstruction
2. Constrictive pericarditis
3. Budd Chiari syndrome
4. Veno occlusive disease

**Complications of portal hypertension**

1. Hypertrophy of porto systemic collaterals
   (i) Oesophageal varices
   (ii) Haemorrhoids
   (iii) Caput medusae
2. Splenomegaly - may lead to hypersplenism
3. Ascites
4. Hepatic failure

## INDICATIONS FOR SPLENECTOMY

1. Ruptured spleen
2. Part of other operation e.g. radical gastrectomy
3. Blood disorder : ITP, hereditary spherocytosis
4. Staging of Hodgkin's disease
5. Tumours, cysts

## FACTORS PREDISPOSING TO GALLSTONE FORMATION

1. Lithogenic bile
2. Stasis
3. Infection
4. Haemolysis
5. Diabetes
6. Hyperlipidemia
7. Contraceptive pill
8. Parasites- clonorchis, ascaris
9. Crohn's disease

## COMPLICATIONS OF SPLENECTOMY

1. Haemorrhage
2. Gastric dilatation
3. Haematenesis
4. Left basal Atelectasis
5. Damage to Tail
6. Leukocytosis of Pancreas
7. Gastric fistula

# COMPLICATIONS OF GALLSTONES

1. Biliary colic
2. Acute cholecystitis
3. Chronic cholecystitis
4. Perforation of gall bladder and peritonitis
5. Common duct obstruction
6. Cholangitis
7. Fistulisation from biliary tree to stomach, duodenum, small bowel or colon
8. Gall stone ileus
9. Increased incidence of pancreatitis
10. Carcinoma of gall bladder

**Asymptomatic stones are likely to cause complications in over 50% of patients eventually**

# MCQ's OF HEPATOBILIARY SYSTEM (LIVER, SPLEEN, PANCREAS)

## What is important in Hepatobiliary System

Liver (Hepatomegaly, Tumors, Cirrhosis, Abscess), Spleen (Splenomegaly, Splenectomy), Gall bladder Cholelithiasis, Cholecystectomy, Charcot triad), Pancreas (Pancreatitis Tumors).

1. **E.R.C.P. is helpful in the diagnosis of following except : Bihar 1989**
   A. Cancer of the liver
   B. Level of obstruction in the biliary tract
   C. Pancreatitis
   D. Pseudopancreatic cyst
2. **P.T.C. is helpful in the diagnosis of : UP 1993**
   A. Cancer of the liver
   B. Level of obstruction in the biliary tract
   C. Pancreatitis
   D. Pseudopancreatic cyst
3. **Conservative surgery for splenic rupture is indicated because of the risk of : DNB 1990**
   A. Sepsis in splenectomised children
   B. Anaemia
   C. High mortality after splenectomy
   D. Post-operative purpura
4. **The afferent lobe syndrome is associated with all of the following, except : UPSC 1985**
   A. Post-cibal vomiting.
   B. Develop more frequently in gastric ulcers that in duodenal ulcer.
   C. Vit $B_{12}$ deficiency.
   D. Emesis without bile is characteristic.
   E. Rarely total obstruction.
5. **True about medical treatment of gallstones are all except : AI 1992**
   A. Gall bladder should be functioning
   B. Gall stones should be radiolucent
   C. Gall stones should be radioopaque
   D. Useful in patients unfit for surgery
6. **The commonest cause of external biliary fistula is : BHU 1987**
   A. Injury to the common bile duct during cholecystectomy.
   B. A leakage after cholecystojejunostomy.
   C. Division of an aberrent right hepatic duct.
   D. A leakage after cholecystoduodenostomy.
   E. Division of a hepaticocystic duct.
7. **Most of the cases of portal hypertension are due to : DNB 1990**
   A. Pre-hepatic causes
   B. Thrombosis of the portal vein
   C. Intrahepatic causes
   D. Constrictive pericarditis
   E. Budd-Chiari sydrome
8. **Tetracycline fluorescence may be used for : AMU 1987**
   A. Standardization of tetracycline samples.
   B. The diagnosis of gastric carcinoma.
   C. The treatment of colloid carcinoma of the stomach.
   D. Detecting tetracycline sensitive micro-organisms.
   E. None of the above
9. **Carcinoma pancreas is most common in : AMU 1988**
   A. The body of pancreas
   B. The tail of pancreas
   C. The periampullary region of head
   D. The head proper
   E. Ampulla of Vater
10. **'Lead paint' appearance of stool in a jaundiced patient indicates : DNB 1991**
    A. Carcinoma of the head proper of pancreas.
    B. Carcinoma of the tail pancreas.
    C. Carcinoma of periampullary region of pancreas.
    D. Cholecystitis along with haemorrhage.
    E. Jaundice with intoxication due to lead paints.

**Ans.** 1. A 2. B 3. A 4. D 5. C 6. A 7. C 8. B 9. D 10. C

**11. The usual treatment of gallstones in the common bile duct is : AIIMS 1988**
A. Cholecystectomy and choledochotomy
B. Cholecystostomy
C. Sphincterotomy
D. Choledochoduodenostomy
E. None of the above

**12. Which of the following is not associated with cirrhosis of the liver: AMU 1985**
A. Dupuytren's contracture
B. Gynaecomastia
C. Testicular atrophy
D. Pale palms
E. All of the above

**13. A choledochus cyst is : Rohtak 1985**
A. Parasitic B. Congenital
C. Symptomless D. Commoner in males

**14. All of the following complications may occur during cholecystectomy, except : BHU 1987**
A. Haemorrhage from cystic artery
B. Damage to hepatic artery
C. Failure to find all duct stones
D. Haemorrhage from cystic vein

**15. Budd Chiari syndrome may be seen in : Rajasthan 1998**
A. IVC B. PNH
C. OC D. All of the above

**16. Indications for endoscopic sphincterectomy include common duct pathology in association with : AMU 1985**
A. Severe cardiovascular or respiratory disease
B. Advanced age
C. Marked obesity
D. Prior post-operative surgical complications
E. All of the above

**17. Which of the following procedures for portal hypertension seem(s) to protect against recurrent bleeding and at the same time cause(s) the least post-operative encephalopathy : UPSC 1986**
A. Side-to-side portocaval shunt
B. Distal splenorenal shunt
C. End-to-side portocaval shunt
D. Mesocaval shunt
E. All of the above are equal

**18. Segmental atrophy of the liver is best diagnosed by : UP 1991**
A. Percutaneous transhepatic cholangiogram
B. Liver scan
C. Angiography
D. Exploration
E. None of the above

**19. Which of the following has lowest sensitivity for the diagnosis of hydatid cyst : DNB 1991**
A. Casoni's test
B. Indirect haemagglutination test
C. Complement fixation test
D. ELISA

**20. Which of the following is not the part of classic triad of symptoms seen in hemobilia : DNB 1991**
A. GI bleeding
B. Right upper quadrant pain
C. Jaundice
D. Fever

**21. Commonest site of gallstone impaction in acute calculous cholecystitis is : TN 1996**
A. CBD
B. Hepatic duct
C. Fundus of gall bladder
D. Neck of gall bladder & cystic duct

**22. All except one are sites of portocaval anastomosis : AI 1989**
A. Umbilicus
B. Anal canal
C. Lower end of esophagus
D. Pylorus

**23. Common bile duct stones will manifest with following except : AIIMS 1984; AI 1989**
A. Distended gall bladder
B. Jaundice
C. Itching
D. Gray coloured stools

**24. Secondaries to liver can arise from the following sites except : Kerala 1998**
A. Lungs B. Kidney
C. Stomach D. Breast

**25. Courvoisier's law is not applicable if there is following, except : AIIMS 1986**
A. Double impactation of stone (Cystic duct and CBD).
B. Oriental cholangiohepatitis.
C. Pancreatic calculus obstructing ampulla of Vater.
D. Chronic recurrent cholecystitis.

**26. Discolouration in the loins in acute pancreatitis is : UPSC 1983, 97; AMC 1984, 85**
A. Gray Turner's sign B. Murphy's sign
C. Cullen's sign D. Homan's sign

| Ans. | 11. A | 12. D | 13. B | 14. D | 15. D | 16. E | 17. B | 18. D | 19. C | 20. D |
|---|---|---|---|---|---|---|---|---|---|---|
| | 21. D | 22. D | 23. A | 24. B | 25. D | 26. A | | | | |

27. **Membrane damage in pancreatitis is caused by : TN 1996**
A. Amylase B. Lysolecithin
C. Peptidase D. Elastase

28. **Splenectomy is sometimes indicated in : AIIMS 1996**
A. Portal hypertension B. Myelofibrosis
C. Amyloidosis D. Angioma

29. **Splenosis means : AIIMS 1985**
A. Infection of spleen
B. Presence of accessory spleens
C. Rupture of spleen and distribution of its parts on peritoneum
D. Non-functioning spleen

30. **The commonest pancreatic tumour is : AMC 1983**
A. Ductal adenocarcinoma
B. Cystadenoma
C. Insulinoma
D. Non-islet cell tumour

31. **Spontaneous rupture of the liver occurs in : PGI 1981**
A. Hepatoma B. Portal hypertension
C. Spherocytosis D. Secondary depositE

32. **Following are true about CBD stones except : JIPMER 1997**
A. Lipid soluble substance may be used to treat
B. Surgically removed
C. Distention of GB seldom occurs
D. Stones have origin always in GB

33. **In all of the following conditions, there is localised swelling of liver except : AIIMS 1981**
A. Riedel's lobe
B. Hydatid cyst
C. Cholangio hepatoadenoma
D. Amoebic abscess

34. **The length of the common bile duct is : PGI 1983, 85**
A. 5 cm B. 7.5 cm
C. 8.0 cm D. 9 cm

35. **Best investigative modality for detecting gall bladder stone is : PGI 1985, 88**
A. OCG
B. PTC
C. Ultrasound
D. Intravenous cholangiogram

36. **Following are true of Pseudopancreatic cyst except : JIPMER 1993; PGI 2000**
A. Raised amylase level
B. Surgery after 6-8 weeks
C. Drains into duodenum
D. Follows Acute duodenum

37. **Investigation of choice in Acute cholangitis is : JIPMER 1993**
A. HIDA scan B. I.V. Cholangiogram
C. USG D. Plain X-ray

38. **Cholangiocarcinoma histological resembles : Delhi 1993**
A. Sq. cell type B. Colloid cell type
C. Schirrhous type D. Columnar cell type

39. **Causes of massive splenomegaly are following except : Delhi 1993**
A. Kala Azar B. Gaucher's disease
C. CML D. CLL

40. **During management of obstructive jaundice, renal failure can be prevented by : Delhi 1992**
A. Adequate hydration
B. Low dose dopamine infusion
C. Blood transfusion
D. Vit K administration

41. **The hepatic artery supplies approximately —— % of blood flow to the liver. DNB 1990**
A. 15% B. 25%
C. 45% D. 60%
E. 75%

42. **The most common cause of Hemobilia is : Delhi 1989; JIPMER 1992**
A. Trauma B. Liver abscess
C. Gall stone D. Cholangitis

43. **Most common complication of splenectomy is : AIIMS 1992; Delhi 1994; JIPMER 1997**
A. Haemorrhage
B. Pulmonary complication
C. Pancreatic leak
D. Pneumococcal infection

44. **Splenunculi most commonly occurs at : AIIMS 1992, 95; PGI 1993**
A. Tail of pancreas B. Hilum of spleen
C. Lesser omentum D. Greater omentum

45. **Splenunculi should also be removed when splenectomy is done for : JIPMER 1993**
A. Portal hypertension B. Hypersplenism
C. Lymphoma D. Trauma

| Ans. | | | | | | | | | |
|---|---|---|---|---|---|---|---|---|---|
| 27. A | 28. B | 29. C | 30. A | 31. A | 32. D | 33. A | 34. B | 35. C | 36. C |
| 37. A | 38. C | 39. D | 40. A | 41. B | 42. A | 43. B | 44. B | 45. B | |

**46. Following is not a complication of acute pancreatitis: UPSC 1985; AIIMS 1988**

A. Left sided pleural effusion
B. Hypocalcaemia
C. Hyperglycaemia
D. Pancreatic pseudocyst

**47. Chemotherapeutic agent of choice in Ca. pancreas is : AIIMS 1990, 92**

A. Mitomycin-C
B. 5-FU
C. Adriamycin
D. Streptozocin

**48. Post-splenectomy infection is commonly caused by : PGI 1993, 2000**

A. Pneumococcus
B. H. influenzae
C. Meningococcus
D. Gram negative rods

**49. While doing cholecystectomy, common bile duct exploration is indication in following, except : AIIMS 1985**

A. Common bile duct is turbid
B. White, thick-walled duct
C. Single large gall stone
D. Presence of jaundice
E. Dilated common duct

**50. Post-operative cholongiography is usually to be done ——— days later. UPSC 1987**

A. 1-2
B. 3-5
C. 5-7
D. 10-14

**51. Encephalopathy secondary to portal canal shunt is caused by : Delhi 1983**

A. Starvation
B. Bleeding from G.I. tract
C. Ammonia intoxication
D. All of the above

**52. Upto how much of liver may be resected before a major change in liver functions takes place : AIIMS 1985**

A. 20%
B. 40%
C. 60%
D. 80%
E. 90%

**53. The most dangerous anomally in the arterial supply of the gall bladder is : DNB 1989**

A. When the main trunk of hepatic artery takes a tortuous course in front of the origin of the cystic duct.
B. Presence of double cystic arteries.
C. When right hepatic artery crosses in front of the common bile duct.
D. When cystic artery crosses in front of the common bile duct.

**54. Hepatic abscess ruptures most commonly into the : UPSC 1986**

A. Peritoneal cavity
B. Intraabdominal viscus
C. Pericardial cavity
D. Pleuropulmonary area
E. All have equal incidence

**55. The most common nodule found in the liver is : AIIMS 1985; AI 1992**

A. Haemangioma
B. Hamartoma
C. Cholangioadenoma
D. Hepatoadenoma

**56. All of the following are true about mucoviscidosis of the pancreas, except : AIIMS 1986**

A. Causes intestinal obstruction.
B. Causes excessive loss of sodium chloride in the sweat.
C. Accompanies congenital cystic disease of the kidney.
D. Encourages staphylococcal infection.
E. Is a manifestation of hereditary congenital anomally of mucus secretion

**57. All of the following pathological features may be found in Pancreatic Pseudocyst except : Delhi 1994**

A. Mucinous epithelial lining
B. Haemorrhage
C. Fistulisation is stomach
D. Amylase rich fluid

**58. Liver biopsy may be attempted in : Delhi 1991, 94**

A. Bleeding disorders
B. Ascites
C. Hydated liver disease
D. Hepatoma

**59. Pus in empyema of Gall bladder is : Delhi 1994**

A. Greenish
B. Anchovy sauce
C. Creamy
D. Yellow

**60. The word 'Cirrhosis', which is derived from Greed word 'kirrhosis', relates to which of the following : AMU 1986**

A. Orange-yellow discoloration of liver
B. Shrinkage of liver
C. Hardening of liver
D. Scarring of liver

**61. Which of the following is not a presinosoidal cause of portal hypertension : AMU 1986**

A. Schistosomiasis
B. Toxin injury from vinyl chloride
C. Primary biliary cirrhosis
D. Non-cirrhotic nodular regeneration

**Ans.** 46. C 47. D 48. A 49. C 50. D 51. C 52. D 53. A 54. D 55. A
56. C 57. A 58. D 59. C 60. A 61. D

62. **For recurrent variceal bleeding which of the following is surgery of choice : Delhi 1983**
A. Total portocaval shunt
B. Side-to-side protocaval shunt
C. Proximal splenorenal shunt
D. Distal splenorenal shunt

63. **Which of the following does not precipitate hepatic encephalopathy : AIIMS 1985**
A. GI bleeding B. Infection
C. Diuretic D. Diarrhoea

64. **Which of the following is not a possible etiological factor in the case of hepatocellular carcinoma : PGI 1983**
A. Mycotoxin B. Plant alkaloid
C. Oral contraceptive D. Androgens
E. Aspirin

65. **Which of the following histological type of hepatocellular carcinoma carries the best prognosis : AIIMS 1985**
A. Trabecular type B. Pseudoglandular type
C. Schirrhous type D. Pleomorphic type
E. Fibrolamellar type

66. **Which of the following is the principal liver tumor associated with vinyl chloride injection : PGI 1984**
A. Hepatocellular carcinoma
B. Cholangiocarcinoma
C. Leiomyosarcoma
D. Fibrosarcoma
E. Angiosarcoma

67. **Liver cell adenoma and focal nodular hyperplasia of liver have following similarities except : AMU 1985**
A. Occur primarily in women
B. Occur predominantly at older age group
C. Have relation with oral contraceptive intake
D. Both are composed of hepatocytes

68. **The treatment of choice of an accessory cholecystohepatic duct is : AMC 1985**
A. Nothing
B. Cholecystostomy
C. Total cholecystectomy
D. Choledochojejunostomy

69. **The commonest presentation of mucoviscidosis (Fibocystic disease) of the pancreas at birth is : AMU 1987**
A. Intestinal obstruction B. Steatorrhoea
C. Bronchiolitis D. Cirrhosis of liver

70. **In Mucoviscidosis of the pancreas, the commonest defect is in the : PGI 1986**
A. Jejunum B. Ileum
C. Ascending colon D. Descending colon

71. **Banti's syndrome is characterized by the following except : Rohtak 1986**
A. Splenomegaly B. Ascites
C. Pancytopenia D. Purpuric rash

72. **The differential diagnosis of jaundice in neonate includes hepatitis and biliary atresia. Which of the following will differentiate the two disease states : DNB 1990**
A. 5-Nucleotidase is higher in hepatitis.
B. Alkaline phosphatase is higher in atresia.
C. 5-Nucleotidase is higher in atresia.
D. Transaminase is elevated in neonatal hepatitis.
E. Alkaline phosphatase and transaminase are higher in hepatitis.

73. **In insulinoma, following are seen, except : Rajasthan 1998**
A. Hypoglycenoid
B. Loss of body weight
C. Cardiac arrythmias
D. Relieved with I/V glucose

74. **The presence of segmental and/or lobar atrophy of the liver should cause of the surgeon to do : UPSC 1984**
A. Biopsy the atropine protein
B. Biopsy the normal appearing portion
C. Exploration of the common duct and cholangiography
D. Nothing

75. **Which of the following factors may confuse the diagnosis of pancreatic ascites: DNB 1990**
A. 20% of cirrhotics have elevated serum amylase and serum lipase without evidence of pancreatic disease
B. Tuberculous peritonitis
C. Nephrosis
D. Cirrhotic ascites
E. All of the above

76. **Following ligation of the pancreatic duct, which of the following is primarily affected : AIIMS 1985**
A. Alpha islet cells B. Acinar tissue
C. Delta islet cells D. All of the above
E. None of the above

77. **Following resection of 2/3 of the liver, regeneration is complete within : AIIMS 1984**
A. 2—3 months B. 8—10 months
C. 4—6 months D. 4—5 weeks

| Ans. | | | | | | | | | |
|---|---|---|---|---|---|---|---|---|---|
| 62. D | 63. D | 64. E | 65. E | 66. E | 67. B | 68. B | 69. A | 70. B | 71. D |
| 72. C | 73. B | 74. C | 75. E | 76. B | 77. C | | | | |

**78. A 40-years old male presents with a painless cystic liver enlargement of four years duration without fever or jaundice. The most likely diagnosis is : UPSC 1996**

A. Amoebic liver abscess
B. Hepatoma
C. Hydatid cyst of liver
D. Choledochal cyst

**79. A 20-years old football player received a hard kick in the epigastrium. A large cystic swelling appeared in the epigastrium two weeks later. The most likely diagnosis is : UPSC 1996**

A. Hydatid cyst of liver
B. Amoebic liver abscess
C. Pseudopancreatic cyst
D. Haematoma of rectus sheath

**80. Splenectomy is done in young for : Kerala 1998**

A. ITP B. Elliptocytosis
C. Hodgkin's D. None

**81. The spleen contains about ——% of the total blood volume. AIIMS 1984; PGI 1985**

A. 1 B. 2
C. 5 D. 7

**82. Gall stones are likely to impact at : PGI 1983; AMC 1986, 90**

A. Duodenum B. Jejunum
C. Ileum D. Sigmoid colon

**83. Shunt operation is done in portal Hypertension because of : Delhi 1982; PGI 1982, 84; AIIMS 1983, 87; UPSC 1982, 83; ESI 1989;**

A. Ascites
B. Deteriorating liver functioning
C. Splenomegaly
D. Haemorrhage

**84. If pancreas is crushed against vertebral bodies, best treatment is : AIIMS 1983, 85, 86; ESI 1989**

A. Remove distal part and suture proximal end
B. Total pancreatectomy
C. Drain proximal and distal ends into jejunum
D. Simple closure of both ends

**85. Budd Chiari syndrome can be caused by : AIIMS 1985**

A. Thrombosis of hepatic veins
B. Polycythemia
C. Drinking herbal tea
D. Membranous webs of IVC
E. All of the above

**86. Pigment stones are common is : PGI 1982; Delhi 1983; AIIMS 1983, 87; ESI 1989**

A. Chronic pancreatitis
B. Hereditary spherocytosis
C. Idiopathic thrombocytopenic purpura
D. Cirrhosis

**87. Accidental, small, splenic rupture is treated with : UPSC 1986, 96**

A. Catgut suture
B. Silk sutures
C. Omental patch
D. Catgut suturing with omental patch
E. Splenectomy

**88. Zollinger Ellison syndrome is caused by : UPSC 1986**

A. Non-Beta cells
B. Beta cells
C. Alpha cells
D. Non-Alpha Non-Beta cells

**89. Bile is concentrated in the gall bladder by —— times. AIIMS 1986**

A. 5 B. 10
C. 20 D. 50

**90. ——% of the cardiac output flows through the liver. PGI 1985**

A. 10 B. 20
C. 30 D. 40

**91. In cholangitis, the organism mostly responsible is : PGI 1981**

A. E. coli B. Streptococcus
C. E. histolytica D. Clostridium

**92. The gall bladder is capable of distending —— times : PGI 1983**

A. 10 B. 20
C. 40 D. 50

**93. Hepatocellular carcinoma may be a complication of following except : Delhi 1988; PGI 1988; UPSC 1989**

A. Pain last for several hours
B. Serum amylase levels corelates with severity of attack
C. Common in alcoholics
D. Low serum calcium levels indicate good prognosis

**94. Regarding hepatic artery ligation which statement is false : Karnataka 1996**

A. The best results are obtained in case of haembilia.
B. Not useful in primary hepatoma.
C. Can cure secondary carcinoma.
D. Must be covered by massive antibiotic administration.

**Ans.** 78. C 79. D 80. B 81. A 82. C 83. D 84. A 85. E 86. B 87. B 88. A 89. B 90. D 91. A 92. D 93. C 94. C

**95. The triad of intermittent attacks of upper abdominal pain, jaundice and fever in a 40 years old male is seen in : UPSC 1982, 85; ESI 1985, 86; AI 1989**
A. Cystic duct stones
B. Common bile duct stone
C. Chronic recurrent pancreatitis
D. Carcinoma pancreas

**96. Splenomegaly and hematemesis are usually present in : UPSC 1981; ESI 1986**
A. Gastric carcinoma
B. Gastric ulcer
C. Portal hypertension
D. Common bile duct stone

**97. Best treatment of acute suppurative cholangitis : Delhi 1989**
A. Gall bladder stone removal
B. Common bile duct patency
C. Cholecystectomy
D. Dialysis

**98. Function of gall bladder is to increase : Delhi 1983, 89**
A. Alkalinity of bile B. Concentration
C. Intrabiliary pressure D. Phosphate level

**99. An ultrasound examination shows dilated intrahepatic biliary channels with a small gall bladder. The most likely possibility is : Karnataka 1996**
A. Gall bladder stone
B. Pancreatic calculus
C. Common bile duct stone
D. Carcinoma of the head of the pancreas

**100. Stone in ampulla of Vater with obstructive Jaundice is best diagnosed by : Delhi 1987**
A. ERCP B. PTC
C. IVC D. OCG

**101. Splenic vein thrombosis is best treated by : UPSC 1997**
A. Splenectomy
B. Portacaval shunt
C. Splenorenal shunt
D. Mesenterico-caval shunt

**102. One of the following is not a complication of following liver biopsy : AIIMS 1986**
A. Biliary peritonitis
B. Haemorrhage
C. Infective hepatitis
D. Abdominal/shoulder pain

**103. Gall-stones in ultrasound are : DNB 1989**
A. Sonolucent B. Echogenic
C. Opaque D. Not recognisable

**104. In acute pancreatitis serum amylase level reaches : DNB 1990**
A. 160 somogyl units B. 1000 somogyl units
C. 200 somogyl units D. 300 somogyl units

**105. Morphine is not advisable in biliary colic because : AMU 1990; DNB 1991**
A. Relief of pain is inadequate
B. It causes spasm of sphincter of Oddi
C. It does not control infection
D. Surgery is the best method

**106. In obstructive jaundice, the gall bladder is not enlarged if there is : AMU 1990**
A. Double-impactation by stone
B. Obstruction at the porta-hepatis
C. Stone in the common bile duct
D. Stone at the ampulla of Vater

**107. Which of the earliest post-operative sign of common-duct injury : AP 1989**
A. Obstructive jaundice
B. Excess bile leakage from wound
C. Peritonitis
D. Fever

**108. The barium-meal picture in a pseudo-pancreatic cyst shows : Rohtak 1990**
A. Filling defect in stomach
B. Stomach displaced forwards
C. Contracted stomach
D. Ulcer crater

**109. The commonest manifestation of carcinoma head of pancreas is : Rohtak 1989, 93**
A. Palpable mass B. Obstructive jaundice
C. Steatorrhoea D. Pain

**110. All of the following are causes of post-hepatic portal hypertension except : PGI 1985**
A. Constrictive percarditis
B. Tricuspid valvular incompetence
C. Budd Chiari syndrome
D. Schistosomiasis

**111. Foaming liver is produced by : Rohtak 1986**
A. Cirrhosis of liver
B. Gas gangrene
C. Hepatic amoebiasis
D. Pyaemic abscess of liver
E. All of the above

| Ans. | 95. B | 96. C | 97. B | 98. B | 99. C | 100. A | 101. A | 102. C | 103. B | 104. B |
|---|---|---|---|---|---|---|---|---|---|---|
| | 105. B | 106. A | 107. B | 108. B | 109. B | 110. D | 111. B | | | |

**112. All of the following are features of splenunculi (accessory spleens) except : AIIMS 1984**

A. They are common among adults.
B. They are present usually near the hilum.
C. After splenectomy the symptoms reappear.
D. These may also be found behind the tail and body of the pancreas.

**113. Acute pancreatitis : UPSC 1986**

A. May often be associated with gall stones.
B. Has no predilection for stout people.
C. Usually presents in people over-40 years of age.
D. All of the above.

**114. Air in Biliary tract is seen in following except : AIIMS 1995**

A. Sclerosing cholangitis
B. Gallstone ileus
C. Endoscopic papillotomy
D. Ca Gall bladder

**115. Presence of white bile indicates : TN 1987**

A. Viral hepatitis
B. Obstruction of cystic duct
C. Obstruction of common bile duct
D. Less intake of cholesterol
E. Disturbed bile salts and cholesterol ratio

**116. Asiatic cholangio-hepatitis is due to : AMU 1989**

A. Infection with trematodes
B. Australia antigen infection
C. Congenital malformation
D. Extraintestinal amoebiasis
E. All of the above

**117. Commonest type of gall stones are : DNB 1989**

A. Cholesterol stones B. Pigment stones
C. Pure phosphate stones D. Mixed stones
E. All occur with same frequency

**118. In the living person, pyloric canal is distinguished from first part of the duodenum by : DNB 1989**

A. Its sharp curvature B. Veins of Mayo
C. Consistency D. Decrease in thickness
E. Right gastric artery

**119. The left side boundary for the Calot's triangle is formed by : UPSC 1994**

A. Cystic duct B. Common bile duct
C. Common hepatic duct D. Inferior vena cava

**120. In idiopathic bile duct perforation, the treatment most preferred is : PGI 1985**

A. Simple drainage
B. Cholecystectomy
C. Choledochojejunostomy
D. Choledochoileostomy

**121. Non-correctable biliary atresia should perferable be operated before the age of : PGI 1984**

A. 3 months B. 6 months
C. 12 months D. 18 months

**122. Alpha foetoproteins in hepatoblastoma are seen in about : AIIMS 1988**

A. One third cases B. Two third cases
C. 90% D. 100%

**123. Drainage tube after draining the amoebic liver abscess should be kept for. AP 1987**

A. 7 days B. 10 days
C. 14 days D. 21 days
E. None of the above

**124. The peak of jaundice in congenital atresia of bileduct appears ——— days of life : DNB 1990**

A. At birth B. 2-3 days
C. 1-2 weeks D. 2-4 weeks

**125. Roux-en Y or Hepaticodochojejunostomy is recommended when there is : AIIMS 1985**

| | Gall bladder | Hepatic duct | Bile duct |
|---|---|---|---|
| A. | Present | Distended | Atresia (lower third) |
| B. | Functionless or absent | Distended | Atresia (lower third) |
| C. | Absent | Alone present | Absent |
| D. | Absent | Absent | Absent |

**126. Klatskin tumour is situated at : TN 1996; Rajasthan 1996**

A. At ehe junction of Right & left hepatic duct
B. At the lower end of common hepatic duct
C. At the lower end of common bile duct
D. At porta hepatis

**127. Which of the following is not seen in rupture of spleen : PGI 1986**

A. Kehr's sign B. Ballance's sign
C. Fall of B.P D. Murphy's sign

**128. Necrolytic erythema is a feature of : Rajasthan 1996**

A. Gastrinoma B. Glucagonoma
C. Insulinoma D. VIPoma

**129. If a patient known to have an abdominal aortic aneurysm complaints of severe back pain it usually means : AIIMS 1986**

A. Associated pancreatitis
B. Pressure on spinal cord
C. Impending rupture
D. Enlargement of sac

**Ans.** 112. A 113. D 114. D 115. C 116. A 117. D 118. B 119. C 120. A 121. A
122. B 123. E 124. B 125. C 126. A 127. D 128. B 129. C

**130. The age group most often present with jaundice due to Omphalitis in infants is : Kerala 1990**

A. At birth B. 24-72 hours
C. 1-3 weeks D. 3-6 weeks

**131. In congenital hemolytic anaemia (Hereditary spherocytosis or Acholuric familial jaundice), there is ——— permeability of the RBCs to ———. AMU 1983**

A. Increased sodium
B. Decreased sodium
C. Increased calcium
D. Increased all electrolytes

**132. The optimum time of splenectomy in a child with hereditary spherocytosis is : AIIMS 1985**

A. At birth B. 1-2 years of age
C. 3-4 years of age D. At puberty

**133. Differential diagnosis of chylous ascites include all of the following except : Karnataka 1994**

A. Lymphoma B. Nephrotic syndrome
C. TB D. CHF

**134. Carcinoma of pancreas attains greatest size when it is located in : Rohtak 1988**

A. Head B. Body and tail
C. Ampullary region D. Ampulla of Vater

**135. In one of the following condition, the ruptured spleen produces irreversible shock : DNB 1991; Delhi 1996**

A. Malaria B. Typhoid
C. Tuberculosis D. Haemophilia

**136. Patient with a large liver and glass eye is likely to be suffering from : DNB 1991**

A. Hepatic carcinoma B. Intra-ocular melanoma
C. Teratoma D. Carcinoma of prostate

**137. Following are complications of hydatid cyst in the liver except : AP 1997**

A. Jaundice B. Suppuration
C. Cirrhosis D. Rupture

**138. The common predisposing factor in Saint's triad is : DNB 1984**

A. Gall stones B. Obesity
C. Trauma D. Congenital defect

**139. The commonest cause of cirrhosis of liver among infants is : TN 1988**

A. Atresia of the bile duct
B. Marasmus
C. Infections
D. Erythroblastosis foetalis

**140. Congenital absence of the spleen is near always associated with the congenital abnormality in the : AMU 1985**

A. Anal region B. Heart
C. Kidney D. Spine

**141. Strawberry Gall bladder is : AP 1997**

A. Adenoma gall bladder
B. Acute cholecystitis
C. Cholesterosis
D. Carcinoma Gall Bladder

**142. Honeycomb liver is seen in : AMU 1990**

A. Micronodular cirrhosis
B. Dubin Johnson's syndrome
C. Actinomycosis
D. Hydatidosis

**143. When splenic injury is suspected, do : DNB 1991**

A. Exploration
B. Four quadrant aspiration
C. Ultrasonography
D. Clinical observation

**144. Which of the following carries better prognosis : AIIMS 1986**

A. Carcinoma gall bladder
B. Carcinoma head of pancreas
C. Hepatoma
D. Periampullary carcinoma

**145. Leukocytic infiltration in islet cells of pancreas is characteristically seen in some cases of : AMU 1987**

A. Juvenile diabetes
B. Diabetic ketosis
C. Systemic mucoviscidosis
D. Haemorrhagic pancreatic necrosis

**146. Floating gall bladder means : AMC 1984**

A. Gall bladder without concentrating function
B. Gall bladder with a mesentery
C. Double gall bladder
D. None of the above

**147. All of the following are clinical manifestations of chronic hepatic failure of the cirrhotic type except : AIIMS 1985**

A. Loss of axillary and pubic hair
B. Gynaecomastia and testicular atrophy
C. Personality changes
D. Jaundice

**148. In portal hypertension the portal venous pressure is usually above : Karnataka 1998**

A. 4 mm Hg B. 20 mm Hg
C. 40 mm Hg D. 12 mm Hg

| Ans. | | | | | | | | | |
|---|---|---|---|---|---|---|---|---|---|
| 130. D | 131. A | 132. C | 133. D | 134. B | 135. A | 136. B | 137. C | 138. B | 139. A |
| 140. B | 141. C | 142. C | 143. C | 144. D | 145. A | 146. B | 147. B | 148. B | |

**149. Treatment of choice for recurrent common bile duct stones is : AIIMS 1984, 87; UPSC 1984, 91**
A. Cheynodeoxycholic acid
B. Choledocholithotomy
C. Operative liver flushing
D. Endoscopic sphincterostomy

**150. Which of the following is not an indication of operative cholangiogram : PGI 1982; AIIMS 1984**
A. Gall bladder stones
B. Common bile duct stones
C. To study biliary tree
D. To study sphincter of Oddi

**151. Indication of surgery in chronic pancreatitis is : AIIMS 1984, 86**
A. Diabetes mellitus
B. Malabsorption
C. Risk of malignancy
D. Pain or Jaundice

**152. Commonest complication of pseudocyst of the pancreas is : UPSC 1985; AIIMS 1987**
A. Rupture into the peritoneum
B. Rupture into colon
C. Haemorrhage
D. Infection

**153. A 30-years old person met with a roadside accident. On admission, his pulse rate was 120/minute, BP was 100/60 mm Hg. Ultrasonography examination revealed location of the lower pole of spleen and haemoperitoneum. He was resuscitated with blood and fluid. Two hours later, his pulse was 84/minute and BP was 120/70 mm Hg. The most appropriate course of management in this case would be : CSE 1998**
A. Exploring the patient followed by splenectomy.
B. Exploring the patient followed by excision of the lower pole of spleen.
C. Splenorrhaphy.
D. Continuation of conservative treatment under close monitoring system and subsequent surgery if further indicated.

**154. A 20 years old man comes with sudden pain abdomen after meals is found to be in shock. Diagnosis is : AIIMS 1987**
A. Haemorrhagic pancreatitis
B. Gangrenous cholecystitis
C. Ruptured Appendix
D. Diverticulosis

**155. After surgery, a small left over stone in the CBD is best treated by : Kerala 1997**
A. ERCP
B. ESWL
C. Heparinised saline through T-tube
D. Repeat surgery

**156. Saint's triad is : PGI 1988**
A. Gall stone, diverticulitis, hiatus hernia.
B. Gall stone, diverticulitis, renal stones.
C. Bronchiectasis, diverticulitis, gall stones.
D. Gall stones, hiatus hernia, oesophagitis.
E. Hiatus hernia, gall stones, duodenal atresia.

**157. Hepatic artery ligation can be useful in the following except : Karnataka 1994**
A. Hepatoma
B. Secondary carcinoma
C. Haemobilia
D. Cirrhosis

**158. Line of surgical division of liver is : PGI 1989**
A. One inch to the Rt. of gall bladder
B. Falciform ligament to diaphragm
C. Gall bladder bed to IVC
D. Hepatic vein to IVC

**159. Absolute indications of choledochotomy are following except : PGI 1990, 94**
A. Past H/O Jaundice
B. Palpable stone in duct
C. Dilated cystic duct
D. Multiple stones in gall bladder
E. Multiple stones demonstrated by operative cholangiography

**160. Which of the following is not a constituent of gallstone : AMC 1985; UPSC 1989; AP 1990**
A. Protein
B. Bile
C. Carbonate
D. Oxalate

**161. Following are features of glucagonoma except : Delhi 1998**
A. Erythematous hillous rash
B. Mild diabetes
C. Angular cheilitis
D. Arginine enhances serum glucagon

**162. The highest level of serum amylase in acute pancreatitis is reached : PGI 1987; UPSC 1994**
A. Within first 12 hours
B. In 12 to 24 hours
C. In 24 to 48 hours
D. After 48 hours

**163. The most important radiological sign of splenic rupture is : JIPMER 1986, 87**
A. Obliteration of psoas shadow
B. Obliteration of splenic shadow
C. Indentation of the left side air bubble
D. Fracture one or more lower ribs on left side

**Ans.** 149. A 150. A 151. D 152. D 153. A 154. A 155. B 156. A 157. D 158. C
159. A 160. D 161. A 162. A 163. B

**164. Normal portal venous pressure is : PGI 1984**
A. 5—8 mm Hg B. 6—12 mm Hg
C. 13—15 mm Hg D. 30—45 mm Hg

**165. Features of emphysematous cholecystitis include following except : JIPMER 1987**
A. Elderly male patient
B. Diabetic
C. Cl. welchi is the infecting organism
D. Gas in the gall bladder
E. Good prognosis

**166. Round worm may cause the following except : PGI 1997**
A. Gall stone B. Cholangitis
C. Haematobilia D. Pancreatitis

**W167. Length of cystic duct is about —— cm. AIIMS 1986**
A. 2 B. 4
C. 8 D. 12

**168. Pain continuing after cholecystectomy may be due to any of the following except : UPSC 1994**
A. Retained stone in the common bile duct
B. Unsuspected subacute or chronic pancreatitis
C. Dyskinesia or spasm of sphincter of Oddi
D. Biliary cirrhosis

**169. In pancreatic cholera, following are seen, except : AIIMS 1986, 89**
A. Achlorhydria B. Watery diarrhoea
C. Hyperkalemia D. Non-beta cell tumour

**170. Acute hepatocellular failure in cirrhosis of liver is precipitated by : AIIMS 1984, 89**
A. Thrombosis of portal vein
B. Albumin infusion
C. Acute GI bleeding
D. High carbohydrate diet

**171. Urinary ascites is due to : PGI 1998**
A. Injury to bladder during birth
B. Ureteric obstruction
C. Congenital urethral atresia
D. Urethral valves

**172. Whipples triad, useful in the diagnosis of insulinoma of the pancreas consist of : AIIMS 1985**
A. Central nervous system symptoms, fasting blood sugar of 50 mg per 100 ml, relief following ingestion of glucose.
B. Central nervous system symptoms, fasting blood sugar of 60 mg per 100 ml, relief following intravenous glucagon.
C. Abdominal pain, fasting blood sugar of 50 mg per 100 ml, relief following ingestion of glucose.
D. Abdominal pain, high serum insulin, relief following the ingestion of glucose.
E. Fasting nausea and vomiting, positive tolbutamide test, relief following intravenous glucagon.

**173. The commonest tumour in liver is : AIIMS 1982; PGI 1983, 88; AMC 1987, 88**
A. Secondaries B. Hepatoma
C. Haemangioma D. None of the above

**174. Investigation of choice in Ca ampulla of vater is : Punjab 1997**
A. Ba meal follow through
B. ERCP
C. Enzyme essay
D. Radionuclide pancreatic scan

**175. Percentage of gall stones which are radio-opaque : JIPMER 1986**
A. 10% B. 20%
C. 30% D. 50%
E. 80%

**176. Least irritating substance in peritoneum : AI 1999**
A. Blood B. Bile
C. Pancreatic fluid D. Gastric content

**177. The complication least likely to occur in a pseudocyst of the pancreas is : Kerala 1990**
A. Haemorrhage B. Torsion
C. Infection D. Carcinomatous change

**178. A 52-years old man presents with profuse vomiting of blood. Prior to the onset of hematemesis, he had severe bouts of vomiting after imbibing alcohol. The most likely diagnosis is : AIIMS 1994**
A. Cirrhosis liver with bleeding oesophageal varices
B. Acute bleeding peptic ulcer
C. Alcoholic gastritis
D. Mallory-Weiss syndrome

**179. Threatening complication of operation in a patient with jaundice is: AIIMS 1994**
A. Haemorrhage B. Septic shock
C. Renal failure D. Encephalitis

**180. Best prognosis in acute pancreatitis is seen with —— pancreatitis. PGI 1989, 96**
A. Gall stones B. Viral
C. Post-operative D. Alcoholic

| Ans. | 164. B | 165. E | 166. C | 167. NONE | 168. D | 169. C | 170. B | 171. A | 172. A | 173. A |
|---|---|---|---|---|---|---|---|---|---|---|
| | 174. D | 175. A | 176. A | 177. D | 178. D | 179. A | 180. A | | | |

**181. Liver biopsy is contraindicated in the following except : Karnataka 1987; JIPMER 1998; MAHE 1998**

A. Severe jaundice B. Secondaries in the liver
C. Haemangioma D. Hydatid cyst

**182. The following are indications for splenectomy, except: PGI 1983; AI 1999**

A. Splenic rupture
B. Splenorenal shunt
C. Idiopathic thrombocytopenic purpura
D. Non-thrombocytopenic purpura
E. Primary splenic tumour

**183. Fluid thrill alone is elicited without any shifting dullness in ascites in the following situations : Karnataka 1987**

A. Massive fluid B. Short mesentary
C. Peritoneal adhesions D. All of the above

**184. The diagnosis of gall stone ileus can be suspected when there is : Karnataka 1987**

A. Paralytic ileus
B. History of dyspepsia
C. Air in the biliary tract in plain X-ray
D. Distension of C-curve of duodenum

**185. Treatment of choice for Annular pancreas is : AIIMS 1993**

A. Whipples operation B. Duodeno-jejunostomy
C. Gastro-jejunostomy D. Conservative

**186. Gall stone is common in : AIIMS 1993; AI 1998**

A. Ileal resection B. Subtotal gastrectomy
C. Jejunal resection D. Partial Hepatectomy

**187. Treatment of choice of a CBD stone of 2.5 cms size, diagnosed 2 years cholecystectomy : AI 1999**

A. Choledochotomy & T-tube
B. Dormia basket
C. Transduodenal sphincterotomy
D. Supraduodenal choledochotomy

**188. Which is not true regarding choledochal cyst : PGI 1994**

A. Presents in elderly females
B. May cause cirrhosis
C. May turn malignant
D. Cause of obstructive jaundice

**189. Commonest cause of surgical obstructive jaundice in India : AIIMS 1994**

A. Carcinoma head of pancreas
B. Carcinoma gall bladder
C. Periampullary carcinoma
D. Fibrosarcoma

**190. Best treatment modality for CBD stones is : AIIMS 1994**

A. Percutaneous removal
B. Endoscopic sphincterotomy and removal
C. Chenodeoxycholic acid
D. Observation only

**191. Regarding injuries to pancreas, which is not true : AIIMS 1994**

A. Fracture is common at junction of head and body.
B. Associated commonly with vascular injuries.
C. Peritoneal lavage is a good diagnostic modality.
D. Majority of post-operative complications are true due to missed duct injury.

**192. Ectopic pancreas rarely occurs in : AP 1993**

A. Greater curvature of stomach
B. Duodenal bulb
C. Meckel's diverticulum
D. Appendix

**193. A common complication of porcelain gall bladder is : AP 1993**

A. Gangrene B. Perforation
C. Scleroderma D. Malignancy

**194. The commonest site for obstructive jaundice is : AP 1993**

A. Intrahepatic duct
B. Distal hepatic duct
C. Distal common bile duct
D. Distal pancreatic duct

**195. Gallstones are not frequently seen in : AP 1993**

A. Multiple Myeloma B. Thalassemia
C. Sickle cell disease D. Hyperlipidemia

**196. Fistula in bile duct is best diagnosed by : Delhi 1996**

A. CT scan
B. OCG
C. Transhepatic cholangiography
D. Ultrasound

**197. Wrong about Pseudopancreatic cyst is : PGI 1996**

A. Normally diagnosed by sustained β amylase.
B. Transphincteric duodenal drainage is commonly used.
C. Cystogastrectomy is done.
D. Collection of fluid in lesser sac.

**198. In acute pancreatitis, which of the following increases after rise of amylase : PGI 1996**

A. Lipase B. Glucagon
C. Ca++ D. Gastrin

**199. Pancreatitis may be produced by : PGI 1996**

A. Colchicine B. L-Asparaginase
C. Ciprofloxacin D. Nalidixic acid

| Ans. | | | | | | | | | |
|---|---|---|---|---|---|---|---|---|---|
| 181. A | 182. D | 183. D | 184. C | 185. B | 186. A | 187. C | 188. A | 189. B | 190. B |
| 191. C | 192. D | 193. D | 194. C | 195. A | 196. C | 197. B | 198. A | 199. B | |

**200. In Portosystemic shunt, prognosis depends on :** **AIIMS 1996**

A. Albumin level B. Bilirubin level
C. Type of shunt D. Nutritional status

**201 True about hepatocellular carcinoma is following except :** **AIIMS 1996**

A. Uncommon in Asians
B. Aflatoxin
C. Hepatitis B & C markers increased
D. Fibrolamellar type has better prognosis

**202. Liver biopsy is done at 5th intercostal space mid-axillary line, because :** **AI 1995**

A. To avoid pleura
B. To avoid lungs
C. There has bare area of liver
D. There is asparate in Morrison's pouch

**203. Cholangiocarcinoma is seen in following except :** **AI 1997**

A. Sclerosing cholangitis B. Chlonorchiasis sinensis
C. Gall stones D. Ulcerative colitis

**204. Small and soft splenomegaly is found in :** **Punjab 1997**

A. Enteric fever B. Portal hypertension
C. Hodgkin's lymphoma D. Early CML

**205. After cholecystectomy, there is increased chance of carcinoma of :** **Delhi 1996**

A. Pancreas B. Stomach
C. Bile duct D. Liver

**206. Acute Pancreatitis is a type of ——— necrosis.** **JIPMER 1997**

A. Coagulative B. Liquefactive
C. Caseous D. Enzymatic fat

**207. Gall stones are seen in the following except :** **AI 1996**

A. Hypercholesterolemia B. Primary biliary cirrhosis
C. Clofibrate therapy D. Hypothyroidism

**208. Portosystemic anastomosis is seen at :** **AI 1996**

A. Sup. and inf. mesenteric veins
B. Sup. and Inf. rectal veins.
C. Portal and inf. mesenteric veins
D. Ant. and middle cerebral veins

**209. Lithogenic bile has :** **AI 1996**

A. ↑ Bile/cholesterol ratio
B. ↓ Bile/cholesterol ratio
C. Equal bile cholesterol ratio
D. Only ↑ in bile concentration

**210. In Pancreatitis, prognosis depends on following except :** **UPSC 1989, 91; AI 1996; AIIMS 2000**

A. Serum amylase B. Old age
C. Total count D. Serum calcium

**211. Following are seen in chronic calcific pancreatitis except :** **Kerala 1996**

A. Diabetes mellitus
B. Fat malabsorption
C. Hypercalcemia
D. Recurrent abdominal pain
E. Increased incidence of pancreatic carcinoma

**212. Commonest site of amoebic liver abscess is :** **Kerala 1996**

A. Postero-superior portion of lobe of liver
B. Left lobe of liver under surface
C. Under surface of lobe of liver
D. Upper surface of lobe of liver

**213. Most common indication of splenectomy in India is :** **Punjab 1997; AI 1992, 96**

A. Trauma
B. CML
C. Hereditary spherocytosis
D. Hodgkin's lymphoma

**214. A four-week old baby presents with jaundice and clay-coloured stools. Which of the following should be included in the differential diagnosis :** **UPSC 1997**

1. Rh factor incompatibility
2. Neonatal hepatitis
3. Choledochal cyst
4. Extra-hepatic biliary atresia
5. Intra-hepatic biliary atresia
6. Hepatoblastoma

**Select the correct answer using the codes given below:**
**Codes :**

A. 1, 2 and 3 B. 1, 2, 3, 4, 5 and 6
C. 2, 3, 4 and 5 D. 4, 5 and 6

**215. Amoebic Liver Abscess is caused by :** **Karnataka 1999**

A. Trophozoites of EH
B. Cysts of EH
C. Both Trophozoites and cysts of EH
D. All of the above

**216. A cirrhotic presented with upper GI bleed. On examination he was hypotensive with pallor, tachycardia and cold clammy extremities. What is the ideal treatment :** **AIIMS 1999**

A. Whole blood B. Packed cell
C. Crystalloids D. I/V fluids

**Ans.** 200. C 201. A 202. A 203. C 204. A 205. D 206. D 207. B 208. B 209. B
210. A 211. C 212. A 213. A 214. C 215. A 216. A

**217. A 60 years old man suffering from obstructive jaundice. What is the initial investigation of choice : AIIMS 1999**

A. MRI B. USG
C. Radionucleotide scan D. CT Scan

**218. All are true about gall stones except : AIIMS 1999**

A. Predisposed by DM
B. Predisposes to Ca gall bladder
C. Most common b/w 30-40 weeks
D. Gall stones may be asymptomatic

**219. A cirrhotic with massive bleed of 6 hours duration presents with hematemesis. What should be done : AIIMS 1999**

A. Insert Ryle's tube
B. Endoscopy
C. Labelled RBC
D. Surgical intervention contraindicated in young patient

**220. Feature common to carcinoma pancreas, lungs, stomach is : TN 1999**

A. Thrombophlebitis
B. Migratory thrombophlebitis
C. Ascites
D. DIC

**221. In acute calculus cholecystitis all are true except : Kerala 1999**

A. Ultrasound is indicated for diagnosis
B. Hypoasthesia is seen above 9-11 ribs
C. Surgical Rx done
D. Oval cholecystogram is useless

**222. Commonest malignancy of spleen is : AI 2000**

A. Lymphoma B. Metastatic Ca colon
C. Metastatic Ca kidney D. Splenic hemangioma

**223. Consider the following procedures: UPSC 2000**

1. Percutaneous transhepatic cholangiography.
2. Intravenous cholangiography.
3. Endoscopic retrograde cholangiopancreatography.

The procedure used in investigating a case of obstructive jaundice would include:

A. 1, 2 and 3 B. 1 and 3
C. 1 and 2 D. 2 and 3

**224. A 48-years old lady, a known case of gall stone disease presents with a history of severe pain in the epigastrium radiating to the back, accompanied with repeated vomiting, and abdominal distension. She is found to have oliguria and hypotension. The most likely diagnosis is : UPSC 2000**

A. Pancreatitis B. Acute cholecystitis
C. Cholangitis D. Gall stone ilieus

**225. Treatment of choice in chronic pancreatitis with "chain of lakes" appearance on ERCP is : Rohtak 2000**

A. Pancreatico duodenectomy
B. Longitudinal pancreatojejunostomy
C. Pancreatic resection
D. Medical treatment

**226. True about idiopathic cholestasis of pregnancy is, except: Rohtak 2000**

A. Clotting abnormalities
B. ERCP is required
C. Jaundice
D. Usually intrahepatic cholestasis

**227. Indication of cholangiogram are following except : Rohtak 2000**

A. Mucocele of GB
B. ↑ Alk. Phosphatase
C. Past history of pancreatitis
D. Sclerosing cholangitis

**228. Which one of the following statements regarding meconium peritonitis is not correct: UPSC 2000**

A. It is a septic peritonitis.
B. It develops in later intrauterine life or during or just after delivery.
C. This condition should always be considered when a baby is born with tense abdomen.
D. Plain X-ray of abdomen of this condition reveals calcification on liver and spleen.

**229. Gold standard test in insulinoma : PGI 2000**

A. CT scan B. Ultrasound
C. MRI D. Arteriography

**230. Mucinous ascites is seen in : PGI 2000**

A. Stomach Ca B. TB
C. Nephrotic syndrome D. Cirrhosis

**231. Patient with pancreatitis undergoes sudden loss of vision, possible cause is : AI 2001**

A. Methanol toxicity
B. Ethanol toxicity
C. Methanol toxicity followed by ethanol therapy
D. Purtschers retinopathy

**232. Calcified hydatid cyst of the liver should be managed by : TNPSC 1998**

A. Chemotherapy B. Excision
C. No treatment D. Radiation

**233. Causes of choledochal cyst are all except : UP 1999**

A. Pancreatico-biliary anatomical anomaly
B. Inspissated bile
C. Congenital anomaly of bile duct
D. Due to both, intrinsic defect & obstruction

| Ans. | | | | | | | | | |
|---|---|---|---|---|---|---|---|---|---|
| 217. B | 218. A | 219. B | 220. B | 221. B | 222. A | 223. A | 224. A | 225. B | 226. A |
| 227. D | 228. A | 229. D | 230. A | 231. D | 232. C | 233. B | | | |

**234. Which of the following regarding pancreatic carcinoma is false :** **Kerala 2000**

A. Most frequent symptoms are weight loss, pain and anorexia.

B. More than 75 percent of all cases are Adenocarcinomas of ductal cell origin.

C. The ratio of the Head & Neck tumors compared to body and tail is 1 : 2.

D. The prevalence of jaundice varies with the position in the pancreas where the tumour is situated.

E. At the time of presentation disease is beyond surgical resection in over 80 percent of cases.

**235. Regarding stones in gall bladder the following are true except :** **Kerala 2000**

A. Mixed stones are common in the west.

B. In Saints Triad diverticulosis of colon and hiatus hernia coexist.

C. Is a risk factor in the development of GB carcinoma.

D. 90% of gall stones are radio-opaque.

E. A mucocele of GB is caused by a stone impacted in the Hartmann's pouch.

**236. The following are true regarding Ascites except :** **Kerala 2000**

A. Only when the amount of fluid present exceeds 1500 ml. it can be recognised clinically.

B. Shifting dullness is absent when there is a very large accumulation of fluid.

C. In cirrhosis there is obstruction to be venous outflow of the liver due to obliterative fibrosis of the Intra hepatic venous bed.

D. A transudate has a protein content of greater than 30 gms. of protein per litre.

E. In Meig's syndrome it is associated with pleural effusion and solid fibroma of ovary.

**237. A child presents with history of blunt injury abdomen associated with splenic trauma. On examination the child is stable. Which of the following is the treatment of choice :** **AI 2000**

A. Splenorrhaphy B. Observation
C. Splenectomy D. Arterial embolisation

**238. Most common malignant tumor of spleen is :** **UP 2000**

A. Lymphoma B. Haemangioma
C. Adenocarcinoma D. Sq. cell carcinoma

**239. Pancreatic Ca is caused by :** **AI 2001**

A. Fasciola B. Clonorchiasis
C. Paragonimus D. Granulosus

**240. Indication of medical treatment of gall stone is :** **AI 1998**

A. Size < 15 mm B. Ca. bilirubinate stone
C. Radio-opaque D. Non-functioning GB

**241. Pt. with recurrent abd. pain, normal serum bilirubin, Ehrlich test positive diagnosis :** **JIPMER 2001**

A. Choledocholithiasis B. Porphyria
C. Renal stones D. Abd. Koch's

**242. Ramu, 8 years old boy presents upper GI bleeding. On examination, splenomegaly, no ascites, no hepatomegaly; esophageal varices present and UGIE. Diagnosis is :** **AI 2001**

A. Budd Chiari syndrome
B. Non-cirrhotic portal fibrosis
C. Cirrhosis
D. Venoocclusive disease

**243. A Young patient presents with jaundice. Bilirubin is 21, direct is 9 and SAP 84 KA units. Diagnosis is :** **AI 2001**

A. Hemolytic jaundice
B. Viral hepatitis
C. Chronic active hepatitis
D. Obstructive jaundice

**244. All the following are true regarding fibrolamellar carcinoma of the liver except :** **AIIMS 2001**

A. AFP levels > 1000
B. It occurs in younger individuals
C. More common in females
D. Better prognosis as compared to HCC

**245. Which of the following is the most common cause of suppurative cholangitis :** **SGPGI 2002**

A. Hepatic vein B. CBD stone
C. Sepsis D. Empyema

**246. Caput medusa is obvious in all of the following, except :** **SGPGI 2002**

A. Budd Chiari syndrome
B. Extra hepatic portal vein thrombosis
C. Non-cirrhotic peri portal fibrosis
D. Alcoholic cirrhosis

**247. After splenectomy earliest changes seen are increase in :** **SGPGI 2002**

A. Lymphocytes B. Monocytes
C. Platelets D. Neutrophils

**248. Insulinoma most commonly occurs in :** **AIIMS 2002**

A. Head of pancreas
B. Body of pancreas
C. Tail of pancreas
D. Equally distributed in head, body and tail

**Ans.** 234. E 235. D 236. D 237. B 238. A 239. B 240. A 241. B 242. B 243. D
244. C 245. B 246. B 247. C 248. C

**249. A case of portal hypertension has Serum Bilirubin 2.5 mg/dl. Albumin 3.5 gm/dl and minimal ascites. The patient never had haemetemisis. Which one of the following statements is correct : UPSC 2002**

A. Patient is grouped as child's grade-A and treated by selective shunt.
B. Patient is grouped as child's grade-B and treated conservatively.
C. Patient is grouped as child's grade-B and treated selective shunt.
D. Patient is grouped as child's grade-A and treated conservatively.

**250. Which one of the following parasites may cause Suppurative Cholangitis : UPSC 2002**

A. Ankylostoma duodenale
B. Ascaris lumbricoides
C. Necator americanus
D. Trichuris trichura

**251. A 22 years old man presents with a solitary 2 cm space occupying lesion of mixed echogenicity in the right lobe of liver on ultrasound examination. The rest of the liver is normal. Which of the following tests should be done next : AIIMS 2002**

A. Ultrasound guided biopsy of the lesion
B. Hepatic Scintiography
C. Hepatic angiography
D. Contrast enhanced CT scan of the liver

**252. A 70 years old male patient presented with history of chest pain and was diagnosed to have coronary artery disease. During routine evaluation, an ultrasound of the abdomen showed presence of gall bladder stones. There was no past history of biliary colic or jaundice. What is the best treatment advice for such a patient for his gall bladder stones : AI 2003**

A. Open cholecystectomy
B. Laparoscopic cholecystectomy
C. No surgery for gall bladder stones
D. ERCP and removal of gall bladder stones

**253. An increased incidence of cholangiocarcinoma is seen in all of the following except : AI 2003**

A. Hydatid cyst of the liver
B. Polycystic disease of liver
C. Sclerosing cholangitis
D. Liver fluke

**254. Surgical intervention is not indicated in which one of the following conditions in acute pancreatitis : UPSC 2003**

A. Acute fluid collection
B. Pseudocyst
C. Infected pancreatic necrosis
D. Pancreatic abscess

**255. The most common cause of stricture in the bile duct is due to : JIPMER 2003**

A. Ascending cholangitis
B. Post-surgery-Cholecystectomy
C. Malignancy
D. Sclerosing cholangitis

**256. Which one of the following is not true about laparoscopic cholecystectomy as compared to conventional cholecystectomy : UPSC 2003**

A. Shorter hospital stay
B. Better evaluation of CBD
C. Early return to work
D. Decreased requirement of post-operative analgesia

**257. A patient comes with jaundice, dilated intrahepatic biliary raddicles and small gall bladder. Which of the following is most likely diagnosis : CUPGME 2003**

A. Gall bladder stone
B. Common Bile Duct Stone
C. Pancreatic Calculus
D. Carcinoma of head of pancreas

**258. The Couinaud's segmental nomenclature is based on the position of the : AI 2004**

A. Hepatic veins and portal vein
B. Hepatic veins and biliary ducts
C. Portal vein and biliary ducts
D. Portal vein and hepatic artery

**259. In neonatal cholestasis, if the serum gamma-glutamyl-transpeptidase (gamma GTP) is more than 600 IU/L the most likely diagnosis is: AI 2004**

A. Neonatal hepatitis
B. Choledochal cyst
C. Sclerosing cholangitis
D. Biliary atresia

**260. In patients with cirrhosis of the liver the site of obstruction in the portal system is in the: AI 2004**

A. Hepatic vein
B. Post-sinusoidal
C. Extra hepatic portal vein
D. Sinusoids

**261. In Budd Chiari syndrome, the site of venous thrombosis is : AI 2004**

A. Infrahepatic inferior vena cava
B. Infrarenal inferior vena cava
C. Hepatic veins
D. Portal vein

**Ans.** 249. B 250. B 251. A 252. C 253. B 254. A 255. B 256. B 257. B 258. A 259. D 260. D 261. C

**262. Which of the following types of pancreatitis has the best prognosis: AI 2004**

A. Alcoholic pancreatitis
B. Gall stone pancreatitis
C. Post-operative pancreatitis
D. Idiopathic pancreatitis

**263. In patients with cirrhosis of the liver the site of obstruction in the portal system is in the : AI 2004**

A. Hepatic vein
B. Post-sinusoidal
C. Extra hepatic portal vein
D. Sinusoids

**264. During surgical exploration for hydatid cyst of the liver, any of the following agents can be used as scolicidal agent except : UPSC 2004**

A. Hypertonic sodium chloride
B. Formalin
C. Cetrimide
D. Povidone iodine

**265. Which one of the following treatment modalities is NOT used for management of acute blood loss due to ruptured esophageal varices : UPSC 2004**

A. Endoscopic sclerotherapy
B. Endoscopic band ligation
C. Octreotide
D. Propranolol

**266. Tender hepatomegaly is NOT seen in : UPSC 2004**

A. Viral hepatitis B. Typhoid fever
C. Right heart failure D. Liver abscess

**267. In a patient with spontaneous biliary-enteric fistula the most common site of communication with gall bladder is : UPSC 2005**

A. Duodenum B. Jejunum
C. Ileum D. Transverse colon

**268. A 30-years-old lady is found to have gall stones. She is asymptomatic and has never had any jaundice or dyspeptic symptoms in the past. The best course of management for her would be : UPSC 2005**

A. Dissolution therapy
B. Extra corporeal lithotripsy
C. Cholecystectomy
D. To wait till she becomes symptomatic

**269. A 17-years-old boy is admitted to hospital after road traffic accident. Per abdomen examination is normal. After adequate resuscitation his pulse rate is 80/min. and blood pressure is 110/70 mm Hg. Abdominal CT reveals 1 cm deep laceration in left lobe of the liver extending from the dome more than half way through the parenchyma. Appropriate management at this time would be : UPSC 2005**

A. Conservative treatment
B. Abdominal exploration and packing of hepatic wound
C. Abdominal exploration and ligation of left hepatic artery
D. Left hepatectomy

**270. Consider the following : UPSC 2005**

1. Alcohol
2. Cholelithiasis
3. Insulinoma
4. Hyperparathyroidism

Which of the above are etiological factors for acute pancreatitis :

A. 1 and 3 B. 1, 2 and 3
C. 1, 2 and 4 D. 2 and 4

**271. Complications of chronic pancreatitis include the following except : UPSC 2005**

A. Portal hypertension
B. Obstructive jaundice
C. Duodenal obstruction
D. Renal artery aneurysm

**272. Patient with pancreatic transplant with urinary drainage. Monitoring will be done by : AI 2009**

A. Blood amylase B. Urine amylase
C. Serum glucose levels D. Serum lipase levels

**273. A gall blader with a poly, what is not a risk factor for development of Carcinomas : AI 2009**

A. Presence of gall stones
B. Age > 60 years
C. Polyp > 5 mm in length
D. Sudden increase in size of polyp

**274. Which of the following is not a component of Reynold's Pentad in tonic chalangitis : Delhi 2009**

A. Right upper quadrant pain
B. Congusion
C. Septic shock
D. Markedly elevated transaminases

**275. Which of the following liver tumors always merit surgery? Delhi 2009**

A. Hemangioma
B. Hepatic adenoma
C. Focal nodular hyperplasia
D. Peliosis hepatis

| Ans. | 262. B | 263. D | 264. D | 265. D | 266. B | 267. A | 268. D | 269. A | 270. C | 271. D |
|---|---|---|---|---|---|---|---|---|---|---|
| | 272. B | 273. C | 274. D | 275. B | | | | | | |

# EXPLANATIONS OF HEPATOBILIARY SYSTEM (LIVER, SPLEEN, PANCREAS)

1. Ans.— A. **Cancer of the liver**
2. Ans.— B. **Level of obstruction in the biliary tract.**
3. Ans.— A. **Sepsis in splenectomised children**
4. Ans.— D. **Emesis without bile is characteristic**
5. Ans.— C. **Gall stones should be radioopaque**

   Bile acids, chenodeoxycholic acid and uredeoxycholic acid taken orally will dissolve gall stones as long as they are radioluscent and gall bladder is not "non-functioning".
6. Ans.— A. **Injury to the common bile duct during cholecystectomy.**
7. Ans.— C. **Intrahepatic causes**

   Alcoholic cirrhosis is the commonest cause.
8. Ans.— B. **The diagnosis of gastric carcinoma**
9. Ans.— D. **The head proper**
10. Ans.— C. **Carcinoma of periampullary region of pancreas.**
11. Ans.— A. **Cholecystectomy and choledochotomy.**
12. Ans.— D. **Pale palms**
13. Ans.— B. **Congenital**
14. Ans.— D. **Haemorrhage from cystic vein**
15. Ans.— D. **All of the above**

    It is due to obstruction of hepatic veins and may result due to polycythemia, OCP and infertility. Congenital cause is also present. Hepatocellular carcinoma is a common cause.
16. Ans.— E. **All of the above**
17. Ans.— B. **Distal splenorenal shunt**
18. Ans.— D. **Exploration**
19. Ans.— C. **Complement fixation test**
20. Ans.— D. **Fever**

    This is a triad of haemobilia and the commonest cause is trauma (surgical).
21. Ans.— D. **Neck of gall bladder & cystic duct**
22. Ans.— D. **Pylorus**
23. Ans.— A. **Distended gall bladder**

    As stated by Courvoisiers law, if in a case of obstructive jaundice there is distended Gall Bladder it can not be due to gall stones. Features of itching is due to bile salts & clay coloured stools are due to lack of bile pigments & steatorrhea.
24. Ans.— B. **Kidney**
25. Ans.— D. **Chronic recurrent cholecystitis**
26. Ans.— A. **Gray Turner's sign**
27. Ans.— A. **Amylase**
28. Ans.— B. **Myelofibrosis**
29. Ans.— C. **Rupture of spleen and distribution of its parts on peritoneum.**
30. Ans.— A. **Ductal adenocarcinoma**
31. Ans.— A. **Hepatoma**
32. Ans.— D. **Stones have origin always in GB**
33. Ans.— A. **Riedel's lobe**
34. Ans.— B. **7.5 cm**
35. Ans.— C. **Ultrasound**
36. Ans.— C. **Drains into duodenum**

    It is often single (85%), has persistent rise in serum amylase and cystogastrostomy is treatment of choice. Infection is commonest complication.
37. Ans.— A. **HIDA scan**
38. Ans.— C. **Schirrhous type**
39. Ans.— D. **CLL**
40. Ans.— A. **Adequate hydration**

41. Ans.— B. 25%

42. Ans.— A. Trauma

43. Ans.— B. Pulmonary complication

That is why it is avoided in children.

44. Ans.— B. Hilum of spleen

45. Ans.— B. Hypersplenism

46. Ans.— C. Hyperglycaemia

47. Ans.— D. Streptozocin

48. Ans.— A. Pneumococcus

Splenectomised patients are at increased risk of septicemia. Children who are splenectomised are at increased risk of pneumococcus and should receive Pneumococcal vaccine and antibiotics (Erythromycin) cover until 18 yrs of age.

49. Ans.— C. Single large gall stone

50. Ans.— D. 10-14

51. Ans.— C. Ammonia intoxication

52. Ans.— D. 80%

53. Ans. A. When the main trunk of hepatic artery takes a tortuous course in front of the origin of the cystic duct.

54. Ans.— D. Pleuropulmonary area

Hepatic pain is commonest presentation.

55. Ans.— A. Haemangioma

Haemangioma occurs more commonly in the lives than in any other internal organ and is usually of cavernous type. It is small solitary and well defined. It is treated only when they are causing a large AV shunting that embarrass the heart or suspicion of malignant vascular tumor. Treatment is by embolization or exceptionally removal of liver segment.

56. Ans.— C. Accompanies congenital cystic disease of the kidney.

57. Ans.— A. Mucinous epithelial lining

58. Ans.— D. Hepatoma

59. Ans.— C. Creamy

60. Ans.— A. Orange-yellow discoloration of liver.

61. Ans.— D. Non-cirrhotic nodular regeneration

62. Ans.— D. Distal splenorenal shunt

63. Ans.— D. Diarrhoea

64. Ans.— E. Aspirin

65. Ans.— E. Fibrolamellar type

66. Ans.— E. Angiosarcoma

67. Ans.— B. Occur predominantly at older age group.

68. Ans.— B. Cholecystostomy

69. Ans.— A. Intestinal obstruction

70. Ans.— B. Ileum

71. Ans.— D. Purpuric rash

72. Ans.— C. 5-Nucleotidase is higher in atresia

73. Ans.— B. Loss of body weight

74. Ans.— C. Exploration of the common duct and cholangiography.

75. Ans.— E. All of the above

76. Ans.— B. Acinar tissue

77. Ans.— C. 4—6 months

78. Ans.— C. Hydatid cyst of liver

79. Ans.— D. Haematoma of rectus sheath

80. Ans.— B. Elliptocytosis

81. Ans.— A. 1

82. Ans.— C. Ileum

It is most often seen in women, average age is 70. Obstruction occurs if stone is more than 2.5 cm size. It can cause perforation.

83. Ans.— D. Haemorrhage

84. Ans.— A. Remove distal part and suture proximal end.

85. Ans.— E. All of the above

86. Ans.— B. Hereditary spherocytosis

Gall stones in hemolytic anemia are due to excessive bilirubin due to hemolysis & hence are pigment stones.

87. Ans.— B. Silk sutures

88. Ans.— A. Non-Beta cells

89. Ans.— B. 10

90. Ans.— D. 40

91. Ans.— A. E. coli

92. Ans.— D. 50

93. Ans.— C. Common in alcoholics

94. Ans.— C. Can cure secondary carcinoma

**95. Ans.— B. Common bile duct stone**

**Stones in the bile duct causes pain, jaundice and fever. Ch. cholecystitis causes only pain in Rt. hypochondria and flatulence dyspepsia.**

**96. Ans.— C. Portal hypertension**

**97. Ans.— B. Common bile duct patency**

**98. Ans.— B. Concentration**

**99. Ans.— C. Common bile duct stone**

**100. Ans.— A. ERCP**

**101. Ans.— A. Splenectomy**

**102. Ans.— C. Infective hepatitis**

**103. Ans.— B. Echogenic**

**104. Ans.— B. 1000 somogyl units**

**105. Ans.— B. It causes spasm of sphincter of Oddi.**

**106. Ans.— A. Double-impactation by stone**

**107. Ans.— B. Excess bile leakage from wound**

**108. Ans.— B. Stomach displaced forwards**

**109. Ans.— B. Obstructive jaundice**

**110. Ans.— D. Schistosomiasis**

**111. Ans.— B. Gas gangrene**

**112. Ans.— A. They are common among adults**

**113. Ans.— D. All of the above**

**40% cases of pancreatitis are associated with gallstone disease. It may be due to Alcohol, hyperparathyroidism, hyperlipidemia, familial protein deficiency, post-operative, obstructive and drug induced (corticosteroids, oral contraceptives, azathioprine, thiazides and tetracycline).**

**114. Ans.— D. Ca Gall bladder**

**115. Ans.— C. Obstruction of common bile duct**

**116. Ans.— A. Infection with trematodes**

**117. Ans.— D. Mixed stones**

**Mixed stones 90% and cholesterol stones 6%. These are commonest nipple pathology.**

**118. Ans.— B. Veins of Mayo**

**119. Ans.— C. Common hepatic duct**

**120. Ans.— A. Simple drainage**

**121. Ans.— A. 3 months**

**122. Ans.— B. Two third cases**

**Alpha fetoproteins are present in plasma long before clinical features appear.**

**123. Ans.— E. None of the above**

**124. Ans.— B. 2-3 days**

**125. Ans.— C. Absent Alone present Absent**

**126. Ans.— A. At the junction of Right & left hepatic duct.**

**127. Ans.— D. Murphy's sign**

**128. Ans.— B. Glucagonoma**

**129. Ans.— C. Impending rupture**

**130. Ans.— D. 3-6 weeks**

**131. Ans.— A. Increased sodium**

**132. Ans.— C. 3-4 years of age**

**133. Ans.— D. CHF**

**134. Ans.— B. Body and tail**

**135. Ans.— A. Malaria**

**136. Ans.— B. Intra-ocular melanoma**

**137. Ans.— C. Cirrhosis**

**138. Ans.— B. Obesity**

**139. Ans.— A. Atresia of the bile duct**

**140. Ans.— B. Heart**

**141. Ans.— C. Cholesterosis**

**142. Ans.— C. Actinomycosis**

**143. Ans.— C. Ultrasonography**

**144. Ans.— D. Periampullary carcinoma**

**145. Ans.— A. Juvenile diabetes**

**146. Ans.— B. Gall bladder with a mesentery**

**147. Ans.— B. Gynaecomastia and testicular atrophy**

**148. Ans.— B. 20 mm Hg**

**149. Ans.— A. Cheynodeoxycholic acid**

**150. Ans.— A. Gall bladder stones**

**151. Ans.— D. Pain or Jaundice**

**152. Ans.— D. Infection**

**Marsupialization or internal drainage is the treatment of choice.**

**153. Ans.— A. Exploring the patient followed by splenectomy.**

**154. Ans.— A. Haemorrhagic pancreatitis**

**155. Ans.— B. ESWL**

**156. Ans.— A. Gall stone, diverticulitis, hiatus hernia.**

157. Ans.— D. Cirrhosis

158. Ans.— C. Gall bladder bed to IVC

159. Ans.— A. Past H/O Jaundice

160. Ans.— D. Oxalate

Incidence of Gall stones are - truncal vagotomy, Ileal resection, OCP, bypass surgery pregnancy.

161. Ans.— A. Erythematous hillous rash

162. Ans.— A. Within first 12 hours

163. Ans.— B. Obliteration of splenic shadow

164. Ans.— B. 6—12 mm Hg

165. Ans.— E. Good prognosis

166. Ans.— C. Haematobilia

167. Ans.— NONE

168. Ans.— D. Biliary cirrhosis

169. Ans.— C. Hyperkalemia

170. Ans.— B. Albumin infusion

171. Ans.— A. Injury to bladder during birth

172. Ans.— A. Central nervous system symptoms, fasting blood sugar of 50 mg per 100 ml, relief following ingestion of glucose.

173. Ans.— A. Secondaries

Among primaries, hemangioma is commonest benign and hepatocellular carcinoma is commonest malignant tumor.

174. Ans.— D. Radionuclide pancreatic scan

175. Ans.— A. 10%

176. Ans.— A. Blood

177. Ans.— D. Carcinomatous change

178. Ans.— D. Mallory-Weiss syndrome

179. Ans.— A. Haemorrhage

180. Ans.— A. Gall stones

181. Ans.— A. Severe jaundice

182. Ans.— D. Non-thrombocytopenic purpura

Splenectomy is also done in splenic rutpure, hereditary elliptocytosis, pyruvate kinase deficiency, thalassaemia, as part of radical gastrectomy, staging for Hodgkins, in association with variceal surgery.

183. Ans.— D. All of the above

184. Ans.— C. Air in the biliary tract in plain X-ray.

185. Ans.— B. Duodeno-jejunostomy

186. Ans.— A. Ileal resection

187. Ans.— C. Transduodenal sphincterotomy

It is done when stone is impacted near ampulla of Vater and cannot be retrieved from above.

188. Ans.— A. Presents in elderly females

189. Ans.— B. Carcinoma gall bladder

190. Ans.— B. Endoscopic sphincterotomy and removal.

191. Ans.— C. Peritoneal lavage is a good diagnostic modality.

192. Ans.— D. Appendix

193. Ans.— D. Malignancy

194. Ans.— C. Distal common bile duct

Jaundice is present in 2/3 cases of Ca head.

195. Ans.— A. Multiple Myeloma

196. Ans.— C. Transhepatic cholangiography

197. Ans.— B. Transphincteric duodenal drainage is commonly used.

198. Ans.— A. Lipase

199. Ans.— B. L-Asparaginase

200. Ans.— C. Type of shunt

201. Ans.— A. Uncommon in Asians

202. Ans.— A. To avoid pleura

203. Ans.— C. Gall stones

Question is wrong as it is found in all and choledochal cyst and Caroli's disease also have an increased incidence.

204. Ans.— A. Enteric fever

205. Ans.— D. Liver

206. Ans.— D. Enzymatic fat

207. Ans.— B. Primary biliary cirrhosis

Question is wrong (Bailey & Love pp 823 & Harrison's pp 1728). It is also seen in fasting, pregnancy, high calorie high fat diet, drugs e.g. Octreotide etc.

208. Ans.— B. Sup. and Inf. rectal veins

209. Ans.— B. $\downarrow$ Bile/cholesterol ratio

It predisposes to Gallstone formation.

210. Ans.— A. **Serum amylase**

**Criteria which determine high risk patients have been identified by Ranson are—old age, extent of rise in blood sugar, WBC count, LFT, Blood urea and base deficit. Extent of fall in Calcium, haematocrit, arterial $O_2$ tension and vol. of fluid accumulated in extravascular space (third space collection).**

211. Ans.— C. **Hypercalcemia**

212. Ans.— A. **Postero superior portion of lobe of liver**

213. Ans.— A. **Trauma**

**Pneumococcal, H. influenzae and babesia infections are commonest after it. Trauma is another common indication.**

214. Ans.— C. **2, 3, 4 and 5**

215. Ans.— A. **Trophozoites of EH**

216. Ans.— A. **Whole blood**

217. Ans.— B. **USG**

218. Ans.— A. **Predisposed by DM**

219. Ans.— B. **Endoscopy**

220. Ans.— B. **Migratory thrombophlebitis**

221. Ans.— B. **Hypoasthesia is seen above 9-11 ribs**

222. Ans.— A. **Lymphoma**

**Commonest benign tumor is haemangioma**

223. Ans.— A. **1, 2 and 3**

224. Ans.— A. **Pancreatitis**

225. Ans.— B. **Longitudinal pancreatojejunostomy**

226. Ans.— A. **Clotting abnormalities**

227. Ans.— D. **Sclerosing cholangitis**

228. Ans.— A. **It is a septic peritonitis**

229. Ans.— D. **Arteriography**

230. Ans.— A. **Stomach Ca**

231. Ans.— D. **Purtschers retinopathy**

**It is a complication of pancreatitis, Grey Turner's sign (Echymotic discolouration of blanks) and Cullen's sign (Discoluration in periumbilical area) are also seen in acute pancreatitis.**

232. Ans.— C. **No treatment**

233. Ans.— B. **Inspissated bile**

234. Ans.— E. **At the time of presentation disease is beyond surgical resection in over 80 percent of cases.**

235. Ans.— D. **90% of gall stones are radio-opaque.**

236. Ans.— D. **A transudate has a protein content of greater than 30 gms. of protein per litre.**

237. Ans.— B. **Observation**

238. Ans.— A. **Lymphoma**

239. Ans.— B. **Clonorchiasis**

**A western diet (high in protein and fat), smoling and chronic pancreatitis are other predisposing factors. More than 75% are adenocarcinoma of duct cell origin.**

240. Ans.— A. **Size < 15 mm**

**Chenodeoxycholic acid (15 mg/kg/d) or ursodeoxycholic acid are used which expands the bile salt pool and their effect is noticed in 6-9 months. The drugs are ineffective if pigment stones, calcified stones, nonopacifying GB on OCG, large (> 17 mm) gallstones, obesity or choledocholithiasis. Drugs are contraindicated in severe symptoms, pregnancy, liver disease or advanced atherosclerosis.**

241. Ans.— B. **Porphyria**

242. Ans.— B. **Non-cirrhotic portal fibrosis**

243. Ans.— D. **Obstructive jaundice**

244. Ans.— C. **More common in females**

245. Ans.— B. **CBD stone**

246. Ans.— B. **Extra hepatic portal vein thrombosis**

247. Ans.— C. **Platelets**

248. Ans.— C. **Tail of pancreas**

249. Ans.— B. **Patient is grouped as child's grade-B and treated conservatively.**

250. Ans.— B. **Ascaris lumbricoides**

251. Ans.— A. **Ultrasound guided biopsy of the lesion**

252. Ans.— C. **No surgery for gall-bladder stones**

253. Ans.— B. **Polycystic disease of liver**

**Predisposing factors for cholangio carcinoma are :**

| | |
|---|---|
| **U- Ulcerative colitis** | **Hydatid cyst** |
| **P- Psc (Primary sclerosing cholengitis,** | **parasitic infection** |
| **S - Scleroderma** | |
| **C - Clonorchiasis sinensis** | |

**254. Ans.— A. Acute fluid collection**

* The only indication for operative intervention in acute pancreatitis is the presence of an abscess related to necrosis in or around the pancreas.
* Acute fluid collection occurs early in course of acute pancreatitis and is located in or near the pancreas. The wall of the collection is ill defined.
* Infected pancreatic necrosis should be treated by surgical debridement because the solid component of the infected pancreas is not amenable to effective radiologically guided percutaneous evacuation.
* Pancreatic abscess can be treated surgically or in selected cases by percutaneous drainage.

**255. Ans.— B. Post-surgery-Cholecystectomy**

**256. Ans.— B. Better evaluation of CBD**

Laparoscopic cholecystectomy is a minimal-abcess approach for the removal of the gall-bladder together with its stones. Because of a markedly shortened hospital stay as well as decreased cost and a mortality rate of < 1 percent. It is the procedure of choice for most patients referred for elective cholecystectomy. The advantages to the patient derived from removing the gall bladder by the laparoscopic method, in contrast to other cholecystectomy removal procedures are:

* Reduced pain
* Shorter hospital stay (out-patient or 1 day stay)
* Earlier return to full activity and work
* Less pain and less medication requirement
* Less visible abdominal scars

**257. Ans.— B. Common Bile Duct Stone**

**258. Ans.— A. Hepatic veins and portal vein**

**259. Ans.— D. Biliary atresia**

**260. Ans.— D. Sinusoids**

**261. Ans.— C. Hepatic veins**

**262. Ans.— B. Gall stone pancreatitis**

The prognosis is best in patients with recurrent acute pancreatitis caused by a remediable condition such as :

- Cholelithiasis (gallstone)
- Choledocholithiasis
- Stenosis of sphincter of oddi
- Hyperparathyroidism

**263. Ans.— D. Sinusoids**

**264. Ans.— D. Povidone iodine**

**265. Ans.— D. Propranolol**

**266. Ans.— B. Typhoid fever**

**267. Ans.— A. Duodenum**

**268. Ans.— D. To wait till she becomes symptomatic.**

**269. Ans.— A. Conservative treatment**

**270. Ans.— C. 1, 2 and 4**

**271. Ans.— D. Renal artery aneurysm**

**272. Ans.— B. Urine amylase**

* Pancreas allograft rejection in dogs with pancreaticocystostomy can be predicted in advance of hyperglycemia by monitoring the urinary amylase (UA) concentration (U/L)

**273. Ans.— C. Polyp > 5 mm in length**

* Polyps larger than 1 centimeter are more likely to be malignant.

**274. Ans.— D. Markedly elevated transaminases**

Reynold's Pentad of Toxic cholangitis (bacterial cholangitis) include abdominal pain; jaundice; fever and chills; mental confusion or lethargy and shock.

**275. Ans.— B. Hepatic adenima**

Adenomas have malignant potential and surgery is treatment of choice.

# 11

# IMPORTANT TEXT OF INTESTINES

* The only living part of hydatid cyst is a single layer of cells (germinal epithelium) lining the cyst (endocyst).
* **Goodsall's Rule**—*Fistula-in-ano*
  — Fistulae with an external opening in relation to the anterior half of the anus tend to be of the direct type and those with an external opening or opening in relation to the posterior half of the anus usually have curving tracks, with the internal opening in the midline, and may be of the horseshoe variety.
* **Dukes' Staging :** (A staging system to predict the prognosis of cancer of the rectum)

***Stage-A*** : Growth is extended to the extra rectal wall (15%)—Prognosis excellent.

***Stage-B*** : Growth is extended to the extra rectal tissues, but no metastasis to the regional lymphnodes (35%)—Prognosis good.

***Stage-C*** : Regional lymphnode metastasis regardless the depth of invasion (50%)—Prognosis bad.

C-1 Local pararectal lymph nodes alone are involved (2/3rd of stage-C.)

C-2 The nodes accompanying the supplying blood vessels are implicated upto the point of division (1/3rd of stage-C).

***Stage-D*** : (Not described by Dukes) Cancer with distant metastasis (usually hepatic) or with adjacent organ involvement.

**Aster-Coller Staging :** (Modification of Dukes) for **Carcinoma rectum.**

***Stage-A-1***—Lesions limited to the mucosa

***Stage-B-1***—Lesions limited to the muscularis propria with negative nodes.

***Stage-C-1***—Lesions limited to the wall with positive nodes.

***Stage-C-2***—Lesions that have extended through the wall with positive nodes.

**Bowen's Disease :** *Intraepidermal carcinoma* or *carcinoma in situ of perineum.*

— **Pruritus, dull, red spreading, irregular plaque like eczematoid lesion. Biopsy reveals carcinoma in situ.**

*Treatment :* Local excision with adequate margins or topical use of fluorouracil.

**Extra mammary Paget's Disease of the anus**

— A pale gray, plaque like lesion with surrounding induration & sometimes underlying mass. Diagnosis by biopsy.

*Treatment :* Local excision if tumour is absent. More radical excision, chemotherapy & radiotherapy for presence of Cancer.

**Buschke-Lowenstein tumour**—Giant, perianal condyloma associated with carcinoma (rare).

## DIFFERENTIAL DIAGNOSIS OF CROHN'S DISEASE

| *Feature* | *Ischaemic colitis* | *Ulcerative colitis* | *Crohn's disease* |
|---|---|---|---|
| Age incidene: | Elderly | Young | Middle-aged |
| Presentation | Always acute | Acute or chronic | Chronic |
| Part involved | Splenic flexure (rectum rare, anus never) | Left-side or total (rectum always) | Any where (rectum usual, commonly) |
| Radiology | Thumb prints<br>Stricture | Shortening<br>Ulceration | Spicules<br>Skip lesions |
| Pathology | Fibrosis<br>Haemosiderosis | Mucosal loss<br>Crypt abscess | Fissures<br>Granulomas |
| Associated conditions | Claudication<br>Angina<br>Stroke | Iritis<br>Arthritis<br>Pyoderma | Enteric fistula<br>Megaloblastic anaemia<br>Malignant change |

# MCQ's OF INTESTINES

## What is important in Intestines

Intestine (Obstruction, Crohn's disease, Ulcerative colitis, Diverticulitis, Amoebiasis, TB, Intussusception Tumors)

1. **The following are usual complications of Meckel's diverticulum except : UPSC 1986**
   A. Perforation B. Peptic ulcer
   C. Carcinoid tumour D. Adenocarcinoma
2. **Pathognomonic finding of intussusception in infants is: Rohtak 1986**
   A. Distension
   B. Sausage shaped mass in epigastrium and empty right iliac fossa
   C. Free fluid
   D. Mass in left iliac fossa
3. **All of the following produce a stricture of the small bowel, except : BHU 1987**
   A. Tuberculosis B. Tumour
   C. Typhoid enteritis D. Crohn's disease
   E. Prolonged oral potassium supplementation
4. **Small bowel perforation in tropics is due to : DNB 1991**
   A. Meckel's diverticulum
   B. Typhoid
   C. Crohn's disease
   D. Carcinoma
5. **The most common mesenteric cyst is : Delhi 1983**
   A. Gas containing cyst
   B. Enterogenous cyst
   C. Dermoid cyst
   D. Chylolymphatic cyst
6. **A chronic alcoholic with epigastric pain was submitted to ERCP which showed "chain of lakes" appearance of main pancreatic duct. Treatment of choice is : MAHE 1998**
   A. Lateral pancreaticojejunostomy
   B. Distal pancreaticojejunostomy
   C. Proximal pancreaticojejunostomy
   D. Pancreatectomy
7. **Which of the following is not true about acute small bowel obstruction : UPSC 1984**
   A. Is often associated with a raised serum amylase.
   B. Is usually caused by post-operative adhesions.
   C. Generally produces abdominal distension within 2-4 hours of onset.
   D. Associated with signs of peritonitis, suggests bowel strangulation.
8. **Features of a left sided colonic cancer frequently include all of the following, except : UPSC 1984**
   A. Rectal bleeding
   B. Anaemia
   C. Abdominal pain
   D. Intestinal obstruction
9. **All of the followIng are true about the treatment of duodenal fistula, except : AIIMS 1985**
   A. Skin should be protected from chemical erosion.
   B. Nasoduodenal suction shuld be done.
   C. Jejunostomy tube feeding may be required.
   D. Immediate operative closure is advised.
   E. Tract should be kept empty and dry by stump drainage.
10. **The extra-intestinal complication which is seen more often in Ulcerative colitis than in Crohn's disease is : PGI 1993**
    A. Pyoderma gangrenosum
    B. Cholangiocarcinoma
    C. Uveitis
    D. Cirrhosis
11. **Double-bubble appearance is seen in : PGI 1993**
    A. Duodenal atresia
    B. Infantile pyloric stenosis
    C. Chronic duodenal ulcer with pyloric stenosis
    D. All of the above

**Ans.** 1. D 2. B 3. C 4. B 5. D 6. B 7. C 8. B 9. A 10. B 11. A

12. **The primary aim in Duodenal ulcer management is : JIPMER 1993**
A. To rule out malignancy
B. To decrease acid output
C. To prevent complications
D. To excise ulcerogenic mucosa

13. **All the following are features of Mesenteric cyst except : JIPMER 1993**
A. Common in infants
B. Swelling near umbilicus
C. Painless swelling
D. Can present as acute abdomen

14. **Following conditions predispose to Abdominal wall dehiscence, except : JIPMER 1992**
A. Old age
B. Malignancy
C. Raised intra-abdominal pressure
D. Faulty surgical technique

15. **The ganglion spared in Lumbar sympathectomy is : UPSC 1987; JIPMER 1992; UPSC 1999**
A. L1 B. L2
C. L3 D. L4

16. **Most common cause of Acute intestinal obstruction of neonates is : AIIMS 1992**
A. Duodenal atresia B. Jejunal atresia
C. Acute intussuSception D. Malrotation

17. **Most common site for Intra-Abdominal abscess following laparotomy is : AIIMS 1992**
A. Subphrenic B. Subhepatic
C. Paracolic D. Pelvic

18. **Most common site for Intraperitoneal abscess is : AIIMS 1992; PGI 1993**
A. Subphrenic B. Subhepatic
C. Paracolic D. Pelvic

19. **The treatment of choice in Multiple intestinal strictures of a segment of jejunum is : AIIMS 1992**
A. Stricturoplasty
B. Resection and end-to-end anastomosis
C. Nobel's procedure
D. End-to-side anastomosis

20. **Which of the following is true regarding Ulcerative colitis : AIIMS 1992, 95**
A. Rectum is always involved
B. Skip lesions are seen
C. Fistula are common
D. String sign is positive

21. **Diagnosis of superior mesenteric arterial embolism can be made by : AMC 1989**
A. Leucocytosis
B. Elevated serum amylase
C. Plain X-ray
D. Superior mesenteric arteriogram

22. **Aganglionic megacolon is characterized by : AIIMS 1983**
A. Usually normal growth
B. Normal bowel movements
C. No distension of abdomen
D. Rectum not dilated and usually empty of stool

23. **The period, in which the duodenal stump blow out most likely develops following gastrectomy with a Billroth-II anastomosis, is : UPSC 1987**
A. 2nd to 7th day B. 8th to 14th day
C. 14th to 21st day D. Over 21 days

24. **After bowel is handled at laparotomy, the normal period of paralytic ileus is about : AMU 1987**
A. 6 hours B. 12 hours
C. 24 hours D. 30 hours
E. 48 hours

25. **Which of the following is not true about childhood intussusception: AIIMS 1985**
A. Rarely required surgical treatment.
B. Is frequently ileocolic.
C. Usually presents during the first year of life.
D. Can usually be diagnosed without X-ray examination of the abdomen.

26. **All of the following should be done for successful operation for duodenal ulcer, except : UPSC 1984**
A. Overcome any obstructive mechanism.
B. Remove or cover surfaces which might bleed.
C. Leave motor and secretory function intact.
D. Permanently control the acid factor.
E. Leave a gastric pouch sufficient for physiological needs.

27. **Wind sock deformity is a type of : . AIIMS 1986**
A. Anorectal anomaly
B. Meconium
C. Congenital emphysema
D. Duodenal atresia

28. **Earliest sign of ulcerative colitis after a barium enema is : AMU 1986**
A. Pseudopolypsis
B. Pipe stem colon
C. Loss of haustrations, especially in the distal colon
D. Undermining of the mucosa
E. None of the above

**Ans.** 12. C 13. A 14. A 15. A 16. A 17. A 18. D 19. B 20. A 21. D
22. D 23. A 24. E 25. A 26. C 27. D 28. C

**29. Barium meal X-ray in cases of regional ileitis may show following, except : AMU 1990**
A. Lack of segmentation
B. Cobble stone reticulation
C. 'String' sign of Kantor
D. None of the above

**30. A patient of perforated duodenal ulcer of 12 hours duration should have : UPSC 1986**
A. Subtotal gastrectomy
B. Vagotomy and hemigastrectomy
C. Vagotomy plus pyloroplasty
D. Plication of ulcer with omental reinforcement
E. Surgeon's discretion

**31. The most common cause of bleeding from small bowel lesions are : AIIMS 1984**
A. Myxomas B. Fibromas
C. Leiomymas D. Haemangiomas

**32. Kulchitsky cells are commonly found in : Delhi 1987**
A. Peutz-Jegher's syndrome
B. Gardner's syndrome
C. Meckel diverticulum
D. Carcinoid

**33. The surgical treatment of choice of idiopathic ulcerative colitis is : UPSC 1987**
A. Sub-total colectomy and ileostomy
B. Bypass ileoctomy
C. Total proctocolectomy and ileostomy
D. All of the above
E. None of the above

**34. The treatment of pseudomembranous enterocolitis includes following, except : Delhi 1987**
A. ACTH
B. Discontinuation of all antibiotics
C. Retention enemas of saline with faecal suspension
D. Azulfidine
E. If pseudomonas is the cause, sodium colistimethate is used

**35. Apple-peal bowel is a term used for : AIIMS 1985**
A. Congenital pyloric stenosis
B. Congenital volvulus
C. Absence of mesentry
D. Absence of anal sphincter

**36. In intestine, lipoma is commonest in : PGI 1985**
A. Rectum B. Sigmoid colon
C. Calcum D. Ileum

**37. Stiffening of the bowel wall and fibrosis is frequent in which of the following : AIIMS 1985**
A. Amoebiasis B. Regional enteritis
C. Ulcerative colitis D. Typhoid ulcers

**38. The rationale for operation in case of duodenal ulcer includes all of the following, except : PGI 1985**
A. Obstruction
B. Massive haemorrhage
C. Perforation
D. Fear of developing pancreatic penetration
E. Inability to follow medical regimen

**39. Following procedures (except one) are done for correction of Hirschsprung's disease : AIIMS 1987**
A. Duhamel's B. Soave's
C. Swenson's D. Bayar's

**40. All of the following may cause 'chemical peritonitis', except : PGI 1984**
A. Injury to cisterna chyli
B. Haemoperitoneum
C. Perforation of peptic ulcer
D. After a barium enema
E. Rupture of gall bladder

**41. Following massive resection of the small bowel which of the following is not common: UPSC 1986**
A. Lowered serum protein
B. Hypercalcaemia
C. Loss of weight
D. Loss of protein & fat
E. Intractable diarrhoea

**42. Meckel's diverticulum is congenital anomaly of : Delhi 1994**
A. Oesophagus B. Stomach
C. Ileum D. Colon

**43. In case of Ectopia vesicae, umbilicus is : Delhi 1994; Rajasthan 1994**
A. Normally situated B. Pushed cranially
C. Usually abscent D. Pushed laterally

**44. Following signs may be present in a case of ileocolic intussusception except : Delhi 1994**
A. Palpable lump B. Distended caecum
C. Visible bowel loops D. Blood in stool

**45. The most common cause of Intestinal obstruction in adults is : Delhi 1993; PGI 1993, 96**
A. Volvulus
B. Hernia
C. Post-operative adhesions
D. Intussusception

| Ans. | | | | | | | | | |
|---|---|---|---|---|---|---|---|---|---|
| 29. D | 30. D | 31. D | 32. D | 33. C | 34. D | 35. C | 36. C | 37. B | 38. D |
| 39. D | 40. B | 41. B | 42. C | 43. C | 44. B | 45. C | | | |

**46. Commonest complication of diverticulosis of sigmoid colon : JIPMER 1997**

A. Adhesions  B. Perforation
C. Intussusception  D. Bleeding PR

**47. Most common indication for laparotomy in Intestinal T.B. is : PGI 1993; Delhi 1993**

A. Doubtful diagnosis  B. Intestinal obstruction
C. Peritonitis  D. Lower GI bleeding

**48. Commonest site of Amoebiasis in the gut is : TN 1993**

A. Ileum  B. Caecum
C. Ascending colon  D. Sigmoid colon

**49. Meconium ileus in the neonate is best treated by : MAHE 1994**

A. Enzyme replacement
B. Irrigation of the gut with N-acetyl cysteine
C. Phosphate enema
D. Surgery

**50. All of the following are characteristic findings in the irritable bowel syndrome, except : MAHE 1996**

A. Normal or less than normal stool weight
B. Absence of blood in the stools
C. Normal ESR
D. Diagnostic appearances in a barium enema

**51. Recognised features of the carcinoid syndrome include all of the following except : MAHE 1996**

A. Constipation
B. Pellagra
C. Precipitation of attacks by alcohol ingestion
D. Wheezing

**52. Treatment of choice of umbilical adenoma (2.5 x 1.5 cm) in a new born is : Delhi 1993**

A. Occlusion with a coin
B. Strapping
C. Surgery
D. Leave as such as regression occurs

**53. In acute intestinal obstruction the investigation of choice is : Delhi 1992**

A. Plain X-ray abdomen  B. Ultrasonography
C. Barium enema  D. CT scan

**54. A patient with angiomatous malformation in the colon, the electrolyte abnormality likely is : Bihar 1998**

A. Hyponatremia  B. Hypokalemia
C. Hypercalcemia  D. Metabolic alkalosis

**55. Prognosis in a perforated chr. duodenal ulcer does not depend upon : Delhi 1992**

A. Previous H/O duodenal ulcer
B. Duration of perforation
C. General condition of the patient
D. Presence of septicaemia

**56. The mesenteric attachments most often affected with tumor development is : Delhi 1983**

A. Jejunal  B. Ileal
C. Ascending colon  D. Sigmoid colon

**57. In patients with idiopathic retroperitoneal fibrosis which of the following structures is usually involved first : AMC 1984**

A. Aorta  B. Vena cava
C. Ureter  D. Duodenum

**58. The most common cause of secondary perotonitis is : DNB 1989**

A. Perforated peptic ulcer
B. Acute appendicitis
C. Strangulation of small bowel due to incarcerated hernia
D. Mesenteric vascular accident
E. Gonococcal salpingitIs

**59. What percentage of small intestine can be removed in an adult without causing extensive digestive disabilities : AIIMS 1984, 87**

A. 30%  B. 50%
C. 70%  D. 90%
E. 100%

**60. 'Peutz-Jegher's syndrome is characterized by following, except : AIIMS 1986**

A. It is an inherited disease.
B. They do not undergo malignancy.
C. Melanin spots on lips and buccal mucosa.
D. Polyps are not present throughout G.I. tract.
E. These are hamartomas consisting of normal intestinal epithelium and smooth muscle.

**61. Anastomotic leaks are more common in the large bowel because of all of the following reasons, except : CSE 1995**

A. The colon is prone to gaseous distension.
B. The contents of the colon are infected and semisolid.
C. The blood supply of colon is poorer than that of the small bowel and stomach.
D. Massive colonic peristalsis disrupt the anastomosis.

| Ans. | | | | | | | | | |
|---|---|---|---|---|---|---|---|---|---|
| 46. D | 47. B | 48. B | 49. D | 50. D | 51. A | 52. B | 53. A | 54. B | 55. A |
| 56. B | 57. C | 58. A | 59. C | 60. D | 61. D | | | | |

**62. Tumours which have a tendency towards direct extension through tissue spaces including following, except : PGI 1985**

A. Adenocarcinoma of oesophagus
B. Adenocarcinoma of stomach
C. Hodgkin's disease
D. Soft tissue sarcomas

**63. Which of the following is not true concerning retroperitoneal haematoma : AMU 1985**

A. 80% have gross haematuria.
B. Intraperitoneal abdominal tap may be positive.
C. Retroperitoneal bleeding is self-limiting and exploration is not warranted.
D. Shock is present in about 40% of cases.
E. The Gray-Turner's sign develops within few hours.

**64. Ischemic colitis is least likely to involve : AIIMS 1984**

A. Splenic flexure B. Transverse colon
C. Ascending colon D. Descending colon
E. Sigmoid colon

**65. Vesicointestinal fistulae are most often due to : AMU 1985**

A. Carcinoma of the colon
B. Post-abdominoperitoneal resection
C. Crohn's disease
D. Diverticulitis
E. Direct rectal trauma

**66. Which one of the following physical signs/laboratory aids is helpful in the diagnosis of bowel strangulation: UPSC 1998**

A. Marked abdominal distension
B. Persistent local tenderness
C. Profuse vomiting
D. Multiple air fluid levels on X-ray

**67. The patient vitello-intestinal duct most often discharges : AIIMS 1985**

A. Mucus B. Pus
C. Urine D. Faces

**68. "Respberry tumour" is another name for : BHU 1987**

A. Umbilical fistula
B. Umbilical granuloma
C. Umbilical adenoma
D. Meckel's diverticulum

**69. Umbilical adenoma is most commonly seen in : BHU 1988**

A. Infants B. Adolescents
C. Middle age D. Old age

**70. Liver metastasis of carcinoid tumour most frequently arise from a primary in the : Bihar 1990**

A. Appendix B. Jejunum
C. Ileum D. Rectum

**71. Which of the following is not true about a discharge from the umbilicus: Rohtak 1985**

A. In the neonate is of no immediate clinic significance.
B. May indicate an anomaly of the urachus.
C. May indicate a patent vitello-intestinal duct.
D. At the time of menstruation may indicate endometriosis.

**72. Prune belly syndrome consists of the following, except: AIIMS 1983**

A. Deficiency of abdominal wall musculature
B. Hydroureteronephrosis
C. Cryptorchidism
D. None of the above

**73. Gastrointestinal duplications are most often found in the : PGI 1993**

A. Jejunum B. Ileum
C. Stomach D. Ascending colon
E. Transverse colon

**74. A 35-years old woman complains of attacks of breathlessness, cyanosis and flushing. Apart from occasional diarrhoea, she has no abdominal symptoms. Abdominal examination reveals an enlarged nodular liver. If laparotomy is done, one would expect to find : UPSC 1998**

A. An ovarian tumour
B. A multicentric hepatoma
C. An appendicular carcinoid
D. Crohn's disease

**75. The cause of perforation in colon cancer is : AIIMS 1985**

A. Tumour slough
B. Intussusception
C. Volvulus
D. Pressure of impacted faeces
E. Tension gangrene

**76. Consider the following statements regarding bowel preparation for patients undergoing colonic surgery: CSE 1995**

1. It is not necessary in the case of patients undergoing right hemicolectomy.
2. Mechanical cleansing of the bowel is not important after the advent of the new generation of broad spectrum antibiotics.
3. Rapid bowel preparation may be done using polyethylene glycol electrolyte solution.
4. "On table wash out" of the colon is recommended in emergencies after the abdomen has been opened.

**Of these statements**

A. 1, 2, 3 and 4 are correct B. 2 and 3 are correct
C. 1 and 4 are correct D. 1, 3 and 4 are correct

**Ans.** 62. C 63. C 64. C 65. D 66. B 67. A 68. C 69. A 70. C 71. A
72. D 73. B 74. C 75. E 76. D

**77. Which of the following are least affected in a jejunal bypass for obesity: Rohtak 1986**

A. Serum carotene B. Serum $B_{12}$
C. Serum vitamin-C D. Serum vitamin-A
E. Serum vitamin-E

**78. In ulcerative colitis, the inflammatory process is usually confined to : UPSC 1998**

A. Mucosa alone
B. Mucosa and submucosa
C. Mucosa, submucosa and muscularis
D. Mucosa, submucosa, muscularis and serosa

**79. Internal fistulas with colonic diverticulitis are most often : PGI 1989**

A. Colovesical B. Coloneric
C. Colocolonic D. Colovaginal
E. Coloureteral

**80. The procedure of choice in attempting to identify the bleeding point of colonic disease is : AIIMS 1985**

A. Barium enema
B. Fluorescent string test
C. Selective arteriography
D. A gastrointestinal series with flow through
E. Colonoscopy

**81. Acute toxic megacolon may develop in which of the following : PGI 1996**

A. Ulcerative colitis
B. Acute amebic colitis
C. Granulomatous colitis
D. All of the above
E. None of the above

**82. The appearance of anastomotic leakage following a low colonic anastomosis most often manifests on : AIIMS 1985**

A. 1-4 days B. 5-10 days
C. 11-15 days D. 16-20 days
E. None of the above

**83. The CAT scan in preoperative evaluation of colon carcinoma : AIIMS 1986**

A. Is valuable for spread of disease into pelvic area and should be confined to pelvis only.
B. Is valuable for determining tumor spread outside of pelvis-therefore, it should be limited to abdomen, above pelvic brim.
C. Is valuable for primarily liver metastases.
D. Should be performed through liver, midabdomen, and pelvis, except where primary lesions are proximal to the sigmoid.
E. None of the above.

**84. Which of the following is most dangerous form of obstruction : PGI 1993**

A. Adhesion bands
B. Internal herniation
C. Mesenteric vein thrombosis
D. Intestinal strictures

**85. Primary peritonitis with pneumococcus is associated with : PGI 1982**

A. Lymphomas B. Nephrotic syndrome
C. Carcinoids D. None of the above

**86. Treatment of choice in desmoid tumours is : AIIMS 1985**

A. Irradiation
B. Wide excision
C. Local excision
D. Local excision following radiation

**87. Match List-I with List-II and select the correct answer: CSE 1996**

| List-I (Clinical condition) | List-II (Gross characteristics) |
|---|---|
| A. Juvenile polyp | 1. Multiple, varying sizes and pubertal age |
| B. Metastatic polyp | 2. Large frond-like and solitary |
| C. Villous adenoma | 3. Oedematous bossellated mucous membrane pedunculated |
| D. Familial adenomatous polyposis | 4. Solitary, red and found in children |
| | 5. Small pinkish, multiple and sessile |

| | A | B | C | D |
|---|---|---|---|---|
| A. | 4 | 5 | 2 | 1 |
| B. | 4 | 5 | 1 | 2 |
| C. | 1 | 4 | 3 | 2 |
| D. | 1 | 2 | 4 | 5 |

**88. Thromboembolism after pelvic surgery is usually from the ——— veins except. AI 1989**

A. Iliac B. Calf
C. Femoral D. Pelvic

**89. Haemorrhage from a bleeding duodenal ulcer is due to the erosion of ——— artery. AI 1989**

A. Superior pancreatic duodenal
B. Gastroduodenal
C. Right gastric
D. Left gastric

**Ans.** 77. B 78. B 79. A 80. C 81. D 82. B 83. D 84. C 85. B 86. B 87. A 88. B 89. B

**90. Treatment of choice for stab injury caecum : AI 1989**

A. Caecostomy
B. Ileo-transverse anastomosis
C. Transverse colostomy
D. Sigmoid colostomy

**91. All of the following statements are true regarding burst abdomen, except : UPSC 1985**

A. Peak incidence is between 6th to 8th day after operation.
B. Infection, persistent cough and leakage of pancreatic enzymes predispose to this condition.
C. Lower abdominal incisions disrupt more than upper abdominal incisions.
D. Poor suturing technique and the too early removal of deep tension sutures predispose to this condition.

**92. Diagnostic of Hirschsprung's disease is : JIPMER 1985, 87**

A. Barium enema B. Rectal examination
C. Manometry D. Rectal biopsy

**93. Small intestine is sutured by : PGI 1986, 88**

A. Non-absorbable in 2 layers
B. Absorbable in 2 layers
C. Inner absorbable and outer non-absorbable
D. Inner non-absorbable and outer absorbable

**94. A patient with Crohn's disease was opened for an inflammed appendix. The treatment of choice is : PGI 1986, 88**

A. Appendicectomy
B. Ileocolic resection and anastamosis
C. Close the abdomen and start medical treatment
D. None of the above

**95. Carcinoid syndrome occurs only if there is metastasis to : PGI 1987**

A. Lung B. Liver
C. Brain D. Bone

**96. Match List-I (Types of patients) with List-II (Causes of intestinal obstruction) and select the correct answer: CSE 1997**

| List-I | List-II |
|---|---|
| A. Neonatal | 1. Acute intusseusception |
| B. Infant | 2. Meconium ileus |
| C. Old persons | 3. Tubercular stricture |
| D. Middle-aged females | 4. Carcinoma colon |

| | A | B | C | D |
|---|---|---|---|---|
| A. | 2 | 1 | 4 | 3 |
| B. | 1 | 2 | 3 | 4 |
| C. | 1 | 2 | 4 | 3 |
| D. | 2 | 1 | 3 | 4 |

**97. The narrowest part of the small intestine is : AMC 1985**

A. 60 cms proximal to ileocaecal valve.
B. 60 inches proximal to ileocaecal valve.
C. 90 cms proximal to ileocaecal valve.
D. 90 inches proximal to ileocaecal valve.

**98. Common causes of acute intestinal obstruction in India are following except : PGI 1994**

A. Adhesions
B. Internal hernia
C. Obstructed internal hernia
D. Volvulus

**99. Thumb printing sign is seen in : PGI 1985, 87**

A. Ulcerative colitis B. Ischaemic colitis
C. Crohn's disease D. Toxic megacolon

**100. Commonest cause of intestinal obstruction in children is : PGI 1984, 86; AIIMS 1994**

A. Congenital bands B. Volvulus
C. Hernia D. Adhesions

**101. In pneumoperitoneum, following are seen except : PGI 1997**

A. Hypertension B. Bradycardia
C. Tachycardia D. Hypercapnia

**102. The following is true of mesenteric artery thrombosis, except : AMC 1984; PGI 1988**

A. Mostly embolic in nature
B. Shock is present
C. Extensive infarction of whole of small bowel and cecum is seen
D. Good prognosis

**103. In the abdomen, aneurysms of the —— commonly occur next only to the aorta. AIIMS 1986**

A. Internal iliac artery
B. External iliac artery
C. Splenic artery
D. Inferior mesentric artery

**104. Acute large intestinal obstruction should be operated as early as possible because of : PGI 1994; AIIMS 1995; UPSC 1995**

A. Risk of caecal perforation with closed loop obstruction
B. Severe electrolyte imbalance
C. Loss of fluids
D. Septicaemia

**105. Predisposing factors for colonic carcinomas are following, except : PGI 1981, 88**

A. Familial polyposis
B. Gardner's syndrome
C. Juvenile polyp
D. Chronic ulcerative colitis

**Ans.** 90. B 91. C 92. D 93. C 94. C 95. B 96. A 97. A 98. A 99. B 100. A 101. B 102. D 103. C 104. A 105. C

**106. In carcinoma caecum, commonest surgery done is : Delhi 1988**

A. Total colectomy B. Left hemicolectomy
C. Right hemicolectomy D. Ileostomy

**107. Not seen in ulcerative colitis : Delhi 1988; AI 1990; Rajasthan 1998**

A. Perforation B. Bleeding
C. Pseudopolyposis D. Toxic megacolon

**108. Large bowel obstruction has to be operated urgently because of the risk of the following, except : Delhi 1988**

A. Caecum perforation
B. Electrolyte imbalance
C. Absorption of toxic metabolites
D. Gangrene

**109. Commonest intussusception is : Delhi 1986; 99**

A. Ileocolic B. Ileocaecal
C. Colocolic D. Colorectal

**110. All of the following statements are true regarding carcinoid tumour, except : PGI 1986**

A. Is commonest in distal third of appendix.
B. Is ten times more than other forms of carcinoma of appendix.
C. It is bright red in colour.
D. Hemicolectomy is indicated if it invades mesoappendix.

**111. Best diagnostic method for Meckel's diverticulum includes : TN 1996**

A. Barium study
B. Tc99 scan
C. Tc99 pertechnitium scan
D. Endoscopy

**112. Which of the following is not peritoneal tumour : Rohtak 1988**

A. Lipoma B. Sarcoma
C. Enterogenous cyst D. Ganglioneuroma

**113. Which of the following is not true as underlying cause of 'Dynamic intestinal obstruction': DNB 1989**

A. Adhesion B. Volvulus
C. Paralytic ileus D. Bolus of food

**114. The following is true of a subphrenic abscess, except : PGI 1987**

A. Irregular pyrexia
B. Air-fluid level in X-ray
C. Ultrasound is diagnostic
D. Leucopenia occurs

**115. Regarding Meckel's diverticulum, which is not true : AMU 1989**

A. Seen in 2% of population
B. 2 feet from ileocaecal junction
C. Seen on the mesenteric border
D. Carcinoid can occur in it

**116. The treatment of choice in a duodenal ulcer without complication is : AMU 1989**

A. Medical treatment
B. Gastrojejunostomy (GJ)
C. GJ + HSV
D. GJ + Truncal vagotomy

**117. In paralytic ileus, the following are used except : AIIMS 1987**

A. Naso-gastric suction
B. Administration of I/V fluids
C. Sedatives
D. Immediate laparotomy

**118. Acute intussusception occurs most frequently in age group of : PGI 1994**

A. 3 months-6 years B. 6 months-9 months
C. 2 years-6 years D. 10 years-12 years

**119. Common complication of typhoid fever is : DNB 1990**

A. Cholecystitis
B. Osteomyelitis
C. Intestinal perforation
D. Paralytic ileus

**120. Typhoid ulcer perforation usually occurs during : DNB 1991, 94**

A. Ist week B. 2nd week
C. 3rd week D. 4th week
E. 5th week

**121. Most common presentation of Ileocaecal TB is : Delhi 1984, 88; AIIMS 1986, 89, 94**

A. Pain
B. Lump
C. Change in bowel habits
D. Malaena

**122. Spastic ileus is noticed in : AMC 1986**

A. Hypokalaemia B. Porphyria
C. Pancreatitis D. None of the above

**123. Transmural inflammation with skip lesions in colon is seen in : AIIMS 1994**

A. Ischaemic colitis B. Regional enteritis
C. Ulcerative colitis D. Non-specific colitis

**124. The usual therapy for acute obstruction of the large bowel is : TN 1990**

A. Gastro-duodenal suction
B. An emergency decompression with a colostomy
C. Watch and heavy cover with antibiotics
D. Surgical lysis of adhesive bands

| Ans. | | | | | | | | | |
|---|---|---|---|---|---|---|---|---|---|
| 106. C | 107. A | 108. D | 109. A | 110. C | 111. C | 112. C | 113. C | 114. D | 115. C |
| 116. A | 117. D | 118. B | 119. D | 120. C | 121. C | 122. B | 123. B | 124. B | |

**125. At least 50% of the carcinomas of the colon are found in the : PGI 1987**
A. Sigmoid region B. Caecum
C. Splenic flexure D. Transverse colon

**126. The malignant tumour of the colon that most frequently occurs with ulcerative colitis is : AIIMS 1986**
A. Villous adenoma
B. Carcinoid
C. Adenocarcinoma
D. Squamous cell carcinoma

**127. Radiology after a barium enema in ulcerative colitis does not show one of the following: DNB 1989**
A. A narrow contracted colon
B. Alternation is mucosal outline
C. Pseudopolyposis
D. Saw tooth appearance

**128. Volvulus occurs most frequently in the : AMU 1990**
A. Sigmoid colon B. Jejunum
C. Transverse colon D. Ileum

**129. Which of the following is a feature of generalised peritonitis : UPSC 1986**
A. Pulse rate falls progressively
B. Patient lies still
C. Patient is in agony and rolls in bed
D. None of the above

**130. Which site is not involved in Goting disease : AIIMS 1994**
A. Whole small intestine
B. Whole of large intestine without effects
C. Rectosigmoid region
D. Colon

**131. The commonest retroperitoneal tumour is : TN 1989**
A. Lymphosarcoma B. Liposarcoma
C. Pheochromocytoma D. Neuroblastoma

**132. Carcinoma of right colon is most commonly : AI 1989; AIIMS 1994**
A. Ulcerative B. Fungating
C. Stenosis (Annular) D. Tubular

**133. Regarding adhesional intestinal obstruction, which is true : AIIMS 1994**
A. Operate after minimum 10 days of conservative treatment
B. Avoid surgery for initial 48-72 hours
C. Never operate
D. Operate immediately

**134. Commonest site of Ischaemic colitis : AIIMS 1995, 97; MAHE 1998**
A. Splenic flexure B. Descending colon
C. Hepatic flexure D. Ascending colon

**135. The first to appear in a case of acute intestinal obstruction is : DNB 1990**
A. Constipation B. Colicky pain
C. Vomiting D. Distension

**136. In short bowel syndrome following are seen except : AI 1998**
A. Electrolyte imbalance B. Hypogastrinemia
C. Diarrhoea D. None of the above

**137. Which of the following is a cause of a dynamic intestinal obstruction : DNB 1991**
A. Volvulus B. Intussusception
C. Peritonitis D. Inspissated faeces

**138. Patients with chronic ulcerative colitis may develop carcinoma. Regarding this, the following statements are correct, except : AP 1989**
A. Growths are multiple, flat and infiltrating.
B. Carcinoma arises from pseudopolyps.
C. Age at onset determines frequency of cancer.
D. Incidence increases with duration of disease.

**139. Clinical feature of ischaemic colitis depend on the following, except : TN 1988**
A. Duration of occlusion
B. Efficiency of collateral circulation
C. Extension of vascular occlusion
D. Degree of inflammation

**140. The most frequent cause of massive bleeding from the colon is : AP 1988, 92**
A. Multiple polyposis
B. Cancer of the left colon
C. Cancer of the right colon
D. Diverticular disease

**141. In Hirschsprung's disease in the male, the operation of choice is : Kerala 1989**
A. Presacral plus inferior mesenteric neurectomy
B. Lumbar ganglionectomy
C. Colostomy
D. Colectomy

**142. Ureter sigmoidostomy causes : AIIMS 1995**
A. Bladder Ca
B. Colonic Ca
C. Hyperchloremic alkalosis
D. Hyperchloremic acidosis

| Ans. | | | | | | | | | |
|---|---|---|---|---|---|---|---|---|---|
| 125. A | 126. C | 127. D | 128. A | 129. B | 130. B | 131. A | 132. B | 133. B | 134. A |
| 135. B | 136. D | 137. C | 138. B | 139. D | 140. D | 141. B | 142. D | | |

**143. Which about pneumatosis cystoides intestinalis is incorrect : AIIMS 1995**
A. Surgical resection indicated in all cases.
B. Spontaneous regression seen.
C. May cause tension pneumo-peritoneum.
D. May cause severe rectal bleeding.

**144. In which of the following abdominal incision there is least risk of wound rupture : AIIMS 1984**
A. Midline upper abdominal
B. Paramedian (Upper)
C. Mc Burney's incision
D. Paramedian (Lower)

**145. The most likely cause for suture leak after colon resection and anastomosis for cancer sigmoid colon is : Delhi 1983**
A. Subclinical malnutrition
B. Infection of anastomotic site
C. Mechanical disruption due to colonic pressure and contractility
D. Ischaemia

**146. Active substances involved in the functioning carcinoid tumour includes all of the following except : AP 1989**
A. ACTH B. Parathormone
C. Serotonin D. 5-hydroxytryptamine

**147. The most frequent indication for surgery in Crohn's disease is : Kerala 1989**
A. Abdominal mass
B. External fistula
C. Intestinal obstruction
D. Internal fistula

**148. In blunt abdominal injuries one of the following part of the intestine is commonly injured : AIIMS 1985**
A. Duodenojejunal junction
B. Pyloric end of stomach
C. Ileocecal junction
D. Transverse colon

**149. All of the following are steps in the management of diverticulosis except : UPSC 1987**
A. High residue diet
B. Repeated administration of liquid parafin and other purgatives
C. Antispasmodics
D. Morphine or opiates to relieve pain

**150. One of the following statement is not true regarding sigmoidoscopic examination of ulcerative colitis : PGI 1983**
A. Mucosa is hyperemic and bleeds on touch.
B. Considerable degree of exudate is present.
C. Large deep ulcerations are present with intervening mucosa comparatively healthy.
D. Tiny ulcers may be seen and appear to coalesce.

**151. True about intestinal lymphoma is : Delhi 1995**
A. Most commonly found in jejunum.
B. May follow idiopathic malabsorption and steatorhoea.
C. Pain and constipation are chief complaints.
D. May be associated with pulm. and tricuspid stenosis.

**152. Colonic Carcinoma is associated with : Delhi 1995**
A. Fatty food B. Silicon
C. PVC D. Steel

**153. In Peutz-Jeghers syndrome, polyps are seen in : AI 1995**
A. Colon B. Small bowel
C. Rectum D. Stomach

**154. About six to eight hours after peptic perforation, the disappearance of abdominal wall rigidity is due to : UPSC 1995**
A. Cessation of acid secretion in the stomach.
B. Revival from initial shock.
C. Dilution of acid in the peritoneal cavity.
D. Fatigue of the reflex arc.

**155. Umbilical adenoma is most often in : DNB 1989, 93, 96**
A. Completely obliterated vitello intestinal duct.
B. Partially obliterated vitello intestinal duct.
C. Complete patent vitello intestinal duct.
D. Infection of umbilicus.

**156. Sacrococcygeal teratoma is commonly seen in : AP 1989**
A. Males
B. Females
C. Equally common
D. No predistable sex ratio

**157. The commonest cause of intussusception in infancy is: DNB 1989**
A. TB B. Worms
C. Meconium ileus D. Idiopathic

**158. The following are the indications of operation in necrotizing enterocolitis, except : UPSC 1986, 89**
A. Pneumoperitoneum
B. Non-responsive metabolic acidosis
C. Persistently low platelet
D. Portal gas

| Ans. | | | | | | | | | |
|---|---|---|---|---|---|---|---|---|---|
| 143. A | 144. C | 145. D | 146. B | 147. C | 148. A | 149. B | 150. C | 151. B | 152. A |
| 153. C | 154. C | 155. B | 156. B | 157. D | 158. D | | | | |

**159. The treatment of choice in duodenal atresia : DNB 1989; AIIMS 1997; AI 1998**

A. Gastro jejunostomy
B. Duodeno jejunostomy
C. Bishop Koop procedure
D. Duodenostomy

**160. Most common tumour of duodenum is : AP 1993**

A. Lymphoma B. Leiomyoma
C. Villous tumor D. Adenocarcinoma

**161. Villous tumors of the gastrointestinal tract are least common in : AP 1993**

A. Oesophagus B. Duodenum
C. Caecum D. Rectum

**162. Meckel's diverticulum is a part of : Delhi 1989**

A. Foregut B. Fore and midgut
C. Midgut D. Hindgut

**163. The pain of chronic peptic ulceration in Meckel's diverticulum is felt at : AMU 1989**

A. Epigastrium B. Right hypochondrium
C. Right iliac fossa D. Umbilicus

**164. The following may be affected by the pneumatosis cystoides intestinalis, except : DNB 1990**

A. Oesophagus B. Ileum
C. Colon D. Rectum

**165. The commonest presentation of adenoma of small intestine is : DNB 1990**

A. Intussusception B. Intestinal bleeding
C. Vomiting D. Loss of appetite

**166. The adenomatous polypi of large bowel are most often situated in : AMU 1989**

A. Ascending colon B. Transverse colon
C. Descending colon D. Sigmoid colon

**167. The following are the common presenting features of duodenal atresia, except : UPSC 1987**

A. Persistent vomiting
B. Distension of abdomen
C. Visible peristasis
D. Abdominal pain

**168. Ileal atresia differs from jejunal atresia by : AIIMS 1987**

A. Early abdominal distension (within 24 hours of life)
B. Early vomiting
C. Passage of meconium
D. Marked abdominal pain

**169. Features of necrotising enterocolitis are following except : AI 1996**

A. Abdominal distension B. Vomiting
C. ↑ Bowel sounds D. Constipation

**170. Exomphalos major should be operated at : PGI 1986**

A. Birth B. 3 months of age
C. 1 year D. 3 years

**171. Exomphalos minor, firm strapping is done : AMU 1986**

A. Never B. For 1 week
C. For 2 weeks D. For 3 months

**172. Urinary excretion of 5 hydroxy indole acetic acid is more than ——— in diagnostic of carcinoid syndrome. PGI 1984, 86**

A. 9 mg B. 15 mg
C. 20 mg D. 25 mg

**173. All of the following structures are covered by peritoneum, except. AP 1993**

A. Appendix B. Pancreas
C. Ureters D. Bladder

**174. First muconium is said to be formed during the ——— month of foetal life : AIIMS 1984**

A. Second B. Fourth
C. Seventh D. Ninth

**175. Intussusception is characterized by following except : UPSC 1986**

A. Facial pallor and undistended abdomen
B. Red-current jelly stool
C. Persistent vomiting
D. Common in male child

**176. The most common age of child presenting with intussusception is : UPSC 1986**

A. 0-4 weeks B. 1-6 months
C. 6-9 months D. 2-3 years

**177. On X-ray, intussusception is characterized by following, except : UPSC 1988**

A. Increased gas shadow in small intestine
B. Absence of caecal gas shadow
C. Multiple fluid levels
D. Gas ulcer diaphragm

**178. Best colostomy repair is : AP 1994**

A. With rod B. With enteroferone
C. Intraperitoneal D. Extraperitoneal

**179. Umbilical granuloma is : Kerala 1990**

A. Infected umbilical cicatrix
B. Adenoma
C. Obliterated vitellointestinal duct
D. Hydrocele

**180. Patent vitello-intestinal duct should preferably be operated at : AMU 1985, 89**

A. Birth B. 6 months of age
C. 12 months of age D. 3 years of age

**Ans.** 159. B 160. D 161. A 162. C 163. D 164. D 165. A 166. D 167. B 168. A 169. D 170. A 171. C 172. B 173. A 174. B 175. C 176. C 177. D 178. C 179. A 180. B

**181. Per rectal examination in Hirschsprung's disease shows all of the following except : AP 1988**
A. Anus is free from fissures or excoriations
B. Rectum is empty
C. No perianal soiling
D. Rectum does not grip the examination finger

**182. The operative treatment in Hirschsprung's disease is only undertaken when child : TN 1989**
A. Is a 2 years of age
B. Is atleast 8 kg in weight and thriving
C. Has no distension of abdomen
D. Has failed to respond to conservative treatment

**183. Meckel's diverticulum arises from anti-mesenteric border of : TN 1989**
A. Duodenum B. Ileum
C. Jejunum D. Transverse colon

**184. All of the following statements are true regarding jejunal diverticulam except : Kerala 1987**
A. More often several are present
B. Clinically they may be symptom less
C. Produce malabsorption
D. Are prone to rupture

**185. Abdominal aneurysm should be operated when it is : Rajasthan 1989**
A. 1 cm B. 3 cms
C. 5 cms D. 7 cms

**186. In Jejunum, most common malignant tumor is : Delhi 1996**
A. Adenocarcinoma B. Lymphosarcoma
C. Carcinoid D. Peutz Jegher's syndrome

**187. Scar carcinoma is common in : Delhi 1996**
A. TB pneumoconiosis B. Interstitial fibrosis
C. Pneumoconiosis D. Pulmonary infarction

**188. Malignant potential is rare in following except : Delhi 1996**
A. Peutz Jegher's syndrome
B. Adenomatous polyp
C. Hamartomatous polyp
D. Familial Adenomatous polyposis

**189. The commonest parts of duodenum having congenital atresia are : Delhi 1986**
A. I or II B. II or III
C. III or IV D. IV or I

**190. The commonest site of congenital atresia of duodenum is : AI 1989**
A. Junction of fore-and mid gut
B. Midpoint of midgut
C. Junction of mid and hind gut
D. Any of the above

**191. Trifoliate duodenum is commonest in which part of the duodenum : DNB 1990**
A. I B. II
C. III D. IV

**192. Commonest site of a subdiaphragmatic abscess is : Delhi 1987**
A. Right posterior intraperitoneal sub-diaphragmatic space.
B. Left anterior intraperitoneal space.
C. Right anterior intraperitoneal sub-diaphragmatic space.
D. Left anterior intraperitoneal sub-diaphragmatic space.

**193. The least malignant form of carcinoma colon is : DNB 1990**
A. Annular B. Tubular
C. Ulcerative D. Cauliflower

**194. Ulcerative colitis starts in : PGI 1995**
A. Ileum B. Transverse colon
C. Descending colon D. Rectum

**195. Right-sided colonic cancer commonly presents with : TN 1989**
A. Mobilisation of gall bladder during cholecystectomy.
B. Mobilisation of 2nd part of duodenum.
C. Mobilisation of pancreas during pancreatotomy.
D. Mobilisation of ascending colon.

**196. The following signs and symptoms of paralytic ileus are common, except : UPSC 1989**
A. Hyperactive bowel sounds
B. Abdominal distension
C. Absence of colicky pain
D. Patients may be afebrile

**197. Wrong about amoebiasis is : PGI 1995**
A. In hepatic amoebiasis, serology is important.
B. Ascending colon is commonly involved.
C. May involve small intestine.
D. Stool examination is an essential investigation.

**198. The most common congenital anomaly accompanying duodenal atresia is : Delhi 1986**
A. Mongolism
B. Imperforate anus
C. Congenital heart disease
D. Tracheooesophageal fistula

| Ans. | 181. D | 182. B | 183. B | 184. D | 185. C | 186. A | 187. D | 188. B | 189. B | 190. A |
|---|---|---|---|---|---|---|---|---|---|---|
| | 191. A | 192. A | 193. D | 194. D | 195. C | 196. A | 197. C | 198. A | | |

**199. Minimum amount of bleeding to produce malaena is : UPSC 1987**

A. 50 ml B. 100 ml
C. 150 ml D. 200 ml

**200. Common cause of triad of symptoms of Epigastric pain, haematmesis and malena is : PGI 1985**

A. Duodenal ulcer B. Meckel's diverticulum
C. Haemorrhoids D. Anal fissure

**201. Regarding Meckel's diverticulum, which is correct : Kerala 1989**

A. Arises from jejunum
B. Possesses all three coats of the intestinal wall
C. Usually asymptomatic
D. Is a band connecting to the umbilicus

**202. Bile stained peritoneal exudate may be found in following except : AMC 1987; TN 1990**

A. Perforated gall bladder
B. Perforated duodenal ulcer
C. Spontaneous bile peritonitis
D. Bursting of amoebic liver abscess

**203. One of the following is a late feature seen in peritonitis: UPSC 1988**

A. Vomiting
B. Pain
C. Muscular rigidity
D. Absence of bowel sounds

**204. A 60-years old male presents with acute onset of pain in lower abdomen followed by repeated rectal bleeding. Examination revealed pulse rate of 100/minute, BP-160/96 mm of Hg and a localised tenderness in the left hypochondrium. Stool examination revealed only a few pus cells and sigmoidoscopy was normal. Which one of the following is the most likely diagnosis : UPSC 1996**

A. Idiopathic ulcerative colitis
B. Bacillary dysentery
C. Ischaemic colitis
D. Amoebic colitis

**205. Which of the following complications occur within 48 hours after abdominal surgery : AIIMS 1985**

A. Wounds infection B. Chest infection
C. Deep vein thrombosis D. Pulmonary embolism

**206. Immediate surgery is not indicated in : AIIMS 1985**

A. Ruptured ectopic pregnancy
B. Penetrating duodenal ulcer
C. Acute appendicitis
D. Strangulated hernia

**207. Which of the following is not true about resberry tumour of umbilicus : AMU 1987**

A. Tumour of infant age group.
B. Rich in goblet cells.
C. Treatment in early stages consists of tying of ligature around it.
D. Arises from the skin near umbilicus.

**208. All of the following are clinical features of primary megacolon except : UPSC 1983**

A. There is familial tendency.
B. Infant fails to pass meconium during the first two or three days of life.
C. On examination rectum is full of faecal matter.
D. Abdominal distension is seen on thrice day.

**209. "Lead paint" stools are characteristic of : AIIMS 1986**

A. Lead poisoning
B. Shigellosis
C. Carcinoma of pancreas
D. Carcinoma of rectum

**210. In peptic ulcer prostaglandin important is: Rajasthan 1998**

A. $PGI_2$ B. $PGE_2$
C. $PGI_1$ D. $PGF_2$

**211. Consider the following statements regarding colo-rectal carcinoma : CSE 1998**

1. The 5-years survival in Dukes A stage is 80%.
2. The survival rate for patients with carcinoma colon has not changed in the last three decades.
3. Radiotherapy is quite helpful in treating recurrent disease that is confined to the bowel wall.

**Of these statements**

A. 1 alone is correct B. 2 and 3 are correct
C. 1, 2 and 3 are correct D. 1 and 2 are correct

**212. Tratment of choice for Stage-III a Hodgkins lymphoma : PGI 1987**

A. Chemotherapy
B. Radiotherapy
C. Combination of chemotherapy and Radiotherapy
D. Excision

**213. A driver with seat belt had GI injury and developed colicky pain because of bleeding in GIT, cause is : Rohtak 1996**

A. Haematobilia B. Duodenal perforation
C. Acute pancreatitis D. Volvulus

**Ans.** 199. A 200. A 201. B 202. D 203. D 204. C 205. B 206. B 207. D 208. C
209. C 210. B 211. A 212. B 213. B

**214. Abdominal tuberculosis, true is : Delhi 1995; PGI 1996**
A. Mostly caused by pulmonary TB
B. Pulmonary X-ray diagnostic
C. Mostly perforates
D. Involves appendix mostly

**215. In lumbar sympathectomy (removal of upper ganglion), impotence is because of : UPSC 1983; AIIMS 1984, 85**
A. Defective ejaculation
B. Decreased testicular function
C. Transient erectile impotence
D. Permanent erectile impotence

**216. In acute mechanical obstruction, treatment of choice is : PGI 1996**
A. Gastroduodenal suction
B. Replacement of fluids
C. Relief of obstruction by operation
D. Relief of obstruction by drugs

**217. A young man has haematemesis, evidence that it is because of cirrhosis in : AMC 1993**
A. Caput medusae B. Ascites
C. Oesophageal varices D. Rectal varices

**218. Commonest complication after resection of abdominal aortic aneurysm is : AIIMS 1986**
A. Paralytic ileus
B. Declamping syndrome
C. Atelectasis
D. Leakage from anastomosis site

**219. The most definitive indication of malignant transformation of a benign polyp of colon : AIIMS 1986**
A. Infiltration of fibrous core
B. Infilteration of base of polyp
C. Ulceration at the tip of polyp
D. Lymphatic permeation

**220. Meckel's diverticulum contains following, except : AMC 1993**
A. Colonic mucosa B. Liver tissue
C. Pancreatic tissue D. Gastric mucosa

**221. 'Melanosis coli' presents clinically as : AIIMS 1986, 88**
A. Intussusception B. Asymptomatic
C. Bleeding P/R D. Intestinal obstruction

**222. Cause of upper GI bleeding include following, except : PGI 1996**
A. Peptic ulcer B. Erosive gastritis
C. Oesophageal varices D. Ca stomach

**223. Prognostic factors of Duodenal ulcer perforation include following, except : PGI 1996**
A. Age of 45-55 years B. Nutritional status
C. Duration of ulcer D. Site of ulcer

**224. Most pancancerous for carcinoma colon is : Kerala 1989; AI 1995**
A. Familial polyposis
B. Hamartomatous polyps
C. Adenomatous polyps
D. Peutz Jeghers syndrome

**225. Persistent paralytic ileus is treated by : JIPMER 1997**
A. Tube insertion B. Surgical reopening
C. Protanetic drugs D. None of the above

**226. The following can be diagnosed by intestinal biopsy, except : PGI 1984; AIIMS 1988**
A. Whipple's disease
B. Blind loop syndrome
C. Eosinophilic gastroenteritis
D. Tropical sprue

**227. Pseudopolyposis is seen in : Delhi 1983, 90; AIIMS 1986**
A. Ulcerative colitis B. Crohn's disease
C. TB abdomen D. Carcinoma colon

**228. Tumor marker for colonic cancer is : JIPMER 1997**
A. CEA B. AFP
C. HCG D. Alpha antitrypsin

**229. Consider the following statements : CSE 1998**
**Paralytic ileus could be :**
1. Post-operative
2. Hyperkalemic
3. Uraemic
4. Infective

**Of these statements**
A. 1 and 2 are correct B. 2, 3 and 4 are correct
C. 3 and 4 are correct D. 1, 3 and 4 are correct

**230. Most common cause of meconium ileus is : AI 1995, 96**
A. Fibrocystic disease of pancreas
B. Cirrhosis
C. Liver aplasia
D. Malnutrition

**231. Commonest site of peptic ulcer perforation is : PGI 1985, 89**
A. Anterior aspect of Ist part of duodenum
B. Anterior aspect of 2nd part of duodenum
C. Greater curvature of stomach
D. Meckel's diverticulum

**Ans.** 214. A 215. A 216. C 217. B 218. C 219. A 220. B 221. B 222. D 223. B
224. C 225. B 226. D 227. A 228. A 229. D 230. A 231. A

**232. True about colonic organisms is : PGI 1998**
A. Distal ileum $10^3$-$10^5$ organisms
B. Colon — $10^5$ - $10^7$ organisms
C. First organisms in newborn are coliform, streptococci
D. Chyme in jejunum contains many bacteria

**233. Most common cause of small intestine obstruction is : AI 1996**
A. Intussusception B. Carcinoma
C. Hernia D. Stricture

**234. Prolonged post-operative ileus is best treated with : PGI 1998**
A. Long tube insertion
B. Calcium pantothenate
C. Laprotomy and explore
D. Peristaltic stimulants

**235. True about acute ulcerative colitis in pregnancy is : UPSC 1984; AMC 1986**
A. Increase in severity in 3rd trimester
B. Increase in severity in Ist trimester
C. Remains as such
D. Becomes quiescent

**236. Pseudomyxoma peritoneil is seen with : AIIMS 1986**
A. Thecoma ovary
B. Carcinoid syndrome
C. Mesothelioma
D. Mucocele of appendix or mucinous cystadenoma ovary

**237. Symptomatic intestinal tuberculosis in India has following manifestations except : PGI 1985, 90**
A. Stricture formation
B. Ulcerative is present
C. Tabes mesenterica
D. Ileocaecal involvement commonest
E. Constipation is usual

**238. In Whipple's procedure, following are cut, except AIIMS 1998**
A. Portal vein B. CBD
C. Duodenum D. Head of pancreas

**239. Tenesmus occurs in lesions of : AMC 1986**
A. Ileum B. Right side of colon
C. Descending colon D. Sigmoid colon

**240. All of the following are true about Meckel's diverticulum, except : AI 1996**
A. Arises from mesenteric border
B. Often bleeds
C. May ulcerate
D. Intussusception

**241. Apex of volvulus of sigmoid colon in plain X-ray abdomen is at the : AIIMS 1987, 89, 90**
A. Left iliac fossa B. Right iliac fossa
C. Right hypochondrium D. Left hypochondrium

**242. All of the following are indications for surgery in a case of duodenal ulcer, except : UPSC 1996**
A. Acute perforation of ulcer
B. Pyloric stenosis
C. Massive haemorrhage
D. Typical periodicity

**243. Volvulus is an : UPSC 1996**
A. Internal herniation of the intestine.
B. Invagination of the proximal segment of intestine into the distal segment.
C. Obstruction of the sigmoid.
D. Axial rotation of a loop of intestine around its own axis.

**244. Which is mesentric cyst whose removal entrails removal of part of gut : TN 1995**
A. Chylolymphatic cyst B. Enterogenous cyst
C. Dermoid D. All

**245. Pseudobowel obstruction is found in following except: AIIMS 1987, 89**
A. Hyperthyroidism B. Diabetes mellitus
C. Scleroderma D. Dermatomyositis

**246. When rectal washouts are given to Hirschsprung's disease, the following fluid is used : Karnataka 1995**
A. 5% dextrose B. Normal saline
C. Soap solution D. Tap water

**247. In the diagnosis is MEA Type-II, which of the following confirmatory findings would be least likely: AIIMS 1988**
A. Elevated serum thyrocalcitonin
B. Elevated urinary metanephrins
C. Elevated serum calcium
D. Low serum phosphorus
E. Elevated T4

**248. The best route to drain pelvic abscess is in : AIIMS 1982; AMC 1987, 88**
A. Rectum B. Ponch of Douglas
C. Abdomen D. Any of the above

**249. The commonest cause of bleeding from lower GIT is : AIIMS 1982, 86; Delhi 1987; AMC 1987, 89**
A. Diverticulosis
B. Diverticulitis
C. Meckel's diverticulum
D. Carcinoma

| Ans. | | | | | | | | | |
|---|---|---|---|---|---|---|---|---|---|
| 232. B | 233. A | 234. C | 235. B | 236. D | 237. E | 238. A | 239. D | 240. A | 241. A |
| 242. D | 243. D | 244. B | 245. A | 246. B | 247. E | 248. A | 249. A | | |

250. **String sign of Kantor is seen in :** **UPSC 1982, 86, 87; AIIMS 1983 Delhi 1986; AMC 1987, 89**
A. Regional ileitis B. Ulcerative colitis
C. Diverticulitis D. Ileocaecal TB

251. **In necrotising enterocolitis, earliest change seen in X-ray abdomen is :** **Kerala 1996**
A. Non-specific bowel dilatation
B. Gas in the intestinal wall
C. Gas in splenic flexure
D. Ground glass appearance
E. None

252. **In Intussusception, following are true, except :** **Rajasthan 1994**
A. Common in male child between 6-9 months of age.
B. Ileocolic is the commonest site.
C. Recurrent intussusception may be caused by Peutz Jegher's syndrome.
D. In ileoileal intussusception claw sign is positive.

253. **Christmas tree deformity is seen in :** **Rohtak 1985**
A. Duodenal atresia
B. Jejunal atresia
C. Hirschsprung's disease
D. Volvulus

254. **'Duodenal blow out' is :** **AP 1997**
A. Perforation of duodenal ulcer
B. Iatrogenic
C. Complication of partial gastrectomy
D. Due to trauma

255. **Paul Mikulicz operation is done for :** **AMC 1986**
A. Paraumbilical hernia B. Ileal atresia
C. Intussusception D. Hirschsprung's disease

256. **Water loss is severe if intestinal obstruction occurs at:** **JIPMER 1986, 90**
A. First part of duodenum
B. Third part of duodenum
C. Midjejunum
D. Ileum

257. **Coffee bean sign is usually seen in :** **Karnataka 1988, 89**
A. Volvulus B. Pyloric obstruction
C. Intussusception D. Intestinal obstruction

258. **The following are complications of ulcerative colitis except :** **AI 1990**
A. Peptic ulceration B. Arthritis
C. Sclerosing cholangitis D. Toxic megacolon

259. **In omphalitis, jaundice is most commonly seen in :** **AIIMS 1986**
A. 4-7 days B. 7-14 days
C. 3-6 weeks D. 9-12 weeks

260. **Triple bubble sign is present in :** **DNB 1991**
A. Duodenal atresia B. Jejunal atresia
C. Splenic rupture D. Hepatic rupture

261. **"Peritoneal mice" is :** **AP 1997**
A. Pseudomyxoma peritonei
B. Appendices epiploicae
C. Peritoneal seedings of tumor
D. Endometriosis

262. **A 35-years woman complains of attacks of breathlessness, cyanosis and flushing. Apart from occasional diarrhoea, she has not abdominal symptoms. Abdominal examination reveals an enlarged nodular liver. If laparotomy is done on this patient, one would expect to find :** **UPSC 1994**
A. An ovarian tumour
B. A yellow nodule in the ileum
C. Crohn's disease
D. A tumour in the adrenal gland

263. **In strangulation of intestine, not seen is :** **AIIMS 1994**
A. Shock is early feature
B. Exaggeration of bowel sounds
C. Generalized pain is not present
D. Spasmodic contraction with pain present

264. **In angiodysplasia, which of the following is most common in lesions :** **DNB 1995**
A. An early filling vein
B. A vascular tuft
C. A delayed-emptying vein
D. Thrombosed vei

265. **The most common abdominal tumour in a child is :** **PGI 1983, 85, 96; AMC 1986; AIIMS 1996**
A. Embryoma of the kidney (Wilm's tumour)
B. Neuroblastoma
C. Malignant melanoma
D. Benign sacrococcygeal teratoma

266. **In obstruction of the large gut, rupture occurs at the _____.** **PGI 1989**
A. Ceacum B. Ascending colon
C. Transverse colon D. Descending colon

267. **A patient with umbilical bleed monthly has :** **AI 1994**
A. Umbilical adenoma
B. Endometriosis
C. Meckel's diverticulum
D. All of the above

| Ans. | 250. A | 251. A | 252. D | 253. B | 254. C | 255. B | 256. B | 257. A | 258. A | 259. C |
|---|---|---|---|---|---|---|---|---|---|---|
| | 260. B | 261. B | 262. B | 263. C | 264. C | 265. B | 266. A | 267. B | | |

268. **Troublesome bleeding during lumbar sympathectomy is due to injury to :** **TNPSC 1997**
A. Testicular vessels B. Lumbar veins
C. Lumbar arteries D. Aorta

269. **One of the following is false regarding sliding hiatus hernia :** **Karnataka 1987**
A. Often strangulates
B. Often asymptomatic
C. Commonly associated with reflux oesophagitis
D. Oesophageal hiatus enlarges

270. **In meconium ileus:** **TNPSC 1997**
A. Surgery is always advised primarily.
B. Bilious vomiting is an early feature.
C. There is impaction of meconium in the distal part of duodenum.
D. Upright straight abdominal film shows enormously distended small bowel without gas or fluid levels.

271. **The best investigation for colorectal carcinoma is :** **Kerala 1997**
A. Colonoscopy & biopsy
B. Double contrast barium enema
C. Exfoliative cytology
D. Barium meal follow through

272. **The blind loop syndrome following side-to-side intestinal anastomosis may result in :** **Karnataka 1987**
A. Macrocytic anaemia B. Tetany
C. Hyoproteinemia D. All of the above

273. **In which of the following operative procedures drainage of the peritoneal cavity most necessary :** **Karnataka 1989**
A. Gastrectomy
B. Closure of duodenal perforation
C. Appendicectomy for acute appendicitis
D. Gastrojejunostomy

274. **Most common means by which TB causes peritonitis :** **Kerala 1997**
A. Mesenteric lymph node involved
B. Hematogenous
C. Rupture of cisterna chyli
D. Rupture of small intestine

275. **Most common cause of small intestinal fistula is :** **JIPMER 1998**
A. Post-operative
B. Inflammatory bowel disease
C. Spontaneous
D. Post-inflammatory

276. **A routine gastrojejunostomy without undue contamination of the wound is described as a :** **Karnataka 1993**
A. Clean wound
B. Clean contaminated wound
C. Contaminated wound
D. Dirty wound

277. **A new-born is brought with history suggestive of intestinal obstruction. An upright X-ray of the abdomen shows multiple air fluid levels with area of calcification. The most likely diagnosis is :** **UPSC 1994**
A. Meconium ileus
B. Meconium peritonitis
C. Meconium plug syndrome
D. Hirschsprung's disease

278. **Over 75% of the strength of the intact abdominal wall lies in :** **Karnataka 1993**
A. The skin B. Subcutaneous tissue
C. Aponeurosis D. Peritoneum

279. **"Pseudo G.I. obstruction" is seen in all of the following, except :** **Karnataka 1993; AI 1999**
A. Diabetes Mellitus
B. Hypothyroidism
C. Progressive systemic sclerosis
D. Addison's disease

280. **Bleeding P/R is present in the following, except :** **AIIMS 1994**
A. Sigmoid volvulus B. Meckel's diverticulum
C. Rectal carcinoma D. Ulcerative colitis

281. **Hodgkins disease with single cervical and bilateral inguinal node is stage :** **Kerala 1994**
A. IV B. III
C. IIa D. IIb

282. **In Crohn's disease which extra intestinal manifestation is more common than ulcerative colitis :** **PGI 1993, 94**
A. Bile duct obstruction B. Pyoderma gangrenosum
C. Conjuctivitis D. Finger clubbing

283. **Following are true regarding burst abdomen, except:** **JIPMER 1998**
A. Occurs in early post-operation period
B. Penitonitis rarely seen
C. There is no pain or shock
D. Second dehiscence is common

| Ans. | | | | | | | | | |
|---|---|---|---|---|---|---|---|---|---|
| 268. D | 269. A | 270. A | 271. A | 272. A | 273. B | 274. B | 275. A | 276. A | 277. A |
| 278. C | 279. D | 280. A | 281. B | 282. A | 283. D | | | | |

**284. Lumbar sympathectomy by extraperitoneal approach, the following structures should be protected from damage : PGI 1983, 89, 90, 93**

A. Ureter
B. Gonadal vessels
C. A + B
D. Aorta and IVC

**285. Mesenteric artery embolism is characterized by : PGI 1993**

A. Peritonium
B. Chronic post-prandial pain
C. Shock
D. Air fluid levels on plain X-ray abdomen

**286. Preferential diagnosis aid in Blunt injury abdomen is: PGI 1994**

A. 4 quadrant aspiration
B. Peritoneal lavage
C. Ultrasound
D. X-ray abdomen

**287. Haemoporitoneum occurs in following except : PGI 1994**

A. Kidney (Left) rupture
B. Penetrating injury in Right Hypochondrium
C. Perforation of colon
D. Rupture ectopic

**288. Sigmoid carcinoma with acute intestinal obstruction, treatment of choice : PGI 1994**

A. Proximal colostomy
B. Resection and end-to-end anastomosis
C. Paul-Mickulicz operation
D. Temporary colostomy

**289. Inflammatory bowel disease causes : PGI 1994**

A. Chronic active hepatitis
B. Hepatocellular carcinoma
C. Sclerosing cholangitis
D. Cholangiocarcinoma

**290. Which of the following is not influencing factor for abdomino-perineal resection : PGI 1994**

A. Age of patient
B. Fixity of surrounding stricture
C. Liver metastasis
D. Distance from anal canal

**291. Surgery is not a treatment for : PGI 1994**

A. Lymphoma
B. Neuroblastoma
C. Carcinoma colon
D. Carcinoma stomach

**292. Transmural inflammation with granulomas are a feature of : JIPMER 1998**

A. Ulcerative colitis
B. Amoebic colitis
C. Crohn's disease
D. Irritable bowel syndrome

**293. Gastrointestinal TB is commonest in the ileocaecal region because of : JIPMER 1998**

A. Abundant lymph follicles in that region
B. Stasis of chyme in ileum
C. Alkaline pH of bowel contents
D. All of the above

**294. Intussusceptiens is : PGI 1997**

A. Outer layer
B. Entering layer
C. Protruding layer
D. All of the above

**295. True about ulcerative colitis progressing to malignancy is following except : PGI 1997**

A. ↑ es with the time
B. Prognosis worst
C. Prognosis depends on duration
D. Best treated with chemotherapy

**296. A young lady has been admitted with complaints of acute pain in abdomen, vomiting, abdominal distension and constipation. Clinically she has been diagnosed to be a case of acute intestinal obstruction. The most appropriate investigation would be : CSE 1999**

A. Plain X-ray of abdomen
B. Ultrasound examination of abdomen
C. Upper G.I. endoscopy
D. C.T. examination of abdomen

**297. On exploratory laparotomy for acute intestinal obstruction, a patient was found to have a tubercular stricture, 8 cm proximal to ileocaecal junction in the ileum. The most appropriate surgical procedure would be : CSE 1999**

A. Right hemicolectomy
B. Resection of stricture and end-to-end anastomosis
C. Stricturoplasty
D. Ileo-transverse anastomosis bypassing stricture

**298. Match List-I with List-II and select the correct answer using the codes given below the lists : CSE 1999**

| List-I (Disorders producing intestinal obstruction) | List-II (Clinical features associated with the given disorders) |
|---|---|
| A. Intussusception | 1. Extreme abdominal distension |
| B. Sigmoid volvulus | 2. Red current jelly stool |
| C. Duodenal atresia | 3. Bells at evening pealing |
| D. Acute appendicitis | 4. Rovsing's sign |
| | 5. Double-bubble sign |

| Ans. | | | | | | | | | |
|---|---|---|---|---|---|---|---|---|---|
| 284. C | 285. B | 286. A | 287. C | 288. C | 289. C | 290. C | 291. A | 292. C | 293. A |
| 294. A | 295. D | 296. A | 297. B | 298. C | | | | | |

Codes :

| | a | b | c | d |
|---|---|---|---|---|
| A. | 3 | 4 | 5 | 1 |
| B. | 1 | 2 | 3 | 4 |
| C. | 2 | 1 | 5 | 4 |
| D. | 2 | 1 | 3 | 5 |

**299. 68 years old Chanda presented with bilious vomiting, crampy abdominal pain and a 2 weeks history of constipation. Plain X-ray abdomen revealed no fluid levels or distended bowel loops. The diagnosis could be : AIIMS 1999**

A. Pseudoobstruction
B. Adynamic ilius
C. Duodenal obstruction
D. Total colonic aganglionosis

**300. A 1 year old child presents with Hirschsprung's disease. Which of the following is true regarding further investigations : AIIMS 1999**

A. Ultrasound segment Ba enema is most accurate.
B. Suction biopsy is contraindicated in infant.
C. Giant ganglion cells are sine qua non of diagnosis.
D. Normal manometry rules out diagnosis.

**301. A 26 days old child presented with non-bilious vomiting and passed rabbit-pellet like faeces. The diagnosis is : AIIMS 1999**

A. Duodenal atresia
B. Volvulus
C. Infantile hypertrophic pyloric stenosis
D. Intussusception

**302. Which is false regarding familial adenomatous polyposis : AIIMS 1999**

A. Definitely progresses to malignancy
B. Early appearance of rectal polyps
C. Males and females affected equally
D. Males transmit the disease more

**303. 12 years old girl who swims frequently comes with H/o pain abdomen, rigidity, guarding, tenderness with liver dullness spared, the cause is : AIIMS 1999**

A. Primary peritonitis
B. Enteric Perforation
C. Intussusception
D. Biliary tree obst. with peritonitis

**304. Severity of 75 years old patient with descending Ca colon with acute obstruction treatment of choice : AIIMS 1999**

A. Hartman's pouch
B. Defunctioning colostomy
C. Hemicolectomy
D. A.P. resection

**305. Broders criteria refers to : MAHE 1999**

A. Classification of Ca Colon.
B. Staging of Ca breast by using clinical signs.
C. Classifying Hodgkin's lymphoma.
D. Classifying Head injury.

**306. Dukes classification of Ca colon true is : MAHE 1999**

A. Stage-A with involvement of wall even when lymph nodes are involved.
B. Mitosis in the cells is considered.
C. Distant organ metastasis is considered.
D. Stage-A tumour of wall upto muscularis propria.

**307. Pancreaticoduodenectomy is the treatment of choice for : TN 1999**

A. Duodenal carcinoma
B. Pancreatic carcinoma
C. Gall Bladder carcinoma
D. Gastric carcinoma

**308. About Duodenal ulcar, all are true except : Kerala 1999**

A. Periodicity is prevent
B. Nocturnal pain
C. Good appetite
D. Hematemesis is more common than malaena

**309. Intestinal gangrene is seen in all except : AI 2000**

A. Shock
B. Tricuspid endocarditis
C. Mesenteric atherosclerosis
D. PAN

**310. Superior mesenteric artery syndrome, all are true, except : AI 2000**

A. Recurrent mid abdominal pain after food
B. Common in females of 15 years of age
C. Compression of duodenum
D. Aggravated by a gain in wt.

**311. In acute diverticular haemorrhage, bleeding occurs from : AI 2000**

A. Gastroduodenal art.
B. Inf. Mesenteric art. Left colic branch
C. Haemorrhoidal artery
D. Superior mesenteric art. rt. colic branch

**312. The commonest site of perforation during colonoscopy is : UPSC 2000**

A. Caecum
B. Hepatic flexure
C. Splenic flexure
D. Sigmoid colon

**Ans.** 299. A 300. A 301. A 302. A 303. A 304. B 305. A 306. D 307. A 308. D 309. B 310. B 311. B 312. B

313. **All of the following complications are more common in ulcerative than Crohn's disease, except: JIPMER 2000**
A. Fistula formation
B. Toxic megacolon
C. Malignancy
D. Bleeding per rectum

314. **Non-movement of neural crest to its specific place leads to : Rohtak 2000**
A. Volvulus
B. Megaureter
C. Cong. aganglionic megacolon
D. Intussusception

315. **True about diverticulitis is : Rohtak 2000**
A. Mostly asymptomatic
B. Surgery is treatment of choice
C. 50% people have malignancy
D. Episodic abdominal pain

316. **Pt. recurrent diarrhoea, pseudopolyp, lead pipe appearance on Ba. enema has : PGI 2000**
A. Ulcerative colitis
B. Crohn's
C. Irritably bowel syndrome
D. Short bowel syndrome

317. **In blind loop syndrome all are true except : UP 2000**
A. Surgery is the treatment of choice
B. Antibodies relieves temporarily
C. Anemia in high loop and steatorrhea in low loop
D. Due to proliferation of abnormal bacterial flora

318. **A patient with 8 year history of diarrhoea and blood in stool presents with multiple fistulae in perineum, was evaluated and found to have multiple strictures in small intestine, most likely cause is : AIIMS 2000**
A. Ulcerative colitis
B. Crohn's disease
C. Ischemic bowel disease
D. Radiation enteritis

319. **The following are true regarding Hirschsprung's disease, except : Kerala 2000**
A. Major feature is the absence of ganglion cells in the neural plexus of the intestinal wall.
B. More common in females than in males.
C. Confirmation of the diagnosis depends on the histology.
D. Rectal examination should not be performed before radiology.
E. Faecal soiling is not usually a feature of the condition.

320. **The following regarding colostomy are true except : Kerala 2000**
A. A colostomy is an artificial opening made in the Large Bowel to divert the faeces to the exterior.
B. Temporary colostomy is established to defunction an Anastomosis.
C. Permanent colostomy is formed after the resection of Rectum by the abdominoperineal technique.
D. Double Barrelled colostomy is commonly done now-a-days.
E. Colostomy hernia is a common complication.

321. **The following statements are true regarding intestinal obstruction, except : Kerala 2000**
A. Increased peristalsis continues for a period from 48 hours to several days
B. As the obstruction progresses, the character of the vomitus alters
C. In infants under two years a few fluid levels in the small intestine are diagnostic of obstruction
D. Intussusception commonly occurs in a male child between 6 to 9 months of age
E. In the obstruction of small intestine the caecum is collapsed

322. **Kalloo, 65-years-old, presents with complaints of abdominal pain. On examination there was distension of abdomen and the stools were maroon coloured. He gives a past history of Cerebral vascular accident and myocardial infarction. What would be the probable diagnosis : AIIMS 2000**
A. Ulcerative colitis
B. Crohn's disease
C. Acute mesenteric ischemia
D. Irritable bowel syndrome

323. **Which of the following is true about carcinoma colon: AIIMS 2000**
A. Lesion on the left side of the colon presents with features of anemia.
B. Solitary metastasis in liver is not a contraindication for surgery.
C. Mucinous carcinoma has a good prognosis.
D. Duke's A stage should receive adjuvant chemotherapy.

324. **Bowel does not get strangulated in which of the following : AI 2000**
A. Rectouterine pouch
B. Omental bursa
C. Ileo-colic recess
D. Para-duodenal and peritoneal recess

Ans. 313. A 314. C 315. D 316. A 317. C 318. B 319. B 320. D 321. C 322. C 323. B 324. A

**325. What is the management of in a case of bullet injury to left side of the colon presenting at 12 hrs after the incident : AIIMS 2000**

A. Primary closure
B. Proximal colostomy and bringing out the distal part as a mucus fistula
C. Resection and primary anastomosis
D. Proximal defunctioning colostomy

**326. A man aged 60 yrs has h/o IHD and atherosclerosis. He presents with abdominal pain and maroon stools : AI 2001**

A. Acute intestinal obstruction
B. Acute mesenteric ischemia
C. Peritonitis
D. Appendicitis

**327. True about afferent loop syndrome is : NIMHANS 2000**

A. Pain and diarrhoea most common symptom
B. Present after 6 months
C. Diagnosed on X-ray as barium filled loop
D. Total obstruction constitutes emergency

**328. Post-prandial pain, abdominal distension, hypovolemia, leukocytosis and diarrhoea. Diagnosis is : NIMHANS 2000**

A. Crohn's disease B. Amaebiasis
C. Worms D. Mesenteric angina

**329. A 8-months old infant is admitted with history of excessive crying with pain abdomen. The child is pale and pain is recurrent. An hour before hospitalisation, the child was passing blood and mucus per rectum. The most likely diagnosis is : UPSC 2001**

A. Acute amoebic colitis
B. Acute Crohn's disease
C. Acute bacillary dysentery
D. Acute intussusception

**330. Transverse colostomy is indicated in all except : AI 1992**

A. Third degree perineal tear
B. High anal fistula
C. Recto sigmoid carcinoma
D. Rectal trauma

**331. Most common cause of spontaneous bacterial peritonitis : JIPMER 2001**

A. E. coli
B. Staph. aureus
C. Anaerobic streptococci
D. Streptococcus

**332. Suspected subphrenic obscess is diagnosed by : JIPMER 2001**

A. Plane X-ray abd.
B. USG
C. Laparoscopy
D. Scanning with labelled leucocytes

**333. Milky spots on omentum is composed of : JIPMER 2001**

A. Lymphocytes B. Neutrophils
C. Macrophages D. Eosinophils

**334. Most common indication for operation in tuberculosis of intestine is : Kerala 2001**

A. Obstruction B. Perforation
C. Mass abdomen D. GI symptoms

**335. False regarding hyperplastic tuberculosis of GI : AIIMS 2001; AI 2001**

A. Mass right iliac fossa
B. Barium meal shows pulled-up caecum
C. Most common site is ileocecal
D. ATT alone can be used as treatment

**336. 56 yearS old woman has passed on stools for 14 days. X-ray shows fluid levels. Probable diagnosis is : AI 2001**

A. Paralytic ileus
B. Aganglionosis of the colon
C. Intestinal pseudo obstruction
D. Duodenal obstruction

**337. An elderly man has abdominal pain, found to have fusiform dilated descending aorta. Likely cause is : AI 2001**

A. Mycotic aneurysm
B. Atherosclerosis
C. Right ventricular failure
D. Syphilitic aortitis

**338. Primary peritonitis is more common in females because : AI 2001**

A. Ostia of Fallopian tubes communicate with abdominal cavity
B. Peritoneum overlies the uterus
C. Rupture of functional ovarian cysts
D. Fallopian tubes lie in broad ligament

**339. True regarding familial adenomatous polyposis are all the following except : SGPGI 2002**

A. 100% chances of malignancy over a period of time.
B. Adenomatous polyps occur in colon.
C. Equal incidence in males and females.
D. Total colectomy early in childhood is the treatment of choice.

| Ans. | | | | | | | | | |
|---|---|---|---|---|---|---|---|---|---|
| 325. B | 326. B | 327. D | 328. D | 329. D | 330. A | 331. D | 332. B | 333. C | 334. A |
| 335. D | 336. C | 337. B | 338. A | 339. D | | | | | |

340. **All of the following are causes of steatorrhea, except :** **SGPGI 2002**
A. Chronic pancreatitis
B. Tropical sprue
C. Whipple's disease
D. Intestinal amebiasis

341. **In post operative ileus, last part of GIT to recover is :** **Delhi 2001**
A. Stomach B. Small intestine
C. Large intestine D. Rectum and anal canal

342. **A newborn presenting with intestinal obstruction showed, on abdominal X-ray, multiple air fluid levels. The diagnosis is not likely to be :** **AI 2002**
A. Pyloric obstruction
B. Duodenal atresia
C. Ileal atresia
D. Ladd's bands

343. **A 9 months old infant presents with features of intestinal obstruction. On barium enema, the diagnosis was confirmed to be intussusception. The most likely etiology would be :** **MAHE 1999; AI 2002**
A. Meckel's diverticulum
B. Hypertrophic Peyer's patch
C. Mucosal polyp
D. Lipoma

344. **The most appropriate route for the administration of significant proteins and calories to a patient comatose for a long period after an automobile accident is by :** **AI 2002**
A. Nasogastric tube feedings
B. Gastrostomy tube feedings
C. Jejunostomy tube feedings
D. Total parenteral nutrition

345. **A patient operated for carcinoma colon 4 months back now presents with a 2 cm solitary mass in the liver. The best line of management is :** **AI 2002**
A. Radiotherapy B. Radiofrequency ablation
C. Resection D. CT scan

346. **Constricting type of colonic carcinoma is seen in :** **Maharashtra 2000**
A. Left colon B. Right colon
C. Transverse colon D. Caecum

347. **A infant presented with abdominal lump, non-bilious vomiting and visible peristalsis, likely diagnosis is :** **UP 2002**
A. Congenital megacolon
B. CHPS
C. Ladds band
D. Electrolyte imbalance

348. **Maximum amount of which of the following gas accumulates in the intestine after intestine obstruction :** **BHU-2002**
A. Oxygen B. Carbon dioxide
C. Nitrogen D. Sulphur dioxide

349. **Which one of the following is not considered as precancerous lesion for carcinoma of the large bowel:** **UPSC 2002**
A. Familial intestinal polyposis
B. Vilious adenoma
C. Chronic ulcerative colitis
D. Peutz-Jegher's polyposis

350. **All of the following statements regarding malignant potential of colo-rectal polyps are true except :** **AIIMS 2002**
A. Polyps of familial polyposis coli could invariably undergo malignant change.
B. Pseudopolyps of ulcerative colitis has high risk of malignancy.
C. Villous adenoma is associated with high risk of malignancy.
D. Juvenile polyps has little or no risk.

351. **An eight year old boy had abdominal pain, fever with bloody diarrhoea for 18 months. His height is 110 cms and weight is 14.5 kg. Stool culture was negative for known enteropathogens. The sigmoidoscopy was normal. During the same period, child had an episode of renal colic and passed urinary gravel. The mantoux test was 5 x 5 mm. The most probable diagnosis is :** **AI 2003**
A. Ulcerative colitis
B. Crohn's disease
C. Intestinal tuberculosis
D. Strongyloidosis

352. **Failure to pass meconium within 48 hours of birth in a new born with no obvious external abnormality should lead to the suspicion of :** **AIIMS 2002**
A. Anal atresia
B. Congenital pouch colon
C. Congenital aganglionosis
D. Meconium ileus

353. **All of the following are significant risk factors for colonic carcinoma in an adenomatous polyp, except :** **AI 2004**
A. Pedunculated polyp
B. Villous histology
C. Size > 2 cms
D. Atypia

| Ans. | 340. D | 341. D | 342. C | 343. B | 344. C | 345. C | 346. A | 347. A | 348. C | 349. D |
|---|---|---|---|---|---|---|---|---|---|---|
| | 350. B | 351. C | 352. C | 353. A | | | | | | |

**354. The short bowel syndrome is characterized by all of the following except : AI 2004**

A. Diarrhoea B. Hypogastrinemia
C. Weight loss D. Steatorrhoea

**355. Lower gastrointestinal bleeding is defined as : UPSC 2004**

A. Bleeding distal to junction of proximal 1/3rd and distal 2/3rd of transverse colon.
B. Bleeding distal to junction of proximal 2/3rd and distal 1/3rd of transverse colon.
C. Bleeding from large bowel beyond ileocaecal junction.
D. Bleeding from small bowel from beyond ligament of Tretiz.

**356. In which one of the following conditions is gas under diaphragm not seen : UPSC 2005**

A. Perforated duodenal ulcer
B. Typhoid perforation
C. After laparotomy
D. Spontaneous rupture of oesophagus

**357. The structures removed, while carrying out radical gastrectomy for a 2 x 2 cm antral adenocarcinoma, would include the following except : UPSC 2005**

A. Distal 2/3rd of stomach with a centimetre cuff of duodenum.
B. Lesser and greater omentum.
C. Lymph nodes along left and right gastric common hepatic and splenic arteries.
D. Spleen.

**358. A 1 cm x 1 cm squamous cell carcinoma of anal canal is best treated initially by : UPSC 2005**

A. Abdominoperineal resection
B. Localised resection followed by irradiation
C. Proximal colostomy followed by interstitial radiation
D. Chemo-radiotherapy

**359. The most useful investigation for profuse lower gastrointestinal bleeding is : UPSC 2005**

A. Proctosigmoidoscopy
B. Colonoscopy
C. Double contrast barium enema
D. Selective arteriography

**360. Non-propulsive peristalsis is a feature of : Karnataka 2004**

A Paralytic ileus
B Impacted faeces
C Mesenteric vascular occlusion
D Incarceration

**361. Which of the follwing is protective against carcinoma colon : AI 2009**

A. High fibre diet
B. High fat
C. High selenium diet
D. Low protein diet

**362. Gold standard to diagnosis insulinoma is :**

A. 72 hours fasting blood glucose levels and insulin levels
B. C-peptide
C. Insulin levels > 5mmol
D. Glucose < 3mmol

**363. Regarding pancreatic cancer, all are true except :**

A. More than 75 % have p53 mutations
B. More common in people with famillal pancreatitis
C. 3-6 m survival in stage 3
D. 15-20 % survival on 5 years

**364. Most common type of parastomal hernia :**

A. Loop colostomy
B. End colostomy
C. Loop ileostomy
D. End ileostomy

**365. The commonest cause of significant is lower gastrointestinal bleed in a middle aged person with unknown reason is : Delhi 2009**

A. Signoid diverticula B. Angio dysplasia
C. Ischemic colitis D. Ulcerative colitis

**366. Which of the following statement about sigmoid volvulus is in correct : Delhi 2009**

A. More common with lascative abuse
B. None operative treatment has no role
C. Recurrence rate around 40%
D. Sigmoid resection is definative treatment

**367. Which of the following statement about Crohn's disease is incorrect ? Delhi 2009**

A. Granulomas present freqeuntly
B. It is separate and distinct from ulcerative colitis
C. Cigratte smoking is a risk factor
D. Rectum spared in 50% patients

**Ans.** 354. B 355. D 356. D 357. D 358. D 359. B 360. C 361. A 362. A 363. D
364. B 365. A 366. B 367. NONE

# EXPLANATIONS OF INTESTINES

1. Ans.— D. Adenocarcinoma
2. Ans.— B. Sausage-shaped mass in epigastrium and empty right iliac fossa.
3. Ans.— C. Typhoid enteritis
4. Ans.— B. Typhoid
5. Ans.— D. Chylolymphatic cyst
6. Ans.— B. Distal pancreaticojejunostomy
7. Ans.— C. Generally produces abdominal distension within 2-4 hours of onset.
8. Ans.— B. Anaemia
9. Ans.— A. Skin should be protected from chemical erosion.
10. Ans.— B. Cholangiocarcinoma
11. Ans.— A. Duodenal atresia

    It is also typically seen in Annular Pancreas.
12. Ans.— C. To prevent complications
13. Ans.— A. Common in infants
14. Ans.— A. Old age
15. Ans.— A. L1
16. Ans.— A. Duodenal atresia
17. Ans.— A. Subphrenic
18. Ans.— D. Pelvic
19. Ans.— B. Resection and end-to-end anastomosis
20. Ans.— A. Rectum is always involved
21. Ans.— D. Superior mesenteric arteriogram
22. Ans.— D. Rectum not dilated and usually empty of stool.
23. Ans.— A. 2nd to 7th day
24. Ans.— E. 48 hours
25. Ans.— A. Rarely required surgical treatment

    Gangrene development is earliest in ileocolic type of obstruction.
26. Ans.— C. Leave motor and secretory function intact.
27. Ans.— D. Duodenal atresia
28. Ans.— C. Loss of haustrations, especially in the distal colon.
29. Ans.— D. None of the above
30. Ans.— D. Plication of ulcer with omental reinforcement.

    Splenic artery is involved in cases of gastric ulcers whereas Gastroduodenal artery is involved in Duodenal ulcer.
31. Ans.— D. Haemangiomas
32. Ans.— D. Carcinoid
33. Ans.— C. Total proctocolectomy and ileostomy
34. Ans.— D. Azulfidine
35. Ans.— C. Absence of mesentry
36. Ans.— C. Calcum
37. Ans.— B. Regional enteritis
38. Ans.— D. Fear of developing pancreatic penetration.
39. Ans.— D. Bayar's
40. Ans.— B. Haemoperitoneum
41. Ans.— B. Hypercalcaemia
42. Ans.— C. Ileum

    Meckel's diverticulum is present in 2% population and situated on antimesenteric border of SI, commonly 60 cm from ileocaecal valve and is usually 3-5 cm long (Mnemonic - 2% - feet - inches).
43. Ans.— C. Usually abscent
44. Ans.— B. Distended caecum
45. Ans.— C. Post-operative adhesions
46. Ans.— D. Bleeding PR

    Diverticulam of the colon are acquired herniation of colonic mucosa, protruding through the circular muscle at the pts. where the blood vessels penetrate the colonic wall. The condition is most often localised to one part of the colon usually the sigmond (95%). Rectum with its muscle layer is not affected.

47. Ans.— B. Intestinal obstruction

The most common site is ileocaecal junction (Hyperplastic variety) & Terminal part of ileum (ulcerative variety).

48. Ans.— B. Caecum

49. Ans.— D. Surgery

50. Ans.— D. Diagnostic appearances in a barium enema.

51. Ans.— A. Constipation

52. Ans.— B. Strapping

53. Ans.— A. Plain X-ray abdomen

54. Ans.— B. Hypokalemia

55. Ans.— A. Previous H/O duodenal ulcer

56. Ans.— B. Ileal

57. Ans.— C. Ureter

58. Ans.— A. Perforated peptic ulcer

59. Ans.— C. 70%

60. Ans.— D. Polyps are not present throughout G.I. tract.

Peutz-Jeghers syndrome consists of hamarto-matous polyps and occur in colon as solitary or multiple lesion. They have minimum malignant potential.

61. Ans.— D. Massive colonic peristalsis disrupt the anastomosis.

62. Ans.— C. Hodgkin's disease

63. Ans.— C. Retroperitoneal bleeding is self-limiting and exploration is not warranted.

64. Ans.— C. Ascending colon

65. Ans.— D. Diverticulitis

Among choices given, Crohn's disease is a common cause in adults otherwise diverticulitis is the most common cause (occurs in 2-4% cases), Ca Colon (in people above 50), radiation bowel injury, external trauma, foreign bodies, and idiopathic are other causes.

66. Ans.— B. Persistent local tenderness

67. Ans.— A. Mucus

68. Ans.— C. Umbilical adenoma

69. Ans.— A. Infants

70. Ans.— C. Ileum

71. Ans.— A. In the neonate is of no immediate clinic significance.

72. Ans.— D. None of the above

73. Ans.— B. Ileum

74. Ans.— C. An appendicular carcinoid

75. Ans.— E. Tension gangrene

76. Ans.— D. 1, 3 and 4 are correct

77. Ans.— B. Serum $B_{12}$

78. Ans.— B. Mucosa and submucosa

79. Ans.— A. Colovesical

80. Ans.— C. Selective arteriography

81. Ans.— D. All of the above

82. Ans.— B. 5-10 days

83. Ans.— D. Should be performed through liver, midabdomen, and pelvis, except where primary lesions are proximal to the sigmoid.

84. Ans.— C. Mesenteric vein thrombosis

85. Ans.— B. Nephrotic syndrome

86. Ans.— B. Wide excision

87. Ans.— A. 4 5 2 1

88. Ans.— B. Calf

89. Ans.— B. Gastroduodenal

Anteriorly placed ulcers tend to perforate whereas posteriorly placed ulcers tend to bleed.

90. Ans.— B. Ileo-transverse anastomosis

Proximal colostomy is required for the rest of injured/Inflammed bowel which in this case is caecum and hence caecostomy is the only feasible solution in the available choices.

91. Ans.— C. Lower abdominal incisions disrupt more than upper abdominal incisions.

92. Ans.— D. Rectal biopsy

93. Ans.— C. Inner absorbable and outer non-absorbable.

94. Ans.— C. Close the abdomen and start medical treatment.

95. Ans.— B. Liver

96. Ans.— A. 2 1 4 3

97. Ans.— A. 60 cms proximal to ileocaecal valve

98. Ans.— A. Adhesions

99. Ans.— B. Ischaemic colitis

100. Ans.— A. Congenital bands

Congenital atresia and stenosis are the most common cause of intestinal obstruction in the new born. The site of these obst are—Duodenum 33%, Jejunum 15%, Ileum 25%, ascending colon 10%, Multiple sites 17%.

101. Ans.— B. Bradycardia

102. Ans.— D. Good prognosis

103. Ans.— C. Splenic artery

104. Ans.— A. Risk of caecal perforation with closed loop obstruction.

105. Ans.— C. Juvenile polyp

106. Ans.— C. Right hemicolectomy

107. Ans.— A. Perforation

Complications of ulcerative colitis are — Pseudopolyposis (15%), carcinoma (35%), fibrous stricture 6%, common sites are rectosigmoid and anal canal. Toxic dilatation 1.5%, Massive haemorrhage 3%, Rectovaginal fistula (3%), Fistula in ano (4%), Ischiorectal abscess 4%, haemorrhoids 20%, arthritis and cholongitis.

108. Ans.— D. Gangrene

109. Ans.— A. Ileocolic

Second commonest is ileocecolic. Colocolic is least common.

110. Ans.— C. It is bright red in colour

111. Ans.— C. Tc99 pertechnitium scan

112. Ans.— C. Enterogenous cyst

113. Ans.— C. Paralytic ileus

114. Ans.— D. Leucopenia occurs

115. Ans.— C. Seen on the mesenteric border

116. Ans.— A. Medical treatment

117. Ans.— D. Immediate laparotomy

118. Ans.— B. 6 months-9 months

119. Ans.— D. Paralytic ileus

120. Ans.— C. 3rd week

121. Ans.— C. Change in bowel habits

122. Ans.— B. Porphyria

123. Ans.— B. Regional enteritis

It was first reported by Crohn, Ginzburg and Oppenheimer (1932). String sign of Kantor is seen on Ba enema.

124. Ans.— B. An emergency decompression with a colostomy.

125. Ans.— A. Sigmoid region

126. Ans.— C. Adenocarcinoma

127. Ans.— D. Saw tooth appearance

128. Ans.— A. Sigmoid colon

129. Ans.— B. Patient lies still

130. Ans.— B. Whole of large intestine without effects

131. Ans.— A. Lymphosarcoma

132. Ans.— B. Fungating

25% cases of Ca right colon present as emergencies with intestinal obstruction or peritonitis. Most frequent presentation is abdominal pains 78%, Altered bowel habit 30%, loss of wt. 50% Lumb 67%.

133. Ans.— B. Avoid surgery for initial 48-72 hours

134. Ans.— A. Splenic flexure

135. Ans.— B. Colicky pain

136. Ans.— D. None of the above

Also called 'short gut syndrome'. Extensive small bowel resection, diarrhoea, steatorrhoea and malnutrition are essential for diagnosis.

137. Ans.— C. Peritonitis

138. Ans.— B. Carcinoma arises from pseudopolyps

139. Ans.— D. Degree of inflammation

140. Ans.— D. Diverticular disease

141. Ans.— B. Lumbar ganglionectomy

142. Ans.— D. Hyperchloremic acidosis

143. Ans.— A. Surgical resection indicated in all cases

144. Ans.— C. Mc Burney's incision

145. Ans.— D. Ischaemia

146. Ans.— B. Parathormone

147. Ans.— C. Intestinal obstruction

148. Ans.— A. Duodenojejunal junction

149. Ans.— B. Repeated administration of liquid parafin and other purgatives.

150. Ans.— C. Large deep ulcerations are present with intervening mucosa comparatively healthy.

151. Ans.— B. May follow idiopathic malabsorption and steatorhoea.

152. Ans.— A. Fatty food

153. Ans.— C. Rectum

154. Ans.— C. Dilution of acid in the peritoneal cavity.

155. Ans.— B. Partially obliterated vitello intestinal duct.

156. Ans.— B. Females

157. Ans.— D. Idiopathic

158. Ans.— D. Portal gas

159. Ans.— B. Duodeno jejunostomy

Stenosis at the fusion of foregut & Midgut near the ampulla of vater. The vomiting contains bile. Treatment of choice is Duodenojugonostomy.

160. Ans.— D. Adenocarcinoma

161. Ans.— A. Oesophagus

162. Ans.— C. Midgut

163. Ans.— D. Umbilicus

164. Ans.— D. Rectum

165. Ans.— A. Intussusception

166. Ans.— D. Sigmoid colon

167. Ans.— B. Distension of abdomen

168. Ans.— A. Early abdominal distension (within 24 hours of life).

169. Ans.— D. Constipation

There is constipation and ↓ bowel sounds. Terminal ileum and right colon are affected first and then transverse and descending colon, appendix, jejunum, stomach, duodenum and esophagus are affected in descending order.

Second commonest is ileoileo colic. Colocolic is least common.

170. Ans.— A. Birth

171. Ans.— C. For 2 weeks

172. Ans.— B. 15 mg

173. Ans.— A. Appendix

174. Ans.— B. Fourth

175. Ans.— C. Persistent vomiting

In Intussusception usually the child is a male of 6 to 9 months age and ileoileal is the commonest type.

In order of frequency, the symptoms are (i) Severe haemorrhage (ii) Meckel's diverti cultis (iii) Chr. peptic ulceration (iv) Intestinal obstruction.

176. Ans.— C. 6-9 months

177. Ans.— D. Gas ulcer diaphragm

178. Ans.— C. Intraperitoneal

179. Ans.— A. Infected umbilical cicatrix

180. Ans.— B. 6 months of age

181. Ans.— D. Rectum does not grip the examination finger.

182. Ans.— B. Is atleast 8 kg in weight and thriving

183. Ans.— B. Ileum

184. Ans.— D. Are prone to rupture

185. Ans.— C. 5 cms

186. Ans.— A. Adenocarcinoma

187. Ans.— D. Pulmonary infarction

188. Ans.— B. Adenomatous polyp

189. Ans.— B. II or III

190. Ans.— A. Junction of fore- and mid gut

191. Ans.— A. I

192. Ans.— A. Right posterior intraperitoneal subdiaphragmatic space.

193. Ans.— D. Cauliflower

194. Ans.— D. Rectum

195. Ans.— C. Mobilisation of pancreas during pancreatotomy

196. Ans.— A. Hyperactive bowel sounds

197. Ans.— C. May involve small intestine

198. Ans.— A. Mongolism

199. Ans.— A. 50 ml

200. Ans.— A. Duodenal ulcer

201. Ans.— B. Possesses all three coats of the intestinal wall.

202. Ans.— D. Bursting of amoebic liver abscess

203. Ans.— D. Absence of bowel sounds

204. Ans.— C. Ischaemic colitis

205. Ans.— B. Chest infection

206. Ans.— B. Penetrating duodenal ulcer

207. Ans.— D. Arises from the skin near umbilicus

208. Ans.— C. On examination rectum is full of faecal matter.

209. Ans.— C. Carcinoma of pancreas

210. Ans.— B. $PGE_2$

211. Ans.— A. 1 alone is correct

212. Ans.— B. Radiotherapy

213. Ans.— B. Duodenal perforation

214. Ans.— A. Mostly caused by pulmonary TB

215. Ans.— A. Defective ejaculation

216. Ans.— C. Relief of obstruction by operation

217. Ans.— B. Ascites

218. Ans.— C. Atelectasis

219. Ans.— A. Infiltration of fibrous core

220. Ans.— B. Liver tissue

Cysto sarcoma phylloides also called serocystic disease of Brodie appears in females over 40. Central softening and ulcer may be present. Remains mobile over the chest wall. Treatment of benign. Type is by wide local excision with a surrounding rows of normal breast lining. Massive tumors may require simple mastectomy. Full Thickness Graft (FTG) is used to cover selective small areas.

221. Ans.— B. Asymptomatic

222. Ans.— D. Ca stomach

223. Ans.— B. Nutritional status

224. Ans.— C. Adenomatous polyps

Multiple rectal polyps develop in puberty.

225. Ans.— B. Surgical reopening

226. Ans.— D. Tropical sprue

227. Ans.— A. Ulcerative colitis

228. Ans.— A. CEA

229. Ans.— D. 1, 3 and 4 are correct

230. Ans.— A. Fibrocystic disease of pancreas

231. Ans.— A. Anterior aspect of Ist part of duodenum

232. Ans.— B. Colon — $10^5$ - $10^7$ organisms

233. Ans.— A. Intussusception

Ileocolic is most common.

234. Ans.— C. Laprotomy and explore

235. Ans.— B. Increase in severity in Ist trimester

236. Ans.— D. Mucocele of appendix or mucinous cystadenoma ovary.

237. Ans.— E. Constipation is usual

238. Ans.— A. Portal vein

239. Ans.— D. Sigmoid colon

240. Ans.— A. Arises from mesenteric border

241. Ans.— A. Left iliac fossa

242. Ans.— D. Typical periodicity

243. Ans.— D. Axial rotation of a loop of intestine around its own axis.

244. Ans.— B. Enterogenous cyst

245. Ans.— A. Hyperthyroidism

246. Ans.— B. Normal saline

247. Ans.— E. Elevated T4

248. Ans.— A. Rectum

249. Ans.— A. Diverticulosis

250. Ans.— A. Regional ileitis

251. Ans.— A. Non-specific bowel dilatation

252. Ans.— D. In ileoileal intussusception claw sign is positive.

253. Ans.— B. Jejunal atresia

254. Ans.— C. Complication of partial gastrectomy

255. Ans.— B. Ileal atresia

256. Ans.— B. Third part of duodenum

257. Ans.— A. Volvulus

258. Ans.— A. Peptic ulceration

259. Ans.— C. 3-6 weeks

260. Ans.— B. Jejunal atresia

261. Ans.— B. Appendices epiploicae

262. Ans.— B. A yellow nodule in the ileum

263. Ans.— C. Generalized pain is not present

264. Ans.— C. A delayed-emptying vein

265. Ans.— B. Neuroblastoma

266. Ans.— A. Ceacum

267. Ans.— B. Endometriosis

268. Ans.— D. Aorta

269. Ans.— A. Often strangulates

270. Ans.— A. Surgery is always advised primarily

271. Ans.— A. Colonoscopy & biopsy

272. Ans.— A. Macrocytic anaemia

273. Ans.— B. Closure of duodenal perforation

274. Ans.— B. Hematogenous

275. Ans.— A. Post-operative

276. Ans.— A. Clean wound

277. Ans.— A. Meconium ileus

278. Ans.— C. Aponeurosis

279. Ans.— D. Addison's disease

In pseudoobstruction, there is no mechanical cause. The colon is the organ most commonly affected but occasionally ileum is involved. Colonoscopy is indicated.

280. Ans.— A. Sigmoid volvulus

281. Ans.— B. III

282. Ans.— A. Bile duct obstruction

283. Ans.— D. Second dehiscence is common

284. Ans.— C. A + B

285. Ans.— B. Chronic post prandial pain

286. Ans.— A. 4 quadrant aspiration

287. Ans.— C. Perforation of colon

288. Ans.— C. Paul-Mickulicz operation

289. Ans.— C. Sclerosing cholangitis

290. Ans.— C. Liver metastasis

291. Ans.— A. Lymphoma

292. Ans.— C. Crohn's disease

293. Ans.— A. Abundant lymph follicles in that region.

294. Ans.— A. Outer layer

295. Ans.— D. Best treated with chemotherapy

296. Ans.— A. Plain X-ray of abdomen

297. Ans.— B. Resection of stricture and end-to-end anastomosis.

298. Ans.— C. 2 1 5 4

299. Ans.— A. Pseudoobstruction

300. Ans.— A. Ultrasound segment Ba enema is most accurate.

301. Ans.— A. Duodenal atresia

302. Ans.— A. Definitely progresses to malignancy

303. Ans.— A. Primary peritonitis

304. Ans.— B. Defunctioning colostomy

305. Ans.— A. Classification of Ca Colon

306. Ans.— D. Stage-A-tumour of wall upto muscularis propria.

307. Ans.— A. Duodenal carcinoma

308. Ans.— D. Hematemesis is more common than malaena.

309. Ans.— B. Tricuspid endocarditis

Possible sources are from left auricle (AF), mural MI atheroma of aortic aneurysm, vegetation from mitral valve, pulmonary vein thrombosis due to septic infarct, left atrial myxoma, TAU, Portal HT, Portal pyaemia, Sickle cell disease and OCP's.

310. Ans.— B. Common in females of 15 years of age

311. Ans.— B. Inf. Mesenteric art. Left colic branch

It is the main artery supplying sigmoid colon (commonest site of diverticulosis). It should be differentiated from angiodysplasia. Colonoscopy is used to localize site of bleeding.

312. Ans.— B. Hepatic flexure

313. Ans.— A. Fistula formation

314. Ans.— C. Cong. aganglionic megacolon

315. Ans.— D. Episodic abdominal pain

316. Ans.— A. Ulcerative colitis

317. Ans.— C. Anemia in high loop and steatorrhea in low loop.

318. Ans.— B. Crohn's disease

319. Ans.— B. More common in females than in males

320. Ans.— D. Double Barrelled colostomy is commonly done now-a-days.

321. Ans.— C. In infants under two years a few fluid levels in the small intestine are diagnostic of obstruction.

322. Ans.— C. Acute mesenteric ischemia

323. Ans.— B. Solitary metastasis in liver is not a contra-indication for surgery.

324. Ans.— A. Rectouterine pouch

325. Ans.— B. Proximal colostomy and bringing out the distal part as a mucus fistula.

326. Ans.— B. Acute mesenteric ischemia

Treatment is arteriography followed by percutaneous transluminal angioplasty or surgical bypass.

327. Ans.— D. Total obstruction constitutes emergency.

328. Ans.— D. Mesenteric angina

329. Ans.— D. Acute intussusception

330. Ans.— A. Third degree perineal tear

Indications for colostomy are obst. of sigmoid colon either by Ca or diverticula, vesicocolic fistula, protection of low colorectal anastomosis. Trauma to rectum or colon, operative Rx of high fistula in ano. Transverse colon is most commonly.

331. Ans.— D. Streptococcus

332. Ans.— B. USG

333. Ans.— C. Macrophages

334. Ans.— A. Obstruction

335. Ans.— D. ATT alone can be used as treatment

336. Ans.— C. Intestinal pseudo obstruction

337. Ans.— B. Atherosclerosis

338. Ans.— A. Ostia of Follopian tubes communicate with abdominal cavity.

339. Ans.— D. Total colectomy early in childhood is the treatment of choice.

340. Ans.— D. Intestinal amebiasis

341. Ans.— D. Rectum and anal canal

342. Ans.— C. Ileal atresia

Ileal atresia is not the cause.

343. Ans.— B. Hypertrophic Peyer's patch

Hypertrophic Peyer's patch in terminal ileium is the usual cause.

344. Ans.— C. Jejunostomy tube feedings

It will prevent regurgitation and aspiration.

345. Ans.— C. Resection

Resection is therapeutic and diagnostic. It must be done without delay.

346. Ans.— A. Left colon

347. Ans.— A. Congenital megacolon

348. Ans.— C. Nitrogen

349. Ans.— D. Peutz-Jegher's polyposis

350. Ans.— B. Pseudopolyps of ulcerative colitis has high risk of malignancy.

351. Ans.— C. Intestinal tuberculosis

Option-A :

* Ulcerative colitis involve sigmoid colon & Rectum Sigmoidoscopy can't be normal.

Option-B :

* Crohn's disease
* It involves small bowels and colon so sigmoidoscopy should not be normal. In 50% cases colon & rectum are spared (But mantoux 5 x 5 cm going against the diagnosis).

Option C

* Child had fever Mantoux 5 x 5 cm Bloody diarrhoea, abdominal pain (Sigmoidoscopy normal because MC site of intestinal tuberculosis is ileocaecal region).

Option-D :

* Strongyloids stercoralis usually not cause bloody diarrhoea.

*Conclusion :* so the diagnosis goes in the favour of intestinal Tuberculosis.

352. Ans.— C. Congenital aganglionosis

353. Ans.— A. Pedunculated polyp

354. Ans.— B. Hypogastrinemia

Patients with short-bowel syndrome may have gastric acid hypersecretion, which is often transient.

Short-Bowel Syndrome

- Malabsorptive condition that arises secondary to removal of significant segment of small intestine.

Most common causes in adults are —

- Crohn's disease
- Mesenteric infarction
- Radiational enteritis
- Trauma
- Resection of 4–50% of total length of small intestine usually well tolerated.
- Type and degree of malabsorption depends upon the length and site of resection.
- Characterised by weight loss and diarrhoea.

Terminal ileal resection cause —

- Malabsorption of bile salt and vit. $B_{12}$
- Malabsorption of fat soluble vitamins (result in steatorrhoea)

- Unabsorbed fatty acid bind with $Ca^{++}$, reducing its absorption and enhancing the absorption of oxalate (oxalate renal stone may develop).
- Cholesterol gallstone due to ↓ed bile salts
- Duodenal resection may result in folate, iron or calcium malabsorption.
- Gastric hypersecretion usually complicate intestinal resections.

355. Ans.— D. Bleeding from small bowel from beyond ligament of Tretiz.

356. Ans.— D. Spontaneous rupture of oesophagus

357. Ans.— D. Spleen

358. Ans.— D. Chemo-radiotherapy

359. Ans.— B. Colonoscopy

360. Ans.— C. Mesenteric vascular occlusion.

361. Ans.— A. High fiber diet

* Fiber : Diets high in fiber and low in fat help reduce the amount of estrogen circulating in the blood. Fiber is also important in preventing colon cancer, as it helps move food waste, extra-hormones, and carcinogens out of the body. Fiber may even help the immune system function properly. Building a diet from fiber-rich plant foods is important for cancer prevention and survival, as well as overall health.

362. Ans.— A. 72 hours fasting blood glucose levels and insulin levels

* The presence of hypoglycemia in the face of inappropriately elevated levels of insulin is the key to diagnosis of insulinoma.

363. Ans.— D. 15-20% survival on 5 years

Mutations in K-ras and p53 genes are common in pancreatic cancer. p53 mutations may occur more frequently in metastatic lesions than in primary tumors, although further work is necessary to investigate this point.

364. Ans.— B. End colostomy

Incidence

* Wide range depending on duration of follow-up and use of imaging

| *Type* | *Range* | *Average* |
|---|---|---|
| End colostomy | 4-48% | 15.3% |
| Loop colostomy | 0-31% | 4% |
| End ileostomy | 2-28% | 6.7% |
| Loop ileostomy | 0-6% | 1.3% |

365. Ans.— A. Sigmoid diverticula

Diverticulosis occurs in age group above 40 but angiodysplasia occurs in age above 60.

366. Ans.— B. None operative treatment has no role

High residue diet, chronic constipation alongation of sigmoid and rectosigmoid (with abuse laxative) are important factors. Decompression (percutaneous) is first tried. Endoscopic decompression is contraindicated if there is evidence of strangulation or perforation. Recurrence rate is 40-50%. Resection is definitive treatment. If entire colon is megocolon, abdominal colectomy is considered.

367. Ans.— None.

Crohn's disease is also called granuloma. Granulomas (Non caseating) occur in 60% smoking increases chances by 3 fold. It is separate and distinct from ulcerative colitis. Rectum is spared in 50% with Crohn's colitis. (Current Surgical Diagnosis and Treatment) and Bailey & Love's Short Practice of Surgery) The Question is incorrect. All the choices are correct. Ans is none.

# 12

# IMPORTANT TEXT OF APPENDIX

## DRUGS USED IN THE MANAGEMENT OF CARCINOID SYNDROME

| *Compounds produced in carcinoid tumours* | *Possible pharmacological treatment prior to surgery* | |
|---|---|---|
| 5-Hydroxytryptamine (5HT, serotonin) | 1. Nicotinamide for associated pellagra | |
| Bradykinin (following kallikrein activation) | | |
| Histamine (esp. gastric carcinoid) | 2. Codeine phosphate | |
| Prostaglandins | Diphenoxylate/atropine | for 5 HT induced diarrhoea |
| Neurotensin | Loperamide | |
| Substance P | 3. Cyproheptadine | specific 5 HT antagonists |
| Enteroglucagon | Methysergide | (NB : methysergide and associated retroperitoneal fibrosis) |
| | 4. Phenoxybenzamine or Phenothiazines with α-adrenergic blocking activity (e.g. chloropromazine) | to control flushing |
| | 5. Parachlorophenylalanine—tryptophan hydroxylase inhibitor (NB: high incidence allergic reaction) | |
| | 6. Antihistamines. $H_1 + H_2$ receptor blockers—esp. in gastric carcinoid | |
| | 7. Somatostatin—continuous i.v. infusion—do not stop before surgery | |

# MCQ's OF APPENDIX

## What is important in Appendix

Appendix (Appendicitis and Management, Carcinoid)

1. **All of the following are indications for opening an appendix abscess except : AIIMS 1984**
   A. When swelling is not reducing in size after 5th day of treatment.
   B. When the body temperature is swinging above 37.8° for several days.
   C. Pelvic position of the appendix.
   D. Copious gastric aspiration.
2. **Indications for operating upon an appendicular abscess is/are : AIIMS 1984**
   A. Persistant hyperpyrexia (above 100°F) for several days.
   B. Development of pelvic abscess.
   C. No regression in size of swelling after 5th day of conservative treatment.
   D. All of the above.
3. **For an appendicular abscess, one should : AIIMS 1983**
   A. Drain it
   B. Perform appendicectomy immediately
   C. Wait and watch
   D. Do nothing
4. **It is generally accepted the appendicectomy is the choice of treatment in all of the following situations except : Karnataka 1987**
   A. Acute appendicitis in children
   B. Ruptured appendicitis with general peritonitis
   C. Ruptured appendicitis with abscess
   D. Ruptured appendicitis with local peritonitis
5. **The first surgeon to perform deliberate appendicectomy was : AIIMS 1985**
   A. McArthur
   B. Lawson Tait
   C. Rutherford Morrison
   D. Sir William Lane
6. **All of the following are early complications arising after appendicectomy for acute appendicitis except : Rohtak 1988**
   A. Ileus
   B. Sterlity in the female
   C. Intestinal obstruction
   D. Pulmonary complications
7. **5 H. indole acetic acid in urine is seen in : PGI 2000**
   A. Carcinoid B. Pheochromocytoma
   C. Hirschsprung's disease D. Wilm's tumor
8. **The appendix was removed in a young girl of 13 for acute appendicitis. Four days later, the patient had generalized peritonitis and paralytic ileus. The best line of treatment would be : UPSC 1987**
   A. Intestinal intubation and continuous suction.
   B. Immediate reoperation and ileostomy to drain the obstructed intestine.
   C. Prompt laparotomy to search for any local abscess and to place multiple drains.
   D. None of the above.
9. **Which of the following is not true of appendicitis : UPSC 1988**
   A. Obstruction of the appendix is the primary cause.
   B. It is a very common acute condition.
   C. It is most frequent in old people.
   D. The higher the amount of lymphoid tissue in the appendix, the greater the likelihood of incidence of the condition.
10. **Carcinoid of the appendix requires : PGI 1993**
    A. Appendicectomy
    B. Chemotherapy
    C. Segmental resection of right colon
    D. Chemotherapy followed by radiotherapy

| Ans. | 1. D | 2. D | 3. A | 4. D | 5. B | 6. B | 7. A | 8. A | 9. C | 10. A |
|---|---|---|---|---|---|---|---|---|---|---|

**11. In caes of rupture of appendix, the following statement is correct : AMC 1985**

A. Incidence is higher at extremes of age.

B. Is confined to the areas nearby (i.e. periappendicular) in most of the cases.

C. Appendix should be removed immediately.

D. All the above statements are correct.

**12. A fistula following appendicectomy will not heal under the following conditions : Bihar 1998**

A. Hb < 9 gm%

B. Serum albumin < 3 gm/dl

C. Rectal stricture

D. Vit. K deficiency

**Directions : The following given items consist of two statements, one labelled the Assertion 'A' and the other labelled the Reason 'R'. You are in examine these two statements carefully and decide if the Assertion 'A' and the Reason 'R' are individually true and if so, whether the Reason is a correct explanation of the Assertion. Select your answer to these items using the codes given below and mark your answer sheet accordingly.**

**Codes :**

A. Both A and R are true and R is the correct explanation of A.

B. Both A and R are true but R is not a correct explanation of A.

C. A is true but R is false.

D. A is false but R is true.

13. Assertion (A) : Appendicectomy should not be done in the presence of appendicular lump.

Reason (R) : Appendicectomy is difficult, dangerous and may lead to the formation of faecal fistula.

**14. Visible appendix on USG indicates : JIPMER 2001; Kerala 2001**

A. Acute appendicitis B. Normal appendix

C. Retro caecal appendix D. Gas under peritoneum

**15. A 30 years old lady who has undergone appendicectomy develops urinary retention in the post-operative period. Which of the following is most appropriate management: Delhi 2001**

A. Do suprapubic cystostomy.

B. Perform Foley's catheterization.

C. Reassure the patient and give analgesics to decrease pain.

D. Do suprapubic aspiration of urine under aseptic conditions.

**16. A pregnant lady presents with abdominal pain. She is diagnosed to have appendicitis. You will advice her : Kerala 2001**

A. Early Surgery

B. MTP & appendicectomy

C. Conservative treatment

D. Surgery after delivery

**17. Which of the following should make one question the clinical diagnosis of acute appendicitis: AMU 1986**

A. A patient who remains hungry

B. Temperature above 101°F

C. Cutaneous hyperaesthesia in the levels of T10 to T12

D. A history of vomiting preceding pain

E. Both A and D

**18. Pain in the acute appendicitis is commonly referred to : JIPMER 1992**

A. Right shoulder B. Right groin

C. Umbilicus D. External genitalia

**19. Most common location of appendix is : UPSC 1986; Delhi 1986; AIIMS 1992; JIPMER 1997**

A. Retrocaecal B. Sub-caecal

C. Para-caecal D. Pelvic

E. Pre-ileal

**20. Most common site for carcinoid syndrome : AI 1993**

A. Appendix B. Small intestine

C. Bronchus D. Adrenal

**21. A major complication of gangrenous appendicitis resulting in chills, spiking fever and jaundice : Delhi 1982; PGI 1985**

A. Haemolytic crisis B. Pyelonphlebitis

C. Subphrenic abscess D. Subhepatic abscess

E. All of the above

**22. An appendix abscess should be opened : UPSC 1983**

A. When the swelling is not diminishing in size after the fifth day of treatment.

B. When the temperature remains above 100°F for several successive days.

C. If a pelvic abscess develops.

D. All of the above.

**23. In acute appendicits, board-like rigidity develops due to : AMU 1986**

A. Local periotonitis B. Perforation

C. Faecoliths D. Pelvic appendicitis

**Ans.** **11. D** **12. C** **13. A** **14. A** **15. C** **16. A** **17. E** **18. C** **19. A** **20. A**
**21. B** **22. D** **23. B**

24. **In a suspected case of acute appendicitis, the most dangerous thing one can order :** **AMC 1984; Rohtak 1989, 2001**
A. Laparotomy B. Antibiotics
C. Catharsis or enemas D. Ice bags
E. Hot packs

25. **The most common obstructing agent for appendix is :** **UPSC 1984, 87**
A. A foreign body B. A round worm
C. Thread worms D. None of the above

26. **A patient of appendicular lump on Ochsner-Sherren regimen should be operated if there is :** **BHU 1986; AMC 1987; UPSC 1990**
A. Rising pulse rate
B. Diarrhoea
C. Passage of mucus in stools
D. Increasing or spreading abdominal pain
E. Presence of any of the above

27. **McBurney's point lies at the junction of :** **UPSC 1986**
A. Lateral and medial halves of the joining the anterior superior iliac spine and umbilicus.
B. Lateral 2/3 and medial 1/3 of the above line.
C. Lateral 2/5 and medial 3/5 of the above line.
D. Lateral third and medial 2/3 of the above line.
E. None of the above.

28. **Epidemic appendicitis is due to :** **AMU 1990**
A. Faecoliths
B. Worms of ileo-caecal region
C. Streptococcal infections
D. Abuse of purgatives
E. None of the above

29. **Gangrene in acute appendicitis usually starts at :** **AIIMS 1983; UPSC 1987**
A. Base of appendix
B. Proximal half of appendix
C. Distal half of appendix
D. Tip of appendix

30. **Mucocele of the appendix is :** **Delhi 1984; AI 1989; Kerala 1990**
A. Benign tumour B. Low grade malignancy
C. Retention cyst D. Infective process

31. **All of the following are clinical features of non-obstructive acute appendicitis except :** **PGI 1983**
A. Colicky abdominal pain
B. Protective pylorospasm
C. Tenderness over Mc Burney's point
D. Vomiting of short duration

32. **Appendicectomy is not advised in :** **UPSC 1981, 83, 88; Delhi 1981, 94; AMC 1986**
A. Recurrent type with abscess
B. Recurrent type without abscess
C. Gangrene
D. Crohn's disease

33. **Faecal fistula after appendicectomy is due to :** **Delhi 1983, 87; PGI 1983, 88, 90; AIIMS 1984, 89; ESI 1989**
A. Electrolyte imbalance
B. Undiagnosed disease of caecum and Ileum
C. Indiscriminate use of antibiotics
D. Postoperative infection

34. **Appendicular stump is obtained by :** **Delhi 1986, 88**
A. Crushing B. Ligation and inversion
C. Inversion D. Ligation

35. **The frequent mechanism in perforation of appendix is :** **DNB 1989**
A. Impacted faecolith
B. Tension gangrene due to the accumulating secretions
C. Necrosis of lymphoid patch
D. Retrocaecal function

36. **True about appendix are following except :** **Rajasthan 1998**
A. Retrocaecal in position
B. Develop from caecum
C. Has mesentry
D. Covered by peritoneum

37. **Which of the following is not true regarding acute appendicitis :** **AIIMS 1988**
A. Abdominal rigidity may be absent if appendix is retrocaecal.
B. Abdominal rigidity may be absent if appendix is pelvic.
C. Vomiting usually preceeds pain.
D. Pain to begin with is around umbilicus.

38. **A large collection of pus in the true pelvis after rupture of acute appendicitis is best drained :** **CSE 1995**
A. Transvaginally B. Trans-rectally
C. Supra-pubically D. Laparotomy

39. **Appendicular abscess is usually treated by :** **CSE 1997**
A. Appendicectomy
B. Oschner-Sherren regime
C. Extra-peritoneal drainage
D. Intra-peritoneal drainage

**Ans.** 24. C 25. D 26. E 27. D 28. C 29. D 30. C 31. A 32. D 33. B 34. B 35. B 36. C 37. C 38. D 39. B

**40. Earliest symptoms in acute appendicitis is : NIMHANS 1986; Kerala 1987**

A. Pain B. Fever
C. Vomiting D. Rise of pulse rate

**41. Interval appendicectomy is usually done——— months after an acute attack. UPSC 1984, 90**

A. 3 B. 6
C. 9 D. 12

**42. All of the following statements are true regarding recurrent acute appendicitis, except : UPSC 1984**

A. It's chronic persistent inflammation of appendix.
B. Dyspepsia which does not respond to alkalis.
C. In most of these cases it is obliterative appendicitis.
D. It ultimately ends in severe acute appendicitis.

**43. In the differential diagnosis of appendicitis in an infant it is important to consider all of the following, except : AIIMS 1994**

A. Basal pneumonia
B. Torsion of an ovarian cyst
C. Henoch-Schonlein purpura
D. Ileo-Ileal intussusception

**44. A 25-years old man presents with 3 days history of pain in the right lower abdomen and vomitings. Patient's general condition is satisfactory and clinical examination reveals a tender lump in right iliac fossa. The most appropriate management in this case would be : CSE 1998**

A. Immediate appendicectomy
B. Exploratory laparotomy
C. Oschner Sherren regimen
D. External drainage

**45. The most frequent neoplastic lesion of appendix is : UPSC 1988**

A. Metastatic B. Carcinoid
C. Haemangiosarcoma D. Lymphosarcoma
E. Adenocarcinoma

**Ans. 40. A 41. A 42. A 43. A 44. C 45. B**

# EXPLANATIONS OF APPENDIX

1. Ans.— D. Copious gastric aspiration
2. Ans.— D. All of the above
3. Ans.— A. Drain it
4. Ans.— D. Ruptured appendicitis with local peritonitis.
5. Ans.— B. Lawson Tait
6. Ans.— B. Sterlity in the female
7. Ans.— A. Carcinoid
8. Ans.— A. Intestinal intubation and continuous suction.
9. Ans.— C. It is most frequent in old people
10. Ans.— A. Appendicectomy
11. Ans.— D. All the above statements are correct
12. Ans.— C. Rectal stricture
13. Ans.— A. Both A and R are true and Ris the correct explanation of A.
14. Ans.— A. Acute appendicitis
15. Ans.— C. Reassure the patient and give analgesics to decrease pain.
16. Ans.— A. Early Surgery
17. Ans.— E. Both A and D
18. Ans.— C. Umbilicus
19. Ans.— A. Retrocaecal

    Retrocaecal in 74%, Plevic -21%. Postileal-5%, Paracaecal-2%, Subcaecal-1.5% and perileal-1%.
20. Ans.— A. Appendix
21. Ans.— B. Pyelonphlebitis
22. Ans.— D. All of the above

    Carcinoid is also called Argentaffinoma which arises in argentaffin tissue (Kubschitzsky cells of crypts of Lieberkuhn) can occur anywhere in GIT but most common in appendix.
23. Ans.— B. Perforation
24. Ans.— C. Catharsis or enemas
25. Ans.— D. None of the above
26. Ans.— E. Presence of any of the above
27. Ans.— D. Lateral third and medial 2/3 of the above line.
28. Ans.— C. Streptococcal infections
29. Ans.— D. Tip of appendix
30. Ans.— C. Retention cyst
31. Ans.— A. Colicky abdominal pain
32. Ans.— D. Crohn's disease

    There is risk of fistula formation.
33. Ans.— B. Undiagnosed disease of caecum and Ileum.
34. Ans.— B. Ligation and inversion
35. Ans.— B. Tension gangrene due to the accumulating secretions.
36. Ans.— C. Has mesentry
37. Ans.— C. Vomiting usually preceeds pain
38. Ans.— D. Laparotomy
39. Ans.— B. Oschner-Sherren regime

    The commonest site is lateral part of right iliac fossa (extension of retrocaecal suppuration) and the second most common is in the pelvis.
40. Ans.— A. Pain
41. Ans.— A. 3
42. Ans.— A. It's chronic persistent inflammation of appendix.
43. Ans.— A. Basal pneumonia
44. Ans.— C. Oschner Sherren regimen
45. Ans.— B. Carcinoid

# 13

# IMPORTANT TEXT OF RECTUM & ANAL CANAL

## MAIN SYMPTOMS OF RECTAL DISEASE

* Bleeding per rectum
* Altered bowel habit
* Mucus discharge
* Tenesmus
* Prolapse

## RECTAL PROLAPSE

* May be partial or complete
* If complete the whole wall of the rectum is induded
* If commences as a rectal intussusception
* In children the prolapse is usually partial and should be treated conservotively
* In the adult, the prolapse is often complete and is associated frequently with incontinence
* Surgery is necessary for complete rectal prolapse
* The operation is performed either via the perineum or via the abdomen

## POLYPS IN THE RECTUM

* Are either single or multiple
* Adenomas are the most frequent histological type
* Villous adenomas may be extensive and undergo malignant change
* All odenomas must be removed to avoid carcinomatous change
* All patients must undergo colonoscopy to determine if further polyps are present
* Most polyps can be removed by endoscopic techniques but sometimes major surgery is required

## PATHOLOGY AND STAGING OF RECTAL CANCER

* Tumours are adenocarcinomas and are well, average or poorly differentiated
* They spread by local, lymphatic, venous and transperitoneal routes
* Circumferential local spread is the most important as this profoundly affects surgical treatment
* Although lymphatic spread follows the blood supply of the rectum, most occur in an upwords direction via the superior rectal vessels to the para-aortic nodes
* The TNM classification is the internationally recognised staging system

## THREE DEGREES OF HAEMORRHOIDS

* First degree — bleed only, no prolapse
* Second degree — prolapse but will reduce spontaneously or can be reduced digitally and will remain reduced
* Third degree — continuously remain prolapsed

# MCQ's OF RECTUM & ANAL CANAL

## What is important in Rectum & Anal Canal

Rectum and Anal Canal (Haemorrhoids, Fistula, Fissure, Prolapse, Ca.)

### 13 (A) — Rectum

1. **Distal clearance in surgery for carcinoma rectum is : AI 1990**
   A. 2 cm B. 5 cm
   C. 10 cm D. 8 cm
2. **To diagnose rectal growth, important procedure is : AIIMS 1994**
   A. PR examination B. Sigmoidoscopy
   C. Ba enema D. Ultrasound
3. **In a child colicky abdominal pain, early onset of vomiting, palpable mass and bleeding per rectum, most strongly suggests : AMC 1985**
   A. Appendicitis
   B. Intussusception
   C. Ulcerative colitis
   D. Volvulus of the mid gut
4. **Rectal continence is maintained by all except : AI 1995**
   A. Puborectalis
   B. External sphincter of anus
   C. Pudendal nerve
   D. Valves of Houston
5. **Rectal polyposis lead to loss of : PGI 1993, 95**
   A. Na B. K
   C. Mg D. Ca
6. **After anterior resection of Ca rectum, the viability of rectal stump is determined by : PGI 1994**
   A. Superior mesenteric artery
   B. Inferior mesenteric artery
   C. External iliac artery
   D. Internal iliac artery
7. **An elderly patient has been admitted with history of bleeding per retum. Rectal examination revealed a growth at a distance of 2 cm from the anal verge. The correct treatment will be : UPSC 1996**
   A. Excision of the growth
   B. Abdomino-perineal resection
   C. Radiotherapy
   D. Chemotherapy
8. **Regarding Rectal carcinoma the following statements are true except : Kerala 2000**
   A. Adenomas and papillomas are pre-cancerous conditions.
   B. Local spread occurs circumferentially rather than longitudinally.
   C. Lymphatic spread from Carcinoma of Rectum above the peritoneal reflection occurs almost exclusively in an upward direction.
   D. Stage-D in the Duke's classification was originally described by Duke.
   E. Bleeding is the earliest and most constant symptom.
9. **A 22-years-old lady presents with pain in the right iliac fossa. On examination there was tenderness and guarding. Which of the following should not be done in this case : AIIMS 2000**
   A. Put patient nil orally B. Give I.V. glucose
   C. Inj. Pethidine I.M. D. Plain X-ray abdomen
10. **Consider the following statements : UPSC 2001**
    Therapeutic colonoscopy is performed in :
    1. Acute and chronic diarrhoea
    2. Colonic polyposis
    3. Decompression of pseudo obstruction and sigmoid volvulus
    4. Dilatation of colonic stricture
    
    Which of the above statements are correct ?
    A. 1, 2 and 3 B. 2, 3 and 4
    C. 1, 3 and 4 D. 1 and 4

**Ans.** 1. A 2. A 3. B 4. D 5. B 6. B 7. B 8. C 9. C 10. B

11. **Surgery for rectal prolapse depends upon : JIPMER 2002**
A. Extent of prolapse
B. Presence of ulcer
C. Presence of associated haemorrhoid
D. Sphincter function

12. **In Duke's classification, B2 indicates : Delhi 1983**
A. Wall involvement including the muscularis
B. Node involvement
C. Distant metastasis to liver
D. Local periodic fat invasion
E. None of the above

13. **Rectal bleeding is small but recurrent in : PGI 1984, 89, 94**
A. Haemorrhoids
B. Diverticulosis
C. Inflammatory bowel disease
D. Polyps

14. **The boundary between Rectum & anal canal is at the level of : TN 1993**
A. Pelvic diaphragm B. Urogenital diaphragm
C. White line of pelvis D. Base of prostate

15. **Anterior resection of rectum is contraindicated in : PGI 1985, 90; Delhi 1993**
A. Intestinal obstruction
B. Growth within 2 cm from anus
C. Two metastatic nodules in liver
D. Anaemia

16. **Commonest cause of bleeding per rectum in a child is : Delhi 1988, 93**
A. Hirschsprung's disease
B. Foreign body
C. Intussusception
D. Rectal polyp

17. **All of the following statements about partial prolapse of the rectum are true except : MAHE 1993**
A. It occurs in elderly people as well as in children
B. It can occur in whooping cough
C. It is predisposed by alorn perineum
D. It characteristically in plum coloured

18. **All of the following are characteristics of villous adenoma of rectum, except : AMU 1985**
A. Large sessile growth
B. Diarrhoea
C. Rectal bleeding
D. Frequent diagnosis by sigmoidoscopy
E. Hyperkalemia

19. **Common early presentation of carcinoma rectum is : Delhi 1989**
A. Pain
B. Bleeding
C. Increasing constipation
D. Alternate constipation and diarrhoea

20. **Carcinoma of the rectum is characterized by following except : UPSC 1987**
A. Is squamous-celled
B. Can occur in youth
C. Causes bleeding which is slight in amount
D. Simulates internal haemorrhoids

21. **Duhamel operation is done in : UPSC 1988**
A. Congenital pyloric stenosis
B. Hiatus hernia
C. Achlasia cardia
D. Hirschsprung's disease

22. **The initial treatment of choice of rectal prolapse in children is : DNB 1989**
A. Digital reposition
B. Submucous injection
C. Thiersch's operation
D. Excision of prolapsed mucosa

23. **"Cherry tumour" is a term for : AMU 1988**
A. Metastatic polyp in rectum
B. Pseudopolyp in sigmoid colon
C. Juvenile polyp in rectum
D. Adenomatous polyp in stomach

24. **Rectal prolapse is common in children in age group: NIMHANS 1987**
A. 1-6 months B. 8-12 months
C. 1-3 months D. 4-6 months

25. **A 50-years old man is admitted with bright red rectal bleeding. He recently had a barium enema which was normal. Nasogastric suction reveals no blood. The next diagnostic step is : CSE 1997**
A. Repeat Barium enema for missed lesions
B. Gastroscopy for bleeding ulcers
C. Barium meal and follow through
D. Mesenteric angiography

26. **Prognosis in cancer rectum is assessed by : PGI 1989**
A. Size of tumour
B. Histological grading
C. Site of tumour
D. Sex of the patient

Ans. 11. D 12. A 13. A 14. A 15. B 16. B 17. D 18. E 19. B 20. A
21. D 22. A 23. C 24. C 25. D 26. B

## 13 (B) — Anal Canal

**27. In imperforated anus, it may be necessary to wait for ______. AIIMS 1985**

A. 0 hour B. 6 hours
C. 24 hours D. 48 hours

**28. The most common congenital anomalies associated with imperforated anus are of : PGI 1982**

A. Duodenum B. Heart
C. Kidney D. Lungs

**29. The commonest variety of piles is : UPSC 1987**

A. Internal B. External
C. Internal-external D. None of the above

**30. Which is the only acceptable solution here of the injection of haemorrhoids: UPSC 1989**

A. 5% sodium tetradecyl sulphate
B. 5% phenol in almond or arachis oil
C. 5% phenol in water
D. Pure almond or arachis oil

**31. An obstructive stricture of rectum due to lymphogranuloma venereum should be treated by : AIIMS 1986**

A. Colostomy
B. Forcible dilatation
C. Abdominoperineal resection
D. None of the above

**32. Symptomatic piles may be present in all but one of the following conditions : Delhi 1983**

A. During pregnancy B. In carcinoma of rectum
C. Portal hypertension D. Enlarged prostate

**33. All of the following are causes of primary haemorrhoids except : DNB 1990**

A. Inferior rectal veins have no valves.
B. Congenital weakness of vein walls.
C. Collecting radicals of superior rectal veins are unsupported in the loose submucous connecting tissue.
D. High venous pressure in the lower rectum which is unparalleled in the body.

**34. All of the following are the causes of internal piles except : AIIMS 1985**

A. Increased intra-abdominal pressure
B. Portal hypertension
C. Because valves in rectal veins are present
D. Rectal veins lie in connective tissue

**35. False statement regarding anal carcinoma is : PGI 1985, 89**

A. A epidermoid variety of carcinoma
B. Radiotherapy is given
C. Spreads to inguinal LN
D. Surgery is contraindicated

**36. Most common type of imperforated anus is : PGI 1990**

A. Anal agenesis B. Anal stenosis
C. Membranous atresia D. Anorectal agenesis

**37. Five-days self-subsiding pain : AP 1997**

A. Anal fissure
B. Fistula-in-ano
C. Thrombosed ext. haemorrhoids
D. Thrombosed int. haemorrhoids

**38. In the treatment of Fissure-in-ano, following are done except : AIIMS 1996**

A. Lateral sphincterotomy
B. Ext. sphincterotomy
C. Manual dilatation after anaesthesia
D. Conservative treatment

**39. Treatment of intestinal obstruction caused by cancer of the rectosigmoid is best accomplished by : AIIMS 1985**

A. Decompressive colostomy
B. Decompression by passage of a long intestinal tube, subsequent resection
C. Immediate resection
D. None of the above

**40. Below the pectineal line, the lymphatic spreads of malignancy is to ——— nodes. PGI 1990**

A. Superficial inguinal B. Internal iliac
C. External iliac D. Para aortic

**41. Seitz Bath consists of which of the following : Karnataka 1996**

A. Patient bathed in normal saline
B. Bathed in molten wax
C. Sits in a basin containing warm antiseptic lotion
D. Sits in a basin containing molten wax

**42. A neonate has been brought with a single perineal opening through which urine and meconium is passed. The most likely diagnosis is : UPSC 1994**

A. Anorectal malformation with ambiguous gentitalia
B. Rectovesical fistula
C. Rectovaginal fistula
D. Cloacal malformation

| Ans. | 27. C | 28. C | 29. A | 30. B | 31. C | 32. C | 33. A | 34. C | 35. D | 36. D |
|---|---|---|---|---|---|---|---|---|---|---|
| | 37. C | 38. B | 39. C | 40. A | 41. C | 42. D | | | | |

**43. Barber's pilonidal sinus occurs at : NIMS 1996**
A. Sacrococcygeal area B. Clivus
C. Interdigital cleft D. Face

**44. All are false regarding internal haemorrhoids except: AP 1994**
A. Aggravated in pregnancy
B. Seen in 2, 7, 10'O clock position
C. It is clearly felt by rectal examination
D. Complete prolapse is second examination

**45. Recurrent obstruction, mass per rectum and diarrhoea in adult : AIIMS 1985**
A. Intussusception B. Rectal prolapse
C. Internal hernia D. Haemorrhoids

**46. Best treatment of anorectal abscess in a neutropenic patient is : UP 1999**
A. Antibiotics
B. Recurrent aspiration
C. Incision and drainage
D. Total parenteral nutrition with bowel rest

**47. The best surgical management for villous adenoma of the rectum is : AP 1988**
A. Local resection of lesion
B. Repeated sigmoidoscopy
C. Abdomino-perineal resection
D. Electrolyte infusion and chemotherapy

**48. All of the following statements are true regarding proctalgia fugax except : AIIMS 1984**
A. Attacks of severe pain arising in the rectum.
B. Pain is mostly felt during the day and is relieved at night.
C. It is seen in anxious and over stressed patients.
D. Pain is unpleasant, incurable but harmless.

**49. Match List-I with List-II and select the correct answer : CSE 1996**

| List-I Methods of treatment | List-II Indications of carcinoma rectum) |
|---|---|
| A. Anterior resection | 1. Carcinoma rectum causing intestinal obstruction |
| B. Hartman's procedure | 2. Carcinoma of upper 2/3rd rectum |
| C. Abdomino perineal | 3. Carcinoma of lower 1/3rd rectum |
| D. Palliative colostomy | 4. Carcinoma rectum in an aged patient |

| | A | B | C | D |
|---|---|---|---|---|
| A. | 3 | 1 | 2 | 4 |
| B. | 2 | 4 | 3 | 1 |
| C. | 2 | 1 | 3 | 4 |
| D. | 3 | 4 | 2 | 1 |

**50. Most common cause of lower gastrointestinal bleeding is : AIIMS 1992**
A. Typhoid B. Tuberculosis
C. Amoebiasis D. Meckel's diverticulum

**51. Treatment of choice in 2nd degree piles is : AIIMS 1992**
A. Sclerotherapy B. Banding
C. Cryosurgery D. Haemorrhoidectomy

**52. The treatment of choice of fistula in ano is : JIPMER 1993**
A. Fistulotomy B. Fistulectomy
C. Fissurotomy D. Anal dilatation

**53. The site of election of anal fissure is in the : UPSC 1982, 87; Delhi 1983; PGI 1989**
A. Midline anteriorly
B. Lower half of left lateral wall
C. Upper half of right lateral wall
D. Midline posteriorly
E. None of the above

**54. Common clinical presentation of cancer of middle 1/3rd rectum are all of the following except : Delhi 1994**
A. Bleeding per rectum
B. Sense of incomplete evacuation
C. Alteration of bowel habit
D. Acute intestinal obstruction

**55. Internal sphincterotomy is the treatment of choice for : AMC 1985**
A. Piles B. Fistula
C. Fissure-in-ano D. Carcinoma

**56. Villous polyps of rectum manifest with : AI 1989**
A. Bleeding PR
B. Mucus diarrhoea with hypokalemia
C. Prolapsed rectum
D. Obstruction

**57. Sentinel pile indicates : AIIMS 1987; Delhi 1994; DNB 1994**
A. Carcinoma rectum B. Internal haemorrhoids
C. Perianal fistula D. Anal fissure

**58. True about Fissure-in-ano is : Rohtak 1995**
A. Involves anal portion above dentate line
B. Involves anal valves of Ball
C. Circular ulcer in long axis
D. Diarrhoea is common

**Ans.** **43. C** **44. A** **45. A** **46. C** **47. A** **48. B** **49. C** **50. C** **51. B** **52. B**
**53. D** **54. D** **55. C** **56. B** **57. D** **58. B**

**59. Wrong about carcinoma Anus : UPSC 1982, 83, 86; PGI 1987, 89 JIPMER 1987; ESI 1989**

A. Squamous cell carcinoma
B. Spreads to Inguinal lymph nodes
C. Radiosensitive
D. Surgery contraindicated

**60. The commonest variety of anorectal abscess is : AMC 1982**

A. Perianal B. Ischiorectal
C. Submucosal D. Pelvirectal

**61. Best diagnosis of uncomplicated piles (second degree) is by : Delhi 1987**

A. Per rectal examination
B. Proctoscopy
C. Barium enema
D. Aortography

**62. In the injection treatment of haemorrhoids, it is important to inject : PGI 1983; Bihar 1998**

A. Into the lumen of vein
B. Around pedicle of pile mass
C. Into the muscularis of the bowel
D. None of the above

**63. Common type of carcinoma involving the anus is : Delhi 1985**

A. Melanoma
B. Adenocarcinoma
C. Transitional cell carcinoma
D. Epidermoid carcinoma

**64. A pilonidal sinus occurs at the following except : AMU 1990**

A. Commonly in blondes
B. Between the fingers
C. At the umbilicus
D. In the natal cleft

**65. Incorrect about an anal fissure is : DNB 1990**

A. A complication of an anal fistula
B. Sometimes due to carcinoma of the anus
C. Painful during defecation
D. A cause of acquired megacolon

**66. A thrombosed external haemorrhoid is not except : DNB 1990**

A. Painless
B. Capable of self-resolution
C. Unlike a semi-ripe blackcurrent in appearance
D. Best treated by masterly inactivity

**67. An ischiorectal abscess is characterized by following except : AP 1989**

A. May be tuberculous in origin
B. Is an infective necrosis of the fat of the ischiorectal fossa
C. Requires deroofing
D. Should be treated entirely by antibiotics

**68. Malignant tumours of the anus is characterized by following except : UPSC 1986**

A. Include baseloid tumours
B. Primarily spread to the inferior mesenteric lymph nodes
C. May be treated by radiotherapy
D. Simulate anal fissure

**69. Thiersch operation is indicated for : Kerala 1988**

A. Procidentia B. Internal piles
C. External piles D. None of the above

**70. Delorme's operation used in : Rajasthan 1998; UP 2000**

A. Rectal prolapse B. Fistula-in-ano
C. Fissure-in-ano D. Rectum carcinoma

**71. True about anorectal fistula is : UP 2000; AI 2001**

A. High and low fistula by pelvic floor levator ani
B. Intersphincteric type is most common
C. Gutter shaped
D. Ischiorectal fossa above the floor

**72. Tumor presenting 3 cm from anal region is treated by : NIMHANS 2000**

A. Ant. resection of rectum
B. ADR
C. Chemoradiation
D. Chemotherapy only

**73. Fistula-in-ano, what is true : AI 2001**

A. Posterior fistulae have straight tracks.
B. High fistulae can be operated with no fear of incontinence.
C. High and low division is based on pelvic floor.
D. Intersphincteric is the most common.

**74. An AIDS patient presents with fistula-in-ano. His CD4 is below 50. What is the treatment of choice : MAHE 2001**

A. Seton B. Fistulectomy
C. None D. Both

**Ans.** 59. D 60. A 61. B 62. B 63. D 64. A 65. A 66. B 67. D 68. B 69. A 70. A 71. B 72. C 73. C 74. A

75. **A patient with external haemorrhoids develops pain while passing stools. The nerve mediating this pain is : AI 2002**
A. Hypogastric nerve
B. Pudendal nerve
C. Splanchnic visceral nerve
D. Sympathetic plexus

76. **The treatment of choice for cancer of the anal canal is : UPSC 2002**
A. Radiation
B. Abdomino perineal resection
C. Chemoradiation
D. Surgery and radiation

77. **A 50 years old male, working as a hotel cook, has four dependent family members. He has been diagnosed with an early stage squamous cell cancer of anal canal. He has more than 60% chances of cure. The best treatment option is : AI 2003**
A. Abdomino-perineal resection
B. Combined surgery and radiotherapy
C. Combined chemotherapy and radiotherapy
D. Chemotherapy alone

78. **The most common 'surgical' cause for bleeding per rectum in infants and children is due to : UPSC 2003**
A. Haemorrhoids
B. Intussusception
C. Rectal polyp
D. Portal hypertension

79. **Regarding the carcinoid tumor of the rectum, which one of the following is not correct : UPSC 2003**
A. It presents as an ulcer of the rectal mucosa.
B. Large carcinoid tumors are malignant.
C. Local excision of the tumor may be sufficient treatment for small (<2 cm) early tumors.
D. Carcinoid syndrome is rare.

80. **Injection sclerotherapy is ideal for the following: AI 2004**
A. External haemorrhoids
B. Internal haemorrhoids
C. Prolapsed haemorrhoids
D. Strangulated haemorrhoids

81. **For a rectal carcinoma at 5 cms from the anal verge the best acceptable operation is: AI 2004**
A. Anterior resection
B. Abdomino-perineal resection
C. Posterior resection
D. Local resection

82. **During APR for CA rectum in a thyrotoxic female, the pco2 falls from 40 mm Hg to 10mm Hg. The most likely explanations is : AIIMS 2009**
A. High blood pressure
B. Pulmonar embolism
C. Thyrotoxic storm
D. None of the above

83. **Hirschprung's disease is due to : AIIMS 2009**
A. Atrophy of longitudinal muscles
B. Loss of ganglion cells in the sympathetic
C. Failure of migration of neural crest cells from cranial to caudal direction
D. Combination of B & C

84. **Which of the foillowing is not felt with a P/R examination : AIIMS 2009**
A. Anorectal ring
B. Prostate
C. Bulb of pains
D. Ureter

| Ans. | 75. B | 76. C | 77. C | 78. C | 79. A | 80. B | 81. B | 82. C | 83. C | 84. D |
|---|---|---|---|---|---|---|---|---|---|---|

# EXPLANATIONS OF RECTUM & ANAL CANAL

## 13 (A) — RECTUM

**1. Ans.— A. 2 cm**

**A sphincter saving operation (anterior resection) is usually possible for tumors of upper 2/3 rd of rectum. Although, removal of rectum with a permanent colostomy (Abdomino-Perineal excision) is often required for tumor of lower 1/3rd of rectum; minimal distal margin of clearance of 2 cm should be secured for continuation of GIT.**

**2. Ans.— A. PR examination**

**3. Ans.— B. Intussusception**

**4. Ans.— D. Valves of HoustOn**

**5. Ans.— B. K**

**Thread worm infestation can also cause rectal prolapse.**

**6. Ans.— B. Inferior mesenteric artery**

**7. Ans.— B. Abdomino-perineal resection**

**8. Ans.— C. Lymphatic spread from Carcinoma of Rectum above the peritoneal reflection occurs almost exclusively in an upward direction.**

**9. Ans.— C. Inj. Pethidine I.M.**

**10. Ans.— B. 2, 3 and 4**

**11. Ans.— D. Sphincter function**

**12. Ans.— A. Wall involvement including the muscularis.**

**13. Ans.— A. Haemorrhoids**

**14. Ans.— A. Pelvic diaphragm**

**15. Ans.— B. Growth within 2 cm from anus**

**16. Ans.— B. Foreign body**

**17. Ans.— D. It is characteristically is plum coloured**

**18. Ans.— E. Hyperkalemia**

**Rectal bleeding is common. There can be deficiency of Na+, K+ and Cl-**

**19. Ans.— B. Bleeding**

**Alteration in bowel habits is common in Ca Ascending colon.**

**20. Ans.— A. Is squamous-celled**

**21. Ans.— D. Hirschsprung's disease**

**22. Ans.— A. Digital reposition**

**23. Ans.— C. Juvenile polyp in rectum**

**It is a bright red glistening pedunculated sphere ("cherry tumor") found in infants bleeding or pain if it prolapses during defecation.**

**24. Ans.— C. 1-3 months**

**25. Ans.— D. Mesenteric angiography**

## 13 (B) — ANAL CANAL

**26. Ans.— B. Histological grading**

**27. Ans.— C. 24 hours**

**28. Ans.— C. Kidney**

**29. Ans.— A. Internal**

**30. Ans.— B. 5% phenol in almond or arachis oil.**

**31. Ans.— C. Abdominoperineal resection**

**32. Ans.— C. Portal hypertension**

**33. Ans.— A. Inferior rectal veins have no valves.**

**34. Ans.— C. Because valves in rectal veins are present.**

**35. Ans.— D. Surgery is contraindicated**

**36. Ans.— D. Anorectal agenesis**

**37. Ans.— C. Thrombosed ext. haemorrhoids**

**38. Ans.— B. Ext. sphincterotomy**

**39. Ans.— C. Immediate resection**

**40. Ans.— A. Superficial inguinal**

**41. Ans.— C. Sits in a basin containing warm antiseptic lotion.**

**42. Ans.— D. Cloacal malformation**

**43. Ans.— C. Interdigital cleft**

**44. Ans.— A. Aggravated in pregnancy**

45. Ans.— A. Intussusception

46. Ans.— C. Incision and drainage

47. Ans.— A. Local resection of lesion

48. Ans.— B. Pain is mostly felt during the day and is relieved at night

49. Ans.— C. 2 1 3 4

50. Ans.— C. Amoebiasis

This is commonest in developing countries.

51. Ans.— B. Banding

52. Ans.— B. Fistulectomy

53. Ans.— D. Midline posteriorly

54. Ans.— D. Acute intestinal obstruction

55. Ans.— C. Fissure-in-ano

56. Ans.— B. Mucus diarrhoea with hypokalaemia

Villous adenoma causes profuse diarrhoea which leads to Na+ and K+ depletion.

57. Ans.— D. Anal fissure

58. Ans.— B. Involves anal valves of Ball

59. Ans.— D. Surgery contraindicated

60. Ans.— A. Perianal

61. Ans.— B. Proctoscopy

62. Ans.— B. Around pedicle of pile mass

63. Ans.— D. Epidermoid carcinoma

Squamous cell carcinoma is commonest cause of its superficial situation. Basaloid carcinoma, mucoepidermoid, basal cell carcinoma and melanoma are also rarely seen.

64. Ans.— A. Commonly in blondes

65. Ans.— A. A complication of an anal fistula

66. Ans.— B. Capable of self-resolution

67. Ans.— D. Should be treated entirely by antibiotics.

68. Ans.— B. Primarily spread to the inferior mesenteric lymph nodes.

69. Ans.— A. Procidentia

70. Ans.— A. Rectal prolapse

71. Ans.— B. Intersphincteric type is most common.

72. Ans.— C. Chemoradiation

73. Ans.— C. High and low division is based on pelvic floor.

High and low are classified according to opening into anal canal in relation to anorectal ring.

74. Ans.— A. Seton

75. Ans.— B. Pudendal nerve

Pudendal nerve supplies this area. The swelling resembles semiripe black current.

76. Ans.— C. Chemoradiation

77. Ans.— C. Combined chemotherapy and radiotherapy

Carcinoma of Anal Canal :

* Pre-Malignant conditions :

Pagets Dx - It leads to Adenocarcinoma of Anal Canal

Bowen's Dx - K/as Ca in situ - (Treatment - Laser ablation, or Excision)

MC type - Squamous cell carcinoma

Management - In all cases by " chemoradiation"

---

78. Ans.— C. Rectal polyp

Causes of Bleeding Per Rectum

Neonates
* Anal fissure
* Necrotizing enterocolitis
* Volvulus neonatorum
* Polyps in intestine

Infants
* Anal fissure
* Intussusception
* Meckel's diverticulum

Children
* Rectal polyps
* Vascular malformations-(NEC)
* Tumors of GIT

79. Ans.— A. It presents as an ulcer of the rectal mucosa

Carcinoid tumors of the rectum can be looked upon as a gradation between a benign tumor and a carcinoma. Like benign tumors they originate in submucosa with the mucous membrane over it being intact. It seldom produces evidence of its presence in the early stages, when it presents as a small plaque like elevation. The incidence of clinical malignancy (e.g. metastases) is 10%.

80. Ans. — B. Internal haemorrhoids

Treatment of Internal haemorrhoids:

1. Medical therapy – The majority of bleeding first and second degree haemorrhoids respond to the addition of dietary fiber or stool softeners and avoidance of straining.
2. Sclerosis (injection treatment) – May be used to stop bleeding from first and second decree haemorrhoids.
3. Elastic ligation (Banding)–Elastic ligation of second and third–degree hemorrhoids 1-2 cm above the dentate line, is very effective for control of bleeding and prolapse.
4. Hemorrhoidectomy – The excision of hemorrhoids should be limited to large third and fourth degree hemorrhoids.

81. Ans. — B. Abdomino-perineal resection

Treatment Re  l Carcinoma

- Resection of the primary rectal cancer is the treatment of choice for virtually all patients who have resectable lesion and can tolerate general anaesthesia.
- The operative approach depends upon the level of tumor above the anal verge, the size and depth of penetration.

82. Ans. — C. Thyrotoxic storm

83. Ans. — C. Failure of migration of neural crest cells from cranial to caudal direction

84. Ans. — D. Ureter

# 14

# IMPORTANT TEXT OF HERNIA

## TYPES OF HERNIAS

* Reducible - contents can be returned to abdomen
* Irreducible - contents cannot be returned but there are no other complications
* Obstructed - bowel in the hernia has good blood supply but bowel is obstructed
* Strangulated - blood supply of bowel is obstructed
* Inflamed - contents of sac have become inflamed

## NATURAL HISTORY OF HERNIAS

* Irreducible hernias - there is a risk of strangulation at any time
* Obstructed hernias - usually goes on to strangulation
* Strangulated hernias - gangrene can occur within 6 hours

# MCQ's OF HERNIA

## What is important in Hernia

Inguinal, Umbilical, Femoral (contents, surgery), Meckel's diverticulum

1. **Deep inguinal ring :** **UPSC 1985**
   A. Is situated 1.25 cm above and lateral to the pubic tubercle.
   B. Is an opening in the transversus abdominus muscle.
   C. Transmits ileo-inguinal nerve.
   D. Is a deficiency in the transversalis fascia.
2. **Sign present in irreducible femoral hernia is :** **AIIMS 1985, 90**
   A. Whiteside's sign B. Roche's sign
   C. Prehn's sign D. Gaur's sign
3. **Commonest sliding component of direct hernia is :** **PGI 1984, 90, 97**
   A. Bladder B. Calcium
   C. Ascending colon D. Descending colon
   E. None of the above
4. **Vaginal hydrocele is connected to :** **AIIMS 1996**
   A. Cord B. Percutaneous tissue
   C. Scrotum D. Peritoneal cavity
5. **Umbilical hernia is best operated after—— of age.** **DNB 1991**
   A. 9-12 months B. 1-2 years
   C. 3-4 years D. 10-12 years
6. **A—Strangulation is common in femoral hernias**
   **R—The femoral ring is narrow and unyielding** **UPSC 1994**
   **Of these statements**
   A. Both A and R are true and R is the correct explanation of A.
   B. Both A and R are true but R is not the correct explanation of A.
   C. A is true but R is false.
   D. A is false but R is true.
7. **A 30-year old male complains of aching sensation in the right groin with an inguinoscrotal swelling which expands on coughing. It is soft, resonant, reduces with a gurgle and is opaque. The most probable cause is :** **UPSC 1996**
   A. Omentocele B. Enterocele
   C. Hydrocele D. Varicocele
8. **Spigelian hernia is a type of hernia occurring at :** **PGI 1994; AI 1999**
   A. Medial border of rectus abdominis
   B. Lateral border of rectus abdominis
   C. Lumbar region
   D. Femoral canal
9. **True about paraumbilical hernia is :** **Delhi 1995**
   A. Usually asymptomatic
   B. No surgery required
   C. Empty sac
   D. Neck of sac is very small as compared to size of sac
10. **True about strangulated inguinal hernia is :** **Delhi 1995**
    A. Usually seen in large hernia
    B. Seen in young adults (15-25 years of age)
    C. Swollen but non-tender scrotum
    D. Elevation relieves pain
11. **The anatomical structure usually involved in the production of a direct inguinal hernia is :** **Orissa 1999**
    A. Poupart's ligament
    B. Conjoint tendon
    C. External oblique fascia
    D. Transversalis fascia
12. **All are done for investigation of strangulated hernia except :** **Kerala 2001**
    A. Abd. X-ray B. Aspiration
    C. USG D. Angiography

**Ans.** 1. D 2. D 3. A 4. C 5. C 6. A 7. B 8. B 9. B 10. B
11. A 12. D

**13. On performing a hernia operation, a patient develops tingling sensation over the dorsal surface of penis and over the scrotum. The nerve implicated is : AIIMS 2001**

A. Genitofemoral nerve
B. Ileoinguinal nerve
C. Hypogastric plexus
D. Pudendal nerve

**14. A patient following open inguinal hernia repair can be neuralgia due to involvement of any of the following nerves except : UPSC 2002**

A. Ileoinguinal
B. Ileohypogastric nerve
C. Lateral cutaneous nerve of thigh
D. Genitofemoral nerve

**15. A patient is advised to avoid strenuous activity following herniorrhaphy for a period of : AMU 1986**

A. One day
B. One week
C. 3 weeks
D. Six weeks

**16. Majority of direct inguinal hernias contain a sliding component of : AI 1989**

A. Urinary bladder
B. Caecum
C. Sigmoid colon
D. None of the above

**17. Direct inguinal hernia can be differentiated from the indirect one by all of the following points, except : UPSC 1987**

A. It is common in older age group.
B. It appears itself on standing.
C. It has strong impulse on coughing.
D Strangulation is not common.
E. It can be prevented by applying pressure over the internal ring with finger tip after reduction.

**18. Deep inguinal ring is ——— shaped. AMU 1986**

A. Triangular
B. Quardrangular
C. U
D. M

**19. Most common type of hernia to strangulate : AI 1993**

A. Inguinal
B. Obturator
C. Femoral
D. Epigastric

**20. All of the following statements about inguinal hernia in children are true, except : MAHE 1994**

A. They are usually of the indirect type.
B. They may be associated with a hydrococele.
C. They often regress spontaneously before the first birthday.
D. Obstruction is a common complication.

**21. Which is not a factor in the recurrence of inguinal hernia : Rajasthan 1995**

A. Failure to close the Internal Inguinal ring
B. Failure to close the External Inguinal ring
C. Associated hernia
D. Absorbable suture

**22. In a 35 years old female, reducible groin mass is most probably due to : AI 1994; Rajasthan 1995**

A. Femoral Hernia
B. Direct Hernia
C. Indirect Hernia
D. Sliding

**23. Incisional hernia are related to all, except : UPSC 1986**

A. Obesity
B. The use of absorbable suturing materials
C. Wound infections
D. Anaemia and malnutrition

**24. In Moore's classification of omphalocele (examphalos), type-I umbilical defect is less than ——— cm. AIIMS 1986**

A. 0.5
B. 2.5
C. 3.5
D. 4.5

**25. Congenital diaphragmatic hernia is commonest in ——— region : Delhi 1983**

A. Left posterior
B. Left anterior
C. Right anterior
D. Right posterior

**26. Which of the following hernia is also known as W-hernia : AIIMS 1984**

A. Spigelian
B. Lumbar
C. Cloquets
D. Maydl's

**27. Hernia into pouch of Douglas is ——— hernia. PGI 1984**

A. Beclard's
B. Berger's
C. Blandin's
D. Maydl's

**28. Hernia with hydrocele is ——— hernia. AIIMS 1984**

A. Gibbon's
B. Gruber's
C. Dobson's
D. Loebel's

**29. Richter's hernia is commonly associated with : UPSC 2001**

A. Direct inguinal hernia
B. Femoral hernia
C. Indirect inguinal hernia
D. Obturator hernia

**Ans.** 13. B 14. C 15. D 16. C 17. E 18. C 19. C 20. C 21. C 22. C 23. D 24. B 25. A 26. D 27. D 28. A 29. B

30. **The commonest variety of Indirect Inguinal (Oblique) hernia in children is : AIIMS 1986**
A. Bubonocele
B. Funicular
C. Scrotal
D. All are equally common

31. **Impulse on coughing for inguinal hernia is best palpated : TNPSC 1997**
A. At the root of the scrotum
B. At the bottom of the scrotum
C. At the deep inguinal ring
D. At the medial part of inguinal canal

32. **The commonest differential diagnosis of oblique hernia in female is : DNB 1990**
A. Vaginal hydrocele
B. Femoral hernia
C. Encysted hydrocele
D. Hydrocele of the canal of Nuck

33. **The treatment of choice for Inguinal hernia in infants is : AMU 1985; DNB 1990, 2001**
A. Herniotomy B. Herniorrhaphy
C. Truss D. Hernioplasty

34. **In an infant external inguinal ring in comparison to deep inguinal ring lies : PGI 1984; Delhi 1995**
A. Medially and above B. Laterally and below
C. Medially and below D. In superimposition

35. **In exomphalos minor, firm strapping is done : AIIMS 1987**
A. Never B. For 1 week
C. For 2 weeks D. For 3 months

36. **Obstruction or strangulation in umbilical hernia of infants is extremely uncommon below the age of : DNB 1989**
A. 3 years B. 6 years
C. 9 years D. 10 years

37. **Herniorrhaphy in umbilical hernia of infant should preferably be : AP 1990**
A. Not done
B. Done at birth
C. Done at about the age of two years
D. Done at the age of 12 years

38. **The covering over an omphalocele is : AIIMS 1987**
A. Skin B. Amniotic membrane
C. Chorionic membrane D. None of the above

39. **Most important step in the repair of an indirect inguinal hernia is : UPSC 1986**
A. Herniotomy
B. Narrowing of the internal ring
C. Bassini's repair
D. Transfixation of the neck of the sac

40. **All of the following statements are true regarding Narath's femoral hernia except : AIIMS 1986**
A. Occurs only in patients with congenital dislocation of hip.
B. Is usually associated with lipoma.
C. There is lateral dislocation of psoas muscle.
D. Hernia lies behind femoral vessels.

41. **On an average, the distance between femoral ring and saphenous opening (length of femoral canal) is : UPSC 1987; DNB 1994**
A. 1.25 cm B. 2.50 cm
C. 3.75 cm D. 5.00 cm

42. **Which of the following is inguinoproperitoneal hernia : DNB 1997**
A. Hey's hernia B. Rieux hernia
C. Kronlein hernia D. Coopers hernia

43. **In an adult, major predisposing factor for hernia is: UPSC 1992**
A. Muscular weakness
B. Neurological weakness
C. Increased abdominal pressure
D. All of the above

44. **A hernia having Meckel's diverticulum as one of the constituents is : UPSC 1988**
A. Richter's hernia B. Littre's hernia
C. Maydl's hernia D. Pantaloon hernia

45. **The most common form of hernia is: UPSC 1985**
A. Incisional
B. Femoral
C. Direct inguinal
D. Indirect inguinal (oblique)

46. **Of all inguinal hernias ——— % incarcerate during first year of life : AP 1989**
A. 0 B. 2-4
C. 20-30 D. Over 50

47. **All of the following statements are true of incisional hernia except : UPSC 1997**
A. Common in multiparous female patients.
B. More common after paramedian incision than after midline incision.
C. Common after wound infection.
D. Common after tubectomy/hysterectomy/caesarean section.

**Ans.** 30. C 31. C 32. D 33. A 34. D 35. C 36. A 37. C 38. B 39. B
40. B 41. A 42. C 43. A 44. B 45. D 46. B 47. B

**48. One of the following is false regarding sliding Hiatus Hernia : UPSC 1985**

A. Often strangulates
B. Often asymptomatic
C. Commonly associated with reflux oesophagitis
D. Oesophageal hiatus enlarges

**49. In a patient with a strangulated Richer's Hernia has all of the following except : Delhi 1984**

A. A portion of the circumference of the intestine is affected.
B. It usually complicates a femoral hernia.
C. The local signs of strangulation are often not obvious.
D. Absolute constipation and vomiting are pathognomonic.

**50. Which is the 1st sign of strangulation of inguinal hernia : AMU 1986; C.U.P.G.E.E 1996**

A. Tense B. Tender
C. Irreducible D. Redness

**51. Differentiation between femoral and inguinal hernia is done by : AIIMS 1998**

A. Pubic tubercle B. Inguinal ligament
C. Inf. epigastric artery D. Pubic symphysis

**52. The following are true regarding the anatomy of femoral canal except : Kerala 2000**

A. Lies medial to femoral vein.
B. Has inguinal ligament as its anterior border.
C. Has the pectineal ligament as its lateral border.
D. Has the lacunar ligament as its medial border.
E. Contains the lymph node of cloquet.

**53. Oblique hernia is commonest in children : DNB 1991**

| | Age | Sex | Side |
|---|---|---|---|
| A. | First decade | Male | Right |
| B. | First decade | Male | Left |
| C. | Second decade | Female | Right |
| D. | Fourth decade | Male | Left |

**54. In Shouldice procedure done is : UP 1999**

A. Narrowing the ring with lateral displacement of cord
B. Double breasting of transversalis fascia and repair with darning material
C. Combined low & high material
D. None of the above

**55. The hernia which often stimulates a peptic ulcer is : Karnataka 1996**

A. Umbilical hernia
B. Fatty hernia of the Linea alba
C. Incisional hernia
D. Inguinal hernia

**56. Herniotomy refers to : UPSC 1987**

A. Excision of the hernial sac
B. Repair of the internal inguinal ring
C. Reconstruction of posterior wall of inguinal canal
D. Combination of B and C

**57. A hernia in which only a portion of the wall of the intestine is incarcerated is called : UPSC 1996**

A. Littre's hernia B. Richter's hernia
C. Sliding hernia D. Spigelian hernia

**58. Strangulated femoral hernia is differentiated from infected inguinal lymph nodes by : PGI 1983**

A. Ultrasound B. Barium enema
C. Antibiotic therapy D. Surgery

**59. Best treatment for epigastric hernia is : AMC 1985**

A. Surgical repair B. Abdominal binder
C. Sclerotherapy D. Physiotherapy

**60. Which is not seen in complete ectopia vesicae : AIIMS 1982**

A. Umbilical hernia
B. Visible uretero vesical efflux
C. Hypospadias
D. Waddling gait

**61. Clinically a femoral hernia is most likely to be confused with : AP 1994**

A. Saphena varix B. Spermatocele
C. Soft sore D. Baker's cyst

**62. Causes of recurrent hernia are all except : PGI 1987, 88**

A. Absorbable sutures B. Sliding hernia
C. Missed sac D. Infection

**63. Hydrocele is a type of —— cyst. AIIMS 1984**

A. Retention B. Distension
C. Exudation D. Traumatic

**64. All of the following statements are true regarding hydrocele of the canal of Nuck except : PGI 1982**

A. It occur in females
B. It partially or wholly lies in the inguinal canal
C. It is associated with spermatic cord
D. It is found in relation to round ligament

**65. Commonest symptom of diaphragmatic hernia in Children is : Delhi 1986, 89**

A. Dyspnoea
B. Cyanosis
C. Abdominal distension
D. Regurgitation

| Ans. | | | | | | | | | |
|---|---|---|---|---|---|---|---|---|---|
| **48. A** | **49. D** | **50. B** | **51. B** | **52. C** | **53. A** | **54. B** | **55. B** | **56. A** | **57. B** |
| **58. D** | **59. A** | **60. C** | **61. B** | **62. B** | **63. C** | **64. C** | **65. A** | | |

**66. Richter's hernia is seen most commonly in : AIIMS 1986, 91**

A. Direct inguinal hernia B. Femoral hernia
C. Umbilical hernia D. Indirect inguinal hernia

**67. Which should not be advised as the treatment of a femoral hernia : DNB 1989; AMU 1989**

A. Lockwood's operation
B. Lotheisen's operation
C. A truss
D. McEvedy's operation

**68. An epigastric hernia is : UPSC 1988**

A. A Spigelian hernia
B. A fatty hernia of the linea alba
C. A type of umbilical hernia
D. Divarication of the rectus abdominis muscles

**69. Which of the following is false regarding hernia through the foramen of Bochdalek: PGI 1986**

A. It is a pleuro-peritoneal hernia.
B. The hernia may not have a sac.
C. It is situated posteriorly in the diaphragm.
D. Defect lies between sternal and costal attachment of diaphragm.

**70. The most common of the serious problems created by a sliding oesophageal hiatus hernia is : Rohtak 1985, 93**

A. Strangulation
B. Respiratory embarrassment
C. Oesophagitis and structure
D. Bleeding

**71. Strangulation of a hernia implies : UPSC 1985, 91**

A. That the hernia is irreducible.
B. That the hernia has a narrow neck.
C. That there is a impaired blood flow to the contents.
D. That there is torsion of the contents.

**72. Preservation of ilioinguinal nerve is an important step during inguinal hernia operation while : UPSC 1997**

A. Incising the sub-cutaneous tissue
B. Incising the extra-oblique aponeurosis
C. Incising the cremasteric fascia
D. Isolating the sac

**73. Usually the inguinal hernia gets constricted due to : UPSC 1984**

A. External abdominal ring
B. Adhesions within the hernial sac
C. Neck of sac
D. Narrowing of inguinal canal

**74. The ratio of males to females in the incidence of strangulated inguinal hernia in infancy is: Karnataka 2004**

A 5 : 1. B 1 : 2.
C 2 : 1 D 1 : 5

**75. All hernias involving bowel that reach the stage of vascular compromise, do cause symptoms & signs of intestinal obstruction, except : Karnataka 2005**

A. Sciatic hernia B. Littre's hernia
C. Cloquet's hernia D. Scraffini's hernia

**Ans. 66. B 67. C 68. B 69. D 70. C 71. C 72. A 73. C 74. D 75. B**

# EXPLANATIONS OF HERNIA

1. Ans.— D. Is a deficiency in the transversalis fascia.
2. Ans.— D. Gaur's sign
3. Ans.— A. Bladder
4. Ans.— C. Scrotum
5. Ans.— C. 3-4 years
6. Ans.— A. Both A and R are true and R is the correct explanation of A.
7. Ans.— B. Enterocele
8. Ans.— B. Lateral border of rectus abdominis

   It is a type of interparietal hernia occurring commonly at the level of arcuate line. Strangulation may occur due to rigid fascia surrounding neck.
9. Ans.— B. No surgery required
10. Ans.— B. Seen in young adults (15-25 years of age)
11. Ans.— A. Poupart's ligament
12. Ans.— D. Angiography
13. Ans.— B. Ileoinguinal nerve
14. Ans.— C. Lateral cutaneous nerve of thigh
15. Ans.— D. Six weeks
16. Ans.— C. Sigmoid colon

    As a result of sliding of posterior parietal peritoneum on the underlying retroperitoneal stricture the posterior wall of the sac is not formed of the retro peritoneum alone but by the sigmoid colon and mesentery on Lt. caecum on Rt. and on either side by a portion of bladder. Five out of six hernia are situated on Rt. side.
17. Ans.— E. It can be prevented by applying pressure over the internal ring with finger tip after reduction.

    Woman practically never develop a direct inguinal hernia. Predisposing factors are a chronic cough, straining and heavy work. It constitutes 10-15% of inguinal hernias and over half of these are bilateral.
18. Ans.— C. U
19. Ans.— C. Femoral
20. Ans.— C. They often regress spontaneously before the first birthday.
21. Ans.— C. Associated hernia
22. Ans.— C. Indirect Hernia

    Indirect (or oblique) inguinal hernia is the most common of all forms of hernia. It is most common in the young whereas a direct hernia is most common in middle life or after. In the first decade of life, inguinal hernia is more common on the right side in the male. After second decade, it is equally common on both sides.
23. Ans.— D. Anaemia and malnutrition
24. Ans.— B. 2.5
25. Ans.— A. Left posterior
26. Ans.— D. Maydl's
27. Ans.— D. Maydl's
28. Ans.— A. Gibbon's
29. Ans.— B. Femoral hernia
30. Ans.— C. Scrotal
31. Ans.— C. At the deep inguinal ring
32. Ans.— D. Hydrocele of the canal of Nuck
33. Ans.— A. Herniotomy

    Herniotomy is sufficient for the treatment of hernia in infants, adolescents and young fit adults who have good inguinal musculature.
34. Ans.— D. In superimposition
35. Ans.— C. For 2 weeks
36. Ans.— A. 3 years
37. Ans.— C. Done at about the age of two years
38. Ans.— B. Amniotic membrane
39. Ans.— B. Narrowing of the internal ring

40. Ans.— B. Is usually associated with lipoma

41. Ans.— A. 1.25 cm

42. Ans.— C. Kronlein hernia

43. Ans.— A. Muscular weakness

44. Ans.— B. Littre's hernia

45. Ans.— D. Indirect inguinal (oblique)

46. Ans.— B. 2-4%

47. Ans.— B. More common after paramedian incision than after midline incision.

48. Ans.— A. Often strangulates

It does not strangulate commonly.

49. Ans.— D. Absolute constipation and vomiting are pathognomonic.

50. Ans.— B. Tender

Strangulation commonly occurs in oblique inguinal hernia and due to truss worn for a long time and in those with partially reduceable or irreduceable hernia.

51. Ans.— B. Inguinal ligament

52. Ans.— C. Has the pectineal ligament as its lateral border.

53. Ans.— A. First decad Male Right

54. Ans.— B. Double breasting of transversalis fascia and repair with darning material.

55. Ans.— B. Fatty hernia of the Linea alba

56. Ans.— A. Excision of the hernial sac

57. Ans.— B. Richter's hernia

58. Ans.— D. Surgery

59. Ans.— A. Surgical repair

60. Ans.— C. Hypospadias

61. Ans.— B. Spermatocele

62. Ans.— B. Sliding hernia

63. Ans.— C. Exudation

64. Ans.— C. It is associated with spermatic cord

65. Ans.— A. Dyspnoea

66. Ans.— B. Femoral hernia

67. Ans.— C. A truss

68. Ans.— B. A fatty hernia of the linea alba

69. Ans.— D. Defect lies between sternal and costal attachment of diaphragm.

This cyst or hydrocele of canal of neck lies in relation to the round ligament.

70. Ans.— C. Oesophagitis and structure

71. Ans.— C. That there is a impaired blood flow to the contents.

72. Ans.— A. Incising the sub-cutaneous tissue

73. Ans.— C. Neck of sac

Although, inguinal hernia is four times more common than femoral hernia, a femoral hernia is more likely to strangulate becuase of narrowness of neck of sac and its rigid walls.

74. Ans.— D 1 : 5

75. Ans.— B. Littre's hernia

# 15

# IMPORTANT TEXT OF URINARY SYSTEM

## MILESTONES IN HISTORY

| | |
|---|---|
| 1556 | **Franco**—First suprapubic approach for removal of vesical calculus. |
| 1870 | **J. Begelow**—Performed Litholapexy (named by Oliver Wendell Holmes). |
| 1895 | **Hugh Yong**—Performed first prostatectomy. |
| 1986 | **Nitze**—Introduced his operating cystoscope. |
| 1870-1945 | **Huge Hampton Young**—"Father of Modern Urology" |
| 1824-76 | **Gustar Simon**—Pioneer in Renal Surgery performed nephrotomy in 1862. |
| 1881 | **Hahn**—Performed the first two nephropexies. |
| 1950 | **Lawier, West, Mc Nulty, Clancy and Murphy**—Performed the first successful human renal homotransplantation in Chicago (1936 **Voronoy**—transplanted kidney). |

## HAEMATURIA

*Causes*

1. Infection 40%
2. Tumour 20%
3. Obstruction 15% (prostate)
4. Stone 20%
5. Trauma 5%

*Site*

1. Kidney 15%
2. Ureter 15%
3. Bladder 40%
4. Prostate 25%
5. Urethra 5%

Don't Forget

1. Generalised bleeding diatheses
2. Unusual causes : Endocarditis, polyarteritis nodosa, malignant hypertension, glomerulonephritis, mitral stenosis, cystic kidneys
3. Tumours are increasingly common after 40 years.

## CAUSES OF URINARY OBSTRUCTION

1. *Pelvis*
   (i) Congenital pelviureteric junction obstruction
   (ii) Tumour, stone, clot
2. *Ureter*
   (i) Stone/clot
   (ii) Tumour - ureter, bladder, prostate
   (iii) Stricture
   (iv) Uretercele
   (v) Aberrant vessels
   (vi) Cancer colon/rectum, cervix
   (vii) Retroperitoneal fibrosis
3. *Urethra*
   (i) Prostate
   (ii) Stricture
   (iii) Foreign bodies
   (iv) Congenital valves

## RENAL INJURIES COMMONLY ASSOCIATED WITH INJURY TO

1. Spleen
2. Liver
3. Pancreas
4. Diaphragm
5. 11th and 12th rib fractures. Fractures of transverse processes

# HISTORICAL FEATURES DIFFERENTIATING TYPES OF INCONTINENCE IN THE ELDERLY

| | *Urge* | *Stress* | *Functional* | *Overflow* |
|---|---|---|---|---|
| Causes | Uninhibited detrusor activity | Sphincter insufficiency | Musculoskeletal<br>Environmental<br>Psychological | Outlet obstruction<br>Underactive detrusor<br>Impaired sensation |
| ***History*** | | | | |
| Amount of urine loss | Moderate to large | Small to moderate | Variable, often | Small |
| Frequency | Normal or increased | Increased, voids | Normal preventively | Increased |
| Nocturnal | Common; accidents on way to toilet | No | Accidents on way to toilet<br>Restraints<br>IV<br>Bedrails<br>Change in environment or cognition | Common |
| Triggers | Short warning<br>Stress induced | Coughing<br>Laughing<br>Sneezing Exercise | | |
| Associated | Urgency | Obesity<br>Multiparity | Unsuccessful bladder repairs | History of diabetes<br>Symptoms of prostatism |
| Palpable bladder | No | No | No | Yes, when gross retention present |

# MCQ's OF URINARY SYSTEM

## What is important in Urinary System

Polycystic kidney, Horseshoe Kidney, Pyonephrosis, Renal calculi and Tumours (Wilm's Grawitz's), Bladder (Calculi, Diverticulum, Cancer, Rupture of Bladder and Urethra)

1. **Subcapsular nephrectomy is indicated in : UPSC 1986**
   A. Perinephric abscess
   B. Solitary adenocarcinoma
   C. Hydronephrosis
   D. Pyonephrosis

2. **Assuming that the case is a renal cell tumour, the preferred treatment would be : UPSC 1986**
   A. Partial nephrectomy
   B. Intracapsular nephrectomy
   C. Radical nephrectomy
   D. Radiotherapy and chemotherapy

3. **Wilm's tumor is best treated by : JIPMER 1993**
   A. Surgery
   B. Radiotherapy
   C. (A) + (B)
   D. (A) + (B) + Chemotherapy

4. **The Renal collar to prevent spread of malignancy from kidney is put around : JIPMER 1993**
   A. Renal Artery B. Renal vein
   C. Aorta D. IVC

5. **Extravasation of urine in Extraperitoneal rupture of bladder is : AI 1993**
   A. Behind the anogenital diaphragm
   B. Around perivesical space
   C. Into the groin
   D. In the scrotum

6. **Posterior urethral valves are commonly situated : Delhi 1993**
   A. Above verumentanum
   B. At verumentanum
   C. Below verumentanum
   D. Bladder neck

7. **If urine escapes when a patient rises after completion of urination, which of the following should be strongly considered : PGI 1984**
   A. Cystitis B. Neurogenic bladder
   C. Urethral diverticulum D. Stress incontinence
   E. Urge incontinence

8. **The most reliable diagnostic method in rupture of bladder is : AIIMS 1985, 86**
   A. Catheterization
   B. Cystoscopy
   C. Retrograde cystogram
   D. Recovery of injected fluid
   E. Await signs of peritoneal irritation

9. **Anuria is always suggestive of : Karnataka 1998**
   A. Intrinsic renal disease B. Obstructive cause
   C. Pre-renal disorder D. Acute tubular necrosis

10. **Anline, bilharzia, magenta and exfoliative cytology are related in terms of : UPSC 1983, 86**
    A. Carcinoma of the colon
    B. Carcinoma of the cervix
    C. Bronchial tumours
    D. Bladder tumours

11. **In kidney trauma, indication for immediate surgical intervention is : UPSC 1985**
    A. Lump in the flank B. Haematuria
    C. Urinary extravasation D. Hydronephrosis
    E. Hypertension

12. **Nephrectomy for a traumatic lesion should be never performed until : Delhi 1986**
    A. Adequate contralateral function ascertained
    B. Fluid replacement is complete
    C. Antibiotics have been given
    D. The abdomen has been explored
    E. Cystoscopy has been carried out

**Ans.** 1. D 2. C 3. D 4. D 5. B 6. C 7. C 8. C 9. B 10. D
11. C 12. A

**13. Features of tuberculosis epididymitis include all, except : AIIMS 1985**
A. The vas often becomes 'beaded'
B. Usually globus minor is first affected
C. Feels firm and raggy
D. The testis proper is soon involved
E. A lax secondary hydrocele may be present

**14. Haematuria at the beginning of micturition is indicative of : AIIMS 1984**
A. Bladder neck pathology
B. Renal pathology
C. Benign prostatic hypertrophy
D. Urethral pathology
E. None of the above

**15. When renal injury is suspected, intravenous pyelography should be done : UPSC 1987**
A. Immediately in most cases
B. Electively in most cases
C. Only if there is oliguria
D. Only if there is anuria
E. Only if there is haematuria

**16. The principal complaint of a patient with uretheral calculus is : UP 1991**
A. Nocturia
B. Urgency and incontinence
C. Haematuria
D. Renal colic
E. Palpable kidney

**17. Which of the following is not correct about extra-peritoneal rupture of the bladder : UPSC 1985**
A. Shock is present
B. Catheterisation is not allowed
C. Sign of the fracture pelvis usually present
D. The organ is palpable

**18. Match List-I with List-II and select the correct answer : CSE 1996**

| List-I Acute retention of urine in a | List-II Causes |
|---|---|
| A. Man of 65 years | 1. Stricture of urethra |
| B. Man of 35 years | 2. Benign prostatic hypertrophy |
| C. Woman of 50 years | 3. Posterior urethral valve |
| D. New-born neonate | 4. Bladder neck obstruction |

| | A | B | C | D |
|---|---|---|---|---|
| A. | 1 | 2 | 4 | 3 |
| B. | 1 | 2 | 3 | 4 |
| C. | 2 | 1 | 4 | 3 |
| D. | 2 | 1 | 3 | 4 |

**19. Bladder cancer most constantly shows which : Rohtak 1986**
A. Dysuria
B. Urgency
C. Increased frequency
D. Haematuria
E. Persistent & recurrent urinary infection

**20. In haemodialysis, too rapid removal of the following substance, especially in children may lead to convulsions: PGI 1985**
A. Creatine
B. Creatinine
C. Urea
D. Potassium

**21. In renal injury following blunt injury to abdomen, which is not done : AIIMS 1992**
A. IVP
B. Diagnostic peritoneal lavage
C. Exploratory laparotomy
D. Prophylactic nephrectomy

**22. All of the following statements regarding benign prostatic hypertrophy are true except: CSE 1996**
A. Glandular and the stromal components of prostate undergo hypertrophy.
B. Urodynamic measurements help to distinguish obstructive from non-obstructive prostatic hypertrophy.
C. Trans-rectal ultrasonography does not help in differentiating obstructive from non-obstructive prostatic hypertrophy.
D. Middle and lateral lobes of prostate undergo hypertrophy.

**23. Oliguria is excretion of urine less than ——c.c. in 24 hours : UPSC 1992**
A. 300
B. 500
C. 600
D. 1000

**24. Normal capacity of the renal pelvis is: CMC 1986; AIIMS 1987**
A. 7 ml
B. 10 ml
C. 15 ml
D. 20 ml

**25. Dormia basketing is used for removal of renal calculi in the : JIPMER 1985, 87**
A. Pelvic ureteric junction
B. Upper 1\3rd of ureter
C. Middle 1\3rd of ureter
D. Lower 1\3rd of ureter

**26. Earliest symptom of Wilm's tumour is : JIPMER 1986, 88**
A. Hematuria
B. Pyrexia
C. Abdominal tumour
D. Metastasis

**27. Commonest cause for pulsion diverticulum of the urinary bladder is : JIPMER 1984, 86**
A. Benign enlargement of prostate
B. Fibrous prostate
C. Contracture of bladder neck
D. Stricture urethra

**Ans.** 13. D 14. D 15. A 16. D 17. D 18. C 19. D 20. A 21. D 22. C 23. A 24. A 25. D 26. C 27. C

**28. The commonest cause of idiopathic hydronephrosis :** **Delhi 1985, 86, 87; AMC 1985, 88**
A. Duplicate pelvis
B. Stone
C. Redudant pelvis
D. Congenital stenosis of ureteropelvic junction

**29. T2 stage of Ca bladder is :** **Orissa 1998**
A. Mucosal invasion
B. Submucosal invasion
C. Muscularis mucosa involvement
D. Pelvic tissue involvement

**30. Complimentary operation done at the time of prostatectomy is:** **AIIMS 1984, 87**
A. Vasectomy B. Circumcision
C. Hernia repair D. All of the above

**31. The minimal amount of urine required to excrete the end products of metabolism is :** **Delhi 1982**
A. 200 ml B. 400 ml
C. 600 ml D. 750 ml

**32. The classical symptom of urinary bilharziasis is :** **AIIMS 1986**
A. Intermittent, painless, terminal haematuria
B. Continuous painful haematuria
C. Intermittent painful haematuria
D. Haemoptysis + haematuria

**33. The commonest bladder stone is :** **PGI 1984, 86**
A. Tripple phosphate B. Xanthine
C. Uric acid D. Cysteine

**34. Regarding polycystic kidney, one of the following is true :** **TN 1989**
A. Generally bilateral
B. Autosomal recessive inheritance
C. Hypertension occurs in 10% cases
D. Urine of high specific gravity

**35. In a case of pelvic fracture with urethral injury, the most important first step in management is :** **AIIMS 1984**
A. Repair of injured urethra
B. Fixation of pelvic fracture
C. Treatment of shock and haemorrhage
D. Splinting urethra with catheters

**36. The commonest late complication of traumatic rupture of urethra is :** **UPSC 1989; JIPMER 1992**
A. Stricture B. Chordee
C. Diverticulum D. Retrograde ejaculation

**37. Which of the following does not occur in Unilateral renal trauma :** **AIIMS 1992, 94**
A. Uremia
B. Clot formation
C. Perinephric haematoma
D. Hypertension

**38. Following are true of Ureteric stone except :** **AIIMS 1992**
A. Source is almost always kidney
B. Urine is always infected
C. Should be removed immediately
D. Pain is referred to lip of penis in intramural stones

**39. Rupture of Bulbar urethra is associated with all of the following except :** **AIIMS 1992**
A. Perineal haemotoma B. Pelvic fracture
C. Urethral haemorrhage D. Retention of urine

**40. Rupture of membranous urethra occurs more commonly because of :** **AIIMS 1992**
A. Angulation B. Thin unsupported wall
C. Fixity of urethra D. Proximity to bladder

**41. Following are true of Horseshoe kidney except :** **AIIMS 1992**
A. Lower calyx is reserved
B. Spider like appearance
C. Heminephrectomy improves function
D. Ureteral obstruction is common

**42. A persistent urinary specific gravity — mosm/L indicates a failing kidney.** **AMU 1986**
A. 100 B. 150
C. 250 D. 300

**43. Alkalinity of urine is usually taken as pH more than :** **AMU 1986**
A. 7.0 B. 7.4
C. 8.2 D. 10.2

**44. Urine output in a 6 months old child in m/hour :** **PGI 1984**
A. 10 B. 30
C. 35 D. 60

**45. Three glass test is used for :** **AIIMS 1986**
A. Posterior urethritis B. Cystitis
C. Infection of the kidney D. Any of the above

**46. A 45 years old male comes with complaint of flank pain without much dysuria & massive (gross) hematuria; urine M/E shows 5-10 RBCs. Next investigation to be done is :** **Rajasthan 1995**
A. CT abdomen
B. IVP
C. Exploratory Laparotomy
D. MRI

**47. In trauma to kidney, Nephrectomy is indicated only when there is :** **UPSC 1986**
A. Hypertension B. Haematuria
C. Hydronephrosis D. Urinary extravasation

| Ans. | 28. D | 29. C | 30. A | 31. B | 32. A | 33. A | 34. A | 35. C | 36. A | 37. A |
|---|---|---|---|---|---|---|---|---|---|---|
| | 38. B | 39. B | 40. C | 41. C | 42. D | 43. B | 44. A | 45. D | 46. B | 47. D |

**48. Which of the following is most frequently associated with renal artery aneurysm : AMU 1986**

A. Hypertension B. Hematuria
C. Abdominal bruit D. Abdominal pain
E. All of the above

**49. Predisposing factors for pyelonephritis would include all of the following except : CSE 1996**

A. Male sex
B. Bladder autonomic neuropathy
C. Vesico-ureteric reflux
D. Lower tract obstruction

**50. Acute onset of auria in elderly men is seen in : AIIMS 1986; AI 1989**

A. Bilateral infarction of kidneys
B. Obstructive urinary disease
C. Acute tubular necrosis
D. Acute cortical necrosis

**51. Post-gonococcal stricture in urethra is most commonly situated in the : AI 1989**

A. Bulb
B. Penoscrotal Junction
C. Distal part of spongy urethra
D. Just distal to external meatus

**52. Narrowest part of the male urethra is : PGI 1986**

A. External meatus B. Membranous urethra
C. Bulbous urethra D. Internal meatus

**53. After an operation for a perforated bowel an elderly patient develops hypotension and oliguria. If the obliguria persists and the following may be useful except : UPSC 1988**

A. Peritoneal dialysis
B. Hydrochlorothiazide administration
C. Haemodialysis
D. Calcium

**54. About left loin nephrectomy, following are cut except : PGI 1998**

A. Trapezius B. Serratus inf. post.
C. Latissimus dorsi D. Internal oblique

**55. Posterior urethral valves are commonly observed in : AIIMS 1984, 87**

A. Boys B. Girls
C. Adult males D. Adult females

**56. Anterior abdominal approach to kidney is justifiable in: AMC 1985, 87**

A. Pyelonephritis B. TB kidney
C. Tumour D. Polycystic disease

**57. Wrong about papilloma in urinary bladder is : Delhi 1982, 83; AIIMS 1982, 87**

A. Painless haematuria B. Periodic haematuria
C. Clot retention D. Pain in perineum

**58. Pus cell without bacilli in an acid urine indicates: Delhi 1982, 88; AMC 1986**

A. TB kidney
B. Phosphate calculi
C. Multiple myeloma
D. Subacute bacterial endocarditis

**59. Anaemia in Wilm tumour is : AMC 1986; Delhi 1987**

A. Microcytic hypochromic
B. Normocytic normochromic
C. Macrocytic
D. None of the above

**60. The least dilatable part of the Urethra is : WB 1996**

A. Prostatic
B. Membranous
C. Spongy
D. All are equally dilatable

**61. The cause of hypertension sweating, dyspnoea, pallor, tachycardia, headche and bilateral abdominal mass is: AIIMS 1983; UPSC 1986**

A. Bilateral aderenal hyperplasia
B. Polycystic kidney
C. Hydronephrosis
D. Horseshoe kidney

**62. While giving bath mother noticed an abdominal mass (unilateral) in 1.5 year old boy, the mass was not crossing midline and there was hemiatrophy . The diagnosis is : UPSC 1981, 83; ESI 1985**

A. Wilm's tumour
B. Neuroblastoma
C. Adenocarcinoma kidney
D. Horseshoe kidney

**63. Most malignant renal tumuor is : UPSC 1983**

A. Grawitz tumor
B. Papillary tumors
C. Squamous cell carcinoma of renal pelvis
D. Wilm's tumor

**64. In surgery for pheochromocytoma, hypotension is because of : Delhi 1986, 87**

A. Removal of catecholamines
B. Resistance to catecholamines
C. Endogenous substance
D. Decreased blood volume

| Ans. | | | | | | | | | |
|---|---|---|---|---|---|---|---|---|---|
| 48. D | 49. A | 50. B | 51. A | 52. A | 53. B | 54. A | 55. A | 56. C | 57. D |
| 58. A | 59. B | 60. B | 61. D | 62. A | 63. C | 64. A | | | |

**65. All of the following are (relative) contraindications for performing a renal transplantation except : MAHE 1996**

A. Age > 60 years
B. Chronic pyelonephritis
C. Generalised bronchiectasis
D. Oxalosis

**66. In an old patient lying in bed for prolonged period, the cause of pain in right loin referring to testis is : Delhi 1988**

A. Appendicitis B. Amoebiasis
C. Ureteric stone D. Constipation

**67. In Intraperitoneal rupture of urinary bladder, not seen is : Delhi 1986**

A. Agonising pain B. Distension of abdomen
C. Shock D. Desire to micturate

**68. Features of phaeochromocytoma include all except : AIIMS 1986**

A. Pallor
B. Hypoglycemia
C. Increased arterial tension
D. Blurring of vision

**69. Features of vesical papilloma include all except : AP 1988**

A. Pain in perineum B. Intermittent haematuria
C. Painless haematuria D. Clot retention

**70. "Jackstone calculi" are found in : AMU 1989**

A. Kidneys B. Ureters
C. Urinary bladder D. Post. prostatic pouch

**71. The most common complication of polycystic kidney in an adult includes : AIIMS 1987**

A. Hypertension B. Haematuria
C. Infection D. Uraemia

**72. Reflex centre for micturition is located in : AIIMS 1985**

A. Cerebrum B. Sacral region of cord
C. Lumbar region of cord D. None of the above

**73. In case of bilateral renal calculi the kidney to be operated upon first is : UPSC 1986**

A. One with better function
B. One with lesser function
C. Any of the above
D. Both at the same time

**74. Painful haematuria may be due to : PGI 1988**

A. Tuberculosis of the kidney
B. Acute cystitis
C. Renal tumour
D. Bleeding disorder

**75. In a clear cell carcinoma of the kidney with a solitary pulmonary metastasis, proceed with : AP 1989**

A. Symptomatic treatment
B. Removal of the diseased kidney
C. Chemotherapy
D. Radiotherapy of lung and affected kidney

**76. On exertion urine steam increases in : AP 1996**

A. Prostate enlargement
B. Marion's disease
C. Post. Urethral valves
D. Urethral Stricture

**W77. All of the following are contraindications to litholapexy except : DNB 1990**

A. Prostatic obstruction.
B. Urethral stricture that cannot be dilated completely.
C. When the patient is below 10 years of age.
D. A very small stone.

**78. Incontinence of urine is more common when prostatectomy is done by : AIIMS 1985**

A. Trans-vesical route B. Retropubic route
C. Trans-uretheral D. From the perineum

**79. One of the following has greater significance in deciding prognosis of carcinoma bladder : AIIMS 1985**

A. Site of occurrence in the bladder
B. Time onset of haematuria
C. Age of the patient
D. Depth of bladder wall invasion

**80. Which is false regarding Hydronephrosis : Delhi 1986**

A. Can be produced by intermittent urinary obstruction.
B. Can follow phimosis.
C. Nephrectomy should be done in all cases.
D. Dietl's crisis is seen.

**81. Wilm's tumour of the kidney : AIIMS 1984**

A. Occurs predominantly in adults
B. May have both adenomatous and carcinomatous segments
C. Is radioresistant
D. Is usually small

**82. Regarding the Waterhouse-Friderichsen syndrome : UPSC 1985**

A. Most cases occur in adults.
B. Treatment should await the result of blood culture.
C. Adrenalectomy is indicated.
D. It is a complication of meningitis.

| Ans. | | | | | | | | | | |
|---|---|---|---|---|---|---|---|---|---|---|
| Ans. | 65. B | 66. C | 67. D | 68. B | 69. A | 70. D | 71. C | 72. B | 73. A | 74. B |
| | 75. B | 76. D | 77. NONE | 78. B | 79. D | 80. C | 81. B | 82. D | | |

**83. Regarding phaeochromocytoma, incorrect is : UPSC 1987**

A. It is bilateral about 15% of cases.
B. It produces noradrenaline.
C. All patients under 60 years who present with sustained arterial hypertension deserve a routine test to confirm or exclude the condition.
D. Treatment should depend upon antihypertensive drugs.

**84. Which of the following explains strangury : AIIMS 1985**

A. Intense desire to pass urine.
B. Painful micturition.
C. The desire to micturite remains unappeased after the act of micturition and patient tends at painful straining.
D. It is analogue of tenesmus.

**85. Which of the following is not true regarding hydronephrosis : Delhi 1987**

A. It may be due to Dietl's crisis
B. It may be due to phimosis
C. It may be due to ureteric stone
D. It is always due to complete obstruction to outflow of urine from a kidney

**86. Which of the following is not included in the list of acquired urinary fistulas : AMU 1986**

A. Vesico-vaginal B. Uretero-vaginal
C. Vesico-colic D. Ectopia vesicae

**87. Post-gonococcal stricture urethra is most commonly situated in the : AP 1989**

A. Bulb
B. Penoscrotal junction
C. Distal part of spongy urethra
D. Just distal to external meatus

**88. Urinary diversion by operation is indication in all of the following except : UPSC 1987**

A. Following cystectomy
B. In cases of ectopia vesicae
C. In cases of having loss of sphincteric control over urinary bladder
D. As a routine is cases of vesico-vaginal fistula

**89. Which of the following is most useful in distinguishing a renal carcinoma : DNB 1989**

A. Intravenous urogram
B. Retrograde pyelogram
C. Radio-active venogram
D. Renal arteriogram

**90. Renal tuberculosis originates in the : DNB 1990**

A. Renal papilla
B. Renal medulla
C. Afferent tubules
D. Efferent arteriole of glomerulus

**91. Vesical stones occur more commonly in : TN 1988**

A. Males B. Females
C. Equal in both D. Variable occurrence

**92. After the injection of a colored dye intravenously the time for appearance of dye in the ureter is : AIIMS 1984**

A. 5-7 hours B. 20 mts
C. 40 mts. D. 60 mts.

**93. Medical adrenalectomy in recurrent carcinoma breast is done with ; AIIMS 1985, 87**

A. Steroids B. Aminoglutethimide
C. Tamoxifen D. Radiotherapy

**94. Which of the following is not a cause of renal amyloidosis : AIIMS 1985, 87**

A. Recurrent urinary tract infection
B. Tuberculosis
C. Leprosy
D. Rheumatoid arthritis

**95. The following testicular tumour has a benign course : AIIMS 1985**

A. Teratoma B. Choriocarcinoma
C. Seminoma D. Leydig cell tumour

**96. Recognised clinical features of Wilm's tumour include each of the following except : AIIMS 1986, 87**

A. Distant metastasis in lungs
B. Silent renal mass
C. Stripped calcification in tumour mass
D. Distortion of renal pelvis on IVP

**97. The following procedure is not useful in the diagnosis of phaeochromocytomas : AIIMS 1986**

A. Phentolamine test B. Histamine test
C. Glucagon infusion D. Urinary catecholamines

**98. Radiolucent stone is : AIIMS 1986; AI 1990**

A. Oxalate B. Phosphate
C. Urates D. Mixed

**99. Most common form of renal fusion is : AIIMS 1987, 90**

A. Pelvic kidney
B. Horseshoe kidney
C. Sigmoid kidney
D. Crossed ectopia with fusion

Ans. 83. D 84. C 85. D 86. D 87. A 88. D 89. D 90. A 91. A 92. A
93. B 94. A 95. D 96. C 97. B 98. C 99. B

**100. An 82 years old man underwent open prostatectomy. Histology revealed benign nodular hyperplasia with an area of focal adenocarcinoma and following further treatment recommended : UPSC 1985; AIIMS 1987**

A. Deep X-ray therapy B. Stilbestrol therapy
C. No treatment D. Orchidectomy

**101. In phaeochromocytoma, treatment is by : JIPMER 1997**

A. Beta blocker followed by alpha blocker.
B. Alpha followed by beta blocker.
C. Both given together and later on alpha blocker.
D. Both given together and later on beta blocker.

**102. The commonest type of congenital renal anomaly is : AIIMS 1987**

A. Horseshoe kidney B. Polycystic disease
C. Duplication of pelvis D. Duplication of ureter

**103. Retention of urine in an old man is due to all of the following except : AIIMS 1987**

A. BPH B. Ca prostate
C. Post. urethral valve D. Urethral stricture

**104. Commonest type of cancer renal pelvis and upper ureter is : UPSC 1986; AIIMS 1988**

A. Transitional cell carcinoma
B. Adenocarcinoma
C. Nephroblastoma
D. Squamous cell carcinoma

**105. Ureterocele occurs due to : AIIMS 1989, 90**

A. Ureters crossing behind artery
B. Renal calculus
C. Ureteric orifice stenosis
D. Congenital intramural malformation

**106. Triad of renal colic, swelling in loin which disappears after passage of urine : AIIMS 1990**

A. Kocher's triad B. Saint's triad
C. Charcot triad D. Dietl's crisis

**107. Renal stone in cases of massive bowel resection occurs due to : AIIMS 1990**

A. ↑ Absorption of Vitamin-D
B. Increased absorption of oxalates
C. Impaired calcium excretion
D. None of the above

**108. Undescended testis is characterized by all except : PGI 1986; AIIMS 1990**

A. 50% in premature babies
B. Generally descend during 1st year of life
C. To be operated at puberty
D. May be bilateral

**109. The left testicular vein drains into : UPSC 1983; PGI 1986; Delhi 1989**

A. Left renal vein B. Left internal iliac vein
C. Inferior vena cava D. Left common iliac vein

**110. The commonest surgical cause of gross hematuria in children is : PGI 1986**

A. Acute glomerulonephritis
B. Acute pyelonephritis
C. Trauma
D. Calculus

**111. Which does not occur in Adrenal cortical tumors : AI 1993**

A. Striae over body B. DM
C. ↑ ACTH D. Hyperkalemia

**112. Commonest symptom of phaeochromocytoma is : AMC 1985; AIIMS 1990**

A. Palpitation B. Headache
C. Sweating D. Dyspnoea

**113. Ectopic ureter opens into the following except : AIIMS 1998**

A. Bladder neck B. Prostatic urethra
C. Bulbous urethra D. Seminal vesicles

**114. Which of the following is least likely to injure the ureter : MAHE 1996**

A. Abdominoperineal resection
B. Penetrating abdominal trauma
C. Radiation therapy for carcinoma of the cervix
D. Radical hysterectomy

**115. Which of the following is not important for the aetiology of renal calculi : AMC 1983**

A. Malabsorption B. Infection
C. Immobilization D. Urea splitting organism

**116. A 26 years old male was found to be infertile 1 year after marriage. He had a history of retroperitoneal lymphnode removal for embryonal cell ca, right testis, when he was 15 years old. His semen analysis showed...Volume 0.5 ml, no sperm, no fructose. TRUS showed a normal seminal vesicle and vas deferens. Lt. testicular biopsy demonstrated spermatogenesis. Treatment of choice is : AI 1999**

A. Electro ejaculation and artificial insemination.
B. Aspiration from epididymis and intra-cytoplasmic injection into ovum.
C. Surgical removal of ejaculatory duct.
D. Artificial insemination from donor.

**Ans.** 100. C 101. B 102. C 103. C 104. A 105. C 106. D 107. B 108. C 109. A
110. D 111. C 112. B 113. C 114. B 115. A 116. B

**117. Urinary incontinence results from following except :** **AIIMS 1985**

A. Neurogenic bladder B. Vesico vaginal fistula
C. Ectopic ureter D. Rectovesical fistula

**118. Renal calculi are radio opaque in :** **UPSC 1982, 87; AMC 1984**

A. 100% B. 95%
C. 70% D. 30%

**119. "Kiss Cancer" of the urinary bladder is :** **UPSC 1988**

A. Highly malignant B. Malignant
C. Benign D. Pre-malignant

**120. Least likely site for bladder cancer is :** **PGI 1989**

A. Vault B. Lateral wall
C. Posterior wall D. Trigone
E. Ureteric orifices

**121. Ideal approach for renal malignancy is :** **AIIMS 1984, 85, 89**

A. Transperitoneal
B. Retroperitoneal
C. Lumbar incision
D. Abdominothoracic incision

**122. The cause of gross hematuria in a male below 40 years of age is :** **UPSC 1982, 83; AMC 1987**

A. Renal trauma B. Prostatitis
C. Oxalate stone D. Carcinoma prostate

**123. Spider leg appearance in IVP is suggestive of :** **AP 1984; Kerala 1986, 88; JIPMER 1987**

A. Renal cyst B. Renal trauma
C. Renal TB D. Hydronephrosis
E. Chronic renal failure

**124. Staghorn calculus is made up of :** **UPSC 1986**

A. Oxalate B. Phosphate
C. Urate D. Cysteine

**125. Glomerular filtration stops when systolic pressure falls below :** **JIPMER 1986, 87**

A. 90 mm Hg B. 80 mm Hg
C. 70 mm Hg D. 60 mm Hg

**126. Drug used for medical adrenal medullectomy is :** **Kerala 1990**

A. Aminogluethemide
B. Ortho-para methyl benzoic acid
C. Alloxan
D. Methiodobenzo guanidine tagged $I^{131}$

**127. Nephrocalcinosis is seen in all except :** **PGI 1983, 88**

A. Polycystic kidney
B. Hyperparathyroidism
C. Medullary sponge kidney
D. Renal tubular acidosis

**128. Evidence of trauma to kidneys is all except :** **AI 1994**

A. Haematuria
B. Enlarged kidney shadow
C. Hypertension
D. Meteorism

**129. Rupture of perineal urethra causes collection of Blood in :** **AIIMS 1993**

A. Deep perineal pouch B. Sup. Inguinal region
C. Ischiorectal Fossa D. Pelvic diaphragm

**130. In hypernephroma, all are true except :** **AIIMS 1993**

A. Usually adenocarcinoma
B. It is radiosensitive
C. Present with rapidly developing varicocele
D. It arises from cortex, possibly from pre-existing adenoma

**131. All are true about renal cell carcinoma except :** **AIIMS 1994**

A. Arises from PCT
B. Invades renal vein
C. More common in female
D. Hematuria may occur

**132. A 10-years old child develops sudden agonising pain in the right side of the scrotum without history of trauma or fever. The scrotum is swollen and the testicle is situated high in the scrotum. Elevation aggravates the pain and there is not leucocytosis. The most appropriate line of management will be :** **UPSC 1994**

A. Immediate exploration of the scrotum.
B. To give analgesics and wait for 24 hours.
C. To give antibiotics and wait for 24 hours.
D. To give local fomentation to relieve the pain.

**133. A 5-years old child presents with diffuse aches and pain and left flank pain had mass with skeletal survey showing irregular lytic lesions. Most likely diagnosis is :** **UPSC 1994**

A. Wilm's tumour with skeletal metastasis.
B. Neuroblastoma with skeletal metastasis.
C. Lymphoma with secondary LN.
D. Undiagnosed malignancy with diffuse metastasis.

**134. Commonest cause of enterovesical fistula in adult is :** **AI 1999**

A. Carcinoma colon B. Ulcerative colitis
C. Crohn's disease D. AP resectio

**Ans.** 117. D 118. B 119. C 120. A 121. A 122. C 123. A 124. B 125. C 126. A
127. A 128. C 129. A 130. B 131. C 132. A 133. B 134. C

**135. The accurate diagnostic aid in renal artery stenosis is : Karnataka 1994**
A. Selective renal angiography
B. Ultrasound
C. CT Scan
D. Inferior vena cava

**136. Epidermoid carcinoma of renal pelvis is usually associated with : Karnataka 1994**
A. Multiple papillomas B. Pelvic calculus
C. TB kidney D. Filariasis

**137. True about uric acid stone is : AI 1995**
A. Common in alkaline urine
B. Radio opaque
C. 20% of renal stones
D. Common in ulcerative colitis

**138. True about renal trauma is : AI 1995**
A. Urgent IVP
B. Exploration of kidney in majority
C. Lumbar approach to kidney
D. Renal artery aneurysms are common

**139. Malignancy and phaeochromocytoma is diagnosed by : AI 1995**
A. Vascular invasion
B. Anaplasia
C. Increase in nuclear cytoplasmic ratio
D. All of the above

**140. Mechanism of stress incontinence : PGI 1993**
A. Loss of posterior angle between bladder neck and urethra
B. Funneling of bladder neck
C. Raised intravesical pressure (> 60 mm Hg)
D. Decreased bladder size

**141. Most common type of renal transplantation in India is : AI 1999**
A. Allograft B. Autograft
C. Isograft D. Xenograft

**142. Which is not true about aberrant renal vessels : PGI 1994**
A. Bilateral common B. More on left side
C. Common in females D. Causes hydronephrosis

**143. Commonest cause of acute retention of urine is : AMU 1989**
A. Stricture B. BPH
C. Stone D. None

**144. A 12-years-old boy experiences sudden severe pain in the right testis. On palpation there is tenderness. The most likely diagnosis is : PGI 1986**
A. Spontaneous haemorrhage
B. Torsion
C. Strangulated hernia
D. Epididymitis
E. Seminoma of the testis

**145. Which of the following statements regarding ureters is correct : PGI 1994**
A. Cross anteriorly to uterine vessels.
B. There is a dilatation at pelvic ureteric junction.
C. Cross laterally to sacroiliac joint.
D. Blood supply from ant. division of int. iliac artery.

**146. Renal calculi is more often seen in patients with massive bowel resection because : AIIMS 1994**
A. Increased absorption of calcium from gut
B. Increased absorption of oxalate from gut
C. Reduced calcium excretion
D. None of the above

**147. Regarding angiohematomas of kidney which is incorrect : AIIMS 1994**
A. Presents with hypertension
B. Loin pain
C. Nephrectomy is the treatment of choice
D. Bleeding is self- limited

**148. Which is false about Renal cell carcinoma : AIIMS 1995**
A. Polycythemia common
B. F > M
C. Hyperchloremic alkalosis
D. Hyperchloremic acidosis

**149. All are true for TB kidney except : AIIMS 1995**
A. Pyuria seen B. Bacteriuria seen
C. Increased frequency D. Decreased pH of urine

**150. U/L renal agenesis is associated with : AIIMS 1995**
A. Single umbilical artery
B. Polycystic disease of pancreas
C. Hypogonadation
D. Hiatus hernia

**151. Which about renal trauma is not true : AIIMS 1995**
A. Exploration indicated in all cases
B. Observation is best
C. IVP is indicated
D. Haematuria is cardinal sign

**152. All are true regarding Wilm's tumor except : AIIMS 1992**
A. Good prognosis in infants
B. Pre-operative use of Actinomycin-D
C. Post-operative radiotherapy
D. Neuroblastoma is the commonest differential diagnosis

| Ans. | 135. A | 136. B | 137. D | 138. A | 139. A | 140. A | 141. A | 142. A | 143. B | 144. B |
|---|---|---|---|---|---|---|---|---|---|---|
| | 145. D | 146. B | 147. C | 148. B | 149. B | 150. A | 151. A | 152. B | | |

**153. Posterior urethral valves may be associated with : Delhi 1995**

A. Hydronephrosis B. Renal dysplasia
C. Pulm. dysplasia D. All of the above

**154. The commonest tumour of urinary bladder is : AI 1988**

A. Papilloma
B. Adenocarcinoma
C. Transitional cell carcinoma
D. Squamous cell carcinoma

**155. Duke's Stage C2 refers to carcinoma : UPSC 1995**

A. Bladder penetrating the extravesical fat.
B. Bladder with metastasis to internal iliac lymph nodes.
C. With histological features of 75% anaplastic cells.
D. Rectum with metastasis to inferior mesenteric lymph nodes.

**156. A sixty years old male presented with a profuse painless hematuria. He had low grade fever and had lost weight, no clinical symptoms were detected. The IVP showed that the right renal pelvis is deformed and pushed way up above. There is a large soft tissue mass at the lower pole. There is no evidence of dilated renal pelvis. The most likely diagnosis would be: UPSC 1986**

A. Hydronephrosis
B. Chronic pyelonephritis
C. Renal cell carcinoma
D. Stone in the right kidney

**157. Which of the following variants if renal cell carcinoma has the worst prognosis. UPSE 1995**

A. Papillary B. Tubuloalveolar
C. Chromophobe D. Sarcomatoid

**158. One of the following is not a common adrenal gland tumour : AP 1993**

A. Haemangioma B. Myelolipoma
C. Aldosteronoma D. Phaeochromocytoma

**159. Symptoms of Wilm's tumor include all except : PGI 1988; Delhi 1994; Orissa 1994**

A. Haematuria B. Dysuria
C. Pyrexia D. Mass abdomen

**160. Polycystic Kidney has the following features except : Delhi 1994, 95**

A. Spider leg appearance on I.V.P.
B. Haematuria
C. Specific gravity urine above 1020
D. Secondary pyelonephrities

**161. In neuroblastoma, the following are raised except : AP 1993**

A. MHPG B. VMA
C. HVA D. None of the above

**162. Polycystic kidney disease is associated with congenital cysts in the following except : TN 1989**

A. Lungs B. Liver
C. Pancreas D. Spleen

**163. The ureteric stone is usually composed of : Delhi 1987**

A. Calcium phosphate B. Calcium Oxalate
C. Sodium urate D. Calcium carbonate

**164. Infantile polycystic disease is : AMC 1986**

A. Autosomal dominant B. Autosomal recessive
C. Sex linked recessive D. Not known

**165. Aberrant renal vessels are more common in : Delhi 1987**

| | Sex | Side |
|---|---|---|
| A. | Males | Left |
| B. | Males | Right |
| C. | Females | Left |
| D. | Females | Bilateral |

**166. Which of the following factor in Wilm's tumour carries better prognosis : AIIMS 1985**

A. Age below 1 year B. Unilateral type
C. Arises from one pole D. Age above 4 years

**167. The following may be the presentation of Grawitz's tumour except : AMU 1990**

A. Polycythemia B. Nephrotic syndrome
C. Hypertension D. Phaeochromocytoma

**168. The following are the features of ectopia vesicae except : AMU 1989**

A. Umbilicus absent
B. Umbilical and inguinal hernia
C. Laxed rectal sphincter
D. Hydronephrosis

**169. The commonest cause of retention of urine in a male child is : PGI 1983**

A. Urethral stricture B. Meatal ulcer
C. Phimosis D. Urethral calculus

**170. The earliest symptom of bladder calculus in a child is : Delhi 1983; Kerala 1999**

A. Pain B. Acute retention
C. Frequency D. Haematuria

**171. The congenital valves of the posterior urethra are commonest ——— the verumontanum. Delhi 1983**

A. Above B. Just below
C. At D. Any of the above

**172. The commonest congenital malformation of urethra is : PGI 1982**

A. Hypospadias B. Stricture
C. Epispadias D. Duplication

| Ans. | 153. A | 154. C | 155. D | 156. C | 157. D | 158. A | 159. B | 160. C | 161. A | 162. D |
|---|---|---|---|---|---|---|---|---|---|---|
| | 163. B | 164. B | 165. C | 166. A | 167. D | 168. D | 169. B | 170. C | 171. B | 172. A |

**173. All of the following are advantages of uretero-ileostomy except : AIIMS 1986**
A. Incidence of pyelonephritis is less.
B. Uriniferous odour is reduced.
C. Highly successful for epispadias.
D. Highly successful in cases of urinary incontinence associated with spina bifida.

**174. In the above case, all the following investigations are of value except : UPSC 1986**
A. Ultrasonography
B. CAT Scan
C. Arteriography and venacavagraphy
D. Renal scan

**175. Flower "Vase" pattern of the renal pelvis in an Intra-venous urogram is seen in : AIIMS 1984**
A. Polycystic kidney B. Renal carcinoma
C. Horseshoe kidney D. Ectopic kidney

**176. Recent left varicocele in an adult should make one suspect : AMU 1989**
A. Filariasis B. Inguinal hernia
C. Left renal carcinoma D. Portal hypertension

**177. Best palliative procedure in Mid renal carcinoma is : AIIMS 1992**
A. Transverse colostomy
B. Perineal loop
C. Abdomino-perineal resection
D. Anterior resection

**178. The following are more common in the left side except : DNB 1991**
A. Duplication of renal pelvis
B. Aberrant renal vessels
C. Renal extopia
D. Crossed dystopia

**179. The least common site of metastasis of Wilm's tumour is : DNB 1991**
A. Liver B. Lungs
C. Bones D. Brain

**180. The following drugs may be useful in the treatment of Wilm's tumour except : AMU 1989**
A. Actinomycin-D B. Vincristine
C. Cyclophosphamide D. 5-FU

**181. The irradiation of the Wilm's tumour is recommended in the following situations except : AMU 1989**
A. Pre-operatively
B. Post-operatively
C. Alongwith chemotherapy
D. Post-operatively alongwith chemotherapy

**182. In Wilm's tumour, X-ray of abdomen characteristically shows —— type of calcification. PGI 1989**
A. Speckled B. Diffuse
C. Corvilinear D. Any of the above

**183. Medullary sponge kidney is often associated with : DNB 1991**
A. Atresia of bile ducts
B. Congenital hepatic fibrosis
C. Galactosemia
D. Cardiac cirrhosis

**184. Following are the commonest renal calculi : Kerala 1990**
A. Calcium oxalate
B. Uric acid
C. Calcium magnesium phosphate
D. Cystine

**185. Ureteral injuries most often are a result of : PGI 1982**
A. Blunt abdominal trauma
B. Gunshot wounds of the abdomen
C. Stab wound of the abdomen
D. Stab wound of the flank
E. Surgical trauma

**186. Treatment of choice for adenocarcinoma of kidney is : AMU 1987**
A. Surgery B. Radiotherapy
C. Chemotherapy D. Immunotherapy

**187. Most constant feature of Ca bladder is : PGI 1996**
A. ↑ Strangury B. Haematuria
C. Recurrent UTI D. Referred pain

**188. True about phaeochromocytoma is : PGI 1995**
A. A soft blue coloured malignant tumor.
B. Presents as yellowish discolouration of face.
C. Urinary HIAA levels are increased.
D. Hypertension is always paroxysmal.

**189. Renal transplant rejection in less than one month is : Rohtak 1985**
A. Acute B. Chronic
C. Hyperacute D. Any of the above

**190. Treatment of Papillary tumor of base of bladder is : Rohtak 1995**
A. TUR B. Cystodiathermy
C. Bladder removal D. Radiotherapy

| Ans. | 173. C | 174. D | 175. C | 176. C | 177. A | 178. D | 179. D | 180. D | 181. A | 182. C |
|---|---|---|---|---|---|---|---|---|---|---|
| | 183. B | 184. A | 185. E | 186. A | 187. B | 188. B | 189. A | 190. B | | |

**191. Best investigation to differentiate between renal cyst and tumor : Rohtak 1996; TN 1996**

A. Clinical examination B. X-ray
C. Ultrasound D. Arteriography

**192. Following are true about renal vein thrombosis in a neonate except : PGI 1990**

A. Diabetic mother
B. Gross hematuria & kidney palpable
C. Aglycoside treatment
D. In B/L, renal failure not occurs

**193. True about congenital polycystic kidney : PGI 1996**

A. Retention of urine not seen
B. Hypotension common
C. Haematuria in 75%
D. Polycythemia

**194. In ureterovaginal fistula, most common presentation is : PGI 1996**

A. Vaginal swelling
B. Continuous incontinence
C. Fever
D. Uremia

**195. Acute nephrosis is seen in : AIIMS 1993, 94**

A. Enteric fever B. SLE
C. Pneumonia D. Fanconi's syndrome

**196. To localize ureter, best is : AIIMS 1996**

A. Renal vein accomplices B. Arterial plexus
C. Lumbar plexus D. Peristalsis

**197. Following are associated with exostrophy of bladder except : AI 1997**

A. Wide pelvis
B. No ant. abdominal wall
C. Rudimentary testes
D. Cloacal membrane defect

**198. Most common predisposing factor for chronic pyelonephritis is : AI 1996**

A. DM B. Stone
C. PUV D. Vesicoureteric reflux

**199. A 60 years old male has been operated for carcinoma of caecum and right hemicolec-tomy has been done. On the fourth post-operative day, the patient develops fever and pain in legs. The most important clinical entity one should look for is : UPSC 1996**

A. Urinary tract infection
B. Intravenous line infection
C. Chest infection
D. Deep vein thrombosis

**200. A known patient with renal stone disease developed pathological fractures along with abdominal pain and certain psychiatric symptoms. He should be investigated for : UPSC 1996**

A. Polycystic kidney B. Renal tubular acidosis
C. Hyperparathyroidism D. Paget's disease of bone

**201. Consider the following statements : UPSC 1996**

A : Radical nephrectomy for a hypernephroma should be done through the anterior transperitoneal approach.

R : Lumbar incision does not give a good exposure of the kidney.

**Of these statements :**

A. Both A and R are true and R is the correct explanation of A.
B. Both A and R are true but R is not the correct explanation of A.
C. A is true but R is false.
D. A is false but R is true.

**202. Consider the following conditions : UPSC 1996**

1. Hydronephrosis
2. Wilm's tumour
3. Neuroblastoma
4. Pheochromocytoma
5. Tumour in undescended testis

**The common abdominal lumps in children are due to :**

A. 1, 2, 3 B. 1, 4, 5
C. 2, 3, 4 D. 1, 2, 5

**203. Simplest diagnostic aid to differentiate a solid & cystic renal cyst is : TN 1996**

A. USG B. CT Scan
C. MRI D. Plain X-ray

**204. About Pyelonephrosis, not true is : Punjab 1997**

A. Common after ac. pyelonephritis
B. Due to infection of hyphonephrotic sac
C. Follows renal calculi
D. Unilateral as a rule

**205. Following are true of Adult polycystic kidney disease except : AIIMS 1997**

A. Progression to terminal stage renal disease is more with PKDI than with Type-II.
B. Progression to terminal stage renal disease is more in females than in males.
C. Autosomal dominant inheritance is the most common mode of inheritance.
D. Though rarer than infantile form is a more severe type than infantile form.

| Ans. | 191. C | 192. D | 193. A | 194. B | 195. A | 196. D | 197. C | 198. D | 199. D | 200. C |
|---|---|---|---|---|---|---|---|---|---|---|
| | 201. A | 202. A | 203. A | 204. D | 205. D | | | | | |

**206. For renal transplant the kidneys should be removed from the dead body within : Bihar 1998**
A. 30 mins B. 60 mins
C. 2 hours D. 3 hours

**207. A 40 years old male presented with pain in costovertebral angle with radiation to loin. Plain X-ray revealed a ureteric stone. False statement regarding this clinical situation is : MAHE 1998**
A. 90% renal stones are opaque.
B. Rediolucent stones contain uric acid.
C. Staghorn calculi commonly occur in alkaline urine.
D. Radio opaque stones are most commonly due to cystine.

**208. Worst prognosis in renal cell carcinoma is associated with : MAHE 1998**
A. Haematuria B. Size > 5 cm
C. Invasion of renal vein D. Pulmonary secondaries

**209. Emergency nephrostomy is most often done in : Rajasthan 1998**
A. Pyonephrosis
B. Pelviureteral obstruction
C. Carcinoma
D. Colonic obstruction of ureter

**210. Cystine stones are : Rajasthan 1998**
A. Triangular B. Circular
C. Hexagonal D. Rectangular

**211. Which of the following statements about renal transplantation is false : MAHE 1992, 94**
A. The donor and the recipient must be ABO-compatible.
B. To achieve maximal function of the transplanted kidney, the warm ischaemic time should not exceed 30 minutes.
C. The donor kidney is usually placed in the right renal bed.
D. The characteristic signs of acute rejection include pyrexia, hypertension and leucocytosis.

**212. All the following statements about renal trauma are true except : MAHE 1994**
A. It should always be suspected in any patient with blunt abdominal trauma.
B. It commonly presents with loin pain and overt/microscopic haematuria.
C. An urgent intravenous pyelogram is one of the most important investigations.
D. Acute parenchymal failure occurs very often.

**213. Gerota's fascia has surgical importance, it normally envelops : Orissa 1999**
A. Lungs B. Kidney
C. Bladder and prostate D. Ureter

**214. Polycystic kidneys may be associated with all of the following except : AI 1991**
A. Congenital cystic liver
B. Congenital pancreatic cysts
C. Congenital lung cysts
D. Congenital brain cysts

**215. In urodynamic study, normal pressure in males should not exceed ——— cm of $H_2O$ : Kerala 1999**
A. 40 B. 60
C. 80 D. 20

**216. Colour of fluid in Epididymal cyst is : Kerala 1999**
A. Barley Water B. Amber colour
C. Crystal clear D. Yellowish Gray

**217. Urinary stones are associated with : MAHE 1999**
A. Paraplegia
B. Myaesthenia gravis
C. Hypercholesterolemia
D. Primary aldosteronism

**218. Which one of the following features suggests strangulation in an inguinal hernia : UPSC 2000**
A. No change in the hernial swelling on coughing and straining.
B. A tense and tender swelling with no impulse on coughing.
C. Vomiting and diarrhoea.
D. Partial reduction in swelling on manipulation.

**219. During investigation of hydronephrosis, isotope renogram is mainly useful in : UPSC 2000**
A. Detecting vesicoureteric reflux
B. Anatomical definition
C. Distinguishing between non-obstructed and obstructed system
D. Identifying ectopic kidney tissue

**220. Rapid sequence excretory urography is used in : UP 2000**
A. Renovascular hypertension
B. Renal transplant rejection
C. Renal cell carcinoma
D. VUJ obstruction

**221. An X-ray pelvis shows urinary bladder calcification that resembles fetal head in pelvis. The likely cause is : AIIMS 2000**
A. Tuberculosis B. Malignancy
C. Schistosomiasis D. Chronic cystitis

| Ans. | 206. D | 207. D | 208. C | 209. B | 210. C | 211. C | 212. D | 213. B | 214. D | 215. B |
|---|---|---|---|---|---|---|---|---|---|---|
| | 216. C | 217. A | 218. B | 219. C | 220. D | 221. C | | | | |

**222. A patient with renal stone having pain with radiation in medial side of thigh and perineum due to slipping of stone in ureter, most likely position of stone is : AIIMS 2000**

A. Junction of ureter and renal pelvis
B. At pelvic brim
C. Intramural opening of ureter
D. At crossing of gonadal vessels and ureter

**223. A boy presents with one episode of painless gross hematuria. An excretory urogram showed a filling defect towards the lower renal infundibulum 1.5 cm in size. What is the next investigation to be done : AIIMS 2000**

A. Cystoscopy
B. Ultrasonography
C. Retrograde pyelography
D. Urine cytology

**224. An 85-years-old man underwent Transurethral resection of prostate. A histological examination of his specimen showed foci of adenocarcinoma. What is the next step in management : AIIMS 2000**

A. Endocrine therapy B. No further treatment
C. Radical surgery D. Hormone therapy

**225. A 5 years child present with calculus of size 2 cm in the upper ureter and haematuria. On USG no obs is seen. TT of choice : AI 2001**

A. Ureterolithotomy B. Endoscopy
C. ESWL D. Observation

**226. Incidence of renal ectopia is : AI 1992**

A. 1 in 1000 B. 1 in 10,000
C. 1 in 50, 000 D. 1 in 1,00,000

**227. A 5-years old child presents with diffuse aches and pain and left flank pain had mass with skeletal survey showing irregular lytic lesions. Most likely diagnosis is : AI 1994**

A. Wilm's tumor with skeletal metastasis
B. Neuroblastoma with skeletal metastasis
C. Lymphoma with secondary LN
D. Undiagnosed malignancy with diffuse metastasis

**228. Not associated with weight gain : AI 1996**

A. Pheochromocytoma B. Acromegaly
C. Cushing's syndrome D. Myxoedema

**229. Patient presents after trauma, with blood at the tip of urinary meatus and only pass a drop of urine. Next step is : AI 2001**

A. Arrange for dialysis
B. MCU
C. Catherterise, drain bladder, remove foleys catheter
D. Catheterise and retain foleys catheter

**230. Chandu, a 45 years male has calcification on AP view right side of abdomen and lateral view the calcification is seen to overlie the spine. Most likely diagnosis is : AI 2001**

A. Gallstones
B. Calcified mesenteric nodes
C. Renal stones
D. Calcified Rib

**231. Best investigation for trauma of urinary bladder is: Kerala 2001**

A. Retrograde cystography
B. IVP
C. USG
D. Plain X-ray

**232. All are true regarding bladder stones except : AIIMS 2001**

A. Primary bladder stones are rare in Indian children.
B. Small stones can be removed by transurethral endoscopy.
C. KUB gives definitive diagnosis.
D. >90% are radioopaque.

**233. In an infant with congenital PUJ obstruction, all the following are true except : AIIMS 2001**

A. Can be diagnosed antenatally.
B. Congenital PUJ obstruction is more commonly due to vascular aberrations than intrinsic cause.
C. Diuretic renogram is helpful in diagnosis.
D. Retrograde pyloroplasty has to be done to know the type and site of lesion.

**234. A 36-years-old female came with flank pain and was found to have PUJ obstruction. All the following are true regarding this, except : AIIMS 2001**

A. Bilateral in 10-15% of the cases.
B. Dismembered pyloroplasty is the treatment of choice.
C. Endoscopic pyloromyotomy is contraindicated.
D. None of the above.

**235. In a patient with tripple phosphate stones, all of the following are true except : AIIMS 2001**

A. Also known as Struvite stones
B. Prone to occur because of infection
C. Needs acidic urine to precipitate
D. Forms staghorn calculi

**Ans.** **222. B 223. B 224. B 225. C 226. A 227. B 228. A 229. B 230. C 231. A 232. A 233. B 234. C 235. C**

**236. Conservative management is indicated for ureteric stones when : AIIMS 2001**

A. The stones are small (<6mm).
B. Hydronephrosis and infection is present.
C. The stone does not descend for 2 weeks of follow-up.
D. Anatomic anomalies.

**237. True regarding urethral injuries are all except : AIIMS 2001**

A. Uncommon in females.
B. Bladder injury is associated with post-urethral injuries.
C. Blood at the urethral meatus is indicative of injury.
D. Catheterize the patient.

**238. A 6 months old child with recurrent UTI was wound on MCU, have grade IV vesicoureteric reflux. The bladder wall is normal. The treatment of choice would be : AI 2002**

A. Ureteric reimplantation
B. Teflon injection to ureteric orifices
C. Antibiotics and observe
D. Endoscopic ureteric resection

**239. A middle aged diabetic female presented with a history of flank pain and fever. On USG, the kidney was an irregular and showed fat density lesion with calculi. The diagnosis is most likely to be : AIIMS 2001**

A. Renal abscess
B. Chronic pyelonephritis
C. Xanthogranulomatous kidney
D. TB kidney

**240. Distention of abdomen with passage of large amount of urine is known as : Maharashtra 2000**

A. Dietl's crisis
B. Andersons Hynes crisis
C. Meteriorism
D. None

**241. Commonest cause of calcium oxalate stones in renal system is : CMC 2001**

A. Hyperparathyroidism
B. Idiopathic hypercalcuria
C. RTA
D. PCKD

**242. Young boy with h/o severe pain in testis after intercourse & o/e pain not relieved by elevation of testis : CMC 2001**

A. Epididymo-orchitis B. Torsion testis
C. Ca. testis D. Fournier's gangrene

**243. Phosphate supplementation helps to reduce the chances of formation of which renal stones: Maharashtra 2002**

A. Staghorn calculus
B. Cysteine stones
C. Oxalate stones
D. Triple phosphate stones

**244. Consider the following statement :**
**Polycystic disease of the kidneys may present with : UPSC 2002**

1. Chronic renal failure
2. Haematuria and renal colic
3. Hypertension
4. Accidentally on routine examination of abdomen

**Which of these statements are correct :**

A. 1 and 3 B. 2 and 4
C. 1, 3 and 4 D. 1, 2, 3 and 4

**245. Operation of choice for Retro Caval Ureter is : UPSC 2002**

A. Cutting and suturing IVC
B. Cutting and suturing ureter
C. Anderson-Heynes pyeloplasty
D. Uretero cystoplasty

**246. A 30 years old male presents with severe bladder irrition, persistent pyuria, microscopic hematuria and absence of bacteria in usual smears and culture. Which is the probable diagnosis : UPSC 2002**

A. Monilial infection
B. Lower urinary tract obstruction
C. Vesical calculus
D. Genito-urinary tuberculosis

**247. A 30-years old male presents with pain on the right flank and hematuria. A CECT abdomen reveals a large 8 x 8 cm sized solid mass in the right kidney and a 3x3 cm solid mass occupying the upper pole of left kidney. The most appropriate surgical treatment for this patient is : AIIMS 2002**

A. Bilateral radical nephrectomy.
B. Right radical nephrectomy and Biopsy of the mass from opposite kidney.
C. Right radical nephrectomy and left partial nephrectomy.
D. Right radical nephrectomy only.

**248. The following statements are true about germ cell tumours of the testes except : AIIMS 2002**

A. They constitute 90-95% of all primary testicular tumors.
B. Seminoma is the most common tumor developing in patients with cryptorchid testes.
C. Alpha-fetoprotein is markedly raised in all germ cell tumors.
D. High Inguinal Orchidectomy is the initial surgical procedure.

**Ans.** 236. A 237. D 238. A 239. C 240. A 241. A 242. B 243. C 244. D 245. B 246. D 247. C 248. C

**249. A 25-years-old male presents to the Emergency Department following a road traffic accident. On examination there is pelvic fracture and blood at the urethral meatus. The following are true about this patient, except : AIIMS 2002**

A. The anterior urethra is most likely the site of injury.
B. Retrograde urethrography should be done after the patient is stabilized.
C. Foley catheter may be carefully passed if the RGU is normal.
D. Rectal examination may reveal a large pelvic hematoma with the prostate displace superiorly.

**250. The commonest cause of an obliterative stricture of the membranous urethra is : AI 2003**

A. Fall-astride injury
B. Road traffic accident with fracture pelvis & rupture urethra
C. Prolonged catheterization
D. Gonococcal infection

**251. The best time for surgery of hypospadias is : AI 2003**

A. 1-4 months of age
B. 6-10 months of age
C. 12-18 months of age
D. 2-4 yrs of age

**252. A 70 years old patient with benign prostatic hyperplasia underwent transurethral resection of prostate under spinal anaesthesia. One hour later, he developed vomiting and altered sensorium. The most probable cause is : AI 2003**

A. Overdosage of spinal anaesthetic agent
B. Rupture of bladder
C. Hyperkalemia
D. Water intoxication

**253. Which of the following lasers is used for the treatment of benign prostatic hyperplasia as well as urinary calculi : AI 2003**

A. $CO_2$ laser B. Excimer laser
C. Ho-YAG laser D. Nd : YAG laser

**254. Semen analysis of a young man who presented with primary infertility revealed low volume, fructose negative ejaculate with azoospermia. Which of the following is the most useful imaging modality to evaluate the cause of this infertility : AI 2003**

A. Colour duplex ultrasonography of the scrotum
B. Transrectal ultrasonography
C. Retrograde urethrography
D. Spermatic venography

**255. In pheochromocytoma there is increased level of : MAHE 2003**

A. Serum HMA B. Serum bradykinin
C. Urinary VMA D. All of the above

**256. A 10-mm calculus in the right lower ureter associated with proximal hydrouretheronephrosis is best treatment modality of choice will be : AI 2003**

A. Extracorporeal shock wave lithotripsy
B. Antegrade percutaneous access
C. Open ureterolithotomy
D. Ureteroscopic retrieval

**257. A 55-years-old male presented with painless terminal hematuria. Cystoscopic examination revealed a solitary papillary tumor. Histopathological examination of completely resected tumor is suggestive of grade-III transitional cell carcinoma with no muscle invasion. Further management of this patient is best done by : AI 2004**

A. Just follow-up
B. Intravesical chemotherapy
C. Intravesical BCG
D. Cystectomy

**258. Polycystic disease of the kidney may have cysts in all of the following organs except : AI 2004**

A. Lung B. Liver
C. Pancreas D. Spleen

**259. Agent of choice for intravesical therapy for carcinoma in situ of bladder cancer following endoscopic treatment is : UPSC 2004**

A. BCG B. Mitomycin-C
C. Adriamycin D. Thio-TEPA

**260. Radical nephrectomy for renal cell carcinoma does NOT involve the excision of : UPSC 2004**

A. Kidney with Gerota's fascia
B. Pre and Para aortic lymph nodes
C. Adrenal Gland
D. Complete ureter with a cuff of urinary bladder

**261. Anaemia of advanced renal insufficiency is best treated by : UPSC 2004**

A. Blood transfusions
B. Recombinant human erythropoietin
C. Parentral iron therapy
D. Folic acid

**Ans.** 249. A 250. B 251. D 252. D 253. C 254. D 255. D 256. D 257. C 258. A 259. A 260. D 261. B

# EXPLANATIONS OF URINARY SYSTEM

1. Ans.— D. Pyonephrosis
2. Ans.— C. Radical nephrectomy
3. Ans.— D. (A) + (B) + Chemotherapy
4. Ans.— D. IVC
5. Ans.— B. Around perivesical space
   It is due to anatomical connections.
6. Ans.— C. Below verumentanum
7. Ans.— C. Urethral diverticulum
8. Ans.— C. Retrograde cystogram
9. Ans.— B. Obstructive cause
   Anuria is defined as the complete absence of urine production. Oliguria is the excretion of only 300 ml in a 24 hours period. Renal calculus disease is the most common cause of acute obstruction leading to anuria.
10. Ans.— D. Bladder tumours
11. Ans.— C. Urinary extravasation
12. Ans.— A. Adequate contralateral function ascertained.
13. Ans.— D. The testis proper is soon involved
14. Ans.— D. Urethral pathology
15. Ans.— A. Immediately in most cases
16. Ans.— D. Renal colic
17. Ans.— D. The organ is palpable
18. Ans.— C. 2 1 4 3
19. Ans.— D. Haematuria
20. Ans.— A. Creatine
21. Ans.— D. Prophylactic nephrectomy
22. Ans.— C. Trans-rectal ultrasonography does not help in differentiating obstructive from non-obstructive prostatic hypertrophy.
23. Ans.— A. 300
24. Ans.— A. 7 ml
25. Ans.— D. Lower 1\3rd of ureter
26. Ans.— C. Abdominal tumour
27. Ans.— C. Contracture of bladder neck
28. Ans.— D. Congenital stenosis of ureteropelvic junction.
29. Ans.— C. Muscularis mucosa involvement
30. Ans.— A. Vasectomy
31. Ans.— B. 400 ml
32. Ans.— A. Intermittent, painless, terminal haematuria.
33. Ans.— A. Triple phosphate
34. Ans.— A. Generally bilateral
35. Ans.— C. Treatment of shock and haemorrhage
36. Ans.— A. Stricture
37. Ans.— A. Uremia
38. Ans.— B. Urine is always infected
39. Ans.— B. Pelvic fracture
40. Ans.— C. Fixity of urethra
41. Ans.— C. Heminephrectomy improves function
42. Ans. D. 300
43. Ans.— B. 7.4
44. Ans.— A. 10
45. Ans.— D. Any of the above
46. Ans.— B. IVP
47. Ans.— D. Urinary extravasation
   Surgical exploration is necessary in less than 10% of closed injuries and is indicate if either there are signs of progressive blood loss or there is an expanding mass in the loin. If laceration is confined to one pole kidney, partial nephrectomy may be practicable.
48. Ans.— D. Abdominal pain
49. Ans.— A. Male sex

50. Ans.— B. Obstructive urinary disease

51. Ans.— A. Bulb

52. Ans.— A. External meatus

53. Ans.— B. Hydrochlorothiazide administration

54. Ans.— A. Trapezius

55. Ans.— A. Boys

They are usually found just distal to the verumontanum but they may be within the prostatic urethra.

56. Ans.— C. Tumour

57. Ans.— D. Pain in perineum

58. Ans.— A. TB kidney

As a rule no pus or organism are present. Leucocytic count is always raised (20,000/mm$^3$) urine is highly acidic.

59. Ans.— B. Normocytic normochromic

60. Ans.— B. Membranous

61. Ans.— D. Horseshoe kidney

62. Ans.— A. Wilm's tumour

63. Ans.— C. Squamous cell carcinoma of renal pelvis

64. Ans.— A. Removal of catecholamines

65. Ans.— B. Chronic pyelonephritis

66. Ans.— C. Ureteric stone

67. Ans.— D. Desire to micturate

68. Ans.— B. Hypoglycemia

Basis of lab diagnosis is measurement of elevated catecholamines and their metabolites in urine. Confirmation is usually readily made by measurement of free catecholamines vainillylmandelic Acid & meta adrenalines (metanephrins) in 24 hours collection of urine. Pt usually excrete free catecholamines in excess of 100 mg/24 hrs. VMA in excess of 7 mg/24 hrs and metadrenalines in excess of 1.3 mg/24 hrs. False +ve metadrenaline elevation may occur in pt on MAO inhibitors and who have had recent angiographic studies.

69. Ans.— A. Pain in perineum

70. Ans.— D. Post. prostatic pouch

71. Ans.— C. Infection

72. Ans.— B. Sacral region of cord

73. Ans.— A. One with better function

74. Ans.— B. Acute cystitis

75. Ans.— B. Removal of the diseased kidney

76. Ans.— D. Urethral Stricture

77. Ans.— NONE

Question is wrong. All are contraindications.

78. Ans.— B. Retropubic route

79. Ans.— D. Depth of bladder wall invasion

80. Ans.— C. Nephrectomy should be done in all cases.

81. Ans.— B. May have both adenomatous and carcinomatous segments.

82. Ans.— D. It is a complication of meningitis

83. Ans.— D. Treatment should depend upon antihypertensive drugs.

84. Ans.— C. The desire to micturite remains unappeased after the act of micturition and patient tends at painful straining.

85. Ans.— D. It is always due to complete obstruction to outflow of urine from a kidney.

86. Ans.— D. Ectopia vesicae

87. Ans.— A. Bulb

88. Ans.— D. As a routine is cases of vesico-vaginal fistula.

89. Ans.— D. Renal arteriogram

90. Ans.— A. Renal papilla

91. Ans.— A. Males

92. Ans.— A. 5-7 hours

93. Ans.— B. Aminoglutethimide

94. Ans.— A. Recurrent urinary tract infection

95. Ans.— D. Leydig cell tumour

96. Ans.— C. Stripped calcification in tumour mass

97. Ans.— B. Histamine test

98. Ans.— C. Urates

Uric acid and urate calculi are hard and smooth, multiple hence typically faceted, colour varies from yellow to redish. Pure uric acid calculi are not radioopaque to X-ray but absolutely pure uric acid stone is very uncommon, have sufficient calcium deposition to make them radioopaque.

99. Ans.— B. Horseshoe kidney

**100. Ans.— C. No treatment**

**101. Ans.— B. Alpha followed by beta blocker**

**102. Ans.— C. Duplication of pelvis**

**103. Ans.— C. Post. urethral valve**

**104. Ans.— A. Transitional cell carcinoma**

**105. Ans.— C. Ureteric orifice stenosis**

**106. Ans.— D. Dietl's crisis**

**This is seen in hydronephrosis. Ultrasonography, excretion urography, isotope renography and *Whitaker Test* are used.**

**107. Ans.— B. Increased absorption of oxalates**

**108. Ans.— C. To be operated at puberty**

**109. Ans.— A. Left renal vein**

**110. Ans.— D. Calculus**

**111. Ans. C. ↑ ACTH**

**112. Ans.— B. Headache**

**113. Ans.— C. Bulbous urethra**

**114. Ans.— B. Penetrating abdominal trauma**

**115. Ans.— A. Malabsorption**

**116. Ans.— B. Aspiration from epididymis and intracytoplasmic injection into ovum.**

**117. Ans.— D. Rectovesical fistula**

**118. Ans.— B. 95%**

**119. Ans.— C. Benign**

**Reversal is possible if done within 3-4 years of vasectomy. Success rate is 60-80% because of autoantibodies against sequestered sperms.**

**120. Ans.— A. Vault**

**121. Ans.— A. Transperitoneal**

**122. Ans.— C. Oxalate stone**

**123. Ans.— A. Renal cyst**

**It is seen in polycystic kidney. The appearance can also be due to bell-like calyces. Rovsing operation is used.**

**124. Ans.— B. Phosphate**

**125. Ans.— C. 70 mm Hg**

**126. Ans.— A. Aminogluethemide**

**127. Ans.— A. Polycystic kidney**

**128. Ans.— C. Hypertension**

**Hypotension may be seen in many cases, abdominal distension occurs about 24-48 hours after accident. Sudden profuse delayed haematuria can occur between 3rd day and 3rd week after accident. Haematuria is cardinal sign. IVP is done to show that other kidney is normal.**

**129. Ans.— A. Deep perineal pouch**

**130. Ans.— B. It is radiosensitive**

**131. Ans.— C. More common in female**

**132. Ans.— A. Immediate exploration of the scrotum**

**133. Ans.— B. Neuroblastoma with skeletal metastasis.**

**134. Ans.— C. Crohn's disease**

**Among choices given, Crohn's disease is common cause in adults otherwise diverticulitis is the most common cause (occurs in 2-4% cases), Ca Colon (in people above 50) radiation bowel injury, external trauma, foreign bodies, and idiopathic are other causes.**

**135. Ans.— A. Selective renal angiography**

**136. Ans.— B. Pelvic calculus**

**137. Ans.— D. Common in ulcerative colitis**

**It is the commonest calculus (hard, smooth and multiple).**

**138. Ans.— A. Urgent IVP**

**It is done to assess function of opposite kidney. Abdominal mass, clot colic and pyrexia may also be present.**

**139. Ans.— A. Vascular invasion**

**140. Ans.— A. Loss of posterior angle between bladder neck and urethra.**

**141. Ans.— A. Allograft**

**David Hume and Joseph Killy undertook first successful series of kidney transplantations started in 1954.**

**142. Ans.— A. Bilateral common**

**143. Ans.— B. BPH**

**144. Ans.— B. Torsion**

**145. Ans.— D. Blood supply from ant. division of int. iliac artery.**

**146. Ans.— B. Increased absorption of oxalate from gut.**

**147. Ans.— C. Nephrectomy is the treatment of choice.**

148. Ans.— B. F > M

149. Ans.— B. Bacteriuria seen

150. Ans.— A. Single umbilical artery

151. Ans.— A. Exploration indicated in all cases

152. Ans.— B. Pre-operative use of Actinomycin-D

153. Ans.— A. Hydronephrosis

154. Ans.— C. Tránsitional cell carcinoma

Carcinoma arising within the bladder may be of three cell types — Transitional, squamous and adeno carcinoma, out of which 90% are Transitional type.

155. Ans.— D. Rectum with metastasis to inferior mesenteric lymph nodes.

156. Ans.— C. Renal cell carcinoma

157. Ans.— D. Sarcomatoid

158. Ans.— A. Haemangioma

159. Ans.— B. Dysuria

160. Ans.— C. Specfic gravity urine above 1020

It is the most common internal malignancy of childhood. Beck with Wiedemann syndrome is characterized by a midabdominal omphalocele association with a baby who is large for gestational age, macroglossia; visceromegaly of kidneys, adrenals and pancreas, high frequency of hepatoblastoma, Wilms tumor or adrenocortical carcinoma.

161. Ans.— A. MHPG

162. Ans.— D. Spleen

163. Ans.— B. Calcium Oxalate

164. Ans.— B. Autosomal recessive

165. Ans.— C. Females Left

166. Ans. D. Age below 1 year

167. Ans.— D. Phaeochromocytoma

168. Ans.— D. Hydronephrosis

169. Ans.— B. Meatal ulcer

The most frequent cause of acute urinary retention are —in male child (meatal ulcer with scabbing), in the male (bladder flow obstruction, urethral stricture, postoperative) and in the female (retroverted gravid uterus, multiple sclerosis).

170. Ans.— C. Frequency

171. Ans.— B. Just below

172. Ans.— A. Hypospadias

173. Ans.— C. Highly successfu`or epispadias

174. Ans.— D. Renal scan

175. Ans.— C. Horseshoe kidney

176. Ans.— C. Left renal carcinoma

177. Ans.— A. Transverse colostomy

178. Ans.— D. Crossed dystopia

179. Ans.— D. Brain

180. Ans.— D. 5-FU

181. Ans.— A. Pre-operatively

182. Ans.— C. Corvilinear

183. Ans.— B. Congenital hepatic fibrosis

184. Ans.— A. Calcium oxalate

Uric acid and urate calculi are hard and smooth, multiple hence typically faceted, colour varies from yellow to redish. Pure uric acid calculi are not radioopaque to X-ray but absolutely pure uric acid stone is very uncommon, have sufficient calcium deposition to make them radioopaque.

185. Ans.— E. Surgical trauma

186. Ans.— A. Surgery

187. Ans.— B. Haematuria

This is most common symptoms and should be regarded as sign of bladder carcinoma unless proved otherwise. Most common site is lateral wall, followed by trigone.

188. Ans.— B. Presents as yellowish discolouration of face.

189. Ans.— A. Acute

190. Ans.— B. Cystodiathermy

191. Ans.— C. Ultrasound

192. Ans.— D. In B/L, renal failure not occurs

193. Ans.— A. Retention of urine not seen

194. Ans.— B. Continuous incontinence

195. Ans.— A. Enteric fever

196. Ans.— D. Peristalsis

197. Ans.— C. Rudimentary testes

It is also called ectopia vesicae. Epispadiac penis is broad and short. Prostate and seminal vesicles are redementary but testes are normal.

198. Ans.— D. Vesicoureteric reflux
It causes ascending infection.

199. Ans.— D. Deep vein thrombosis

200. Ans.— C. Hyperparathyroidism

201. Ans.— A. Both A and R are true and R is the correct explanation of A.

202. Ans.— A. 1, 2, 3

203. Ans.— A. USG

204. Ans.— D. Unilateral as a rule

205. Ans.— D. Though rarer than infantile form is a more severe type than infantile form.

206. Ans.— D. 3 hours

207. Ans.— D. Radioopaque stones are most commonly due to cystine.

208. Ans.— C. Invasion of renal vein

209. Ans.— B. Pelviureteral obstruction

210. Ans.— C. Hexagonal

211. Ans.— C. The donor kidney is usually placed in the right renal bed.

212. Ans.— D. Acute parenchymal failure occurs very often.

213. Ans.— B. Kidney

214. Ans.— D. Congenital brain cysts
In 18% of cases there is a congenital cystic liver, congenital pancreatic cyst and lung cyst.

215. Ans.— B. 60

216. Ans.— C. Crystal clear

217. Ans.— A. Paraplegia

218. Ans.— B. A tense and tender swelling with no impulse on coughing.

219. Ans.— C. Distinguishing between non-obstructed and obstructed system.

220. Ans.— D. VUJ obstruction

221. Ans.— C. Schistosomiasis

222. Ans.— B. At pelvic brim

223. Ans.— B. Ultrasonography

224. Ans.— B. No further treatment

225. Ans.— C. ESWL

226. Ans.— A. 1 in 1000
Incidence of Renal ectopic 1 : 1000 mostly left kidney, arrested at brim of pelvis. As a rule the other kidney is at normal position with normal function.

227. Ans.— B. Neuroblastoma with skeletal metastasis.
In infants, metastasis confined to liver or subcutaneous fat are frequent and bone metastasis unusual. Prognostic factors include age site of primary, stage, histologic grade (Shimada), elevated serum neurone specific enolase in infants (poor prognosis), elevated serum feritin (poor prognosis); and analysis of the tumor for the presence of more than three copies of N-myc oncogenes (poor prognosis).

228. Ans.— A. Pheochromocytoma
Phaeocchromocytoma rarely causes weight gain. It is also called the 10% tumor because in 10% it is bilateral, malignant, extra-adrenal, multiple, familial and occur in children. Headache is most common symptom.

229. Ans.— B. MCU
MCU (Micturating cystourethrogram) is necessary to rule out urethral/bladder injuries.

230. Ans.— C. Renal stones
Mesenteric lymph nodes (Calcified) are anterior to spine on lateral view.

231. Ans.— A. Retrograde cystography

232. Ans.— A. Primary bladder stones are rare in Indian children.

233. Ans.— B. Congenital PUJ obstruction is more commonly due to vascular aberrations than intrinsic cause.

234. Ans.— C. Endoscopic pyloromyotomy is contra-indicated.

235. Ans.— C. Needs acidic urine to precipitate

236. Ans.— A. The stones are small (<6mm)

237. Ans.— D. Catheterize the patient

238. Ans.— A. Ureteric reimplantation
It will control vesicoureteric reflex.

239. Ans.— C. Xanthogranulomatous kidney

240. Ans.— A. Dietl's crisis

241. Ans.— A. Hyperparathyroidism

242. Ans.— B. Torsion testis

243. Ans.— C. Oxalate stones

244. Ans.— D. 1, 2, 3 and 4

245. Ans.— B. Cutting and suturing ureter

246. Ans.— D. Genito-urinary tuberculosis

247. Ans.— C. Right radical nephrectomy and left partial nephrectomy.

248. Ans.— C. Alpha-fetoprotein is markedly raised in all germ cell tumors.

249. Ans.— A. The anterior urethra is most likely the site of injury.

250. Ans.— B. Road traffic accident with fracture pelvis & rupture urethra.

Membranous urethral injury :

* MC cause - Secondary to Pelvic fractures.

Management :

* Mild to moderate injury - Usually by inserting Suprapubic catheter slowly and retaing it then ascending urogram is done to justify its position.

Complication - MC - Urethral stricture T/t - Sachse Optical Urethrotomy.

251. Ans.— D. 2-4 years of age

252. Ans.— D. Water intoxication

* *Water intoxication* - Because of repeated irrigation of surgical field during BPH Surgery which leads excess water reabsorption which lead to hypervolumia and hyponatremia.

* *Prevention* - Now-a-days 1.5% Isotonic Glycine is use for irrigation.

253. Ans.— C. Ho-YAG laser

* In BPH surgery-Laser ablation is done by Nd YAG laser.

* (According to Journal of endourology- Vol. 13, supplement 1, A-98, September-99).

254. Ans.— D. Spermatic venography

* Diagnosis in this question is obstruction of ejaculatory duct or Seminal vesicle.

* Diagnosis of Seminal vesicle obstruction is done by Venogram.

255. Ans.— D. All of the above

256. Ans.— D. Ureteroscopic retrieval

* Uretric stone usually arises in kidney.

* In 90% cases stone is single.

* In 90% cases stone is located in distal ureter.

* Distal 1/3 Uretric stones are best managed. By stone basketing or ureteroscopic removal.

* Proximal 1/3 & mid 1/3 Uretric stones are managed by ESWL.

* Patients not responsing to expectant, manipulative or ESWL therapy require open surgery.

257. Ans.— C. Intravesical BCG

This is a case of superficial papillary carcinoma (Ta) which are treated with complete transurethral resection of tumour and the selective use of intravesical therapy. (Intravesical BCG is more effective than intravesical chemotherapy).

*Rx Ca Urinary Bladder* (In short)

- *Noninvasive tumour* $T_a$, $T_1$

  Complete transurethral resection + Intravesical therapy

- *Invasive tumour* $T_2$, $T_3$

  Radical cystectomy, Radical radiotherapy or combination.

- *Lymph node or Distal metastasis*

  Systemic chemotherapy initially (Combination of cisplatin, Methotrexate, Adriamycin and Vinblastine = M-VAC)

258. Ans.— A. Lung

This question is also highly controversial.

- Acc. to Harrison, cyst formation has also been observed in the spleen, pancreas and ovaries.

- Acc. to Robbins and LB, lungs are also show cyst formation.

259. Ans.— A. BCG

260. Ans.— D. Complete ureter with a cuff of urinary bladder.

261. Ans.— B. Recombinant human erythropoietin

262. Ans.— D. Surgery

* Rx of Stress incontinence

* Minor degree : Pelvic floor exercise

* If exercise fails then surgery : *Gold standard Rx is Burch Colposuspension* (Blader neck suspension)

* Stamey's modification of colposuspension

* Tension free vaginal tape (TVT) : Recent.

263. Ans.— B. Triple phosphate

* Triple Phosphate—ammonium, magnesium and calcium phosphates in patients whose urine is infected with urea splitting organisms like proteus. Found in alkaline urine.

# 16

# IMPORTANT TEXT OF GENITAL SYSTEM

## INDICATIONS FOR ELECTIVE TREATMENT OF BENIGN DISEASE OF PROSTATE

1. Marked symptoms
2. Large residual volume
3. Diverticula
4. Dilated ureters
5. Calculi
6. Persistent urinary infection

## BENIGN PROSTATE HYPERPLASIA (BPH)

* Occurs in men over 50 years of age; by the age of 60 years 50% of men have histological evidence of BPH
* Is a common cause of significant lower urinary tract symptoms in men and is the most common cause of bladder outflow obstruction in men > 70 years of age

## CONSEQUENCES OF BPH

* No symptoms, no bladder outflow obstruction (BOO)
* No symptoms, but urodynamic evidence of BOO
* Lower urinary tract symptoms, no evidence of BOO
* Lower urinary tract symptoms and BOO
* Others (acute/chronic retention, haematuria, urinary infection and stone formation)

## TESTIS TUMOURS

* A scratal lump that cannot be felt separately from the testis may be a malignant tumour
* Lymphatic spread is to the retroperitoneal and intrathoracic lymph nodes
* Pulmonary metastases suggest that the tumour is a teratoma

**Types of testis tumours**

* Seminoma (40%);
* Teratoma (32%);
* Combined seminoma and teratoma (40%);
* Interstitial tumours (1.5%);
* Lymphoma (7%);
* Other tumours (5.5%).

# MCQ's OF GENITAL SYSTEM

## What is important in Genital System

Prostate (BHP, Carcinoma), Testes (Torsion, Hydrocele, Tumours)

1. **The commonest mode of spread of carcinoma prostate is : Delhi 1985**
   A. Lymphatics B. Blood vessels
   C. Direct D. None of the above
2. **Regarding treatment of prostatic cancer which is incorrect : AIIMS 1985**
   A. Radical prostatectomy has great value.
   B. Treatment with oestrogens plays great role.
   C. Orchidectomy has a role.
   D. Supravoltage X-ray therapy is sometimes used.
3. **In testicular Ca. investigation not done is : PGI 1998**
   A. Aortography B. CT scan
   C. Biopsy D. Serum AF
4. **The appropriate age for orchidopexy is : AMU 1989; AIIMS 1994**
   A. 5-7 years B. Puberty
   C. 20 years D. 25 years
5. **Endogenous prostatic calculi are usually composed of : PGI 1985**
   A. Oxalates B. Calcium phosphate
   C. Mixed D. Uric acid
6. **One of the undermentioned scrotal swellings is not painful : PGI 1988**
   A. Recent haematocele
   B. Torsion of the appendix of the testis (recent)
   C. Torsion of the testis
   D. Gumma of the testis
7. **All of the following constitute part of treatment of acute epididymo-orchitis except : TN 1990**
   A. Tetracyclines
   B. Scrotum to be supported on sling
   C. Urine is rendered acidic
   D. High fluid intake
8. **Which of the following is wrong regarding torsion of testis : AMU 1987**
   A. It does not occur in normal fully descended testis.
   B. Inversion of the testis is the commonest predisposing cause.
   C. Operation is not indicated.
   D. It can mimic stangulated inguinal hernia.
9. **The life of preserved semen for artificial insamination is : AIIMS 1987**
   A. One year B. Two years
   C. Five years D. Ten years
   E. Fifty years
10. **The most important factor in assessing 'Fertility potential' is : UPSC 1989**
    A. Sperm count
    B. Sperm motility
    C. Sperm morphology
    D. Quantity of ejaculated semen
11. **True oligospermia is present when sperm count is less than : AIIMS 1987**
    A. 2 million/ml B. 5 million/ml
    C. 20 million/ml D. 40 million/ml
12. **In semen banks, semen is preserved at low temperature around : DNB 1990**
    A. Dry ice B. Deep freeze
    C. Liquid nitrogen D. Liquid air
13. **Which is not true regarding varicocele : Delhi 1988**
    A. State of varicosity of testicular veins.
    B. More common on the right side.
    C. May be the first feature of a renal tumour.
    D. Feels like a bag of worms.

**Ans.** 1. B 2. A 3. C 4. A 5. B 6. D 7. C 8. C 9. D 10. B 11. D 12. C 13. B

**14. Circumcision during infancy is contraindicated in one of the following : AIIMS 1985**
A. Meatal stenosis
B. Hypospadias
C. Ectopia vesicae
D. Meatal ulcer with scabbing

**15. Vasectomy before prostatectomy is done because of: AIIMS 1985**
A. Getting collateral benefit of family planning.
B. Preventing infection to epididymis.
C. It is not needed.
D. It helps to prevent reactionary haemorrhage.

**16. All of the following are clinical features of chronic tuberculous epididymitis except : AMC 1984**
A. Slight ache in testis.
B. Discrete, indurated, slightly tender nodule mostly in globus major.
C. Lax secondary hydrocele may be present in 30% of cases.
D. Vas is often beaded.

**17. In an incompletely descended testis, the damage starts after an age of : AIIMS 1986**
A. 3 years B. 6 years
C. 8 years D. 12 years

**18. Incompletely descended testis is commonest on : UPSC 1984**
A. Right side B. Left side
C. Both sides D. Right sided only

**19. Grade-I benign prostate with outflow obstruction is best treated with : AIIMS 1987; DNB 1990**
A. Retropubic prostatectomy
B. Transurethral resection
C. Tranvesical prostatectomy
D. Androgen therapy

**20. The most common site for carcinoma of the prostate : AIIMS 1986**
A. Anterior lobe B. Posterior lobe
C. Median lobe D. Right lateral lobe

**21. Commonest testicular malignancy is : AIIMS 1982; AI 1989**
A. Seminoma
B. Teratoma
C. Choriocarcinoma
D. Embryonic cell carcinoma

**22. 80 years old man underwent transurethral prostatectomy biopsy and revealed foci of adenocarcinoma. Next line of management : AI 1989**
A. Radiotherapy B. Hormonal therapy
C. Surgery D. No further treatment

**23. Testicular tumour with cartilage elements is: AMC 1985, 89**
A. Seminoma
B. Teratoma
C. Embryonal cell tumour
D. Interstitial cell tumor

**24. All of the following statement are true regarding acute epididymitis, except : AIIMS 1983**
A. As a rule there is evidence of urethritis.
B. Infection is assumed to be blood borne.
C. It is associated with infection in prostate.
D. E. coli, streptococcus, Staphylococcus and Proteus are the common invading organisms.

**25. Penis is curved in downward direction in all types of hypospadias except : AIIMS 1980**
A. Glandular B. Coronal
C. Penile D. Perineal

**26. What percentage of testicular Ca. is associated with crypto-orchidism : PGI 1998**
A. 10 B. 30
C. 70 D. 90

**27. Peyronie's disease is most common in —— years of age. DNB 1990**
A. Below 20 B. 20-40
C. 40-60 D. 60-80

**28. Disseminated seminoma is treated by: PGI 1988, 89**
A. CT, RT and orchidectomy
B. Only RT
C. Only CT (Chemotherapy)
D. Retroperitoneal lymphnode carcinoma

**29 Regarding spermatocele which is not correct : PGI 1988**
A. Occurs in head of epididymis
B. Contains barly water fluid
C. Tender
D. Contains spermatozoa

**30. The lymph nodes first involved in cancer of the skin of the scrotum are : Karnataka 1996**
A. Superficial inguinal B. External iliac
C. Para aortic D. Gland of Cloquet

**31. A child presents with pain in testis, next management would be : Kerala 1998**
A. Arrange for surgery
B. USS
C. Arrange for band doppler
D. CT Scan

| Ans. | 14. B | 15. B | 16. B | 17. B | 18. A | 19. B | 20. B | 21. A | 22. D | 23. B |
|---|---|---|---|---|---|---|---|---|---|---|
| | 24. A | 25. A | 26. A | 27. C | 28. A | 29. C | 30. A | 31. C | | |

32. **The most important differential diagnosis for Testicular tumor is : Delhi 1993; PGI 1993, 95**
A. Hydrocele B. Spermatocele
C. Varicocele D. Hematocele

33. **The most common testicular tumor of childhood is : PGI 1987, 93**
A. Interstitial cell tumor B. Teratoma
C. Seminoma D. Chorio carcinoma

34. **Osteoblastic secondaries in bone are seen with : Bihar 1990; PGI 1993**
A. Ca. breast B. Ca. stomach
C. Ca. prostate D. All of the above

35. **Which is not true of Hypospadias : AIIMS 1999**
A. Surgical correction has good results
B. Glandular type needs no treatment
C. Chordee is reversed after 5 years
D. Circumcision should not be done in infancy

36. **Fructose in semen is produced : TN 1993**
A. Testis B. Prostate
C. Seminal vesicle D. Epididymis

37. **Circumcision is indicated in the following conditions except : AI 1993**
A. Religious indication B. Recurrent balanitis
C. Phimosis D. Hypospadias

38. **Palpable fibrous plaque on dorsal penile shaft indicates : Karnataka 1995**
A. Paget's disease B. Potter's syndrome
C. Prehn's sign D. Peyronie's disease

39. **Testicular malignancy commonest in undescended testes is : Delhi 1992**
A. Seminoma B. Teratoma
C. Embryonal cell Ca. D. Mixed

40. **The most common complication of acute or chronic prostatitis is : BHU 1988**
A. Sterility B. Epididymitis
C. Orchitis D. Seminal vesiculitis
E. None of the above

41. **The usual cause of death from penile cancer is : AIIMS 1986**
A. Liver metastasis
B. Pulmonary metastasis
C. Colonic penetration
D. Exsanguination from iliac or femoral vessels
E. Obstructive uropathy

42. **Which of the following testicular tumours is the most radiosensitive : UPSC 1986, 88**
A. Teratoma B. Embryoma
C. Terato-carcinoma D. Seminoma
E. Chorio-carcinoma

43. **Adequate treatment of benign prostatic hypertrophy is by : UPSC 1987**
A. Prostatic massage B. Antibiotics
C. Hormone therapy D. Resection
E. Suprapubic drainage

44. **All of the following differentiate hernia from hydrocele, except: Rohtak 1985**
A. Tenderness
B. Percussion and auscultation
C. Transillumination
D. Reducibility

45. **Prostatic cancer metastasizes most frequently to : Delhi 1985; AI 1989**
A. Spine B. Femur
C. Lung D. Rectum
E. Liver

46. **The commonest position of ectopic testis is : AIIMS 1984**
A. At the root of the penis
B. In the femoral triangle
C. In the inguinal canal
D. Near the deep inguinal ring
E. Near the superficial inguinal ring

47. **Which variety of hypospadias does not need treatment : Assam 1996**
A. Glandular B. Coronal
C. Penile D. Peno-scrotal

48. **Which is true regarding seminoma testis : PGI 1993**
A. Occurs in undesceded testis
B. Is radioresistant
C. Occurs in a relatively younger age group
D. Is highly malignant

49. **Indications for surgery in benign prostatic hypertrophy are all except : AI 1989**
A. Prostatism B. Chronic retention
C. Haemorrhage D. Enlarged prostate

50. **Commonest type of hypospadias is : JIPMER 1987**
A. Glandular B. Coronal
C. Penile D. Penoscrotal
E. Perineal

51. **Best treatment for prostatic abscess is : Delhi 1984; AIIMS 1984**
A. Erythromycin only B. Drainage
C. Both A + B D. None of the above

| Ans. | | | | | | | | | | |
|---|---|---|---|---|---|---|---|---|---|---|
| | 32. D | 33. B | 34. C | 35. C | 36. C | 37. D | 38. D | 39. A | 40. B | 41. D |
| | 42. D | 43. D | 44. A | 45. A | 46. E | 47. A | 48. A | 49. D | 50. A | 51. C |

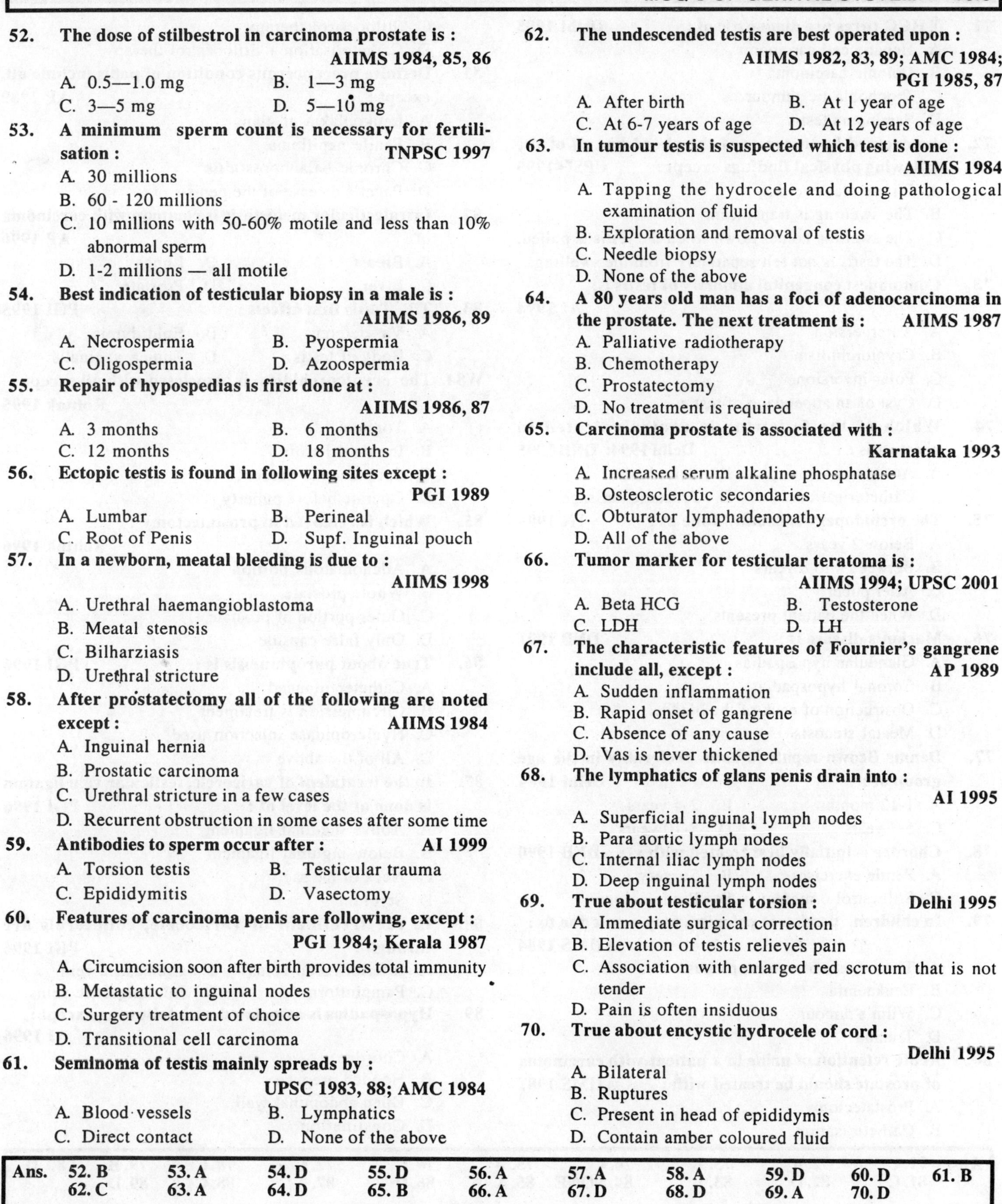

**52. The dose of stilbestrol in carcinoma prostate is :** **AIIMS 1984, 85, 86**

A. 0.5—1.0 mg B. 1—3 mg
C. 3—5 mg D. 5—10 mg

**53. A minimum sperm count is necessary for fertilisation :** **TNPSC 1997**

A. 30 millions
B. 60 - 120 millions
C. 10 millions with 50-60% motile and less than 10% abnormal sperm
D. 1-2 millions — all motile

**54. Best indication of testicular biopsy in a male is :** **AIIMS 1986, 89**

A. Necrospermia B. Pyospermia
C. Oligospermia D. Azoospermia

**55. Repair of hypospedias is first done at :** **AIIMS 1986, 87**

A. 3 months B. 6 months
C. 12 months D. 18 months

**56. Ectopic testis is found in following sites except :** **PGI 1989**

A. Lumbar B. Perineal
C. Root of Penis D. Supf. Inguinal pouch

**57. In a newborn, meatal bleeding is due to :** **AIIMS 1998**

A. Urethral haemangioblastoma
B. Meatal stenosis
C. Bilharziasis
D. Urethral stricture

**58. After prostatecomy all of the following are noted except :** **AIIMS 1984**

A. Inguinal hernia
B. Prostatic carcinoma
C. Urethral stricture in a few cases
D. Recurrent obstruction in some cases after some time

**59. Antibodies to sperm occur after :** **AI 1999**

A. Torsion testis B. Testicular trauma
C. Epididymitis D. Vasectomy

**60. Features of carcinoma penis are following, except :** **PGI 1984; Kerala 1987**

A. Circumcision soon after birth provides total immunity
B. Metastatic to inguinal nodes
C. Surgery treatment of choice
D. Transitional cell carcinoma

**61. Seminoma of testis mainly spreads by :** **UPSC 1983, 88; AMC 1984**

A. Blood vessels B. Lymphatics
C. Direct contact D. None of the above

**62. The undescended testis are best operated upon :** **AIIMS 1982, 83, 89; AMC 1984; PGI 1985, 87**

A. After birth B. At 1 year of age
C. At 6-7 years of age D. At 12 years of age

**63. In tumour testis is suspected which test is done :** **AIIMS 1984**

A. Tapping the hydrocele and doing pathological examination of fluid
B. Exploration and removal of testis
C. Needle biopsy
D. None of the above

**64. A 80 years old man has a foci of adenocarcinoma in the prostate. The next treatment is :** **AIIMS 1987**

A. Palliative radiotherapy
B. Chemotherapy
C. Prostatectomy
D. No treatment is required

**65. Carcinoma prostate is associated with :** **Karnataka 1993**

A. Increased serum alkaline phosphatase
B. Osteosclerotic secondaries
C. Obturator lymphadenopathy
D. All of the above

**66. Tumor marker for testicular teratoma is :** **AIIMS 1994; UPSC 2001**

A. Beta HCG B. Testosterone
C. LDH D. LH

**67. The characteristic features of Fournier's gangrene include all, except :** **AP 1989**

A. Sudden inflammation
B. Rapid onset of gangrene
C. Absence of any cause
D. Vas is never thickened

**68. The lymphatics of glans penis drain into :** **AI 1995**

A. Superficial inguinal lymph nodes
B. Para aortic lymph nodes
C. Internal iliac lymph nodes
D. Deep inguinal lymph nodes

**69. True about testicular torsion :** **Delhi 1995**

A. Immediate surgical correction
B. Elevation of testis relieves pain
C. Association with enlarged red scrotum that is not tender
D. Pain is often insiduous

**70. True about encystic hydrocele of cord :** **Delhi 1995**

A. Bilateral
B. Ruptures
C. Present in head of epididymis
D. Contain amber coloured fluid

| Ans. | | | | | | | | | |
|---|---|---|---|---|---|---|---|---|---|
| 52. B | 53. A | 54. D | 55. D | 56. A | 57. A | 58. A | 59. D | 60. D | 61. B |
| 62. C | 63. A | 64. D | 65. B | 66. A | 67. D | 68. D | 69. A | 70. D | |

**71. ↑ HCG titres are diagnostic of : Delhi 1995**
A. Hepatic cell carcinoma
B. Colonic carcinoma
C. Trophoblastic tumour
D. Seminoma testis

**72. An encysed hydrococele of the chord has all of the following physical findings except : UPSC 1995**
A. It is scrotal swelling.
B. The swelling is translucent.
C. The swelling comes down when the testis is pulled.
D. The testis is not felt separately from the swelling.

**73. Commonest congenital anomaly of testis is: AI 1994**
A. Anterversion
B. Cryptorchidism
C. Polar inversion
D. Cyst of an appendage of testis

**74. Which of the following is contraindicated in prostatitis : Delhi 1994; DNB 1995**
A. Antibiotics B. Seitz bath
C. Catheterisation D. Prostatic massage

**75. The orchidopexy is usually done at : TN 1998**
A. Below 2 years
B. Between 4 to 8 years
C. After puberty
D. When the patient presents

**76. Marion's disease is : DNB 1991**
A. Glandular hypospadias
B. Coronal hypospadias
C. Obstruction of neck of the bladder
D. Meatal stenosis

**77. Dennis Brown repair is done preferably in the age group of : Delhi 1984**
A. 1-12 months B. 2-4 years
C. 5-7 years D. 8-10 years

**78. Chordee is initially best treated with : DNB 1990**
A. Penile exercises B. Surgery
C. Stilbestrol 6 mg/day D. Prednisolone

**79. In children, persistent priapism may result due to : AIIMS 1984**
A. Thrombosis of venous plexus
B. Leukaemia
C. Wilm's tumour
D. Trauma

**80. Acute retention of urine in a patient with carcinoma of prostate should be treated with : AIIMS 1987**
A. Prostatectomy
B. Catheterisation
C. Stilboestrol therapy
D. Catheterisation + Stilboestrol therapy

**81. Definite precancerous condition of penis include all, except : AP 1989**
A. Leukoplakia of glans
B. Penile papilloma
C. Chronic balanoprosthitis
D. Paget's disease of the penis

**82. Intratesticular metastasis is common with carcinoma of : AP 1996**
A. Breast B. Lungs
C. Liver D. Prostate

**83. T.B. Testis first affects : PGI 1995**
A. Vas deferens B. Epididymis
C. Body of testis D. Tunica vaginalis

**W84. The cryptoorchidism is associated with all except : Rohtak 1995**
A. Torsion
B. Inguinal hernia
C. Spontaneous descent
D. Operate before puberty

**85. Which is removed in prostatectomy : Rohtak 1996**
A. Adenomatous portion
B. Whole prostate
C. Outer portion of prostate
D. Only false capsule

**86. True about paraphimosis is : PGI 1996**
A. Catheter induced
B. Circumcision is treatment
C. Hyaluronidase injection used
D. All of the above

**87. In the treatment of varicocele, testicular vein ligation is done at the level of : PGI 1996**
A. Above inguinal ligament
B. Below inguinal ligament
C. Neck of the sac
D. Scrotum

**88. In the treatment of varicocele, collaterals are through : PGI 1996**
A. Inferior rectal veins B. Cremastric vein
C. Pampiniform D. Inf. epigastric veins

**89. Hypospadias is associated with following except : AI 1996**
A. Chordee
B. Hooded prepuce
C. Open abdominal wall
D. Constipation

| Ans. | | | | | | | | | | |
|---|---|---|---|---|---|---|---|---|---|---|
| | 71. C | 72. A | 73. B | 74. C | 75. B | 76. C | 77. C | 78. C | 79. B | 80. D |
| | 81. C | 82. D | 83. B | 84. NONE | 85. A | 86. D | 87. A | 88. C | 89. D | |

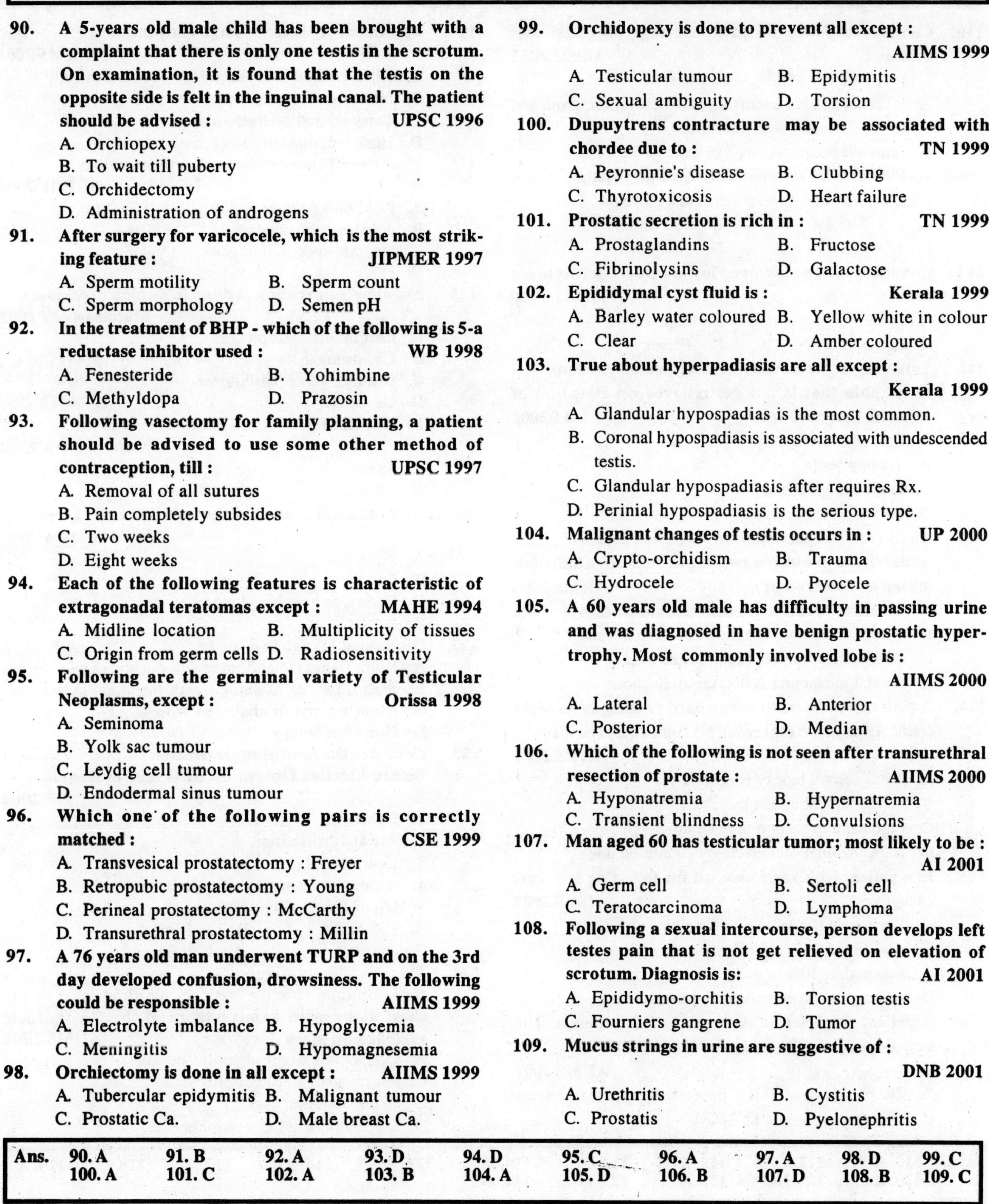

**90. A 5-years old male child has been brought with a complaint that there is only one testis in the scrotum. On examination, it is found that the testis on the opposite side is felt in the inguinal canal. The patient should be advised : UPSC 1996**

A. Orchiopexy
B. To wait till puberty
C. Orchidectomy
D. Administration of androgens

**91. After surgery for varicocele, which is the most striking feature : JIPMER 1997**

A. Sperm motility B. Sperm count
C. Sperm morphology D. Semen pH

**92. In the treatment of BHP - which of the following is 5-a reductase inhibitor used : WB 1998**

A. Fenesteride B. Yohimbine
C. Methyldopa D. Prazosin

**93. Following vasectomy for family planning, a patient should be advised to use some other method of contraception, till : UPSC 1997**

A. Removal of all sutures
B. Pain completely subsides
C. Two weeks
D. Eight weeks

**94. Each of the following features is characteristic of extragonadal teratomas except : MAHE 1994**

A. Midline location B. Multiplicity of tissues
C. Origin from germ cells D. Radiosensitivity

**95. Following are the germinal variety of Testicular Neoplasms, except : Orissa 1998**

A. Seminoma
B. Yolk sac tumour
C. Leydig cell tumour
D. Endodermal sinus tumour

**96. Which one of the following pairs is correctly matched : CSE 1999**

A. Transvesical prostatectomy : Freyer
B. Retropubic prostatectomy : Young
C. Perineal prostatectomy : McCarthy
D. Transurethral prostatectomy : Millin

**97. A 76 years old man underwent TURP and on the 3rd day developed confusion, drowsiness. The following could be responsible : AIIMS 1999**

A. Electrolyte imbalance B. Hypoglycemia
C. Meningitis D. Hypomagnesemia

**98. Orchiectomy is done in all except : AIIMS 1999**

A. Tubercular epidymitis B. Malignant tumour
C. Prostatic Ca. D. Male breast Ca.

**99. Orchidopexy is done to prevent all except : AIIMS 1999**

A. Testicular tumour B. Epidymitis
C. Sexual ambiguity D. Torsion

**100. Dupuytrens contracture may be associated with chordee due to : TN 1999**

A. Peyronnie's disease B. Clubbing
C. Thyrotoxicosis D. Heart failure

**101. Prostatic secretion is rich in : TN 1999**

A. Prostaglandins B. Fructose
C. Fibrinolysins D. Galactose

**102. Epididymal cyst fluid is : Kerala 1999**

A. Barley water coloured B. Yellow white in colour
C. Clear D. Amber coloured

**103. True about hyperpadiasis are all except : Kerala 1999**

A. Glandular hypospadias is the most common.
B. Coronal hypospadiasis is associated with undescended testis.
C. Glandular hypospadiasis after requires Rx.
D. Perinial hypospadiasis is the serious type.

**104. Malignant changes of testis occurs in : UP 2000**

A. Crypto-orchidism B. Trauma
C. Hydrocele D. Pyocele

**105. A 60 years old male has difficulty in passing urine and was diagnosed in have benign prostatic hypertrophy. Most commonly involved lobe is : AIIMS 2000**

A. Lateral B. Anterior
C. Posterior D. Median

**106. Which of the following is not seen after transurethral resection of prostate : AIIMS 2000**

A. Hyponatremia B. Hypernatremia
C. Transient blindness D. Convulsions

**107. Man aged 60 has testicular tumor; most likely to be : AI 2001**

A. Germ cell B. Sertoli cell
C. Teratocarcinoma D. Lymphoma

**108. Following a sexual intercourse, person develops left testes pain that is not get relieved on elevation of scrotum. Diagnosis is: AI 2001**

A. Epididymo-orchitis B. Torsion testis
C. Fourniers gangrene D. Tumor

**109. Mucus strings in urine are suggestive of : DNB 2001**

A. Urethritis B. Cystitis
C. Prostatis D. Pyelonephritis

| Ans. | | | | | | | | | |
|---|---|---|---|---|---|---|---|---|---|
| 90. A | 91. B | 92. A | 93. D | 94. D | 95. C | 96. A | 97. A | 98. D | 99. C |
| 100. A | 101. C | 102. A | 103. B | 104. A | 105. D | 106. B | 107. D | 108. B | 109. C |

**110. Consider the following statements regarding testicular torsion : UPSC 2001**
1. It commonly affects young males.
2. It causes sudden agonising pain in scrotum, groin and lower abdomen with vomiting.
3. Immediate untwisting can relieve the pain.
4. Elevation of scrotum usually relieves pain.

Which of the above statements are correct :

A. 1, 2, 3 and 4 B. 1, 2 and 3
C. 2 and 3 D. 1 and 4

**111. Commonest bone involved in carcinoma prostate is : AI 1990**

A. Spine B. Rips
C. Pelvis D. Femur

**112. Following a sexual intercourse, person develops left testes pain that is not get relieved on elevation of scrotum. Diagnosis is : AI 2001**

A. Epididymo-orchitis
B. Torsion testis
C. Fourniers gangrene
D. Tumor

**113. An 18-years-old patient, Asim Singh, had pain in his right testis following which a swelling developed. All the following are true except : AIIMS 2001**

A. If torsion is present, the other testis also has to be fixed.
B. Pyuria favours the diagnosis of torsion testis.
C. Decreased uptake in radionuclide scan.
D. Scrotal ultrasound is helpful in diagnosis.

**114. A patient was found to have a hard swelling in his right testis. All are true regarding his condition except : AIIMS 2001**

A. Trans-scrotal biopsy is needed
B. Scrotal ultrasound is indicated
C. Inguinal exploration is to be done
D. High inguinal orchidectomy should be done

**115. In a patient with varicocele, all the following are true, except : AIIMS 2001**

A. Varicocele is common in the right side
B. Associated with infertility
C. Bilateral in 10%
D. Association with malignancy described

**116. A patient suspected to have prostatic carcinoma. The best investigation to evaluate him would be : AIIMS 2001**

A. TRUS B. Expressed prostatic secretions
C. CT scan D. MRI

**117. Treatment of choice of stage-I seminoma is : AIIMS 2001**

A. High inguinal orchidectomy with radiotherapy
B. Intravenous chemotherapy
C. Trans-scrotal orchidectomy
D. High inguinal orchidectomy

**118. Most specific tumor marker for prostate is : SGPGI 2002**

A. Acid phosphatase
B. Alkaline phosphatase
C. Prostate specific antigen
D. HCG

**119. Mcknow's operation is done for which carcinoma? Maharashtra 2002**

A. Carcinoma oesophagus
B. Ca. stomach
C. Bronchogenic carcinoma
D. Ca. colon

**120. 16 F circumference of a catheter means : Maharashtra 2002**

A. 48 mm B. 28 mm
C. 84 mm D. 82 mm

**W.121. Minimal Invasive surgery include all except : Maharashtra 2002**

A. FESS
B. Lapcholy
C. Endoscopic sclerotherapy
D. PCNL

**122. Peritoneal lavage is done in : A.P. 2002**

A. Blunt trauma to abdomen without any physical signs
B. Stab injury to abdomen with intestinal laceration
C. Blunt trauma to abdomen with shock
D. Gun shot injury

**123. Consider the following statements :**
**Before Elective Operation ECG may evaluate AP 2002**
1. Heart rate
2. Atrial fibrillations
3. Heart-block
4. Recent myocardial infarction

**Which of these statements are correct :**

A. 1, 2 and 4 B. 2, 3 and 4
C. 1 and 3 D. 1, 2, 3 and 4

**124. The most likely diagnosis in a new born who has a radio-opaque shadow with an air-fluid level in the chest along with hemivertebra of the 6th thoracic vertebra on plain X-ray is : AIIMS 2002**

A. Congenital diaphragmatic hernia
B. Esophageal duplication cyst
C. Bronchogenic cyst
D. Staphylococcal pneumonia

| Ans. | 110. B | 111. C | 112. B | 113. B | 114. A | 115. A | 116. A | 117. A | 118. C | 119. A |
|---|---|---|---|---|---|---|---|---|---|---|
| | 120. A | 121. NONE | 122. A | 123. D | 124. B | | | | | |

125. **Eight years old boy presented with swelling in left eye of 3 months duration. Examination revealed proptosis of left eye with preserved vision. Right eye is normal. CT Scan revealed intraorbital extra conal mass lesion. Biopsy revealed embryonal rhabdomyosarcoma. Metastatic work-up was normal. The standard line of treatment is : AIIMS 2002**
A. Chemotherapy only
B. Wide local excision
C. Enucleation
D. Chemotherapy and Radiation therapy

126. **A 27 years old man presents with a left testicular tumor with a 10 cm retroperitoneal lymph node mass. The treatment of choice is : AI 2003**
A. Radiotherapy
B. Immunotherapy with interferon and interleukins
C. Left high inguinal orchidectomy plus chemotherapy
D. Chemotherapy

127. **Radiation exposure during infancy has been linked to which one of the following carcinoma : AI 2003**
A. Breast B. Melanoma
C. Thyroid D. Lung

128. **Which of the following is most likely to require surgical intervention : CUPGME-2003**
A. Large sliding hernia
B. Hiatal hernia
C. Oesophageal web
D. Oesophageal traction diverticulum

129. **Increased expression of erb2 gene is associated with : CUPGME-2003**
A. Breast cancer B. Hodgkin's lymphoma
C. NHL D. Ca. colon

130. **CEA is elevated in which of the following malignancies : CUPGME-2003**
A. Lung breast testis B. Lung colon pancreas
C. Breast colon testis D. Thyroid breast lung

131. **Which of the following is cut in ectopia vesicae : UP 2003**
A. Symphysis pubis B. Ileum
C. Sacrum D. Coccyx

132. **The most common cause of stricture urethra is : UPSC 2003**
A. Postgonococcal urethritis
B. Congenital
C. Carcinoma penis
D. Instrumentation

133. **Unilateral undescended testis is ideally operated around: AI 2004**
A. ·2 months of age B. 6 months of age
C. 12 months of age D. 24 months of age

**Ans.** 125. D 126. C 127. C 128. A 129. A 130. B 131. A 132. A 133. D

# EXPLANATIONS OF GENITAL SYSTEM

1. Ans.— B. Blood vessels

   Bateson Venous plexus is most common route.
2. Ans.— A. Radical prostatectomy has great value
3. Ans.— C. Biopsy
4. Ans.— A. 5-7 years
5. Ans.— B. Calcium phosphate
6. Ans.— D. Gumma of the testis
7. Ans.— C. Urine is rendered acidic
8. Ans.— C. Operation is not indicated
9. Ans.— D. Ten years
10. Ans.— B. Sperm motility
11. Ans.— D. 40 million/ml
12. Ans.— C. Liquid nitrogen
13. Ans.— B. More common on the right side

    Most varicocele are seen in teens and early adult life. Lt side is effected in 95% cases.
14. Ans.— B. Hypospadias
15. Ans.— B. Preventing infection to epididymes
16. Ans.— B. Discrete, indurated, slightly tender nodule mostly in globus major.
17. Ans.— B. 6 years
18. Ans.— A. Right side
19. Ans.— B. Transurethral resection
20. Ans.— B. Posterior lobe
21. Ans.— A. Seminoma

    The most common malignant testicular tumor is teratoma but the most common tumor (32%) of testis is seminoma (40%).
22. Ans.— D. No further treatment

    The prostatic ca. is increasing diagnosed due to better facility & longer life of people. It is the commonest malignancy in males over 65 yrs. Majority of the incidentally diagnosed do not exhibit disease progression & therefore do not necessary need any therapy except wait & watch policy.
23. Ans.— B. Teratoma
24. Ans.— A. As a rule there is evidence of urethritis.
25. Ans.— A. Glandular
26. Ans.— A. 10
27. Ans.— C. 40-60
28. Ans.— A. CT, RT and orchidectomy
29. Ans.— C. Tender
30. Ans.— A. Superficial inguinal
31. Ans.— C. Arrange for band doppler
32. Ans.— D. Hematocele
33. Ans.— B. Teratoma

    Testicular tumors in children are usually anaplastic teratomas.
34. Ans.— C. Ca. prostate
35. Ans.— C. Chordee is reversed after 5 years

    If biliary obstruction is not relieved before the age of 3 months, biliary cirrhosis supervenes.
36. Ans.— C. Seminal vesicle
37. Ans.— D. Hypospadias
38. Ans.— D. Peyronie's disease
39. Ans.— A. Seminoma
40. Ans.— B. Epididymitis
41. Ans.— D. Exsanguination from iliac or femoral vessels.
42. Ans.— D. Seminoma
43. Ans.— D. Resection
44. Ans.— A. Tenderness
45. Ans.— A. Spine

    Most common site for metastasis is bone. This mostly involves vertebra becaue of vertebral venous plexus (Lower Lumbar).

Order of Metastasis :

1. Bone
2. Breast
3. Kidney
4. Lung
5. Thyroid other bony site to be involved commonly are Femoral head, Rib, Skull.

46. Ans.— E. Near the superficial inguinal ring

47. Ans.— A. Glandular

48. Ans.— A. Occurs in undescended testis

49. Ans.— D. Enlarged prostate

50. Ans.— A. Glandular

51. Ans.— C. Both A + B

52. Ans.— B. 1—3 mg

Progestogens and medroxyprogesterone have been tried. Testosterone levels are reduced by LHRH agonists. Cyproterone acetate, flutamide (a pure antiandrogen) and aminoglutethimide are also used.

53. Ans.— A. 30 millions

54. Ans.— D. Azoospermia

55. Ans.— D. 18 months

56. Ans.— A. Lumbar

57. Ans.— A. Urethral haemangioblastoma

58. Ans.— A. Inguinal hernia

59. Ans.— D. Vasectomy

60. Ans.— D. Transitional cell carcinoma

61. Ans.— B. Lymphatics

62. Ans.— C. At 6-7 years of age

63. Ans.— A. Tapping the hydrocele and doing pathological examination of fluid.

64. Ans.— D. No treatment is required

65. Ans.— B. Osteosclerotic secondaries

66. Ans.— A. Beta HCG

67. Ans.— D. Vas is never thickened

68. Ans.— D. Deep inguinal lymph nodes

Glans penis drain to deep inguinal LN i.e. the gland of Cloquet. Rest of the penis drain into Sup. inguinal LN.

69. Ans.— A. Immediate surgical correction

70. Ans.— D. Contain amber coloured fluid

71. Ans.— C. Trophoblastic tumour

72. Ans.— A. It is scrotal swelling

73. Ans.— B. Cryptorchidism

74. Ans.— C. Catheterisation

75. Ans.— B. Between 4 to 8 years

76. Ans.— C. Obstruction of neck of the bladder

77. Ans.— C. 5-7 years

78. Ans.— C. Stilboestrol 6 mg/day

79. Ans.— B. Leukaemia

80. Ans.— D. Catheterisation + Stilboestrol therapy

81. Ans.— C. Chronic balanoprosthitis

82. Ans.— D. Prostate

83. Ans.— B. Epididymis

84. Ans.— NONE

85. Ans.— A. Adenomatous portion

86. Ans.— D. All of the above

87. Ans.— A. Above inguinal ligament

88. Ans.— C. Pampiniform

89. Ans.— D. Constipation

90. Ans.— A. Orchiopexy

91. Ans.— B. Sperm count

92. Ans.— A. Fenesteride

93. Ans.— D. Eight weeks

94. Ans.— D. Radiosensitivity

95. Ans.— C. Leydig cell tumour

96. Ans.— A. Transvesical prostatectomy : Freyer

97. Ans.— A. Electrolyte imbalance

98. Ans.— D. Male breast Ca.

99. Ans.— C. Sexual ambiguity

100. Ans.— A. Peyronnie's disease

101. Ans.— C. Fibrinolysins

102. Ans.— A. Barley water coloured

103. Ans.— B. Coronal hypospadiasis is associated with undescended testis.

104. Ans.— A. Crypto-orchidism

105. Ans.— D. Median

106. Ans.— B. Hypernatremia

107. Ans.— D. Lymphoma

108. Ans.— B. Torsion testis

109. Ans.— C. Prostatis

110. Ans.— B. 1, 2 and 3

111. Ans.— C. Pelvis

Spread to bones occur by blood. Prostate is the most common source of skeletal metastasis followed inturn by breast, kidney, bronchial tree and thyroid. The bones involved most frequently are pelvis, lower lumbar vertebra, femoral head; rib cage and skull are other favour sites.

112. Ans.—B. Torsion testis

113. Ans.— B. Pyuria favours the diagnosis of torsion testis.

114. Ans.— A. Trans-scrotal biopsy is needed

115. Ans.— A. Varicocele is common in the right side

116. Ans.— A. TRUS

117. Ans.— A. High inguinal orchidectomy with radiotherapy.

118. Ans.— C. Prostate specific antigen

119. Ans.— A. Carcinoma oesophagus

120. Ans.— A. 48 mm

121. Ans.— NONE

122. Ans.— A. Blunt trauma to abdomen without any physical signs.

123. Ans.— D. 1, 2, 3 and 4

124. Ans.— B. Esophageal duplication cyst

125. Ans.— D. Chemotherapy and Radiation therapy

126. Ans.— C. Left high inguinal orchidectomy plus chemotherapy.

Teratoma

* Age (25-35)
* Stages -

*Stage- I* - Testis involved only

*Stage- II* - Nodes below the diaphragm involved only

II a - (Nodes < 2 cm), IIb - (nodes of 2-5 cm)., IIc (Nodes > 5 cm),

*Stage- III* - Nodes above the diaphragm involved

*Stage- IV* - Spread upto lung, liver

*M/m* - "Common denominator in every stage is high inguinal orchidectomy regardless of histology."

* *Stage I* - Watch by serum markers estimation
* *Stage IIa, IIb* - TARPLNO (Total Abdominal Retro-Peritoneal lymph node dissection).

127. Ans.— C. Thyroid

* Papillary carcinoma thyroid frequently follows accidental irradiation in childhood.
* Papillary carcinoma thyroid - Orphan Annie eyed nuclei in histology.
* It is also responsible for lateral abberent thyroid (occult metastasis).
* Spread by a lymphnodes but blood born metastases is unusual so prognosis is good (Best amongst all thyroid carcinoma's).

128. Ans.— A. Large sliding hernia

129. Ans.— A. Breast cancer

130. Ans.— B. Lung colon pancreas

131. Ans.— A. Symphysis pubis

132. Ans.— A. Postgonococcal urethritis

Postgonococcal stricture is most commonly seen in the bulbar urethra. Most strictures appear within 1 year infection but may not cause difficulty in micturition for 10 to 15 years.

133. Ans.— D. 24 months of age

Ideal timing of surgery for surgical condition

| Malformations | Optimal age |
|---|---|
| • Cleft lip* | 3–6 month |
| • Cleft palate* | 6–18 month |
| • Tongue tie* | Around 1 year of age |
| • PDA | At birth |
| • Coarctation of aorta | 3–4 years |
| • ASD | At 2–4 years |
| • TOF | 6–12 months |
| • Undescented testis* | 2 years |
| • Umbilical hernia | After 2–3 years |
| • Inguinal hernia | Any age |
| • Hydrocele | After 6 months |
| • Exostrophy bladder | |
| a) Bladder closure | Within 48 hours |
| b) Bladder neck repair | After 24 years |
| c) Urethroplasty | After achieving continence |
| • Hypospodiasis | |
| a) Meatotomy | Any time after birth |
| b) Chordee correction | Around 6 month (1-1½ years—Schwartz) |
| c) Urethroplasty | 12 month (5-7 years—Schwartz) |
| • Phimosis | |
| a) Prepucial separation | Around 1 years |
| b) Circumcision | After 2-3 years |
| • Sacrococcygeal teratoma | As early as possible |
| • Meningo-myelocele | As early as possible |

# 17

# IMPORTANT TEXT OF MISCELLANEOUS ASPECTS

## TYPICAL HAND AND LESIONS

| | | |
|---|---|---|
| 1. | Accoucheur's hand or Obstetrician hand | in tetany |
| 2. | Ape hand or Simian hand | in Median nerve paralysis |
| 3. | Claw hand | in Ulnar nerve palsy |
| 4. | Trident hand | in Achondroplasia |
| 5. | Frog hand | in deep palmar abscess |
| 6. | Gardener's hand | in Callosity |
| 7. | Wrist drop | in radial nerve palsy |
| 8. | Foot drop | in common peroneal nerve palsy |

## TREATMENT OF CHOICE

* The treatment of choice for incised wound is—*Exploration and Primary suture.*
* Penetrating wounds—*Exploration and Primary suture.*
* Lacerated wounds—*Wound excision and Primary suture of skin.*
* Crushed and Devitalised wounds (Industrial road traffic accidents & war wounds)—*Wound Excision and Delayed Primary suture.*
* Clean incised wounds with skin loss—*Primary grafting.*
* Lacerated wounds with skin loss—*Wound excision and primary grafting.*
* Crushed and devitalised wounds with skin loss—*Wound excision and delayed primary, or occasional secondary grafting.*
* Missile injuries—*Wound excision and left open* —(On 4th or 6th day after injury on inspection if wound looks healthy—*Delayed Primary Suture).*
* Explosive blast injuries—*All blast wounds should be left open at the end of initial operation and delayed primary suture performed 4-7 days later.*
* Scorpion stings—*Local hydrocortisone injection or dehydroemetine injection.*
* Bee venom (alkaline)—*Neutralised by vinegar or lemon juice.*
* A frequent choice for maintenance fluid in the post-operative period—*0.45% sodium chloride in 5% dextrose.*
* Metabolic alkalosis without hypokalaemia—*Seldom requires direct treatment.*
* Hypokalaemic alkalosis—*Infusion of isotonic saline and 20 mmol KCL given* (once urine output is adequate).
* Respiratory alkalosis—*Respiratory suppression is rectified by insufflation of* $CO_2$.
* Metabolic acidosis (Class-I)—*Ringer's lactate solution or slow infusion of dilute sodium bicarbonate solution.*
* Metabolic acidosis due to renal failure with hyperkalaemia—*Calcium resonium enema* (simplest remedy).
* Hyperchloraemic acidosis due to transplantation of ureters into colon—*IV 8.4% sodium bicarbonate* (if necessary IV potassium also).

## 17.2 GENERAL SURGERY

### *HAEMORRHAGE*

- Stop blood loss by—
  - i) Pressure & Packing
  - ii) Position & Rest
  - iii) Operative procedures (ligation repair & excision).
- Restore blood volume by—*Blood transfusion & other I/V transfusions.*

### *SHOCK*

- Neurogenic shock—*Trendelenburg position, rapid administration of fluids and/or a vasopressor drug.*
- Hypovolaemic shock—*Extra cellular fluid replacement* + *Blood transfusion* (SOS).
- Gram-positive sepsis & shock—*Appropriate antibiotics* + *Surgical drainage* (when indicated) + Correction of any fluid deficit.
- Gram-negative sepsis & shock—*Control of infection (by early surgical debridement or drainage + appropriate antibiotics + Fluids replacement + Steroids + Vasoactive drugs).*
- Anaphylactic shock—Adrenaline + Cardiopulmonary resuscitation + Infusion of coloids + Antihistaminics + Steroids.
- Crush Syndrome—*Gradual release of Tourniquet* + *Rheomacrodex or Mannitol* (If necessary Dialysis).
- Wounds infected with anaerobic or microaerophilic organisms (Spreading symbiotic gangrene of abdominal wall) and top free the sloughs of ulcers—*Topical oxygen therapy.*

## CONTRAINDICATIONS

- It is seldom wise to attempts surgical improvement of scar of less than 6 months.
- Contraindications to intravenous therapy are the failing heart and Pulmonary congestion.
- Miliary anti-shock trousers (MAST) are contraindicated in—pulmonary edema, pregnancy, abdominal evisceration, and decreased pulmonary function (pneumothorax).
- Incisions should be made directly across skin creases (unless there is some overriding reason).
- Tourniquets are to be avoided in first aid.
- Chronic haemorrhage patients must not be transfused with normal blood (Packed cells can be given).
- Magnesium ion should not be given to the oliguric patient or in the presence of severe volume deficit unless actual magnesium depletion is demonstrated.
- Topical antibiotics should be reserved for use in eye or ear surgery and skin antibiotics are seldom ever indicated and can lead to severe antibiotic-resistant infections.
- The bubo (of chancroid) should never be incised (since healing is very slow).
- Parenteral nutrition is contraindications to Feeding by tube enterostomy include complete or partial gastric or intestinal obstruction.
- Gastrostomy is contraindicated in gastric disease, impaired gastric emptying, significant gastro-oesophageal reflux, loss of gag reflex.
- Liver transplantation is contraindicated in any patient with irreversible infection, widespread malignancies, concurrent disease (myocardial failure, old age) that would seriously impair survival and a high risk for recurrent disease in the transplant organ.
- Human tetanus antitoxin should never be given intravenously.
- Surgical removal is contraindicated in warts (as it leads to scarring & recurrence).

## EPONYMS

- **Epstein's pearls**—Cell rests at the line of fusion of the palatal shelves occur as a diamond-shaped group of miniature, white cysts seen at the junction of hard and soft palate in neonates (Disappear spontaneously).
- **Vincent's Acute ulcerative gingivitis and stomatitis**—Acute ulceromembranous stomatitis due to *Borrelia vincentii and Fusiformis fusiforms.*

* **Vincent's angina**—Tonsillar infection.
* **Hutchinson's wart**—A secondary syphilitic condyloma is always found in the midline of tongue.
* **Hutchinson's incisor**—Notched incisor with a narrow incistal edge is seen in congenital syphilis.
* **Warthin's tumour**—Adenolymphoma of parotid gland (usually).
* **Cushing response**—Elevated ICP, if severe, will compromise the circulation in the supra-and infratentorial compartments and if the latter is affected, the resultant medullary, ischaemia will produce a rise in systemic blood pressure, a bradycardia and a slowing of the respiratory rate.
* **Kernohan's notch**—Changes due to coning or hernation of brain contents with ICP, produce a deterioration in the level of consciousness, dilatation of the pupil (on the side of the compressing mass, and a hemiparesis on the same side as the mass).

## LYMPHATIC DRAINAGE OF GASTROINTESTINAL VISCERA

| *Viscera* | *Regional Lymph Nodes* | *Central Lymph Nodes* |
|---|---|---|
| Esophagus (abdominal part) | Left gastric | Celiac |
| Stomach | Gastric, gastroomental, pancreatico splenic | Celiac |
| Duodenum | Pancreaticoduodenal | Celiac and Pyloric superior mesenteric |
| Jejunum and ileum | Mesenteric | Superior Mesenteric |
| Pancreas | Pancreaticosplenic, Pyloric | Celiac, Superior mesenteric |
| Liver | Hepatic (mostly) Phrenic (partly) | Celiac, parasternal |
| Gall bladder and bile duct | Cystic, hepatic | Celiac |
| Caecum appendix ascending and transverse colon (prox. two thirds) | Ileocolic, paracolic, middle colic | Superior mesenteric |
| Transverse colon (distal one third), descending and sigmoid colon | Paracolic, Intermediate colic | Inferior mesenteric |

## ANATOMICAL BASIS OF SUNDERLAND'S AND SEDDON'S CLASSIFICATIONS OF NERVE INJURIES

| ***Sunderland grade*** | ***Axon*** | ***Endoneurial tube*** | ***Perineurium*** | ***Epineurium*** | ***Seddon group*** |
|---|---|---|---|---|---|
| First-degree | + | + | + | + | Neurapraxia |
| Second-degree | - | + | + | + | Axonotmesis |
| Third-degree | - | - | + | + | |
| Fourth-degree | - | - | - | + | Neurotmesis |
| Fifth-degree | - | - | - | - | Neurotmesis |

+, Intact; -, severed.

## CLINICAL FEATURES AND NEUROPHYSIOLOGY FINDINGS OF THE THREE TYPES OF NERVE INJURY DEFINED IN SEDDON'S CLASSIFICATION

| | *Neurapraxia* | *Axonotmesis* | *Neurotmesis* |
|---|---|---|---|
| Motor loss | Complete | Complete | Complete |
| Sensory loss | Partial sparing | Complete | Complete |
| Autonomic function | Spared | Absent | Absent |
| Nerve conduction distal to injury | Present | Absent | Absent |
| Fibrillatin on EMG | Absent | Present | Present |
| Recovery | Rapid | 1 mm per day | 1 mm per day |
| | Complete | Good | Always imperfect |

# MCQ's OF MISCELLANEOUS ASPECTS

## What is important in Miscellaneous Aspects

Transplantation of organs, Named signs, Tests, and Operations, Factual data, Recent Advances

1. **Which of the following test is used for pancreatic efficiency : DNB 1990**
   A. Topfer's B. String test
   C. Sahli's test D. Perthes test
2. **Whipple's triad in insulinomia include all except : JIPMER 1985**
   A. Hypoglycemia below 45 mg%
   B. An attack of hypoglycemia in the fasting stage
   C. Symptoms relieved by glucose
   D. ACTH is treatment of choice
3. **von Graefe's sign is : Delhi 1983**
   A. Lagging behind of the upper eyelid.
   B. Retraction of the upper eyelid with infrequent wrinkling.
   C. Absence of wrinkling of the forehead.
   D. Convergence of the eyes in difficult.
4. **Proud flesh is the term used to describe : AIIMS 1986**
   A. Excessive granulation tissue
   B. Muscle protuding through a skin wound
   C. Hypertrophy of the nose
   D. Hypertrophy of the tongue
5. **The nerve of Kuntz is an important landmark in : Delhi 1984**
   A. Lumbar sympathectomy
   B. Cervicodorsal sympathectomy
   C. Splanchniectomy
   D. Herniorrhaphy
6. **Primary malignant neoplasms are rare in the : MAHE 1994**
   A. Oesophagus B. Stomach
   C. Small bowel D. Large bowel
7. **Simon Artz band is present in : DNB 1989**
   A. Hypertrophic pyloric stenosis (congenital)
   B. Aganglionic megacolon
   C. Intussusception
   D. Prealveolar cleft
8. **Arrow headed finger on X-ray is suggestive of : PGI 1983, 85**
   A. Acromegaly B. Hyperparathyroidism
   C. Down's syndrome D. Sarcoidosis
9. **In Sjorgren's syndrome, not seen is : PGI 1986; AMC 1986, 88**
   A. Inflammation of parotid and lacrimal glands
   B. Arthritis
   C. Xerostomia
   D. Diarrhoea
10. **Prehn's sign is typically seen in : Delhi 1982, 83; UPSC 1983, 86; AIIMS 1983**
    A. Ectopic pregnancy B. Ascites
    C. Torsion of testis D. Epididymoorchitis
11. **The Commando operation is : UPSC 1985**
    A. Abdomino-perineal excision of the rectum for carcinoma.
    B. Disarticulation of the hip for gas gangrene of the leg.
    C. Extended radical mastectomy.
    D. Excision of carcinoma of the tongue, the floor of the mouth, part of the jaw and lymph nodes en bloc.
12. **Which of the following test is to know peptic activity in diagnosis of gastric cancer : AIIMS 1985**
    A. Sahli's B. String
    C. Topfer D Edestin
13. **Who is known as father of surgery : AMC 1987**
    A. Joseph Lister B. John Hunter
    C. Ambroise Parey D. Rudlph Matas
14. **Rosenthal's syndrome is seen in deficiency of factor : DNB 1991**
    A. II B. V
    C. IX D. XI

| Ans. | 1. B | 2. D | 3. A | 4. A | 5. B | 6. C | 7. D | 8. A | 9. D | 10. D |
|---|---|---|---|---|---|---|---|---|---|---|
| | 11. D | 12. D | 13. C | 14. D | | | | | | |

**15. Father of Modern surgery is : AMC 1989**

A. Joseph Lister B. John Hunter
C. Rudolph Matas D. Theodore Kocher

**16. Which of the following is also known as falx inguinalis : AMC 1985**

A. Polya's ligament
B. Thomson's ligament
C. Hesselbach's ligament
D. Henle's ligament

**17. Riches technique is used for : BHU 1987**

A. Removal of ureteric stones
B. Suprapubic catheterization
C. Contracture of bladder neck
D. Obstruction of ureter

**18. Bow's sign is seen in : AMU 1988**

A. Hydronephrosis B. Perinephric abscess
C. Varicocele D. Nephrolithiasis

**19. Which of the following sign is seen in Nephrolithias is : AIIMS 1985**

A. Mathe's B. Thronton's
C. Flush-Tanks D. Whiteside's

**20. Heparin was discovered by : PGI 1985**

A. Mosny & Dumont B. Brain & Joboulay
C. Howell & Holt D. Seldinger

**21. Mauriac's syndrome is characterized by the following except : PGI 1986**

A. Diabetes B. Obesity
C. Dwarfism D. Cardiomegaly
E. Hepatomegaly

**22. Parrot's node is seen in : BHU 1988**

A. Congenital syphilis B. Miliary TB
C. Cretinism D. Bacterial endocarditis

**23. Parrot's node is : BHU 1988**

A. Enlarged mediastinal nodes
B. Interstitial keratic nodules
C. Thickening of frontal and parietal bones
D. Enlarged adenoids

**24. Osler's sign is seen in : DNB 1990**

A. Meningitis
B. Intestinal obstruction
C. Bladder stone
D. Malignant endocarditis

**25. Oxygen consumption during anaesthesia and surgery with mild levels of hypothermia in infants less than 12 kg is (35-36°C) : DNB 1990**

A. Unchanged B. Doubled
C. Trippled D. Quadrupled
E. None of the above

**26. The simplest renal transplant to perform technically is : AIIMS 1987**

A. Right kidney on the left side
B. Left kidney on the right side
C. Right kidney on the right side
D. Left kidney on the left side
E. None of the above

**27. Arterial anastomosis in renal transplantation include all except : PGI 1986**

A. Renal artery to renal artery
B. Renal artery to hypogastric artery
C. Renal artery to external iliac artery
D. Renal artery to common iliac artery

**28. Levator syndrome mainly involves : AIIMS 1982**

A. Kidney B. Testes
C. Rectum D. Liver

**29. Lumpectomy followed by irradiation is the treatment of choice in : AIIMS 1984**

A. Adenocarcinoma of breast
B. Early adenocarcinoma
C. Adenocarcinoma of thyroid
D. Liposarcoma

**30. Quant's sign (a T-shaped depression in the occipital bone) may be present in : AIIMS 1984**

A. Down's syndrome B. Head injury
C. Rickets D. Scurvy

**31. The symptom typical in infants suffering from Prader Willi syndrome is : PGI 1986**

A. Obesity B. Short stature
C. Dysphagia D. Mental Retardation

**32. Aaron's sign is seen in : AIIMS 1984**

A. Achlasia cardia
B. Hiatus hernia
C. Mediastinal emphysema
D. Acute appendicitis

**33. When the rectum is inflated with air through a rectal tube, pain and tenderness occur in the right iliac fossa in case of appendicitis. This is known as : AMU 1985**

A. Aaron's sign B. Battle's sign
C. Bastede's sign D. McBurney's sign

**34. Winter bottom's sign is typically seen in : AIIMS 1983**

A. Meconium peritonitis
B. Kala Azar
C. American trypanosomiasis
D. African trypanosomiasis

| Ans. | | | | | | | | | | |
|---|---|---|---|---|---|---|---|---|---|---|
| | 15. A | 16. D | 17. B | 18. C | 19. B | 20. C | 21. D | 22. A | 23. C | 24. D |
| | 25. B | 26. B | 27. A | 28. C | 29. A | 30. C | 31. C | 32. D | 33. C | 34. D |

35. **Water-Gurgle test is typically positive in :** **AIIMS 1985**

A. Achlasia cardia B. Oesophageal stricture
C. Hiatus hernia D. Duodenal atresia

36. **Van Buchem's syndrome is characterized by all except:** **Rohtak 1986**

A. Overgrowth
B. Distortion of mandible
C. Facial palsy
D. Increased acid phosphatase

37. **Nezelof's syndrome is recurrent episode of :** **DNB 1990**

A. Appendicitis B. Cholecystitis
C. Intestinal obstruction D. Pneumonia

38. **Biot's respiration is seen in :** **PGI 1984**

A. Hypnosedative poisoning
B. Appendicitis
C. Cholecystitis
D. Bulbar poliomyelitis

39. **Oesophageal rupture following severe vomiting may result in :** **PGI 1986**

A. Bonnevie-UIlrich syndrome
B. Bloom's syndrome
C. Boerhaave's syndrome
D. Any of the above

40. **Bolognini's symptom (a feeling of crepitation occurring from gradual increasing pressure on the abdomen) is seen in :** **AMU 1986**

A. Congenital pyloric stenosis
B. Gastric polyp
C. Duodenal atresia
D. Measles

41. **Bouchard's nodes are seen in :** **DNB 1990**

A. Juvenile rheumatoid arthritis
B. Syphilic arthritis
C. Rheumatic fever
D. Osteoarthritis

42. **Burton's line is :** **DNB 1990**

A. Fluid level on X-rays indicating intestinal obstruction.
B. Bluish discolouration around umbilicus in pancreatitis.
C. Bluish line on gums in lead poisoning.
D. Line of demarcation between normal abnormal colon in a congenital disorder.

43. **D 'Espine's sign indicates TB of :** **AMU 1986**

A. Liver B. Mediastinal nodes
C. Spleen D. Kidney

44. **Beck's triad consists of :** **AMU 1986**

A. Paradoxial pulse, shock, pulmonary oedema.
B. Low blood pressure, elevated pulse pressure, systolic murmur .
C. Low blood pressure, elevated venous pressure, quiet heart.
D. None of the above.

45. **Dalrymple's sign is seen in :** **AIIMS 1985**

A. Cretinism B. Myxoedema
C. Hyperthyroidism D. Chronic cholecystitis

46. **Edwards syndrome is characterized by the following except :** **AIIMS 1985**

A. Mental retardation
B. Malformed skull, mandible and ears
C. Diaphragmatic or inguinal hernia
D. None of the above

47. **Protrusion of the lips occurring due to tapping the skin at the angle of the mouth (Escherich's sign) is seen in:** **AMU 1986**

A. Frontal lobe damage B. Tuberous sclerosis
C. Tetany D. Hyperparathyroidism

48. **Glasgow's sign (a systolic murmur over the branchial artery) is seen in:** **DNB 1989**

A. Aortic regurgitation B. Tracheo oesophageal
C. Mitral slenosis D. Aortic anurysm

49. **Libman sack's syndrome has the following except :** **AIIMS 1984**

A. Arthritis B. Glomerulonephritis
C. Atypical endocarditis D. Pneumonitis

50. **If rupture marks are to be avoided, skin sutures should be removed in :** **AMC 1989**

A. 72 hours B. 1 week
C. 2 weeks D. 3 weeks

51. **The most common cause of death following renal transplant is :** **JIPMER 1992**

A. Rejection B. Renal failure
C. Infection D. Malignancy

52. **Investigation of choice to detect small paraaortic lymph nodes is :** **JIPMER 1992**

A. CT scan B. Ultrasonogram
C. Arteriograpy D. Lymphangiography

53. **Catgut is made from intestine of :** **Rajasthan 1993; DNB 1993, 95**

A. Cat B. Human
C. Sheep D. All of the above

54. **Metastasis to bone is not a feature of :** **AIIMS 1992**

A. Ca rectum B. Renal cell carcinoma
C. Ca thyroid D. Ca breast

| Ans. | | | | | | | | | |
|---|---|---|---|---|---|---|---|---|---|
| 35. B | 36. D | 37. D | 38. D | 39. C | 40. D | 41. D | 42. C | 43. B | 44. C |
| 45. C | 46. D | 47. C | 48. D | 49. D | 50. B | 51. C | 52. D | 53. C | 54. A |

**55. 5-FU is the chemotherapeutic of choice in the following solid tumors except: PGI 1993**

A. Ca pancreas B. Ca breast
C. Ca colon D. Ca stomach

**56. Beckwith Weidman syndrome is characterised by following except : PGI 1984**

A. Macroglossia B. Omphalocele
C. Dwarfism D. Microcephaly

**57. Following are tests for appendicitis except : AMU 1985**

A. Cope B. Obturator
C. Sahli's D. Psoas

**58. Harvey's sign is : AIIMS 1986**

A. Transmitted pressure wave on coughing in a varicose vein.
B. Related to the speed of venous filling after emptying a length of vein .
C. Loss of hair from eyebrows.
D. None of the above.

**59. Proven tumour specific antigen is for all of the following except : PGI 1987**

A. Gastric carcinoma B. Burkitt's lymphoma
C. Carcinoma of breast D. Neuroblastoma
E. Carcinoma colon

**60. Regarding kidney transplantation each of the following is true, except : UPSC 1987**

A. Bilateral nephrectomy is preferred before transplantation.
B. Any evidence of infection in recipient is a contraindication.
C. Urine formation should be almost immediate after transplantation.
D. Right kidney is preferred because its vessels are longer
E. Early signs of rejection are fever and reduced renal function.

**61. Rejection phenomena include : AIIMS 1986**

A. Lymphocytes in the urine
B. Urine and blood LDH changes
C. Changes in size of kidney
D. Depression of $CO_2$ fraction of complement
E. All of the above

**62. The figure—— are very important to the oesophagoscopist. AIIMS 1986**

A. 10, 20 and 30 B. 15, 25 and 40
C. 20, 30 and 40 D. 25, 35 and 45
E. 25, 35 and 50

**63. Courvoisier's law is related to : AMC 1984**

A. Jaundice
B. Ureteric calculi
C. Portal hypertension
D. The length of skin flap in skin grafting
E. Renal transplantation

**64. The best candidates for hepatic transplantation seem to be : AIIMS 1985; AI 1989**

A. Children with biliary atresia
B. Patients with primary cancer
C. Adults with Laennec's cirrhosis
D. Adults with post-hepatic cirrhosis

**65. Which of the following are operative complications associated with hepatic transplantation : UPSC 1986**

A. Bleeding
B. Ligation of cystic duct along with common duct
C. Paralysis of right diaphragm
D. Hypothermia
E. All of the above

**66. Mercedes Benz or Seagull sign is present in : AIIMS 1986**

A. Cholelithiasis B. Cholecystitis
C. Phrygian cap D. Duodenal atresia

**67. Which one of the following is not APU Domas : UPSC 2003**

A. Pheochromocytoma
B. Medullary carcinoma of thyroid
C. Insulinoma
D. Papillary carcinoma of thyroid

**68. 'Riding Breeches' deformity is collection of fat on : AIIMS 1984**

A. The medial aspect of upper arms
B. On the medial thighs
C. Over the femoral trochanters of the thighs
D. Drooping buttocks

**69. Pressure over the descending colon elicits pain at Mc-Burney point in appendicitis. This is called : PGI 1986**

A. Rotch's sign B. Aron's sign
C. Rovsing'sign D. Rogoff's sign

**70. Palpation on the costovertebral angle produces pain and tenderness in acute adrenal insufficiency. This is: PGI 1986**

A. Rotch's sign B. Rossolimo's sign
C. Rogoff's sign D. Osler's sign

| Ans. | | | | | | | | | |
|---|---|---|---|---|---|---|---|---|---|
| 55. A | 56. C | 57. C | 58. B | 59. A | 60. D | 61. E | 62. B | 63. A | 64. A |
| 65. E | 66. A | 67. D | 68. C | 69. C | 70. C | | | | |

**71. Which of the following are true of lumbar sympathectomy : CSE 1995**

1. It often results in the healing of ischaemic ulcers
2. It improves skin nutrition
3. It opens up the occluded blood vessels
4. It relieves pain

**Select the correct answer**

A. 1, 2 and 3 B. 1, 3 and 4
C. 1, 2 and 4 D. 2, 3 and 4

**72. Emptying sign is seen in : Delhi 1986**

A. Cavernous lymphangioma
B. Haemangioma
C. Hydrocele
D. Arterio-venous fistula

**73. Preoperative shaving is idealy done at : Delhi 1986**

A. Before evening B. Morning of operation
C. Just before operation D. At operation table

**74. Hilton's method of abscess drainage is used for abscess in : Delhi 1985**

A. Breast B. Parotid
C. Gluteal region D. Legs

**75. Estimation of catecholamines help in the diagnosis of: AIIMS 1986**

A. Teratoma B. Neuroblastoma
C. Wilm's tumour D. Carcinoid tumour

**76. Which of the following scientists diagnosed his own gastric cancer by his own sign : UPSC 1986**

A. Charle's Trosier B. Armand Trousseau
C. Ronald Ross D. Domimic Corrigan

**77. Brodie's grading of tumours pertains to : AMU 1987**

A. Size of tumour
B. Histological differentiation
C. Local spread
D. All of the above

**78. Pressure over the left iliac fossa causes pain over the inflammed appendix, this sign is known as : DNB 1989**

A. Murphy's sign B. Rovsing's sign
C. Cope's psoas test D. Cope's obturator test
E. None of the above

**79. The most highly radioresistant tumour of the following is : AIIMS 1986**

A. Squamous cell carcinoma
B. Fibrosarcoma
C. Lymphosarcoma
D. Embryonal carcinoma

**80. Minimal alveolar concentration of cyclopropane (vol percent)to prevent muscular response to skin incision is: DNB 1990**

A. 0.16 B. 0.765
C. 9.2 D. 101

**81. In cryosurgery, the probe is cooled to the extent: AMU 1990**

A. -50° B. -100°
C. -150° D. -200°

**82. Murphy's sign is a diagnostic of : AMC 1984**

A. Gall bladder B. Hepatic disease
C. Pancreatic disease D. None of the above

**83. Kanavel's sign is : AIIMS 1986**

A. Swelling above the flexor retinaculum.
B. Flexion of the thumb when the radial bursa is infected.
C. Flexion of the fingers in a compound palmar ganglion.
D. Tenderness over an infected ulnar bursa between the transverse palmar creases .

**84. Keratin horn is : UPSC 1983**

A. Congenital
B. Due to matting of hair
C. A papilloma with excessive Keritan formation
D. None of the above

**85. The commonest tumor in childhood and infancy is : AIIMS 1985**

A. Ewing's tumour B. Grawitz tumour
C. Nephroblastoma D. Carcinoma prostate

**86. Difficulty in convergence of the eyes in thyrotoxicosis is denoted by : PGI 1987**

A. Stellwig' sign B. Moebius sign
C. von Graefe's sign D. Joffroy's sign

**87. Chvostek's sign is : UPSC 1987**

A. Carpal spasm induced by sphygmomanometer cuff pressure on the upper arm above the systolic blood pressure for not more than two minutes in the normal person.
B. As above, but the person has tetanus.
C. Twitching of facial muscles produced by tapping over the branches of the facial nerve at the angle of the jaw in the normal person.
D. As above, but the person has tetany.

**88. The Brodie- Trendelenburg test is used to detect : AIIMS 1989**

A. The presence of deep femoral vein thrombosis.
B. The integrity of the long saphenous nerve.
C. The presence of an incompetent valve at the saphenofemoral junction.
D. The presence of an incompetent valve at the junction of the short saphenous and popliteal veins.

| Ans. | | | | | | | | | |
|---|---|---|---|---|---|---|---|---|---|
| 71. C | 72. B | 73. C | 74. B | 75. B | 76. B | 77. B | 78. B | 79. B | 80. C |
| 81. D | 82. A | 83. D | 84. C | 85. C | 86. B | 87. D | 88. C | | |

**89. Sistrunk's operation is excision of : TN 1989**

A. Pancreatic adenoma
B. Thyroglossal fistulous tract along with the body of the hyoid bone
C. Gall bladder by the fundus first methodis
D. Branchial fistulous tract excision

**90. Astley Cooper's ligament is : UPSC 1987**

A. Medial ėnd of inguinal ligament
B. Pectineal part of inguinal ligament
C. Fibres along the iliopectineal line
D. Linea semilunaris

**91. Serum alkaline phosphatase is produce from the following except : AI 1988**

A. Liver cells
B. Osteoblasts
C. Polymorphonuclear leucocytes
D. Renal tubular cells

**92. 'Rest pain' occurs : AMU 1985**

A. Anywhere in the body at rest.
B. In the thigh of a patient with Buerger's disease.
C. In the calf of a patient with intermittent claudication.
D. In the foot of a patient with severe vascular disease.

**93. Immunosuppression which is commonly used in organ transplant : PGI 1985, 90; TN 1990, 92**

A. Prednisolone + azathioprine
B. Total lymphocytic irradiation
C. Methotrexate
D. Immunotherapy
E. BCG vaccine

**94. A Seldinger needle is used for : AMC 1987**

A. Liver biopsy B. Suturing skin
C. Arteriography D. Lymphography

**95. Bisgaard's treatment is done for : UPSC 1988**

A. Venous ulcer B. Coarctation of aorta.
C. Complete heart block D. Fallot's tetralogy

**96. Newman and Seabrook's operation is used for : AIIMS 1984**

A. Repair of parotid fistula
B. For parotid calculi
C. For carcinoma of tongue
D. For treatment of recurrent chronic parotitis
E. None of the above

**97. Randall's plaque is seen in: TN 1998**

A. Gall stone B. Renal stone
C. Vesical stone D. Chronic appendicitis

**98. Commonest complication of immunosuppression is : NIMHANS 1986; JIPMER 1987; AI 1988**

A. Malignancy B. Graft rejection
C. Infection D. Thrombocytopenia

**99. A 30 years old man has undergone subtotal gastrectomy for ulcer. On the second post-operative morning he develops a fever of 103 degrees, tachycardia to 180 and is slightly tachypnea. The most likely diagnosis is : UPSC 1982**

A. Wound infection B. Urinary tract infection
C. Thrombophlebitis D. Atelectasis
E. Subphrenic abscess

**100. Site of transplantation in islet cell transplant for diabetes mellitus : PGI 1989**

A. Forearm muscles
B. Pelvis
C. Thigh
D. Injected into the portal vein

**101. Sturge-Weber syndrome is characterized by all of the following except : AIIMS 1985**

A. Mental retardation
B. Visual disturbances
C. Angiomas of choroid and pia mater
D. Renal abnormalities

**102. Pressure over the descending colon elicits pain at McBurney point in appendicitis. This is called : AIIMS 1986**

A. Rotch's sign B. Aaron's sign
C. Rovsing's sign D. Rogoff's sign

**103. Palpation on the costovertebral angle produces pain and tenderness in acute adrenal insufficiency. This is : AIIMS 1987**

A. Rotch's sign B. Rossolimi's sign
C. Rogoff's sign D. Nephrotic syndrome

**104. Giganitism can occur in : Karnataka 1987**

A. Turner's syndrome B. Cohn's syndrome
C. Milroy's disease D. Nephrotic syndrome

**105. Ormond's disease is : Kerala 1998**

A. Idiopathic lymphadenopathy
B. Retractile mesentritis
C. Idiopathic retroperitoneal fibrosis
D. Idiopathic mediastinitis

**106. When administering intravenous antibiotics for antibiotic prophylaxis, the drug should be administered : Karnataka 1993**

A. The night before surgery
B. With premedication
C. With induction of anaesthesia
D. After completion of surgery

**107. Secondaries not responding to chemotherapy are of : PGI 1993**

A. Bone B. Brain
C. Lung D. Lymphatics

| Ans. | | | | | | | | | |
|---|---|---|---|---|---|---|---|---|---|
| 89. B | 90. C | 91. D | 92. D | 93. A | 94. C | 95. A | 96. A | 97. B | 98. C |
| 99. D | 100. D | 101. D | 102. C | 103. C | 104. C | 105. C | 106. A | 107. A | |

**108. Coffee bed sign is usually seen in : PGI 1989, 94**
A. Volvulus B. Pyloric obstruction
C. Intussusception D. Intestinal obstruction

**109. Which is not important for tissue typing in organ transplantation : PGI 1994**
A. MHC B. HLA-B
C. HLA-A D. HLA-D/DR

**110. Solid tumor which responds best to 5-FU is of : PGI 1994**
A. Pancreas B. Thyroid
C. Colon D. Lung

**111. Following electrolyte abnormalities are seen in immediate post-operative period except : AIIMS 1994**
A. Hypokalaemia
B. Hyponatremia
C. Negative nitrogen balance
D. Glucose intolerance

**112. Regarding MHC which is not true : AIIMS 1984**
A. Coded by multiple genes
B. Components for complement system is one part of MHC
C. Responsible for graft rejections
D. Located on chromosome 6

**113. Murphy's sign is seen in the case of : AIIMS 1989**
A. Pancreatitis B. Splenic rupture
C. Cholecystisis D. Appendicitis

**114. Survival of organ\ tissue allograft is longest with: DNB 1991**
A. Skin B. Cornea
C. Kidney D. Lung

**115. Surgery is not useful in : DNB 1989**
A. Cerebral oedema
B. Depressed fracture
C. Extra dural haemorrhage
D. Subdural haemorrhage

**116. Of the following suture material, which causes the least reaction : AIIMS 1986**
A. Plain catgut B. Chromic catgut
C. Monofilament nylon D. Silk

**117. The 'Augmented Histamine Test' is a test for : Delhi 1987**
A. Pheochromocytoma B. Duodenal ulcer
C. Gastric secretion D. Leprosy

**118. Infrequent blinking in thyrotoxicosis is : DNB 1991**
A. Stellwig sign B. Von Graefe sign
C. Mobius sign D. Weider sign

**119. In children with congenital hypertrophic pyloric stenosis, there is increased incidence of—— among family members. UPSC 1986**
A. Down's syndrome B. Marfan's syndrome
C. Anal atresia D. Achlasia cardia

**120. A patient with multiple injuries, developed on the second day high fever, tachycardia, tachyponea, restlessness, low $pO_2$ level and a macular rash around axilla. The most likely diagnosis : UPSC 1995**
A. Meningitis B. Fat embolism
C. Pulmonary embolism D. Drug rash

**121. During nutritional assesment of a surgical patient, the status of muscle protein is indicated by which one of the following parameters: UPSC 1995**
A. Serum albumin
B. Triceps skinfold thickness
C. Mid-arm circumference
D. Haemoglobin level

**122. Buerger's disease involves : CSE 1996**
A. Medium and small size arteries and superficial veins.
B. Medium size arteries and superficial veins.
C. Superficial veins and small size arteries.
D. Medium size and small size arteries.

**123. Pemberton's sign is positive in : AP 1994**
A. Myxoedema B. Thyrotoxicosis
C. Exophthalmos D. Retrosternal goiter

**124. Following are associated with pheochromocytoma except : Kerala 1998**
A. MEN IIa
B. MEN IIb
C. Von Hippel Lindau syndrome
D. Sturge Weber's syndrome

**125. Mauriac's syndrome is characterized by the following except : AIIMS 1986**
A. Diabetes mellitus B. Obesity
C. Dwarfism D. Cardiomegaly

**126. Discolouration around umbilicus relates to : Delhi 1984**
A. Cullen's sign B. Murphy's sign
C. Psoas's sign D. McBurney's sign

**127. In the Matas operation what is reconstructed : AMC 1983**
A. An artery B. A vein
C. A nerve D. A joint

**128. The Hunterian ligature, operation is performed for : AMC 1986**
A. Varicose veins B. Arteriovenous fistula
C. An aneurysm D. A lymph fistula

**Ans.** 108. C 109. C 110. A 111. C 112. A 113. C 114. B 115. A 116. C 117. C 118. A 119. D 120. B 121. B 122. D 123. D 124. B 125. D 126. A 127. A 128. C

**129. Graham Cole test refers to :** **AP 1989**
A. Oral cholecystography
B. Intravenous cholangiography
C. Pre-operative cholangiography
D. Post-operative cholangiography
E. Tomography

**130. Nicoladoni's sign is also known as :** **AIIMS 1984**
A. Harvey's sign B. Grey Turner's sign
C. Murphy's sign D. Branham's sign

**131. Preservative in catgut packing is :** **MP 1993; Delhi 1994**
A. Benzidine B. Ether
C. Tetra zinc D. Isopropyl alcohol

**132. A patient has hypocalcemia which was the result of a surgical complication. Which operation could it possibly have been :** **UPSC 1986**
A. Nephrectomy
B. Thyroidectomy
C. Gastrectomy
D. Vocal cord tumour biopsy

**133. Morris incision is used in the operation of :** **AMU 1987**
A. Appendix B. Kidney
C. Prostate D. Gall bladder

**134. Characteristic of renal allograft rejection is :** **AIIMS 1985**
A. Lymphocytopenia
B. Bradycardia
C. Polyuria
D. Urinary excretion of fibrin degradation products

**135. In the rejection phenomenon after kidney transplant, the primary target for early immunological attack is :** **UPSC 1988**
A. Vascular endothelium B. Renal papillae
C. Glomeruli D. Proximal tubules

**136. The most common indication for kidney transplantation is :** **AI 1989**
A. Hydronephrosis
B. End stage glomerulonephritis or pyelonephritis
C. Tuberculosis
D. Wilm's tumour

**137. Common homograft is :** **DNB 1991**
A. Kidney B. Heart
C. Blood D. Lung

**138. Kehr's sign is :** **DNB 1990**
A. Pain referred to the left shoulder.
B. Shift of the dullness from the right side to left side.
C. Pain referred to right shoulder.
D. Pain referred to between 9th and 11th ribs posteriorly.

**139. Gallard Thomas incision is used for :** **AIIMS 1986, 87**
A. Thyroid adenoma B. Mixed parotid tumor
C. Branchial fistula D. Gynaecomastia

**140. Transplantation of kidney from mother to son is an example of :** **Delhi 1985; AIIMS 1987**
A. Autograft B. Allograft
C. Isograft D. Xenograft

**141. The surgical treatment of abdominal injuries includes all the following except :** **CSE 1997**
A. A generous mid-line incision
B. Obtaining haemostasis as the first priority
C. Kocherization of the duodenum
D. Exploration of pelvic and retro-peritoneal haematoma

**142. Eaton Lanbert syndrome is seen in :** **AIIMS 1987**
A. Bronchogenic Ca B. Pancreatic Ca
C. Ovarian tumors D. Meningiomas

**143. Which of the following test is done for peptic activity in the diagnosis of gastric cancer :** **DNB 1989**
A. Topfer's test B. Edestin test
C. String test D. Gmelin test

**144. Swan-Ganz catheter is used for :** **AIIMS 1986, 87**
A. Cardiac catherterization
B. CVP monitoring
C. Portal veins pressure recording
D. Double lumen endotracheal intubation

**145. Sicca syndrome is associated with :** **UPSC 1987; AIIMS 1990**
A. Rheumatoid arthritis B. Laennec's cirrhosis
C. Scleroderma D. SLE
E. Sarcoidosis

**146. Z-plasty is done in all except :** **AIIMS 1990**
A. Meatal stenosis
B. Ectopic urethral opening
C. Vertical chordee
D. Prepuce deficient vertically

**147. Dance's sign is present in :** **DNB 1989**
A. Duodenal atresia B. Intussusception
C. Hirschsprung's disease D. Hiatus hernia

**148. Benda's sign is present in :** **PGI 1986**
A. Ascites B. Hydrocephalus
C. Hydrothorax D. Intussusception

**149. Cobra head deformity in the lower end of ureter is seen in :** **PGI 1989**
A. Ureterocele
B. Vesical diverticulam
C. Carcinoma of urinary bladder
D. Urethral stricture

| Ans. | | | | | | | | | | |
|---|---|---|---|---|---|---|---|---|---|---|
| | 129. A | 130. D | 131. D | 132. B | 133. B | 134. D | 135. A | 136. B | 137. C | 138. A |
| | 139. D | 140. C | 141. B | 142. A | 143. B | 144. A | 145. A | 146. B | 147. B | 148. B |
| | 149. A | | | | | | | | | |

**150. Surgical treatment can cure following tumours, except:** **AIIMS 1986**
A. Fibrosarcoma
B. Insulinoma
C. Glucagonoma
D. Appendicular carcinoid
E. Phaeochromocytoma

**151. Earliest tumour to appear after birth is :** **JIPMER 1987, 88**
A. Sternomastoid tumour B. Cystic hygroma
C. Branchial cyst D. Lymphoma

**152. Graft from sister to brother is :** **JIPMER 1986, 90**
A. Isograft B. Allograft
C. Autograft D. Heterograft

**153. A 12 years old boy develops exophthalmos nervousness, diarrhoea and weight loss following the death of her mother. His blood pressure is 170/90. The most likely diagnosis is :** **AIIMS 1987**
A. Multiple endocrine adenoma (MEA), Type-II
B. A pheochromocytoma
C. Graves' disease
D. Retroorbital pseudotumor
E. None of the above

**154. Chemotherapy is not indicated in :** **PGI 1995**
A. Teratoma testis B. Ca breast
C. Malignant melanoma D. Adenocarcinoma colon

**155. Tamoxifen may be used in :** **Rohtak 1995**
A. Ca breast B. Ca prostate
C. Ca thyroid D. Ca pancreas

**156. Chemotherapy is not yet effective in :** **PGI 1996**
A. Pancreatic Ca
B. Choriocarcinoma of testis
C. Testicular seminoma
D. Vulval Ca

**157. Match List-I with List-II and select the correct answer using the codes given below the Lists :** **CSE 1997**

| List-I | List-II |
|---|---|
| A. Umbilical secondaries | 1. Blumer's shelf |
| B. Scalene node deposits | 2. Krukenburg's tumour |
| C. Mass in the pouch of Douglas | 3. Sister Josephine node |
| D. Secondaries in the ovaries | 4. Virchow gland |

**Codes :**

| | A | B | C | D |
|---|---|---|---|---|
| A. | 3 | 4 | 2 | 1 |
| B. | 3 | 4 | 1 | 2 |
| C. | 4 | 3 | 1 | 2 |
| D. | 4 | 3 | 2 | 1 |

**158. Child's criteria is used in :** **PGI 1996**
A. Pancreatitis B. Cirrhosis
C. Multiple myeloma D. AIDS

**159. Least effective for prevention of adhesion :** **PGI 1996**
A. Cauterization B. Laproscopy
C. Hyscon D. Phenergan

**160. All of the following are indications for liver transplantation, except :** **Delhi 1996**
A. Biliary atresia
B. Malignancy
C. Cirrhosis
D. Hereditary spherocytosis

**161. In advanced stage of Malignancy, pain to relieved by:** **WB 1996**
A. Radiotherapy B. Chemotherapy
C. Analgesic D. All of the above

**162. The following is Genetically transmitted :** **WB 1996**
A. Cervical Ca B. Colonic Ca
C. Vaginal Ca D. Wilm's tumor

**163. Haemorrhagic telangiectasis is most common in :** **AI 1996**
A. > 60 years B. 40-60 years
C. 20-40 years D. < 20 years

**164. Hormonal treatment is given for which of the following malignancy :** **Kerala 1996; PGI 1996**
A. Chorio carcinoma B. Carcinoma prostate
C. Hepatoma D. Teratoma
E. Granulosa cell tumour

**165. Good results of surgery are obtained following transplantation of :** **UPSC 1996**
A. Heart and kidney
B. Heart only
C. Kidney, heart and liver
D. Kidney only

**166. Commonest problem in Allograft recipients is :** **TN 1996**
A. CMV B. Candidiasis
C. TB D. AIDS

**167. Montgomery's tube is :** **AI 1999**
A. Siliconised rubber T-tube
B. Endotracheal tube
C. Adjustable flanged tube
D. Tracheostomy double tube

| Ans. | 150. A | 151. B | 152. B | 153. C | 154. C | 155. A | 156. B | 157. B | 158. B | 159. D |
|---|---|---|---|---|---|---|---|---|---|---|
| | 160. D | 161. A | 162. D | 163. D | 164. B | 165. A | 166. A | 167. A | | |

**168. Cold ischemic time of the kidney is : JIPMER 1987; AI 1989**

A. 45 minutes B. 2 hours
C. 6 hours D. 12 hours
E. 72 hours

**169. Spontaneous regression, though rare, may be seen in: Delhi 1993**

A. Burkitt's lymphoma B. Wilm's tumour
C. Neuroblastoma D. Malignant melanoma

**170. Test for saphenofemoral incompetence is : PGI 1985**

A. Ochsner-Mahorner test
B. Morrissey's test
C. Gornall's test
D. Bonney's test

**171. Rule of nine to estimate surface area of a burnt patient was introduced by : AIIMS 1984, 85**

A. Mortiz Kaposi B. Alexander Wallace
C. Joseph Lister D. Thomas Barelay

**172. Chagas disease does not involve : JIPMER 1989, 90**

A. Pancreas B. Colon
C. Esophagus D. Heart

**173. Sappey's line denotes a line : Karnataka 1995**

A. Encircling the neck at C6 vertebra level
B. Encircling the trunk just above the umbilicus
C. Encircling the salphigian tubes
D. None of the above

**174. Currently all of the following malignancies are curable except : Karnataka 1996**

A. Choriocarcinoma
B. Wilm's tumour
C. Acute Myeloid leukemia
D. Hairy cell leukemia

**175. In a Kocher's subcostal incision which of the following should not be divided : Karnataka 1996**

A. Rectus abdominis muscle
B. 8th dorsal nerve
C. Oblique muscles
D. 9th dorsal nerve

**176. Cocket & Dodd's operation is for : AP 1996**

A. Saphenofemoral flush ligation
B. Subfascial ligation
C. Deep vein thrombosis
D. Diabetic foot

**177. In a woman aged 57 yrs. metastatic tumour involving cloquet's lymph nodes obstructs the right lymphatic duct before it joins the venous system. Clinical features associated with palpable nodes are : Rajasthan 1995**

A. Swelling of right breast
B. Swelling of right face
C. Swelling of neck
D. All of the above

**178. Post-operative recurrence of varicose veins is due to: Rajasthan 1995**

A. Ligation lower than the level of Saphenofemoral junction.
B. Persistent great Saphenous vein.
C. Large Perforating veins.
D. Presence of accessory Saphenous vein.

**179. Bleeding encountered on division of Gumbernats ligament is from : Rajasthan 1995**

A. Femoral artery
B. Inferior epigastric artery
C. Aberrant obturator artery
D. External iliac vein

**180. Common component in the boundary of Hesselbach's triangle & Femoral triangle is : Rajasthan 1995**

A. Inguinal ligament
B. Conjoint tendon
C. Sartorius muscle
D. Inferior epigastric vessels

**181. After Surgery, patient is shifted to : Rajasthan 1995**

A. Recovery Room B. Ward
C. ICU D. CCU

**182. Post-operative tachycardia may be due to : Rajasthan 1996**

A. Hypothermia B. Chest pain
C. Hypovolemia D. Hypoxia

**183. Isolated hematuria may imply : Rajasthan 1996**

A. Neoplasm B. Stone
C. T.B. D. Buerger's disease

**184. T.B. adenitis most commonly involves : AP 1997**

A. Submaxillary nodes
B. Jugular nodes
C. Posterior Cervical nodes
D. Supraclavicular nodes

**185. The "Sick cell syndrome" is characterized by : AP 1997**

A. Hyponatremia B. Hypernatremia
C. Hypokalemia D. Hyperkalemia

**186. Beevor'e sign is seen in : NIMHANS 1997**

A. Great foe B. Thumb
C. Plantar reflex D. Umbilicus
E. Anal region

| Ans. | | | | | | | | | |
|---|---|---|---|---|---|---|---|---|---|
| 168. E | 169. C | 170. B | 171. B | 172. A | 173. A | 174. B | 175. B | 176. B | 177. D |
| 178. A | 179. C | 180. B | 181. A | 182. A | 183. A | 184. B | 185. A | 186. D | |

**187. Which of the following is a goitrogen : Kerala 1997**

A. Bringal B. Turnip
C. Cabbage D. Sweet potato

**188. BCG is used in the treatment of : JIPMER 1998**

A. Bladder cancer B. Colon cancer
C. Breast cancer D. Thyroid cancer

**189. In diabetic ulcer, following sites are involved, except: PGI 1997**

A. Heel B. Webs
C. Head of metatarsal D. Tip of toes

**190. In esthesio neuroblastoma, which is involved : PGI 1997**

A. Olfactory N. B. Ophthalmic N.
C. Maxillary N. D. Nasociliary N.

**191. In AIDS, lymphadenopathy is mostly due to : PGI 1997**

A. TB
B. Lymphoma
C. Non-specific enlargement of LN
D. Secondary infection

**192. IVC filter is used in the following except : PGI 1997**

A. Massive emboli
B. Negligible size of emboli
C. Repeated emboli
D. Atherosclerotic plaques

**193. Lymphovenous anastomosis is done for : PGI 1997**

A. Filariasis B. Lymphoid cyst
C. Cystic hygroma D. All

**194. In arterial injury, following are done except : PGI 1997**

A. Thromboectomy
B. End-to-end anastomosis
C. Ligation
D. Venous graft

**195. Venous thrombosis is least common in : Punjab 1997**

A. Sea divers
B. Ca pancreas
C. Ca stomach
D. Prolonged immobilization

**196. Alder's sign is used to differentiate pain of : Punjab 1997**

A. Abdomen/outside abdomen
B. Genital/Extragenital region
C. Spine/cord
D. Heart/ribs

**197. Match List-I with List-II and select the correct answer using the codes given below the lists : UPSC 1997**

| List-I | List-II |
|---|---|
| A. Hodgkin's disease | 1. Adriamycin, Mitomycin, 5-fluorouracil |
| B. Breast carcinoma | 2. Cyclophosphamide, Methotrexate, 5-fluorouracil |
| C. Cancer buccal mucosa | 3. Cyclophosphamide, Oncovin, Procarbazine, Prednisolone |
| D. Cancer stomach | 4. Cisplatinum, 5-fluorouracil |

**Codes :**

| | A | B | C | D |
|---|---|---|---|---|
| A. | 3 | 2 | 1 | 4 |
| B. | 2 | 3 | 1 | 4 |
| C. | 3 | 2 | 4 | 1 |
| D. | 1 | 2 | 3 | 4 |

**198. A 25-years old lady, sustained a lacerates wound on the back of right thigh by the horn of a bull. The wound was sutured. Two months later she developed foot drop and an ulcer on the dorsum of the foot. The most likely diagnosis is : UPSC 1997**

A. Chronic ischaemic to limbs due to popliteal artery injury.
B. Partial injury to sciatic nerve.
C. Complete division of sciatic nerve.
D. Injury to hamstring muscles.

**199. Which of the following are athermal effects of diathermy : UPSC 1997**

I. Cutting and coagulation
II. Eddy currents
III. Piezoelectric effect
IV. Dimagnetism of some molecules

**Select the correct answer using the codes given below:**

**Codes :**

A. I, II and III
B. I, III and IV
C. I, II and IV
D. II, III and IV

**Ans.** 187. C 188. A 189. B 190. A 191. C 192. B 193. D 194. C 195. A 196. B 197. C 198. C 199. C

**200. Following trauma in man - inguinal swelling develops and exploration reveals transection of external common femoral vein. Treatment of choice is : WB 1998**

A. End-to-end anastomosis of this vein.
B. Ligation of vein distally with left sympathectomy.
C. Ligation of vein & artery both.
D. Ligation of vein proximal & distally.

**201. Silk is associated with infection because : WB 1998**

A. It has crevices lodging bacteria
B. Can not be properly sterilised
C. Infection goes deeper during bite
D. Unabsorbable

**202. Suture to be removed earliest in : WB 1998**

A. Face B. Abdomen
C. Perineum D. Chest

**203. Following causes distension of abdomen : CMC 1998**

A. Hirschsprung disease B. Hypokalemia
C. Hyperkalemia D. Hypomagnesemia

**204. Suture used in vascular surgery is : UP 1998**

A. Vicryl B. Silk
C. Polypropylene D. Dacron

**205. Most common cause of surgically treatable male infertility is : MAHE 1998**

A. Varicocele B. Cryptoorchidism
C. Stricture urethra D. Epididymitis

**206. The commonest cause of fever within 48 hours of surgery is : Orissa 1998**

A. Atelectasis B. Wound infection
C. Aspiration pneumonia D. Operative trauma

**207. The malignant tumours that spread by predominantly vascular permeation is : Orissa 1998**

A. Carcinoma of the breast
B. Lympho sarcoma
C. Renal cell carcinoma
D. Basal cell carcinoma

**208. The purpose of a drain as used in surgery is to : Orissa 1999**

A. Enhance healing
B. Evacuate collection of fluids
C. Act as a foreign body to stimulate healing fibrosis
D. Seal wounds

**209. Which of the following is not a predisposing factor for aspiration pneumonitis in surgical patients : Orissa 1998**

A. Altered consciousness
B. Dysphagia with oesophageal disorders
C. Mechanical disruption of defense barriers
D. Fever

**210. Morphine when given to an injured person primarily acts as : MAHE 1999**

A. Sedative B. Analgesic
C. Diaphoretic D. Emetic

**211. Which of the following does not predispose to pharyngocutaneous fistula : AIIMS 1999**

A. Radiotherapy
B. Chemotherapy
C. Neck inadequate closure
D. Residual tumor

**212. A patient with P.O.P. spine cast presents with billious vomiting, cause is : AIIMS 1999**

A. Acute dilatation of stomach
B. Acute pancreatitis
C. Duodenal Obs.
D. Peritonitis

**213. True about Mass in abdomen in neonates is following except : AIIMS 1999**

A. 40% constitute hepatic
B. Neuroblastoma & nephroblastoma most common tumor
C. More than 60% malignant
D. USG helps in diagnosis

**214. Complete bowel preparation is not done in all except : AIIMS 1999**

A. Hirschsprung's disease
B. IBD
C. Colonic CA
D. Ulcerative colitis with acute exacerbation

**215. Female on antibiotics, on prolonged IV cannulation with spikes of fever. Most likely cause is : AIIMS 1999**

A. Pseudomonas auerogenosa
B. Coagulate negative staphylococci
C. Streptococci agalactia
D. E. coli

**216. Radical retroperitoneal lymphnode dissection is indicated for all of the following esticular tumours except: TN 1999**

A. Choriocarcinoma B. Teratoma
C. Teratocarcinoma D. Seminoma

**217. Chyluria is seen in : TN 1999**

A. Schistosomiasis B. Ankylostoma
C. Wucheria bancrofti D. Strongyloides

| Ans. | | | | | | | | | |
|---|---|---|---|---|---|---|---|---|---|
| 200. D | 201. A | 202. A | 203. C | 204. C | 205. A | 206. D | 207. C | 208. B | 209. D |
| 210. B | 211. A | 212. A | 213. A | 214. B | 215. B | 216. A | 217. C | | |

**218. Dupuytren's contracture is associated with all except: Kerala 1999**

A. Kmuckle pads B. Peyronie disease
C. Mitral valve prolapse D. Ledder house disease

**219. Parentral fluid therapy can be started in a person with ——% burns or above. Kerala 1999**

A. 20% B. 32%
C. 40% D. 52%

**220. All are true about carpal tunnel syndrome except : Kerala 1999**

A. Flexion of wrist a fingers cause to increase in symptoms.
B. Surgical treatment sometimes do not alleviate the symptoms.
C. Tinels sign is positive.
D. More common in males.

**221. A middle aged man was treated for arthritis with high doses of aspirin. He has been posted for an elective surgery, following is advised : AI 2000**

A. Stop aspirin for 7 days & then do surgery.
B. Surgery can be done without any risk.
C. Keep platelet transfusion ready & do surgery.
D. Keep blood ready & do surgery.

**222. Treatment of carpal tunnel syndrome includes all the following except : UPSC 2000**

A. Neurolysis of median nerve
B. Local injection of steroids
C. Splinting of hand in neutral position
D. Tenosynvectomy

**223. Match List-I (Complains of liver transplantation) with List-II (Features of complications) and select the correct answer using the codes given below the Lists: UPSC 2000**

| List-I | List-II |
|---|---|
| a. Rejection | 1. Peritonitis |
| b. Hepatic artery thrombosis | 2. Delayed liver necrosis |
| c. Bile leak | 3. Graft non-function |
| d. Portal vein thrombosis | 4. Poor graft function |

**Codes :**

| | a | b | c | d |
|---|---|---|---|---|
| A. | 4 | 2 | 3 | 1 |
| B. | 4 | 2 | 1 | 3 |
| C. | 2 | 4 | 3 | 1 |
| D. | 2 | 4 | 1 | 3 |

**224. Following an incised wound in the front of wrist, the subject is unable to oppose the tips of the little finger and the thumb. The nerve(s) involved is/are : UPSC 2000**

A. Ulnar nerve alone
B. Median nerve alone
C. Median and ulnar nerves
D. Radial and ulnar nerves

**225. Gleasen's staging is done in : UPSC 2000**

A. Ca prostate B. Ca Pancreas
C. Ca kidney D. Ca Cx

**226. Dissection of which artery is seen in pregnancy : UPSC 2000**

A. Carotid artery B. Aorta
C. Coronary A D. Femoral artery

**227. What is the line of management of a case of moderate to severe hepatic insufficiency with portal hypertension, according to the modified Pugh's classification : AI 2000**

A. Sclerotherapy
B. Orthotopic liver transplantation
C. Shunt surgery
D. Conservative

**228. While doing below knee amputation which of the following is the most important technical consideration: AI 2000**

A. Posterior flap should be longer than the anterior flap.
B. Anterior flap should be longer than the posterior flap.
C. Stump should be long.
D. Stump should be short.

**229. A patient was undergoing abdominal surgery under local anaesthesia. He suddenly developed sharp severe pain. Which of the following structures will be responsible for his pain : AI 2000**

A. Parietal peritoneum B. Liver parenchyma
C. Colon D. Small intestine

**230. While doing central venous catheterization of a patient through internal jugular vein, the patient suddenly developed respiratory distress and hypoxemia. What would be the likely cause : AIIMS 2000**

A. Pneumothorax B. Cardiac Tamponade
C. Hypovolemia D. Septicemia

**231. Head trauma patient presents four weeks after his injury with features of irritability and altered sensorium. What is the most likely diagnosis : AIIMS 2000**

A. Electrolyte imbalance
B. Chronic subdural hematoma
C. Extradural hematoma
D. Intraparenchymal bleeding

**Ans.** **218. B** **219. A** **220. D** **221. A** **222. C** **223. B** **224. C** **225. A** **226. B** **227. B** **228. C** **229. A** **230. A** **231. B**

**232. Skin graft survival within 48 hrs of transplantation is due to : AIIMS 2000**
A. New vessels growing from the donor tissue
B. Plasma imbibition
C. Amount of saline in graft
D. Connection between donor and recepient capillaries

**233. Primary peritonitis is more common inf emales because : AI 2001**
A. Ostia of Follopian tubes communicate with abdominal cavity
B. Peritoneum overlies the uterus
C. Rupture of functional ovarian cysts
D. All of the above

**234. A 45 yrs old man presents with progressive cervical lymph node enlargement, since 3 months, most appropiate investigation is : AI 2001**
A. X-ray soft tissue B. FNAC
C. Lymph node biopsy D. Peripheral blood smear

**235. A patient is brought with head injury, head on collision and BP 90/60. Tachycardia present. Diagnosis : AI 2001**
A. EDH B. SDH
C. Intracranal hemorrhag D. Intraabdominal bleed

**236. Patient's semen sample reveals 15 million sperms, 60% normal morphology 60% motile, sperm volume is 2 ml, no agglutmation . Diagnosis : AI 2001**
A. Azoospermia B. Aspermia
C. Oligospermia D. Normospermia

**237. A 18 yr old presents with massive hematemesis; history of fever past 14 days; treatment with drugs; moderate spleen present; diagnosis : AI 2001**
A. NSAID induced gastritis
B. Drug induced gastritis
C. Esophageal varices
D. Duodenal ulcer

**238. Babu presents h/o road accident. He is hypotensive. Most likely injured organ is : AI 2001**
A. Spleen B. Mesentry
C. Kidney D. Rectum

**239. All the following statements relating to penetrating injuries of the abdomen are true except: UPSC 2001**
A. The abdomen can be adequately explored.
B. They frequently result in acquired abdominal wall herniae.
C. Exploratory laparotomy only if peritonitis or shock is evident.
D. They can be treated conservatively if the weapon is less than 3 cm in size.

**240. The most important factor which limits the use of the combination of isoniazid, rifampicin and pyrazinamide in tuberculosis patients is: UPSC 2001**
A. Ototoxicity.
B. Nephrotoxicity.
C. Bone marrow suppression
D. Hepatotoxicity

**241. Match List-I (Syndrome) with List-II (Clinical conditions) and select the correct answer using the codes given below the lists : UPSC 2001**

| List-I | List-II |
|---|---|
| A. Leber's Disease | 1. Optic neuropathy |
| B. Whipple's Triad | 2. CBD Stone |
| C. Charcot Triad | 3. Rupture of the lower |
| D. Boerhaeeve's syndrome | 4. Insulinoma |

**Codes :**

| | A | B | C | D |
|---|---|---|---|---|
| A. | 1 | 4 | 2 | 3 |
| B. | 4 | 1 | 2 | 3 |
| C. | 3 | 2 | 1 | 4 |
| D. | 1 | 4 | 3 | 2 |

**242. Which one of the following pairs of names and surgical procedures is not correctly matched : UPSC 2001**
A. Auchinclos : Mastectomy
B. Theodore Kocchar : Splenectomy
C. Sistrunks : Thyroglossal cyst operation
D. Shouldice : Hernia repair

**243. Which type of Hodgkin's disease carries the best prognosis ? AI 1991**
A. Lymphcytic depletion
B. Lymphocytic predominance
C. Nodular sclerosis
D. Mixed cellularity

**244. Most common sarcoma in a person recieving immunosup-pressive treatment is : Kerala 2001**
A. Kaposi's sarcoma B. Lymphoma
C. CA D. Leukemia

Ans. 232. B 233. A 234. C 235. D 236. C 237. A 238. A 239. C 240. D 241. A 242. B 243. B 244. A

**245. Which of the following is not true for angiodysplasia : Kerala 2001**

A. Associated with AS
B. Dialated submucosal vessels seen
C. Commonest site is cecum & ascending colon
D. Commonly treated by injecting sclerosants

**246. All the following need emergency operation except : Kerala 2001**

A. Obstruction due to bands
B. Volvulus of sigmoid colon
C. Appendix perfn with paralytic ileus
D. Strangulation

**247. A lump in Rt iliac fossa due to : Rohtak 2001**

A. Ileococal TB B. Appendicular limb
C. External iliac adenitis D. All of the above

**248. Non-irritant fluid to peritonium : DNB 2001**

A. Bile B. Blood
C. Saline D. Intestinal contents

**249. In IVDP Schmrols node in MRI which is correct : MAHE 2001**

A. Significant B. Not significant
C. Good prognostic D. Not prognostic

**250. A man aged 60 years has h/o IHD and atherosclerosis. He presents with abdominal pain and maroon stools. Diagnosis is : AI 2001**

A. Acute intestinal obstruction
B. Acute mesenteric ischemia
C. Perionitis
D. Appendicitis

**251. A patient presents with mild hemoptysis. He is a chronic smoker for the past 20 years. X-ray chest-normal. Next investigation of choice is : AIIMS 2002**

A. Bronchography B. CT chest
C. USG D. Fibreoptic bronchoscopy

**252. On her third day of hospitalization, a 70 years old woman who is being treated for acute cholecystitis develops increased pain and tenderness in the right upper quadrant with a palpable mass. Her temperature rises to 104 and her BP falls to 80/60. Hemetamesis and malena ensure and petechiae are noted. Laboratory studies reveal thrombocytopenia, prolonged PT, and decreased fibrinogen level. The most important step in the correction of this patients coagulopathy : AI 2002**

A. Administration of heparin
B. Administration of fresh frozen plasma
C. Administration of Epilon amino caproic acid
D. Exploratory laparotomy

**253. A man of 70 kgs is transferred to a burn centre 4 weeks after sustaining a 2nd and 3rd degree burn injury to 45% of his total body surface area. Prior to the accident the patient's weight was 90 kgs. The patient has not been given anything by mouth since the injury, except for antacids because of a previous ulcer history. On examination the patient's burn wound are clean, but only minimal healing is evident and thick adherent eschar present. The patient's abdomen is soft and non-distended and active bowel sounds are heard. His stools are trace positive for blood and he has a reducible right inguinal hernia, which appears to be easily reducible. He has poor range of motion of all involved joints and had developed early axillary and popliteal fossae flexion contractures. In managing this patient at this stage of his injury, top priority must be given to correcting.: AI 2002**

A. The open, poorly healing burn wounds by surgical excision and grafting.
B. The inguinal hernia by surgical repair using local anaestheic.
C. The nutritional status by enteral supplementation or parenteral hyperalimentation.
D. By increasing the dose of antacids and adding cimetidine.

**254. A 16 years old girl who has nonpitting edema of recent onset affecting her right leg but no other symptoms is referred for evaluation. True statements about this patient include all the following except : AI 2002**

A. A lymphangiogram probably will show hypoplasia of the lymphatics.
B. Prophylactic antibiotics are indicated.
C. Elastic support and diuretics will restore the affected limb to normal appearance.
D. A variety of operations will restore the affected limb to a normal appearance.

**255. A previously healthy 45 years old construction worker develops acute low back pain, right leg pain, and weakness of dorsiflexion of the great toe. True statements regarding this case include which of the following : AI 2002**

A. Immediate treatment should include analgesics, muscle relaxants, and back strengthening exercises.
B. The appearance of foot drop would be an early indication for early surgery.
C. Lumbar laminectomy and excision of any herniated nucleus pulposus should be performed if the presenting symptoms should fail to resolve in 1 week.
D. If the neurological signs but not the back pain resolve in 2 to 3 weeks proper treatment would include fusion of affected lumbar vertebrae.

**Ans.** 245. D 246. A 247. D 248. C 249. B 250. B 251. A 252. D 253. C 254. D 255. B

**256. Ten days after a splenectomy for abdominal trauma, a 23 years old man complains of upper abdominal and lower chest pain exacerbated by deep breathing. He is anorectic but ambulatory and otherwise making satisfactoy progress. On physical examination, his temperature is 38.2° rectally, and he has decreased breath sounds at the left lung base. His abdominal wound appears to be healing well, bowel sounds are active, and there are no peritoneal signs. Rectal examination is negative. The white blood cell count is 12,500/mm3 with a shift to the left. Chest X-rays show plate like atelectasis of the left lung field. Abdominal X-rays show a non-specific gas pattern in the bowel and an air fluid level in the left upper quadrant. Serum amylase is 150 Somogyi units per dl. : AI 2002**

The most likely diagnosis :

A. Subphrenic abscess
B. Subfascial wound infection
C. Pancreatitis
D. Pulmonary embolism

**257. Hypergastrinemia with hypochlorhydria is seen in : AI 2002**

A. Zollinger Ellison Syndrome
B. VIPoma
C. Pernicious anemia
D. Glucagonoma

**258. Match List-I (Primary malignancies ) with List-II (Most common site of metastasis and select the correct answer : UPSC 2002**

| List-I | List-II |
|---|---|
| A. Prostatic carcinoma | 1. Left supraclavicular lymph nodes |
| B. Seminoma testis | 2. Lungs |
| C. Carcinoma stomach | 3. Lumbar vertebrae |
| D. Choriocarcinoma | 4. Paraortic lymph nodes |

| | A | B | C | D |
|---|---|---|---|---|
| A. | 3 | 4 | 2 | 1 |
| B. | 4 | 3 | 1 | 2 |
| C. | 4 | 3 | 2 | 1 |
| D. | 3 | 4 | 1 | 2 |

**259. A 20 years old male presented with chronic constipation, headache and palpitati ›. On examination he had marfanoid habitus, neuromas of tongue, medullated corneal nerve fibres and a nodule of 2 ´2 cms size in the left lobe of thyroid gland. This patient is a case of : AI 2004**

A. Sporadic medúllary carcinoma of thyroid
B. Familial medullary carcinoma of thyroid
C. MEN IIA
D. MEN IIB

**260. Which of the following is not an important cause of hyponatremia: AI 2004**

A. Gastric fistula
B. Excessive vomiting
C. Excessive Sweating
D. Prolonged Ryle's tube aspiration

**261. Which is high risk for laparoscopic surgery : AI 2009**

A. Hiatus hernia
B. Obesity
C. Heart diseases
D. Hb <8 gm %

**262. Chemoradiotherapy is not given in : AI 2009**

A. II Ca cervix
B. Anal carcinoma T2 N1 M0
C. T2 N0 M0 glottic Ca
D. Nasopharyngeal Cas

**263. All of the patients presenting with abdominal pain and shock need immidiate laporatomy except : Delhi 2009**

A. Ruptured ectopic pregnancy
B. Haemorrhagic pancreatic
C. Rupture abdominal aortic aneurysm
D. Ruptured liver hemangioma

**264. Lynch syndrome is associated with tumors of : AIIMS 2009**

A. Colon, Breast, Endometrium
B. Breast, Ovary, Endometrium
C. Colon, Breast, Ovary
D. Colon, Endometrium, Ovary

| Ans. | 256. A | 257. C | 258. D | 259. D | 260. A | 261. B | 262. C | 263. B | 264. D |
|---|---|---|---|---|---|---|---|---|---|

# EXPLANATIONS OF MISCELLANEOUS ASPECTS

1. Ans.— B. String test
2. Ans.— D. ACTH is treatment of choice

   Insulinoma is a beta cell tumor. Confirmation is made by fasting hypoglycemia associated by radioimmunoassay. The only curative treatment is extirpation of tumor.
3. Ans.— A. Lagging behind of the upper eyelid
4. Ans.— A. Excessive granulation tissue
5. Ans.— B. Cervicodorsal sympathectomy
6. Ans.— C. Small bowel
7. Ans.— D. Pre-alveolar cleft
8. Ans.— A. Acromegaly
9. Ans.— D. Diarrhoea
10. Ans.— D. Epididymoorchitis
11. Ans.— D. Excision of carcinoma of the tongue, the floor of the mouth, part of the jaw and lymph nodes en bloc.
12. Ans.— D Edestin
13. Ans.— C. Ambroise Parey
14. Ans.— D. XI
15. Ans.— A. Joseph Lister
16. Ans.— D. Henle's ligament
17. Ans.— B. Suprapubic catheterization
18. Ans.— C. Varicocele
19. Ans.— B. Thronton's
20. Ans.— C. Howell & Holt
21. Ans.— D. Cardiomegaly
22. Ans.— A. Congenital syphilis
23. Ans.— C. Thickening of frontal and parietal bones
24. Ans.— D. Malignant endocarditis
25. Ans.— B. Doubled
26. Ans.— B. Left kidney on the right side
27. Ans.— A. Renal artery to renal artery
28. Ans.— C. Rectum
29. Ans.— A. Adenocarcinoma of breast
30. Ans.— C. Rickets
31. Ans.— C. Dysphagia
32. Ans.— D. Acute appendicitis
33. Ans.— C. Bastede's sign
34. Ans.— D. African trypanosomiasis
35. Ans.— B. Oesophageal stricture
36. Ans.— D. Increased acid phosphatase
37. Ans.— D. Pneumonia
38. Ans.— D. Bulbar poliomyelitis
39. Ans.— C. Boerhaave's syndrome

   Full thickness rupture is Boerhaave's syndrome and partial thickness mucosal rupture is Mallory Weiss syndrome. Most common cause of oesophageal rupture is tatrogenic (by instruments).
40. Ans.— D. Measles
41. Ans.— D. Osteoarthritis
42. Ans.— C. Bluish line on gums in lead poisoning
43. Ans.— B. Mediastinal nodes
44. Ans.— C. Low blood pressure, elevated venous pressure, quiet heart.
45. Ans.— C. Hyperthyroidism
46. Ans.— D. None of the above
47. Ans.— C. Tetany
48. Ans.— D. Aortic anurysm
49. Ans.— D. Pneumonitis
50. Ans.— B. 1 week
51. Ans.— C. Infection

   The effect of immunosuppression is susceptibility to infection usually becomes greatest between 1 and 6 months after transplantation and drug side effects are usually also greatest at this time.
52. Ans.— D. Lymphangiography
53. Ans.— C. Sheep

54. Ans.— A. Ca rectum

Ca rectum is fourth most common variety of malignant tumor found in women and its frequency in men is usually surpassed only by Ca bronchus and stomach. It spreads locally (circumferentially) and by lymphatics to LN and by venous system (only late except portion of anal canal) to liver (34%) lungs (22%), adrenals (11%) and rarely to other sites including brain.

55. Ans.— A. Ca pancreas

56. Ans.— C. Dwarfism

57. Ans.— C. Sahli's

58. Ans.— B. Related to the speed of venous filling after emptying a length of vein.

59. Ans.— A. Gastric carcinoma

60. Ans.— D. Right kidney is preferred because its vessels are longer.

61. Ans.— E. All of the above

62. Ans.— B. 15, 25 and 40

63. Ans.— A. Jaundice

64. Ans.— A. Children with biliary atresia

Starzl performed first human liver transplantation in 1903.

65. Ans.— E. All of the above

66. Ans.— A. Cholelithiasis

67. Ans.— D. Papillary carcinoma of thyroid

68. Ans.— C. Over the femoral trochanters of the thighs.

69. Ans.— C. Rovsing'sign

70. Ans.— C. Rogoff's sign

71. Ans.— C. 1, 2 and 4

72. Ans.— B. Haemangioma

73. Ans.— C. Just before operation

This is done not to allow the growth of bacteria.

74. Ans.— B. Parotid

75. Ans.— B. Neuroblastoma

76. Ans.— B. Armand Trousseau

77. Ans.— B. Histological differentiation

78. Ans.— B. Rovsing's sign

79. Ans.— B. Fibrosarcoma

80. Ans.— C. 9.2

81. Ans.— D. -200°

82. Ans.— A. Gall bladder

Murphy's sign is also known as Nauynyn's sign (after Bernard Naunyn 1839-1925 given in 1890, 13 years before Morphy) is seen in chronic calculous cholecystitis.

83. Ans.— D. Tenderness over an infected ulnar bursa between the transverse palmar creases.

84. Ans.— C. A papilloma with excessive Keratin formation.

85. Ans.— C. Nephroblastoma

86. Ans.— B. Moebius sign

87. Ans.— D. As above, but the person has tetany

88. Ans.— C. The presence of an incompetent valve at the saphenofemoral junction.

89. Ans.— B. Thyroglossal fistulous tract along with the body of the hyoid bone.

90. Ans.— C. Fibres along the iliopectineal line

91. Ans.— D. Renal tubular cells

Liver, osteoblasts & Polymorph nuclear Leucocyte secrete serum Alkaline phosphatase, is used in diagnosis of Liver & Bone disorders.

92. Ans.— D. In the foot of a patient with severe vascular disease.

It is the cry of the dying nerves especially seen in Buerger's disease.

93. Ans.— A. Prednisolone + azathioprine

94. Ans.— C. Arteriography

95. Ans.— A. Venous ulcer

96. Ans.— A. Repair of parotid fistula

97. Ans.— B. Renal stone

Randall's plaque or microliths. Randall suggested that the initial lesion in some cases of kidney stone was an erosion at the tip of renal papilla. Deposition of calcium on this erosion produced a lesion which has been called Randall's plaque.

98. Ans.— C. Infection

99. Ans.— D. Atelectasis

100. Ans.— D. Injected into the portal vein

101. Ans.— D. Renal abnormalities

102. Ans.— C. Rovsing's sign

103. Ans.— C. Rogoff's sign

104. Ans.— C. Milroy's disease

105. Ans.— C. Idiopathic retroperitoneal fibrosis

106. Ans.— A. The night before surgery

107. Ans.— A. Bone
Radiotherapy is given to alleviate pain

108. Ans.— C. Intussusception

109. Ans.— C. HLA-A

110. Ans.— A. Pancreas

111. Ans.— C. Negative nitrogen balance

112. Ans.— A. Coded by multiple genes

113. Ans.— C. Cholecystitis

114. Ans.— B. Cornea

115. Ans.— A. Cerebral oedema

116. Ans.— C. Monofilament nylon

117. Ans.— C. Gastric secretion

118. Ans.— A. Stellwig sign

119. Ans.— D. Achlasia cardia

120. Ans.— B. Fat embolism

121. Ans.— B. Triceps skinfold thickness

122. Ans.— D. Medium size and small size arteries
It is common in smokers and gangrene results.

123. Ans.— D. Retrosternal goiter

124. Ans.— B. MEN IIb

125. Ans.— D. Cardiomegaly

126. Ans.— A. Cullen's sign

127. Ans.— A. An artery

128. Ans.— C. An aneurysm

129. Ans.— A. Oral cholecystography

130. Ans.— D. Branham's sign

131. Ans.— D. Isopropyl alcohol
Pressure on artery proximal to A-V fistula causes the swelling to diminish in size, the thrill and bruit to cease, the pulse rate to fall and pulse pressure to return to normal.

132. Ans.— B. Thyroidectomy

133. Ans.— B. Kidney

134. Ans.— D. Urinary excretion of fibrin degradation products.

135. Ans.— A. Vascular endothelium

136. Ans.— B. End stage glomerulonephritis or pyelonephritis.
David Hume and Joseph Kelly undertook the first successful series of human kidney transplantations starting in 1954, Gregoir-Lich technique or Leadbelter-Politano technique are used.

137. Ans.— C. Blood

138. Ans.— A. Pain referred to the left shoulder

139. Ans.— D. Gynaecomastia

140. Ans.— C. Isograft

141. Ans.— B. Obtaining haemostasis as the first priority.

142. Ans.— A. Bronchogenic Ca

143. Ans.— B. Edestin test

144. Ans.— A. Cardiac catherterization

145. Ans.— A. Rheumatoid arthritis

146. Ans.— B. Ectopic urethral opening

147. Ans.— B. Intussusception

148. Ans.— B. Hydrocephalus

149. Ans.— A. Ureterocele
It is also called "adder head" deformity seen on excretory urography. Ureterocele is most common in women, endoscopic diathermy incision is required. In advanced cases with hydronephrosis or pyonephrosis, nephrectomy may be appropriate.

150. Ans.— A. Fibrosarcoma

151. Ans.— B. Cystic hygroma

152. Ans.— B. Allograft

153. Ans.— C. Graves' disease

154. Ans.— C. Malignant melanoma

155. Ans.— A. Ca breast

156. Ans.— B. Choriocarcinoma of testis
Seminomas are radiosensitive and for Teratomas, chemotherapy is used.

157. Ans.— B.

| A | B | C | D |
|---|---|---|---|
| 3 | 4 | 1 | 2 |

158. Ans.— B. Cirrhosis

159. Ans.— D. Promethazine

160. Ans.— D. Hereditary spherocytosis

161. Ans.— A. Radiotherapy

162. Ans.— D. Wilm's tumor

163. Ans.— D. < 20 years

164. Ans.— B. Carcinoma prostate

165. Ans.— A. Heart and kidney

166. Ans.— A. CMV

167. Ans.— A. Siliconised rubber T-tube

168. Ans.— E. 72 hours

Cold storage times (hours) for various organs are

| *Organ* | *Ideal* | *Safe* | *Maximum* |
|---|---|---|---|
| Kidney | Below 24 | 48 | 4 |
| Heart | Below 3 | 5 | 6 |
| Liver | Below 8 | 12 | 24 |
| Pancreas | Below 8 | 12 | 24 |

169. Ans.— C. Neuroblastoma
170. Ans.— B. Morrissey's test
171. Ans.— B. Alexander Wallace
172. Ans.— A. Pancreas
173. Ans.— A. Encircling the neck at C6 vertebra level
174. Ans.— B. Wilm's tumour
175. Ans.— B. 8th dorsal nerve
176. Ans.— B. Subfascial ligation
177. Ans.— D. All of the above
178. Ans.— A. Ligation lower than the level of Sapheno-femoral junction.
179. Ans.— C. Aberrant obturator artery
180. Ans.— B. Conjoint tendon
181. Ans.— A. Recovery Room
182. Ans.— A. Hypothermia
183. Ans.— A. Neoplasm

It may be seen in Ca bladder or kidney.

184. Ans.— B. Jugular nodes
185. Ans.— A. Hyponatremia
186. Ans.— D. Umbilicus
187. Ans.— C. Cabbage
188. Ans.— A. Bladder cancer
189. Ans.— B. Webs
190. Ans.— A. Olfactory N.
191. Ans.— C. Non-specific enlargement of LN
192. Ans.— B. Negligible size of emboli

This is used in Budd Chiari syndrome.

193. Ans.— D. All
194. Ans.— C. Ligation
195. Ans.— A. Sea divers
196. Ans.— B. Genital/Extragenital region
197. Ans.— C. A B C D

3 2 4 1

198. Ans.— C. Complete division of sciatic nerve
199. Ans.— C. I, II and IV
200. Ans.— D. Ligation of vein proximal & distally.
201. Ans.— A. It has crevices lodging bacteria
202. Ans.— A. Face
203. Ans.— C. Hyperkalemia
204. Ans.— C. Polypropylene
205. Ans.— A. Varicocele
206. Ans.— D. Operative trauma

It is most commonly due to operative trauma and tissue.

207. Ans.— C. Renal cell carcinoma
208. Ans.— B. Evacuate collection of fluids
209. Ans.— D. Fever
210. Ans.— B. Analgesic
211. Ans.— A. Radiotherapy
212. Ans.— A. Acute dilatation of stomach
213. Ans.— A. 40% constitute hepatic
214. Ans.— B. IBD
215. Ans.— B. Coagulate negative staphylococci
216. Ans.— A. Çhoriocarcinoma
217. Ans.— C. Wucheria bancrofti
218. Ans.— B. Mitral valve prolapse
219. Ans.— A. 20%
220. Ans.— D. More common in males
221. Ans.— A. Stop aspirin for 7 days & then do surgery.

Anticoagulants or salicylates should be stopped atleast a week before surgery reaction.

222. Ans.— C. Splinting of hand in neutral position
223. Ans.— B. 4 2 1 3
224. Ans.— C. Median and ulnar nerves
225. Ans.— A. Ca prostate
226. Ans.— B. Aorta
227. Ans.— B. Orthotopic liver transplantation
228. Ans.— C. Stump should be long
229. Ans.— A. Parietal peritoneum
230. Ans.— A. Pneumothorax
231. Ans.— B. Chronic subdural hematoma
232. Ans.— B. Plasma inhibition
233. Ans.— A. Ostia of Fallopian tubes communicate with abdominal cavity.

Pneumococcal is an important cause in adolescent girls.

**234. Ans.— C. Lymph node biopsy**

**Biopsy is best to diagnose inflammatory or neoplastic aetiology. FNAC is also becoming increasingly popular.**

**235. Ans.— D. Intra-abdominal bleeding**

**Hypotension is usually due to haemorrhage from extracranial site and most often from abdomen.**

**236. Ans.— C. Oligospermia**

**The findings are suggestive of oligospermia.**

**237. Ans.— A. NSAID induced gastritis**

**238. Ans.— A. Spleen**

**The most commonly injured organ is spleen lying under ribs.**

**239. Ans.— C. Exploratory laparotomy only if peritonitis or shock is evident.**

**240. Ans.— D. Hepatotoxicity**

**241. Ans.— A. A B C D**

**1 4 2 3**

**242. Ans.— B. Theodore Kocchar : Splenectomy**

**243. Ans.— B. Lymphocytic predominance**

**There are 2 varieties of HC, a localised predominantly nonaggressive form; progressive and fatal variety. Histologically inactive disease is lymphocyte predominant clinically stage-I and potentially curable.**

**244. Ans.— A. Kaposi's sarcoma**

**245. Ans.— D. Commonly treated by injecting sclerosants.**

**246. Ans.— A. Obstruction due to bands**

**247. Ans.— D. All of the above**

**248. Ans.— C. Saline**

**249. Ans.— B. Not significant**

**250. Ans.— B. Acute mesenteric ischemia**

**251. Ans.— A. Bronchography**

**252. Ans.— D. Exploratory laparotomy**

**Explorative laparotomy is both diagnostic and curative.**

**253. Ans.— C. The nutritional status by enteral supplementation or parenteral hyperalimentation.**

**Nutritional status has to be restored first.**

**254. Ans.— D. A variety of operations will restore the affected limb to a normal appearance.**

**It may be due to filariae or bacterial infection. Operative procedure are not often successful in restoring normal appearance of limb.**

**255. Ans.— B. The appearance of foot drop would be an early indication for early surgery.**

**Foot drop requires immediate cord decompression.**

**256. Ans.— A. Subphrenic abscess**

**The symptoms and signs of subphrenic infection are frequently non-specific. If suppuration seems probable, intervention is indicated.**

**257. Ans.— C. Pernicious anemia**

**258. Ans.— D. 3 4 1 2**

**259. Ans.— D. MEN IIB**

**Gastrointestinal neuroendocrine tumors (NETs) are derived from neuroendocrine system of GI tract and are composed of amine and acid producing cells with different hormonal profiles, depending on the site of origin. These tumors were originally classified as APUDomas (amine precursor uptake and decarboxylation), as were pheochromocytomas, melanomas and medullary carcinoma thyroid.**

**Marfanoid habitus, neuroma of tongue and thyroid nodule are catch point for diagnosis of MEN IIB.**

***MEN I (Wermer's Syndrome)***

- **Pituitary adenoma**
- **Parathyroid hyperplasia (or adenoma)**
- **Pancreatic islet cell neoplasm**
- **Adrenal cortical hyperplasia**

***MEN II A (Sipple Syndrome)***

- **Medullary carcinoma of thyroid**
- **Pheochromocytoma**
- **Parathyroid hyperplasia (or adenoma)**
- **Hirschsprung disease**
- **Cutaneous lichen amyloidosis**

***MEN II B***

- **Medullary carcinoma of thyroid**
- **Pheochromocytoma**
- **Marfanoid habitus**
- **Mucocutaneous and gastrointestinal neuroma**

**260. Ans.— A. Gastric fistula**

**261. Ans.— B. Obesity**

**The risk of such injuries is increased in patients *who are obese* or have a history of prior abdominal surgery.**

**262. Ans.— C. T2 N0 M0 glottic Ca**

*** In general, early stage glottic cancers (i.e T1 and T2) are managed with a single modality, such as radiation, endoscopic excision, or conservation laryngeal surgery.**

**263. Ans.— B. Haemorrhagic pancreatic**

**Surgery is not indicated in initial period of resuscitation and stabilisation. If patient deteriorates following sucessful stabilization or there is surgical intervention is contemplated. In haemorrhagic type, surgery is not immediately used.**

**264. Ans.— D. Colon, Endometrium, Ovary**

# REVIEW PAPER—I

## (Based on Difficult & Important MCQ's)

**1. In tumor lysis syndrome, there are increased levels of following except :**
A. Potassium B. Calcium
C. Phosphate D. Uric acid

**2. Familial polyposis of colon with gliomas is seen in :**
A. Unna-Thost's syndrome B. Winkel's syndrome
C. Turcot's syndrome D. Vernet's syndrome

**3. Vagoaccessory syndrome is ——— syndrome.**
A. Unna-Thost's B. Univerricht's
C. Schmidt's D. MacLeod's

**4. Cleft lip, cleft palate and cysts of lower lips are seen in —syndrome.**
A. Weingarton's B. Vogt's
C. Villaret's D. Vander Woude's

**5. Beta cell tumors of pancreatic islets and increased levels of VIP are seen in ——— syndrome.**
A. Ullrich Feichtiger B. Verner-Morrison
C. Weingarten's D. Wermer's

**6. Vernet's syndrome differs from Villaret's syndrome that there is non-involvement of—— cranial nerve.**
A. IX B. X
C. XI D. XII

**7. Renal hypoplasia, aplasia anomalies of int. genitalia especially vaginal atresia and anomalies of ossicles of middle ear are seen in —— syndrome.**
A. Wolf Hirshchern B. Wright's
C. Wolfram's D. Winter's

**8. A syndrome of deletion of short arm of chromosome 4 and hypospadias is—— syndrome.**
A. William's B. Wright's
C. Wofl-Hirschhorn's D. Wolfram's

**9. Yellow nail syndrome is due to :**
A. Venous thrombosis B. Arterial thrombosis
C. Lymphoedema D. Congenital jaundice

**10. Cerebrohepatorenal syndrome is —— syndrome.**
A. Wolfram's B. Wright's
C. William's D. Zellweger's

**11. Neurovascular syndrome caused by hyperabduction of arm is ——— syndrome.**
A. Wright's B. Wolfram's
C. William's D. Zinsser-Cole-Engman

**12. Obstructive azoospermia and chronic sinopulmonary infections are seen in ——— syndrome.**
A. William's B. Wolfram's
C. Young's D. Zieve's

**13. Enlargement of spleen due to splenic vein thrombosis is ——— syndrome.**
A. Carpent
B. Cauchois-Eppinger-Fregoni
C. Cairns
D. Cossidy

**14. Infantile Celiac disease is called ——— syndrome.**
A. Gee-Hereter Heubner B. Gardner
C. Gaisboch D. Fraser

**15. To rule out organic cause of backache, test used is :**
A. Aird's test B. Bapat's test
C. Carnett's test D. Cozen's test

**16. Baldwin's method is used for ——— percussion.**
A. Pleural fluid B. Liver
C. Spleen D. Kidney

**17. Which of the following test is also known as bed shaking test to elicit pain due to inflammed peritoneum :**
A. Chiene's test B. Buerger's test
C. Bapat's test D. Carnett's test

**18. Kocher's test is used to confirm enlargement of :**
A. Larynx B. Thyroid
C. Liver D. Kidney

**19. Halo's test can be used to confirm presence of ———.**
A. Blood B. CSF
C. Saliva D. Nasal discharge

**20. Which of the following test is positive in varicose veins of lower limb :**
A. Paget's test B. Schwartz's test
C. Lasegue's test D. Naffegier's test

| Ans. | | | | | | | | | |
|---|---|---|---|---|---|---|---|---|---|
| 1. B | 2. C | 3. C | 4. D | 5. B | 6. D | 7. D | 8. C | 9. C | 10. D |
| 11. A | 12. C | 13. B | 14. A | 15. A | 16. D | 17. C | 18. B | 19. B | 20. B |

**21. Which of the following test is used in thyrotoxicosis :**
A. Chiene's test B. Buerger's test
C. Carnett's test D. Werner's test

**22. A test used to differentiate intraabdominal swelling and swelling of abdominal wall :**
A. Card's test B. Chair test
C. Carnett's test D. Chiene's test

**23. A test used to diagnose pathological condition of hip is ——— test.**
A. Buerger's B. Paget's
C. Chiene's D. Cope's psoas

**24. A test used to diagnose tennis elbow :**
A. Buerger's test B. Compression test
C. Cope's obturator test D. Cozen's test

**25. Flexion and internal rotation causes pain in right iliac fossa in acute appendicitis. This is :**
A. Naffegier's test B. Cope's obturator test
C. Cope's psoas test D. Chair test

**26. Triad of Hand-Schuller Christian syndrome is characterized by the following' except :**
A. Diabetes insipidus B. Exophthalmos
C. Bone destruction D. Optic atrophy

**27. Hanot's syndrome is characterized by :**
A. Cystic fibrosis of pancreas
B. Biliary cirrhosis
C. Hanot-Chauffard syndrome
D. Hanhart's syndrome

**28. T.B. Testis first affects :**
A. Vas deferens B. Epididymis
C. Body of testis D. Tunica vaginalis

**29. Hyperinsulism is seen in :**
A. Hare's syndrome B. Harris syndrome
C. Hanhart's syndrome D. Gruber's syndrome

**30. Hayem Widal syndrome is characterized by :**
A. Idiopathic steatorrhoea
B. Hemolytic anemia
C. Pyelonephritis
D. Recurrent pneumonitis

**31. Intermittent attacks of low temperature and disabling sweating are features of :**
A. Homen's syndrome
B. Hines-Bannick syndrome
C. Howel-Evans syndrome
D. Gruber's syndrome

**32. Gruber's syndrome is also known as :**
A. Gronblad-Strandberg syndrome
B. Holmes-Adie syndrome
C. Hanhart's syndrome
D. Meckel's syndrome

**33. Paralysis of X, XI and XII cranial nerves seen in ——— syndrome.**
A. Jahnke's B. Jackson's
C. Jeune' D. Meckel's syndrome

**34. Which of the following is a variant of Sturge-Weber syndrome :**
A. Jahnke's syndrome B. Jeune's syndrome
C. Kennedy's syndrome D. Kinsbourne's syndrome

**35. Analgesia of perineal nerve, sometimes noticed in Tabes dorsalis is called :**
A. Roser's sign B. Sarboo's sign
C. Saunders' sign D. Schick's sign

**36. Increased pulsation over the cardiac region in intrathoracic tumours is called :**
A. Sternburg's sign B. Stierlin's sign
C Sterles sign D. Strauss sign

**37. Increase in fat following the use of fatty acids in chylous ascites is :**
A. Stierlin's sign B. Sternberg's sign
C. Strauss sign D. Saunders sign

**38. Severe pain in the region of the flanks in nephrolithiasis is —— sign.**
A. Testivin's B. Thompson's
C. Thornton's D. Tournay's

**39. If the dilatation above an oesophageal stricture is conic it is fibrous, if cup shaped, it is malignant. It is known as :**
A. Vedder's sign B. Uhthoff's sign
C. Trimadeau's sign D. Thesilian's sign

**40. The localization of a tumor to an area previously treated with a carcinogen and scarified is called :**
A. Cytopathic B. Deelman effect
C. Donnan effect D. Founder effect

**41. Inhibition of synthesis of thyroid hormone after administration of large doses of iodide is called :**
A. Tyndall effect B. Wolff Chaikoff effect
C. Somogyi effect D. Soret effect

**42. Cubital tunnel syndrome is due to compression of —— nerve.**
A. Ulnar B. Median
C. Radial D. Axillary

**43. Hypertrophy of one side of whole of the body is seen in——— syndrome.**
A. Cyriax B. Danbolt-closs
C. Curtius D. Degos

**Ans.** 21. D 22. C 23. C 24. D 25. B 26. D 27. B 28. B 29. B 30. B
31. B 32. D 33. B 34. A 35. B 36. C 37. C 38. C 39. C 40. B
41. B 42. A 43. C

**44. Syndrome due to slipped rib cartilages pressing on the nerve at interchondral joint is — syndrome.**
A. Conradi B. Cyriax
C. Dennie Marfan D. Del Castillo

**45. Dennie Marfan syndrome is seen in :**
A. Multiple sclerosis B. Porphyria
C. Syphilis D. Sarcoidosis

**46. Myaesthenia like syndrome is :**
A. Eissenmenger's B. Duplay's
C. Eaton-Lambert's D. Epstein

**47. The totality of signs of myaesthenia gravis is seen in ——— syndrome.**
A. Duplay's B. Conradi
C. Erb's D. Faber's

**48. Cleft lip and palate and fistula of lower lip are some of the features of —— syndrome.**
A. Gerhardt's B. Fevre-Languepin
C. Francois D. Fuch's

**49. Painful bruising is seen in —— syndrome.**
A. Gardner-Diamond B. Gasser
C. Golenher's D. Goltz's

**50. Hemolytic uremic syndrome is also called ——— syndrome.**
A. Gardner's B. Gasser's
C. Canradi's D. Duplay's

**51. Immunodeficiency with thymoma is seen in ——— syndrome.**
A. Gopalan's B. Gorlin's
C. Good's D. Goodman's

**52. Vasovagal attack is ———— syndrome.**
A. Gorlin's B. Gower's
C. Goodman's D. Duplay's

**53. A test for thoracic outlet syndrome is.**
A. Allen's test B. Adson's test
C. Allen Doisy test D. Ames test

**54. A test for determining whether the site of bleeding is in the low oesophagus, stomach or duodenum is.**
A. Duke's test B. Dolman's test
C. Elsberg's test D. Einhron string test

**55. A test for contracture of lateral fascia of the thigh is :**
A. Ehrlich's test B. Dugas test
C. Ely's test D. Erhard's test

**56. A test for quick differential diagnosis of acute pancreatitis is :**
A. Fishman-Doubilet test B. Fluhmann's test
C Fouchet's test D. Frankel's test

**57. Glycyl tryptophan test is for detecting :**
A. Nephrotic syndrome
B. Ca stomach
C. Budd Chiari syndrome
D. Mensenteric vein thrombosis

**58. In hourglass stomach, a splashing sound will be heard on auscultation of the pyloric portion after siphonge is known as :**
A. Jansen's test B. Jaworski's test
C. Kaplan's test D. Kantor and Gies's test

**59. Cutaneous hyperthesia in abdominal distension is —— test.**
A. Mac Lean's B. Lyon's
C. Ligat's D. Lieben's

**60. Moynihan's test is for :**
A. Duodenal ulcer B. Hourglass stomach
C. Ac. Cholecystitis D. Nephrolithiasis

**61. Kartagener's syndrome is transmitted as :**
A. Autosomal dominant B. Autosomal recessive
C. Sex linked recessive D. None of the above

**62. Alternating constipation and diarrhoea, abdominal pain, meteorism and gurgling sounds in right iliac fossa are seen in :**
A. Job's syndrome B. Konig's syndrome
C. Karroo's syndrome D. Jeune's syndrome

**63. Ladd's syndrome results due to malrotation of :**
A. Duodenum B. Ileum
C. Caecum D. Kidney

**64. Abnormal localized collections of gas in the colon (splenic flexure) and stomach following acute myocardial infarction is seen in :**
A. Larsen's syndrome
B. Laubry-Soulle syndrome
C. Launois syndrome
D. Lawford's syndrome

**65. Gigantism due to excessive pituitary secretion is seen in :**
A. Launois's syndrome B. Kunkel's syndrome
C. Lichtheim's syndrome D. Leigh's syndrome

**66. Pneumomediastinum is seen in ——— syndrome.**
A. Hamman's syndrome
B. Hamman-Rich syndrome
C. Hanhart's syndrome
D. Homen's syndrome

**67. Characteristic symptoms of Lucey Driscoll syndrome is :**
A. Hemolytic anemia B. Jaundice
C. Cholecystitis D. Hiatus hernia

| Ans. | | | | | | | | | |
|---|---|---|---|---|---|---|---|---|---|
| 44. B | 45. C | 46. C | 47. C | 48. B | 49. A | 50. B | 51. C | 52. B | 53. B |
| 54. D | 55. C | 56. A | 57. B | 58. B | 59. C | 60. B | 61. B | 62. B | 63. C |
| 64. B | 65. A | 66. A | 67. B | | | | | | |

**68. In Mallory-Weiss syndrome, lacerations are usually :**
A. Above oesophagogastric (OG) junction
B. Below OG junction
C. At or below OG junction
D. Only at the OG Junction

**69. Hypertrophic Pulmonary osteoarthropathy is —— syndrome.**
A. Marie B. Marie-Robinson
C. Lutembacher D. Malin

**70. Dwarfism, hepatomegaly, obesity, retarded sexual maturity and diabetes mellitus is seen in :**
A. Melkerson Rosenthal syndrome
B. Mauriac syndrome
C. Moore's syndrome
D. Morel's syndrome

**71. Polycystic kidneys are seen in ——— syndrome.**
A. Mengert's B. Meckel-Gruber's
C. Mohr's D. Moore's

**72. Syringomyelia is seen in ——- syndrome.**
A. Mortan's B. Morvan's
C. Moore's D. Mohr's

**73. Pronation sign is also known as——— sign.**
A. Prehn sign B. Plummer sign
C. Pseudo Babinski sign D. None of the above

**74. Plummer sign is seen in :**
A. Poliomyelitis B. Graves' disease
C. Tabes dorsalis D. Addisons' disease

**75. Raimste sign is seen in ——— paralysis of arm :**
A. Spastic organic B. Flaccid organic
C. Flaccid functional D. Spastic functional

**76. Rising sun sign is seen in ———.**
A. Thyrotoxicosis B. Secondaries in eye
C. Retinoblastoma D. Hydrocephalus

**77. Fremitus felt on palpation and percussion over hydatid cyst is —— sign.**
A. Rovighi B. Rovsing
C. Rucker D. Spurling

**78. Unilateral palpable oedema, conjunctivitis and regional lymphadenopathy occurring and the primary lesion in acute Chagas disease is ——— sign.**
A. Homan B. Romana
C. Rucker D. Ruggeri

**79. Stridor heart during exhalation in an infant with bronchial lymph node tuberculosis is——— sign.**
A. Rucker B. Ruggeri
C. Schick D. Schultz

**80. Which is a rebound sign:**
A. Pastia B. Puddle
C. Steward Holmes D. Riviere

**81. Hodgkin's disease is also known as:**
A. Naffziger's syndrome
B. Murchison-Sanderson syndrome
C. Netherton's syndrome
D. Naegeli's syndrome

**82. Sclenus syndrome is also known as ——— syndrome.**
A. Netherton B. Noone-Milroy-meige
C. Naffziger's D. Naegeli's

**83. A condition simulating colonic obstruction, with persistent contraction of intestinal musculature without evidence of organic disease of colon is —— syndrome :**
A. Oldfield's B. Ogilvie's
C. Naegeli's D. Netherton's

**84. Familial polyposis of the colon associated with extensive sebaceous cysts are seen in :**
A. Naegeli's syndrome
B. Oldfield syndrome
C. Parry-romberg's
D. Netherton's

**85. Juvenile paralysis agitans is known as :**
A. Pfeiffer syndrome B. Pallidal syndrome
C. Picchini's syndrome D. Putnam-Dana syndrome

**86. Unilateral absence of sternococostal head of pectoralis major and ipsilateral syndactyly is seen in :**
A. Poland's syndrome
B. Inemark s syndrome
C. Riegers''s syndrome
D. Richards-Rundle syndrome

**87. Postperfusion syndrome is usually due to :**
A. Legionella B. Brucella
C. Cytomegalovirus D. Toxoplasma

**88. Renal agenesis or hypoplasia and other defects are seen in —— syndrome.**
A. Profichet B. Potter
C. Richards Rundl D. Rieger

**89. Skin stones are seen in —— syndrome.**
A. Richards Rundle B. Profichet
C. Robinow D. Roger

**90. In Prune Belly syndrome, following may be involved except :**
A. Kidney B. Internal oblique
C. Liver D. External oblique

| Ans. | 68. C | 69. A | 70. B | 71. B | 72. B | 73. D | 74. B | 75. B | 76. D | 77. A |
|---|---|---|---|---|---|---|---|---|---|---|
| | 78. B | 79. C | 80. C | 81. B | 82. C | 83. B | 84. B | 85. B | 86. A | 87. C |
| | 88. B | 89. B | 90. C | | | | | | | |

**91. Chorioretinitis and cerebral calcifications similar to the manifestation of toxoplasmosis but having all test of toxoplasmosis negative is seen in —— syndrome.**
A. Russel B. Silver
C. Rud D. Sabin-Feldman

**92. Pseudohypoparathyroidism is seen in —— syndrome.**
A. Seckel B. Senear-Usher
C. Sea bright Bantam D. Schanz

**93. Primary pancreatic insufficiency and bone marrow failure are seen in :**
A. Shwachman B. Sicard syndrome
C. Silver Skiold syndrome D. Sipple

**94. Congenital syndrome of male hypogonadism associated with multiple skeletal abnormalities of cervical spone and ribs and mental retardation are features of .**
A. Stokes syndrome
B. Stewart-Morel syndrome
C. Sohval-Soffer syndrome
D. Sorsby syndrome

**95. Lymphangiosarcoma which occurs as a late complication of severe lymphoedema of the arm following the excision of lymphonodes, usually associated with radical mastectomy is ——— syndrome.**
A. Stokvis-Talma B. Stilling
C. Stewart-treves D. Stewart-Morel

**96. In superior mesenteric artery syndrome there is often compression of —— part of duodenum.**
A. I B. II
C. III D. IV

**97. The unilateral paralysis of tongue and larynx but the venulum palati being unffected is seen in :**
A. Tommaseli syndrome B. Tapia syndrome
C. Torres syndrome D. Thorn syndrome

**98. Tarsal tunnel syndrome is due to compression of —— nerve.**
A. Anterior tarsal B. Posterior tarsal
C. Both D. Any one at a time

**99. Calcinosis is seen in —— syndrome :**
A. Thibierge-Weissenbach
B. Thorn
C. Tommaselli
D. Torres

**100. Pain and tenderness in the lower portion of sacrum and coccyx or in the contigous soft tissue and muscle is seen in ——— syndrome.**
A. Thiele B. Thiemann
C. Tourraine-solente-gole D. Tommaselli

**101. Cullen sign is also known as — sign.**
A. Hellendall B. Hoehno
C. Hochsinger D. Kleist

**102. Homans sign is —— of deep calf vein thrombosis.**
A. Diagnostic B. Suggestive
C. Both D. None of the above

**103. Horn sign is seen in :**
A. Acute Cholecystitis B. Acute Pancreatitis
C. Ureteric colic D. Acute appendicits

**104. Hornnr sign is also known as —— sign.**
A. Hoyne B. Le Gendre
C. Spalding D. Neri

**105. In paralysis of intercostal muscles, the upper chest is drawn in during inspiration instead of the reverse, due to action of diaphragm is —— sign.**
A. Jolly B. Jackson
C. Jiirgensen D. Kleist

**106. In echinococcal liver cyst, a furrow present on deep inspiration below the lowest rib and above the liver cyst is ——— sign.**
A. Laugier B. Lennhoff
C. Mc Clintock D. Nothnagel

**107. Macewan sign is observed in the following except :**
A. Internal hydrocephalus
B. Cerebral abscess
C. Brain oedema
D. None of the above

**108. Moulage sign is observed in :**
A. Acute Pancreatitis B. Ca head of Pancreas
C. Idiopathic steatorrhoea D. Acute orchitis

**109. Murphy sign acute cholecystitis is detected by :**
A. Pulse rate B. Respiratory rate
C. Pain radiation D. Temperature rise

**110. Signe de journal is also known as —— sign.**
A. Neri B. Froment
C. Nothangel D. Ober

**111. Ober sign is an indication of integrity of ———.**
A. Medial cruciate ligament
B. Tenser fascia lata
C. Ant. Cruciate ligament
D. Pleura

**112. Tenderness to abdominal palpation performs while the patient tones his Ant. abdominal musculature showing that the tenderness is Parietal in location is —— sign.**
A. Capps B. Carnett
C. Case's pad D. Chaddock

| Ans. | | | | | | | | | |
|---|---|---|---|---|---|---|---|---|---|
| 91. D | 92. C | 93. A | 94. C | 95. C | 96. C | 97. B | 98. B | 99. A | 100. A |
| 101. A | 102. A | 103. D | 104. C | 105. B | 106. B | 107. C | 108. C | 109. B | 110. B |
| 111. B | 112. B | | | | | | | | |

**113. Cullen sign is seen in :**
A. Acute Haemorrhagic pancreatitis
B. Ruptured ectopic pregnancy
C. Splenic rupture
D. Any of the above

**114. A sign seen in nerve root irritation is :**
A. Dupuy-Dutemps B. Dejerine sign
C. Dennie sign D. Elliot sign

**115. Doublet sign may be seen in :**
A. Acute Pancreatitis B. Acute Cholangitis
C. Tetany D. Milk alkali syndrome

**116. The shortened little finger of congential syphilis —— is sign.**
A. Elliot B. Gobiet
C. Dubois D. Escherich

**117. Echo sign may be heard over :**
A. Hydatid cyst B. Hydronephrosis
C. Pneumothorax D. TB cavity

**118. In acute appendicitis, pain elicited by passive hyperextension of the hip due to irritation of the psoas major muscle is —— sign.**
A. Federici B. Femoral
C. Foerster D. Fuchs

**119. Formication sign is also known as —— sign.**
A. Fuchs B. Tinel
C. Gobiet D. Goodell

**120. Fournier sign is seen in :**
A. Syphilis B. TB
C. Gangrene D. Trauma

**121. Dilatation of transverse colon in acute pancreatitis is ——— sign.**
A. Fuchs B. Gobier
C. Goodell D. Gorden

**122. In tired housewife syndrome, there is hypofunction of :**
A. Thyroid B. Gobier
C. Goodell D. Gorden

**123. Multiple carcinoma, primarily of GIT, in association with a large number of sebaceous gland neoplasms are seen in :**
A. Triparanol syndrome B. Tommaselli's syndrome
C. Torres's syndrome D. Tolosa-Hunt syndrome

**124. Meckel's diverticulum may be associated with trisomy :**
A. 13 B. 18
C. 21 D. 22

**125. Bronzed cachexia associated with diabetes mellitus associated with haemochromatosis is seen in —— syndrome.**
A. Weingarten's B. Vander Woude's
C. Trosier's D. Waardenbrug's

**126. Burning feet syndrome is also called :**
A. Gopalan's syndrome
B. Buerger-Grutz syndrome
C. Brissaud-Sicard syndrom
D. Bristowe's syndrome

**127. Milk-alkali syndrome is also called :**
A. Bart's syndrome B. Burnett's syndrome
C. Barter's syndrome D. Bruns syndrome

**128. Charcot's syndrome is :**
A. Amyotrophic lateral sclerosis
B. Intermittent claudication
C. Intermittent hepatic fever due to cholangitis
D. Any of the above

**129. Carotid sinus syndrome is also called :**
A. Chauffard's syndrome
B. Charcot-Weiss-Baker syndrome
C. Cestan's syndrome
D. Ayerza's syndrome

**130. Interposition of colon between liver and diaphragm is seen in ——— syndrome.**
A. Chotzen's B. Cogan's
C. Chilaiditi's D. Collet's

**131. Lesions of IX, X, XI, XII nerves are seen in — syndrom.**
A. Cogan's B. Collet-Sicard's
C. Chotzen D. Bruns

**132. Rovsing sign is typically seen in :**
A. Hiatus hernia B. Ureteric calculi
C. Ectopic pregnancy D. Appendicitis

**133. Pulsation in the temporal artery, visible during an attack of migraine is called :**
A. Vedder's sign B. Uriolla sign
C. Vermei sign D. Vipond sign

**134. Brodie's sign is present in :**
A. TB spine
B. Chronic osteomyelitis
C. Extravasation of urine into spongiosum
D. Pelvic fracture

**135. Glasgow's sign is present in :**
A. Buerger's disease B. Latent aortic aneurysm
C. Crohn's disease D. Head injury

**136. Guyon's sign is present in :**
A. Splenic rupture B. Appedicular abscess
C. Ectopic pregnancy D. Floating kidney

| Ans. | | | | | | | | | |
|---|---|---|---|---|---|---|---|---|---|
| 113. D | 114. B | 115. C | 116. C | 117. A | 118. B | 119. B | 120. A | 121. B | 122. A |
| 123. C | 124. B | 125. C | 126. A | 127. B | 128. D | 129. B | 130. C | 131. B | 132. D |
| 133. C | 134. C | 135. B | 136. D | | | | | | |

137. **Hail's sign is present in :**
A. Aortic aneurysm B. Tricuspid stenosis
C. Aortic Regurgitation D. Hydronephrosis

138. **Hamman's sign iS present in the following except :**
A. Mediastinitis B. Pneumothorax
C. Pneumomediastinum D. Hiatus hernia

139. **Pfuhl's sign is present in :**
A. Pericardial effusion
B. Pyopneumothorax
C. Int.carotid artery stenosis
D. Cavernous sinus thrombosis

140. **Semon's sign is present in malignant disease of :**
A. Stomach B. Tongue
C. Larynx D. Liver

141. **Augmented histamine sign indicates function of :**
A. Stomach B. GB
C. Liver D. Pancreas

142. **Ayer's test indicates —— block.**
A. Complete heart B. CHF
C. Spinal D. Lower GIT

143. **Which of the following is a test for urethritis :**
A. Thomas test B. Thompsons test
C. Thormahlen's test D. Roser test

144. **Tobey-Ayer test is done when ——— is suspected.**
A. Unilateral Sigmoid sinus thrombosis
B. Bilateral Sigmoid sinus thormbosis
C. Neurocysticercosis
D. Any of the above

145. **A syndrome with double kidney and clubbed fingers, sometimes with facial asymmetry is :**
A. Aldrich syndrome B. Angelucci syndrome
C. Allemann's syndrome D. Alstrom syndrome

146. **Progressive sensorineural deafness with progressive pyelonephritis or glomerulonephritis and occasional ocular defects is known as —— syndrome.**
A. Anton's B. Alport's
C. Alstrom's D. Ascher's

147. **Cystic fibrosis of pancreas, bronchiectasis and vitamin A deficiency is called ——— syndrome.**
A. Asherson's B. Baastrup's
C. Andersen's D. Axenfelds

148. **Cricopharyngeal achlasia is known as ——— syndrome.**
A. Asherson's B. Baastrup's
C. Ascher's D. Balint's

149. **Blepharochalasis occurring with adenoma of thyroid and redundancy of the mucous membrane and submucous tissue of the upper lip is :**
A. Chotzen's syndrome B. Barlow's syndrome
C. Ascher's syndrome D. Ayerza's syndrome

150. **Hakim's syndrome is mainly characterized by :**
A. Hemiparesis
B. Seizures
C. Normal pressure hydrocephalus
D. Mental retardation

151. **A test used to differentiate retractile and undescended testis is :**
A. Compression test B. Oshner's clasping test
C. Drawer's test D. Orr test

152. **Ratio of ankle blood pressure to brachial blood pressure is called ankle pressure index. Normally it is more than :**
A. 0.5 B. 1.0
C. 1.5 D. 2.0

153. **Anterior meningocele is most common in ——— spine.**
A. Cervical B. Thoracic
C. Lumbar D. Sacral

154. **Barlow's arcade is formed by confluence of right and left :**
A. Gastroduodenal artery B. Gastroepiploic artery
C. Splenic artery D. Internal carotid artery

155. **Bird beak (ace of spade) appearance is seen in :**
A. Intussusception B. Volvulus
C. Wilm's tumor D. Ulcerative colitis

156. **Brown's vasomotor index, useful in peripheral vascular disease is calculated by :**
A. Pulse rate B. BP
C. Temperature D. Hair density

157. **Buerger's angle is —— proportional to severity of disease.**
A. Directly B. (Directly)2
C. Three times D. Inversally

158. **Term 'Bubo' literally means :**
A. Ulcer B. Swelling
C. Groin D. Discharge

159. **Angell's sign is important for :**
A. Hydrocele
B. Torsion testis
C. III degree haemorrhoids
D. Carcinoma rectum

160. **Battle's sign most often developes on ——— day.**
A. First B. Second
C. Third D. Fifth

| Ans. | | | | | | | | | |
|---|---|---|---|---|---|---|---|---|---|
| 137. A | 138. D | 139. B | 140. C | 141. A | 142. C | 143. B | 144. A | 145. C | 146. B |
| 147. C | 148. A | 149. C | 150. C | 151. D | 152. B | 153. A | 154. B | 155. B | 156. C |
| 157. D | 158. C | 159. B | 160. B | | | | | | |

**161. Term 'Causalgia' literally means :**

A. Acute Pain B. Colicky pain
C. Heat pain D. Piercing pain

**162. In making rectus muscle taut by head lifting or leg raising. If previously palpable abdominal mass is intra-abdominal else it is extra abdominal, it is :**

A. Cruveilhier's sign B. Coleman's sign
C. Fothergill's sign D. Berry's sign

**163. Imperforate anus of membranous type is treated by :**

A. Sigmoid colostomy
B. Anoplasty
C. Abdominoperineal pull through
D. Sacro-perineal pull through

**164. Most appropriate age for operation of neonatal umbilical hernia is :**

A. At birth B. 1 month
C. 2 months D. 6 months

**165. Scar remodelling occurs :**

A. Only in abdominal scars
B. Only in scars on the face
C. Always in all wounds
D. Only in some after a few months

**166. Human bite infections are specially severe due to :**

A. Anaerobic streptococci
B. Aerobic non-haemolytic streptococci
C. Rabies
D. Tetanus

**167. Packed red cells are prepared by :**

A. Precipitation B. Filtration
C. Centrifugation D. Freeze-drying

**168. Parenterovite is :**

A. A high intravenous lipid for parenteral nutrition
B. A high calorie intravenous fluid
C. A vitamin capsule of oral ingestion
D. A vitamin injection

**169. Wound contraction in the process of wound healing starts :**

A. Immediately
B. After an initial lag period of 2 to 3 days
C. After 4 days
D. After 1 week

**170. Drainage of abscess by incision :**

A. Should be through a small incision without any disturbances to adjacent tissues.
B. Should be undertaken before the signs of fluctuation appear.
C. Should always be dependent.
D. Has been made outdated by antibiotic therapy.

**171. The best treatment of extradural haemorrhage is :**

A. Biparietal burr-holes.
B. Parietal craniotomy to find the haematoma
C. Temporal burr-hole to see the haematoma then tot increase the size of the hole to control the bleeding artery even at the foramen spinosum
D. A flap craniotomy to remove a portion of the temporal bone to find out haemorrhage

**172. What should be the incision when a temporal burr-hole is to be made in case of extradural haemorrhage ?**

A. The incision begins above the external auditory meatus and is extended vertically upwards for 4 cm.
B. Incision begins just in front of the external auditory meatus and is extended upwards for 7 cm.
C. The incision begins at the upper border of the zygomatic arch about 4 cm in front of the external auditory meatus and is extended upwards and slightly backwards for 7 cm.
D. Incision starts from the external auditory meatus and is extended upwards and backwards for 5 cm.

**173. In cerebral contusion the pulse will be :**

A. Slow and bounding
B. Slow and of small volume
C. Rapid, thready and of small volume
D. Slow and high volume

**174. Jacksonian epilepsy in head injury is evident of :**

A. Cerebral concussion
B. Cerebral irritation
C. Cerebral compression
D. Lesion of the cerebral hemisphere

**175. The followings are diagnosed by myelography except :**

A. Prolapse intervertebral disc
B. Spinal tumours
C. Spinal arach noiditis
D. Spinal extradural haematoma

**176. The followings are the ways to bring about surgical relief of pain in a patient with malignant tumour of the pelvis except :**

A. Section of the peripheral nerve
B. Anterolateral chordotomy
C. Thalamotomy
D. Sympathectomy

| Ans. | 161. C | 162. C | 163. B | 164. A | 165. C | 166. B | 167. B | 168. D | 169. C | 170. D |
|---|---|---|---|---|---|---|---|---|---|---|
| | 171. C | 172. D | 173. B | 174. B | 175. B | 176. C | | | | |

**177. The followings are the causes of Macroglossia except :**
A. Lymphangioma B. Haemangioma
C. Neurofibroma D. Lipoma

**178. Pseudo-Babinski sign is present in :**
A. Multiple sclerosis B. Poliomyelitis
C. Tabes dorsalis D. All of the above

**179. Rail road track sign is seen in :**
A. Rupture of urethra B. Pelvic fracture
C. Phlebothrombosis D. Splenic rupture

**180. A yellow colour in the periumbilical region indicating rupture of the common bile duct is ——.**
A. Rasch sign B. Ransohoff sign
C. Remark sign D. Raimiste sign

**181. Roche sign is present in :**
A. Appendicular gangrene
B. Torsion of testis
C. Caecal perforation
D. Kidney rupture

**182. Meralgia paresthetica is also known as ——— syndrome.**
A. Rieder B. Rieger
C. Roth D. Rothmund Thomson

**183. A test for occult blood in urine is :**
A. Purdy's test B. Pyramidon test
C. Preyer's test D. Proetz test

**184. A test to known gastric secretion is :**
A. Rees test B. Rehberg's test
C. Rehfuss test D. Remont's test

**185. For motive and digestive power of stomach, test is :**
A. Sahli's test B. Sakaguchi's test
C. Rosenbach's test D. Rosenthal's test

**186. Sponge test is to know lesion in the :**
A. Tongue B. Liver
C. Face D. Spine

**187. A test for Tuberculous ulceration of intestine is :**
A. Topfer's test B. Trommer's test
C. Triboulet's test D. Torquay's test

**188. Watson Schwartz's test is positive in acute :**
A. Pancreatitis B. Porphyria
C. Cholecystitis D. Gastritis

**189. Sclerotherapy is not indicated in :**
A. Oesophagus varic
B. Varicose veins leg
C. Varicocele
D. Internal haemorrhoids

**190. Most acceptable site of growth from anal verge for sphincter preserving operation for cancer rectum is**
A. 1 cm B. 3 cms
C. 5 cms D. 10 cms

**191. Berry's sign is seen malignancy of :**
A. Larynx B. Thyroid
C. Bronchus D. Stomach

**192. Rebound tenderness is also known as :**
A. Coleman's sign B. Blumberg's sign
C. Javid's sign D. Goblet sign

**193. A sign present in fracture of body of mandible is :**
A. Gaur's sign B. Goblet sign
C. Coleman's sign D. Cruveilhier's sign

**194. Operation is contraindicated in which of the following conditions :**
A. Acute appendicitis
B. Acute pancreatitis
C. Perforated gastric ulcer
D. Reputured ectopic pregnancy

**195. Polycystic kidney has all of the following features except :**
A. Spider leg appearance on I.V.P.
B. Haematuria
C. Specific gravity urine above 1020
D. Secondary pyelonephritis

**196. Pus in empyema of gall bladder is :**
A. Greenish B. Anchovy sauce
C. Orange D. Turbid

**197. Earliest symptoms of Wilm's tumor is :**
A. Haematuria B. Pyrexia
C. Abdominal lump D. Metastasis

**198. The sensitivity of Casoni's test is ——%:**
A. 50 B. 60
C. 75 D. 90

**199. Serological test of choice for the diagnosis of hydatid cyst is.**
A. Casoni's test
B. Immunoelectrophoresis
C. ELISA test
D. Indirect Haemagglutination

**200. The full name of Chvostek sign seen in tetany is Chvostek—— sign.**
A. Thomas B. Weiss
C. Richardson D. Williams

**201. To differentiate between calf haematoma and deep vein thrombosis is —— sign.**
A. Goblet B. Crescent
C. Javid's D. Joffroy's

**202. A sign indicates strangulation or obstruction in femoral hernia is ——— sign.**
A. Goblet B. Gaut's
C. Javid's D. Harvey's

| Ans. | | | | | | | | | |
|---|---|---|---|---|---|---|---|---|---|
| 177. C | 178. B | 179. C | 180. B | 181. B | 182. C | 183. B | 184. C | 185. A | 186. D |
| 187. C | 188. B | 189. C | 190. C | 191. B | 192. B | 193. C | 194. B | 195. C | 196. D |
| 197. C | 198. C | 199. D | 200. B | 201. B | 202. B | | | | |

203. **Which of the following sign is an indication for laparotomy to rule out impact of blunt injury to abdomen :**
A. Kelin sign B. Mose's
C. London's D. Javid's

204. **Which of the following sign is present in Subclavian steal syndrome :**
A. Javid's B. Joffroy's
C. Goblet sign D. Gifford's sign

205. **Gifford's sign is present in :**
A. Thyrotoxicosis B. Addison's disease
C. Pneumoconiosis D. Ac. pancreatitis

206. **Which sign is present in transitional cell carcinoma of ureter :**
A. Goblet B. Mose's
C. Ludloff's D. Kelin's

207. **A sign which may be seen in Meckel's diverticulitis :**
A. Millon's ear sign B. Prehn's sign
C. Kenway's sign D. Rust sign

208. **A sign used to differentiate erysipelas and cellulitis is.**
A. Millon's ear sign B. Prehn's sign
C. Kenway's sign D. Rust sign

209. **A sign seen in deep vein thrombosis :**
A. Mose's sign B. Vermoonten's sign
C. Stewart's sign D. Rust sign

210. **In tuberculosis of cervical spine, with every change of position and when patient is seated he supports his head with the hand. This is called —— sign.**
A. Rust B. Rovsing
C. Stewart's D. Tonyol's

211. **Downward displacement of umbilicus in distended abdomen suggests presence of ascites is called :**
A. Rovsing B. Seagull
C. Tanyol D. Vermoonten's

212. **A sign present in complete intrapelvic rupture of urethra is —— sign.**
A. Rovsing's B. Prehn
C. Vermoonten's D. Victor Harsley's

213. **A sign present in Saphena varix is :**
A. Joffroy's sign B. Klein's sign
C. Cruveilhier's sign D. Mose's sign

214. **A test for GI lesion using Phenolphthalein is :**
A. Wolff-Junghans test B. Woodbury's test
C. Woldman's test D. Wurster's test

215. **A test for HCL in gastric Juice is :**
A. Wehl's test B. Witz's test
C. Worm Muller test D. Wormley's test

216. **A test in which intensive antituberculosis therapy is applied to a patient with ant' -acosis who is suspected of having superimposed tuberculosis :**
A. Bial's test B. Bernard's test
C. Block-Steiger test D. Boyden's test

217. **Pseudoclaudication syndrome is due to compression of :**
A. Femoral artery B. Femoral vein
C. Inferior vena cava D. Cauda equina

218. **Obstruction to wings of basilar artery causing lesions of the pontine region is seen in :**
A. Raymond-Cestan syndrome
B. Reichmann's syndrome
C. Roberts syndrome
D. Robinow's syndrome

219. **Gastrosuccorrhea is seen in :**
A. Roger's syndrome B. Rieger's syndrome
C. Reichmann's syndrome D. Robinow's syndrome

220. **Anal stenosis, hypondontia, facial bones agenesis, hypertelorism and mental retardation are seen in :**
A. Riley Smith syndrome B. Rieger's syndrome
C. Robinow's syndrome D. Roger's syndrome

221. **Macrocephaly without hydrocephalus, multiple haemangioma and pseudopapilloedema are seen in —— syndrome.**
A. Richards-Rundle B. Roberts
C. Robinow's D. Riley-Smith's

222. **Hypogonadism, sterility and gynaecomastia in male are seen in —— syndrome.**
A. Rothmund-Thompson B. Rosewater
C. Rosenthal D. Roussay-Levy

223. **Term `Plastic surgery' was coined by :**
A. Edward Zeis B. Gaspara Tagliacozzi
C. Baronio D. Von Graefe

224. **Graft versus Host reaction is the characteristic of :**
A. Rust's syndrome B. Rud's syndrome
C. Rosenthal's syndrome D. Runting syndrome

225. **Stiff neck is the characteristic feature of —— syndrome.**
A. Rud's B. Rust's
C. Senear-Usher D. Schmidt's

226. **Sarcoidosis is also known as —— syndrome.**
A. Scheie's B. Schafer's
C. Schaumann's D. Schmidt's

227. **Cole's sign is positive in :**
A. Ac. diverticulitis B. Duodenal ulcer
C. Chronic Pancreatitis D. Umbilical adenoma

**Ans.** 203. C 204. A 205. A 206. A 207. A 208. A 209. A 210. A 211. C 212. C
213. C 214. C 215. B 216. B 217. D 218. A 219. C 220. B 221. D 222. B
223. A 224. D 225. B 226. C 227. B

**228. Cope's sign is positive in :**
A. Appendicitis B. Peritonitis
C. Amoebic colitis D. Diverticulosis

**229. Crescent sign is positive in :**
A. Hydatid cyst
B. Chronic hydronephrosis
C. Peritoneal effusion
D. Pleural effusion

**230. Curveilhier sign is positive in :**
A. Thromboangitis obliterans
B. Saphenous vein varices
C. Ac. hydronephrosis
D. Ac. Pancreatitis

**231. Dance sign is indicative of :**
A. Duodenal perforation B. Ileal obstruction
C. Intussusception D. Volvulus

**232. On auscultation of abdomen, heart sounds are audible in cases of intestinal perforation with gas in the peritoneal cavity is known as :**
A. Dubois sign B. Echo sign
C. Federici sign D. Dejerine sign

**233. Femoral sign is positive in :**
A. Femoral hernia B. Direct inguinal hernia
C. Ac. Appendicitis D. Ac. diverticulitis

**234. A fixed dilated pupil on the same side as a subdural haematoma is called :**
A. Grisolle sign B. Gubler sign
C. Gowers sign D. Griesinger sign

**235. In acute appendicitis, pain caused by traction on the right spermatic cord is called :**
A. Hoyne's sign B. Horn sign
C. Hochsinger sign D. Hueter sign

**236. In paralysis of the intercostal muscles, the upper chest is drawn in during inspiration instead of the reverse due to action of the diaphragm is called :**
A. Jolly sign B. Jackson sign
C. Jurgensen sign D. Kerandel sign

**237. A test to study the contrast ability and functional response of the gall bladder is :**
A. Hallipke's sign B. Boyden's test
C. Clark's test D. Chrobak's test

**238. Breath analysis test is used to detect :**
A. Lactose deficiency
B. Bacterial growth in intestine
C. Intestinal absorptive ability and hepatic metabolism
D. All of the above

**239. A variant of extensor plantar response is :**
A. Crafts test B. Caille's test
C. Dreyer's test D. Draize's test

**240. The presence of swallowed vernix cells in the meconium of newborn infants who display symptoms of intestinal obstruction is known as :**
A. Farber's test B. Fahraeus test
C. Feulgen's test D. Fehling's test

**241. Babinski's syndrome is seen in :**
A. Syphilis B. Miliary TB
C. Brucellosis D. Sarcoidosis

**242. Beckwith-Wiedemann's syndrome is :**
A. Autosomal dominant B. Autosomal recessive
C. Sexlinked recessive D. Not known

**243. Boerhaave's syndrome is :**
A. Duodenal perforation B. Oesophageal rupture
C. Ileal perforation D. TB mesenteritis

**244. Mesenteric and retroperitoneal lymphadenitis as a sequel of throat infections is ——— syndrome.**
A. Bruns syndrome
B. Brennemann's syndrome
C. Brunsting's syndrome
D. Bertolotti's syndrome

**245. The pH of the extracellular fluid :**
A. Is increased in hypovolaemic shock.
B. Is maintained entirely by the buffering system of the intra-and extracellular fluids.
C. Is decreased immediately after cardiac arrest.
D. Is between 7.5 and 7.7.

**246. A test for organic arterial occlusion by reactive hyperemia is :**
A. Lewis and Pickering test
B. Luenback Koeppe test
C. Mancini test
D. Manzullo test

**247. A procedure for revealing the presence of slight paresis of an upper or lower limb is :**
A. Mingazzine's test B. Mittel-Meyer test
C. Montenegro's test D. Morton's test

**248. A test for sclenus anterior syndrome is :**
A. Rumpel-Leede test B. Rubino test
C. Naffziger's test D. Paul's test

**249. A test for the patency of deep veins of legs in presence of varicose veins is :**
A. Paul's test B. Perthes test
C. Rubin test D. Stoll test

**250. Asplenia syndrome is also known as :**
A. Ayerza's syndrome B. Ivemark's syndrome
C. Bart's syndrome D. Barter's syndrome

| Ans. | | | | | | | | | |
|---|---|---|---|---|---|---|---|---|---|
| 228. A | 229. B | 230. B | 231. C | 232. C | 233. C | 234. D | 235. B | 236. B | 237. B |
| 238. D | 239. A | 240. A | 241. A | 242. A | 243. B | 244. B | 245. C | 246. A | 247. A |
| 248. C | 249. B | 250. B | | | | | | | |

# REVIEW PAPER—II

## (Based on Difficult & Important MCQ's)

1. **Potter facies is seen in :**
A. Renal agenesis B. Hydronephrosis
C. Polycystis kidney D. Renal colic

2. **Which of the following is also known as "frog like position" :**
A. Albert's position B. Batrachian position
C. Brrickner position D. Bonner's position

3. **Inflammed sacculations between the rectal valves with mucous discharge are—— pouches.**
A. Pavlov B. Kock
C. Heidenhain D. Physick's

4. **Midpoint of epigastric region is ——— point.**
A. Addison's B. Arrhigi's
C. Bolton D. Cannon

5. **Resting venous blood contains ——— mmol lactate/ litre.**
A. 0 B. 0.5
C. 1.0 D. 2.0

6. **A reflex in the female corresponding to the cremastric reflex in the male is ——— reflex.**
A. Loven's B. Kehrer's
C. Haab's D. Giegel's

7. **A point on the abdomen 5 to 7 cm from umbilicus on the line joining it to the right axilla; it lies over the head of pancreas and is ——— point.**
A. Cova's B. Desjardin's
C. Meglin's D. Munra

8. **Which of the following position is used after intubation so that the patient may swallow without danger of fluid entering the tube :**
A. Depage position
B. Casselberry's position
C. Jone position
D. Kraske position

9. **A point of tenderness in gall bladder disease between the heads of the sternocleidomastoid is ——— point.**
A. Ramond's B. Meglin's
C. Lanz's D. Krafft's

10. **Intervals between those parts of the diaphragm which are attached to the ribs and that which is attached to the sternum is ——— space.**
A. Kiernan's B. Lesshaft's
C. Larrey' D. Henke's

11. **A red line observed on the gingivae in pulmonary tuberculosis is ——— line.**
A. Thompson's B. Topinards
C. Poupart's D. Pickerill's

12. **A fold of mucous membrane occasionally seen in the fossa navicularis of the urethra is ——— fold.**
A. Brachet's B. Guerin's
C. Hasner's D. Rindfleisch

13. **Fossa jugularis is also known as ——— space.**
A. Bogros B. Burn's
C. Crookes D. Czermark

14. **A transverse fold of mucous membrane in the rectum, marking the junction of its lower and middle thirds is ——— fold.**
A. Marshall's B. Nelaton's
C. Hasner's D. Schultz's

15. **A fold of extraperitoneal fascia enveloping the obliterated umbilical vein is ——— fascia.**
A. Richet's B. Cruveilhier's
C. Abernethy's D. Buck's

16. **Which of the position is used to irrigate the urethra :**
A. Valentine position
B. Titterington position
C. Rose position
D. Robson position

17. **Omentum minus is also called ——— pouch.**
A. Willis B. Seessel's
C. Prussak D. Troltsc

18. **A point of tenderness in gall bladder disease situated under the right clavicle is ——— point.**
A. Barker B. Chauffard's
C. Keen's D. Krafft

| Ans. | 1. A | 2. B | 3. D | 4. A | 5. C | 6. D | 7. B | 8. B | 9. A | 10. C |
|---|---|---|---|---|---|---|---|---|---|---|
| | 11. A | 12. B | 13. B | 14. B | 15. A | 16. A | 17. A | 18. B | | |

**19. A decrease in BP following vagotomy is ——— reflex.**
A. Loven's B. Lust's
C. Mc Dowall's D. Morley's

**20. A circular mucosal thickening at the opening of the pncreatic duct into the common bile duct is ——— ring.**
A. Maxwell's B. Lowe's
C. Ochsner's D. Duran's

**21. Pouch used in experimental study of gastric physiology is --------- pouch.**
A. Kock's B. Guttural
C. Heidenhain D. Pavlow

**22. The point of greatest tenderness in gall bladder inflammation is :**
A. Boas point B. Ramond's
C. Robson's D. Chauffard's

**23. Rexed laminae is an architectural scheme to classify the structure of the :**
A. Hypothalamus B. Spinal cord
C. Retina D. Acoustic neuroma

**24. Nervus intermedius is ——————— nerve.**
A. Wriberg's B. Tiedemann's
C. Scarpa's D. Back's

**25. An inguinal hernia which has turned outward into the groin is ——— hernia.**
A. Grynfelt B. Holthouse
C. Rieux D. Serafini

**26. After headache and palpitations, which is the most frequent symptom of Phaeochromocytoma :**
A. Sweating B. Dyspnoea
C. Pallor D. Vomiting

**27. Flaps transferred to new sites through a tunnel beneath skin is —— flap.**
A. Transposition B. Island
C. Rotation D. Pedicle

**28. Phaeochromocytoma may occasionally arise from :**
A. Thyroid B. Pancreas
C. Appendix D. Urinary bladder

**29. Length of oesophagus below diaphragm is —— cm.**
A. 1 B. 2
C. 4 D. 7

**30. Soap bubble sign is typically seen in :**
A. Osteoclastoma
B. Nectrosing enterocolitis
C. Meconium ileus
D. None of the above

**31. Among the following, most common site of necrotising enterocolitis is :**
A. Jejunum B. Ascending colon
C. Transverse colon D. Descending colon

**32. In Budd Chiari syndrome, the most preferred treatment is :**
A. Denver shunt B. Lee Veen shunt
C. Warren shunt D. H-mesocaval shunt

**33. Intraperitoneal injection of streptococcal antigen extract (OK-432) is useful in :**
A. Intestinal TB B. Hodgkin's disease
C. Chylous ascites D. Malignant ascites

**34. First Liver transplant was done by :**
A. Shapiro in 1968 B. Calne in 1970
C. Staz in 1971 D. Pichlmayr in 1972

**35. "Watering pot perineum" is seen in :**
A. Gonorrhoea B. Chancroid
C. LGV D. GI

**36. Whitaker test is used in :**
A. Budd chiari syndrome B. Elephantiasis
C. Obstructive uropathy D. Achalasia cardia

**37. Allochiria is a main complication of :**
A. Cordotomy
B. Commisural myelotomy
C. Sacral neurectomy
D. Stereotactic thalamotomy

**38. Mann Bollman fistula is present in :**
A. Anal canal B. Uterus
C. Abdominal wall D. Oesophagus

**39. Kurtzke disability status score is used to assess disability caused by :**
A. Leprosy B. Syphilis
C. Multiple sclerosis D. Alcoholism

**40. Glossitis typical of pernicious anemia is :**
A. Moeller's B. Clarke-Fournier's
C. Hunter's D. Fournier's

**41. Zuelzer-Wilson syndrome is a variant of :**
A. Achlasia cardia B. Hirschsprung's disease
C. Pancreatitis D. Carcinoid syndrome

**42. Birds leak or "Ace of Spades" appearance is seen in :**
A. Ca oesophagus B. Ca rectum
C. Sigmoid volvulus D. Intussusception

**43. Bubbly's appearance in right side of colon may be seen in the following except :**
A. Ileal atresia B. Meconium ileus
C. Ameboma D. Hirschsprung's disease

| Ans. | | | | | | | | | |
|---|---|---|---|---|---|---|---|---|---|
| 19. C | 20. C | 21. C,D | 22. C | 23. B | 24. A | 25. B | 26. D | 27. B | 28. D |
| 29. C | 30. C | 31. B | 32. D | 33. D | 34. B | 35. C | 36. C | 37. A | 38. C |
| 39. C | 40. C | 41. B | 42. C | 43. C | | | | | |

44. **Hua T'O a Chinese surgeon is said to have been first to perform —— in about 190 AD.**
A. Nephrectomy B. Mastectomy
C. Splenectomy D. Skin grafting

45. **All patients, who have undergone splenectomy develop infection with :**
A. S. pneumonia B. H. influenza
C. B. pertusis D. N. meningitis

46. **In blunt trauma to abdomen, positive diagnostic peritoneal lavage is indicated by all except :**
A. RBC count 1 Lac or more
B. WBC 100 lacs or more
C. Presence of bile or blood particles
D. None of the above

47. **Dislocation of knee is often associated with injury to :**
A. Ant. tibial nerve B. Post-tibial nerve
C. Popliteal artery D. Saphenous vein

48. **Struvite is another name for —— renal stone.**
A. Calcium B. Uric acid
C. Phosphate D. Cystine

49. **Renal cell carcinoma sometimes produce following hormones except :**
A. Erythropoietin B. Angiotensin
C. Thyroxine D. Parathormone

50. **In infants, the percent assigned to burns in head and neck is —— than in adult.**
A. Higher B. Same
C. Lower D. Any of the above

51. **A common etiologic factor for basal cell carcinoma, sq. cell carcinoma and melanoma is exposure to UV light in the —— range.**
A. A B. B
C. C D. D

52. **Following factors indicate poor prognosis on Ca breast except :**
A. Medullary type
B. Estrogen receptor negative
C. Aneuploidy and higher number of cells of S-phase
D. Cathepsin-D positive cells

53. **Following are present in MEN-II type-B except :**
A. Pancreatic islet cell tumors
B. Pheochromocytoma
C. Medullary Ca thyroid
D. Mucosal neuromas

54. **Most common endocrine tumor of pancreas is :**
A. VIPoma B. Gastrinoma
C. Insulinoma D. WDHA syndrome

55. **VIPoma is characterized by following except :**
A. Watery diarrhoea
B. Hypokalemia
C. Recurrent pain abdomen
D. Achlorhydria

56. **Parathyroid adenoma in hyperparathyroidism was first removed by :**
A. Williams B. Felix Mandl
C. Theodor Kocher D. W. Halstead

57. **Cribriform or lace-like appearance is seen in —— tumor of salivary glands.**
A. Mucoepidermoid B. Acinic cell
C. Adenoid cystic D. Warthin's tumor

58. **Alpha fetoprotein is a normal component of plasma protein of human fetus older than —— weeks :**
A. 2 B. 4
C. 6 D. 10

59. **Fibrinous adhesions are normally lysed within —— hours after development.**
A. 12-24 hours B. 24-48 hours
C. 48-96 hours D. 1-2 weeks

60. **Which of the following may be most useful in fat embolism syndrome :**
A. Aspirin B. Heparin
C. Corticosteroids D. Cholestyramine

61. **Hunt Lawrence pouch is created in surgery of :**
A. Liver B. Gall bladder
C. Stomach D. Spleen

62. **Percussion test of Chevrier is used to detect :**
A. Minimal ascites B. Varicose veins
C. Polycystic kidneys D. Localized emphysema

63. **Malherbe's epithelioma is most common on :**
A. Face B. Trunk
C. Arm D. Leg

64. **Molluscum sebaceum is most common on :**
A. Upper limb B. Thigh
C. Face D. Scalp

65. **Actinomycosis of liver is most commonly associated with primary focus in :**
A. Faciocervical region B. Stomach
C. Right iliac fossa D. Lungs

66. **Typhitis is inflammation of :**
A. Ileum B. Caecum
C. Descending colon D. Rectum

67. **Leontiasis ossea is :**
A. Congenital anomaly B. Infection
C. Tumor D. Fracture

68. **Third space effect is seen in the following except :**
A. Perforated ulcer
B. Severe peritonitis
C. First degree burns
D. Extensive peritonitis

**Ans.** **44. C** **45. C** **46. B** **47. C** **48. C** **49. A** **50. A** **51. B** **52. A** **53. A**
**54. C** **55. C** **56. B** **57. C** **58. C** **59. C** **60. C** **61. C** **62. B** **63. A**
**64. C** **65. C** **66. B** **67. C** **68. C**

**69. Which is the least common terminal complication of Ca oesophagus :**
A. Dehydration B. Erosion of the aorta
C. Mediastinitis D. Pneumonia

**70. Acanthosis nigricans may be associated with cancer of :**
A. Thyroid B. Breast
C. Bronchus D. None of the above

**71. The name "Eusol" is based on the name of :**
A. Person B. Company
C. University D. Country

**72. Which of the least common connective tissue tumor of urinary bladder is :**
A. Sarcoma B. Fibroma
C. Angioma D. Myoma

**73. Microscopical differences between an incompletely descended testis and a normal testis are not observed upto the age of :**
A. 2 years B. 4 years
C. 6 years D. 8 years

**74. Pheochromocytoma is bilateral in about—— % cases.**
A. 25 B. 15
C. 8 D. 2

**75. Most valid sign of hiatus hernia on oesophagoscopy is :**
A. Inflammation of lower end of esophagus
B. Reflux of gastric juice through cardia
C. Closing of cardia during inspiration
D. Descent of cardia during inspiration

**76. Pancreatitis may be produced by following except :**
A. Alcohol B. Oestrogen
C. ACTH D. Gold

**77. It is advised not to have children after radical mastectomy for carcinoma for :**
A. 1 year B. 2 years
C. 3 years D. Life long

**78. Most common complication of polycystic kidney is :**
A. Haematuria B. Infection
C. Hypertension D. Uremia

**79. Term socia parotids is used for :**
A. Mixed parotid tumor B. Stone
C. Accessory parotids D. Parotid abscess

**80. Necrotising fascitis mostly occurs due to :**
A. Trauma B. Diabetes mellitus
C. Smoking D. Gas gangrene

**81. Human bites can cause following infection except :**
A. Fusobacterium
B. Spirochetes
C. Eikenella corrodens
D. Pseudomonas

**82. Intractable hypotension is seen in :**
A. Hypothyroidism
B. Hypoparathyroidism
C. Adrenal insufficiency
D. Diabetes mellitus

**83. In Ranson's criteria at least —— or more criteria suggest a mortality approaching 100%.**
A. 3 B. 5
C. 7 D. 10

**84. Cholangitis is treated with :**
A. Steroids
B. Antibiotics
C. NSAIDS's
D. Radiotherapy

**85. Best treatment for Carroli's disease is :**
A. Antibiotics
B. Steroids
C. Bile duct transplantation
D. Liver transplantation

**86. About ——% of patients, with uric acid renal stones have gout.**
A. 10 B. 25
C. 50 D. 70

**87. Indications for surgery in infective endocarditis are the following except :**
A. Resistant infection
B. Prosthetic valve carditis
C. Microscopic haematuria
D. Persistent valvular vegetations

**88. Congenital pyloric stenosis most often presents at about the age of —— weeks.**
A. 2 B. 4
C. 6 D. 12

**89. Splenic artery aneurysm is common in :**
A. Diabetes mellitus B. Trauma
C. Crohn's disease D. Pregnancy

**90. Puestow operation is mainly indicated in pancreatitis for :**
A. Diabetes mellitus B. Chronic steatorrhoea
C. Intractable pain D. Malignancy

**91. Most common cause of multiple organ failure is :**
A. Hypotension B. Sepsis
C. Third space effect D. Trauma

**Ans.** 69. B 70. B 71. C 72. C 73. C 74. B 75. B 76. D 77. C 78. B 79. C 80. B 81. D 82. C 83. C 84. B 85. D 86. B 87. C 88. C 89. D 90. C 91. B

**92. A patient is speaking inappropriate but comprehensible words, withdraws from pain, shows eye opening to pain has a Glasgow coma scale score of :**

A. 7 B. 9
C. 11 D. 12

**93. In Child-Pugh-Turcotte classification of adequacy of liver function, following indicates 'C' risk category except :**

A. Bilirubin 5.2 mg/dl
B. Albumin 3.2 g/dl
C. Poorly controlled ascites
D. Poor nutrition

**94. Metastasis to breast is common from following except :**

A. Lymphoma B. Hepatoma
C. Melanoma D. Ovarian cancer

**95. Double arc shadow is seen in :**

A. Aortic aneurysm B. Duodenal atresia
C. Cholecystolithiasis D. Amoeboma

**96. "Floating stones" in gall bladder are usually :**

A. Pigment stones B. Mixed stones
C. Cholesterol stones D. Bilirubin stones

**97. "Starry sky pattern" of portal venules is seen in :**

A. Hepatoblastoma B. Acute hepatitis
C. Haemangioma D. Hemochromatosis

**98. Which of the following disease is known as "Great imitator" :**

A. Sarcoidosis B. Brucellosis
C. Syphilis D. AIDS

**99. Lofgren syndrome is seen in :**

A. Acute Pancreatitis B. Acute appendicitis
C. Acute sarcoidosis D. Pneumoconiosis

**100. Internist's tumor is :**

A. Desmoid B. Renal cell carcinoma
C. Hernia D. Melanoma

**101. Gradual painless enlargement of subhyloid bursa is known as ——— cyst.**

A. Blessig's B. Boyer's
C. Sampson's D. Tarlow's

**102. Traumatic meningocele is also known as ——— disease :**

A. Brown symmer's B. Breisky's
C. Billroth's D. Beauvais's

**103. Linitis plastica is also known as ——— disease.**

A. Barcoo's B. Bannister's
C. Brinton's D. Castellani's

**104. Perinei superficialis is known as——— fascia.**

A. Colles B. Gerota
C. Cruveilheir D. Cooper's

**105. Plicae gastropancreaticae is also known as ——— ligament :**

A. Hey's B. Hueck's
C. Humphry's D. Huschke's

**106. A line from umbilicus to left anterior superior iliac spine is ——— line.**

A. Hensen's B. Helmoholt's
C. Munro's D. Moyer's

**107. Which is a perineural cyst :**

A. Blessig's B. Sampson's
C. Munro's D. Moyer's

**108. Addison's disease is also known as —— disease.**

A. Andes B. Bronzed
C. Durante's D. Filatov's

**109. 'Tell Tale swelling' in groin is due to :**

A. Femoral artery aneurysm
B. Buerger's disease
C. Inferior epigastric artery tearing
D. Superior epigastric artery tearing

**110. Gangrenous balanitis is seen in —— disease.**

A. Chester's B. Corbus's
C. Flajani's D. Erb-Goldflam's

**111. Hypertrophic pyloric stenosis on Barium examination shows following signs except :**

A. Diamond sign B. Triple track sign
C. String sign D. Kirklin's sing
E. Patricks's

**112. Post-traumatic osteoporosis is known as ——— disease.**

A. Leydon's B. Leriche's
C. Lenegre's D. Maliba

**113. A fold of extraperitoneal fascia covering the obliterated umbilical vein is —— fascia.**

A. Sibson's B. Tyrrell's
C. Richet's D. Colle

**114. An occasional peritoneal fold connecting the infundibulpelvic ligament and the mesoappendix is ——— ligament.**

A. Gunz's B. Ferrein's
C. Clado's D. Casser's

**115. Marcy repair is done for :**

A. Hiatus hernia
B. Paraumbilical hernia
C. Inguinal hernia
D. Volvulus

**116. Commonest renal sarcoma is :**

A. Rhabdomyosarcoma B. Fibrosarcoma
C. Leiomyosarcoma D. Liposarcoma

| Ans. | | | | | | | | | |
|---|---|---|---|---|---|---|---|---|---|
| 92. B | 93. B | 94. B | 95. C | 96. C | 97. B | 98. C | 99. C | 100. B | 101. B |
| 102. C | 103. C | 104. C | 105. D | 106. C | 107. C | 108. B | 109. C | 110. B | 111. E |
| 112. B | 113. C | 114. C | 115. C | 116. C | | | | | |

———

**117. Lymphatic spread is most commonly exhibited by :**
A. Osteosarcoma B. Neurolemmoma
C. Ewing's tumor D. Synovial cell sarcoma

**118. Following laparotomy, peristalsis returns fully in left colon by ———.**
A. 24 hours B. 48 hours
C. 72 hours D. 1 week

**119. Following trauma, concentration of fat macroglobules (200mm) reach a peak at —— hours.**
A. 6 B. 12
C. 24 D. 36

**120. Which flap is used for upper lip :**
A. Gullies B. Estlander
C. Eloesser D. Italian

**121. Length of Wharton's duct is —— cm.**
A. 2 B. 3
C. 5 D. 8

**122. Sialosis is seen in following except :**
A. SLE B. Diabetes mellitus
C. Obesity D. Acromegaly

**123. Which is considered to be agent of first choice in recurrent Ca breast :**
A. Oestrogens B. Antioestrogens
C. Androgens D. Progesterones

**124. Highest level of serum amylase is attained in :**
A. 15 minutes B. 60 minutes
C. 12 hours D. 72 hours

**125. High fever, tachycardia and coma may be seen in :**
A. Pheochromocytoma B. Conn's disease
C. Hyperthyroidism D. Hypothyroidism

**126. Retrocaecal hernia is ——— hernia.**
A. Rieux's B. Serafini's
C. Grynfelt D. Barth's

**127. A space containing connective tissue between the vertebral column and the pharynx and oesophagus is ——— space.**
A. Czermark's B. Henke's
C. Lesshaft's D. Kierman's

**128. A groove on the deltoid muscle for the cephalic vein and a branch of the acromiothoracic artery is ——— space.**
A. Nance's leeway B. Nuel's
C. Lesshaft's D. Mohrenheim's

**129. A palmar crease correlated with an increased risk for leukemia and other malignancies in children is ——— line.**
A. Thompson's B. Sydney's
C. Skinne D. Rolando's

**130. Femoral hernia through saphenous opening is ——— hernia.**
A. Barth B. Beclard's
C. Birkett's D. Cloquet's

**131. The space between the pericardium and the beginning of the aorta is ——— space.**
A. Troltsch B. Westberg's
C. Robin 's D. Nuel's

**132. Depressions sometimes seen on the upper surface of the liver from pressure of the ribs generally caused by tight garments or tight lacing of a girdle or corset is ——— furrow.**
A. Sibson's B. Jadelot's
C. Liebermeister's D. Digital

**133. A white line on the abdomen invoked by drawing the finger nail across it; seen in cases of deficient adrenal activity is ——— line.**
A. Retizius B. Sergent's
C. Thompson's D. Voigt

**134. In Denys-Drash syndrome, there are high chances of :**
A. Phaeochromocytoma B. Insulinoma
C. Wilm's tumour D. Neuroblastoma

**135. Femoral hernia infront of femoral vessels is ——— hernia.**
A. Treitz B. Velpeau
C. Hey's D. Kronlein

**136. Homer Wright pseudorosettes are found in :**
A. Insulinoma B. Neuroblastoma
C. Hodgkin's lymphoma D. Medulloblastoma

**137. Currarino's triad consists of the following except :**
A. Scimitar sacrum
B. Flat atlas
C. Presacral ant. meningocele or teratoma or cyst
D. Rectal malformation

**138. The point of greatest tenderness in gall bladder inflammation, situated opposite the junction of the middle and lower third of a line drawn from right nipple to umbillicus is ——— point :**
A. Trigger B. Vogt
C. Voillemier D. Robson

**139. The point of costovertebral angle, tenderness over which points to kidney infection is ——— point.**
A. Bolton B. Keen
C. Brewer D. Ramond's

**140. Marshall Hall's facies is seen in :**
A. Peptic ulcer B. Renal colic
C. Hydrocephalus D. Pulmonary embolism

| Ans. | | | | | | | | | |
|---|---|---|---|---|---|---|---|---|---|
| 117. D | 118. C | 119. B | 120. B | 121. C | 122. A | 123. B | 124. B | 125. C | 126. A |
| 127. B | 128. D | 129. B | 130. B | 131. B | 132. C | 133. B | 134. C | 135. B | 136. B |
| 137. B | 138. D | 139. C | 140. C | | | | | | |

**141. In appendicitis, a triad of hypersensitiveness of skin, reflex muscular contraction and tenderness at Mc Burney's point is ——— triad.**
A. Grancher's B. Charcot's
C. Dieulafoy's D. Jacob's

**142. The point of tendernessing gall bladder disease in the upper segment of the rectus muscle is——— point.**
A. Bolton B. Brewer
C. Mackenzie D. Kraft

**143. THe point indicating the location of vesical of rifice is——point.**
A. Lenzs B. Paul's
C. Piersol's D. Ramond

**144. Which of the following are known as cancer bodies :**
A. Symington's B. Verocay's
C. Plimmer's D. Renaut's

**145. Femorotibial form of progressive muscular atrophy with contraction of the toes is————atrophy.**
A. Hoffman's B. Hunt's
C. Eichhorst's D. Parrot's

**146. Tractus iliotibialis is————band.**
A. Lane's B. Henel's
C. Harris D. Maissiat's

**147. Knee-elbow position is also known as——— position.**
A Edebohls B. Elliot
C. Brickner D. Bozeman's

**148. Cerebellar tumors usually block :**
A. Lateral ventricle right side
B. Lateral ventricle left side
C. III Ventricles
D. IV Ventricles

**149. Adhesions between tight loops of terminal ileum which may extend as ligamentous bands to the right iliac fossa are ——bands.**
A. Ladd's B. Lane's
C. Mata's D. Meckel's

**150. Which of the following position is used in operations on the gall bladder :**
A. English position B. Elliot position
C. Depage position D. Casselberry position

**151. Following are contraindications for Whitaker test except :**
A. Ac. urinary infection
B. VUR without ipsilateral trapping
C. High grade or complete obstruction
D. Ptotic kidney

**152. Increased pulsation of retinal arteries in Grave's disease is—— phenomenon.**
A. Debre B. Cushing
C. Becker D. Collie

**153. String of pearls sign in small bowel atresia is due to :**
A. Congenital band B. Gas
C. Calcification D. Fluid

**154. Pautrier's microabscess is seen in :**
A. DiGeorge syndrome B. Burns
C. Mycosis fungoides D. CML

**155. Munro abscess is seen in :**
A. TB Liver B. Wilm's tumor
C. Splenectomy D. Reiter's disease

**156. Term 'Polycholia' means :**
A. Aberrant secretion of bile
B. Abnormal secretion of bile
C. Multiple bile stones
D. Multiple gall stones

**157. In deep vein thrombosis, following sign is seen :**
A. Kenway B. Kelin's
C. London's D. Mose's

**158. Which of the following sign represents 'pattern' bruising on the skin (imprint of clothing), indication of laparotomy in blunt injury abdomen :**
A. Millon sign B. London's sign
C. Rust sign D. Vermoonten's sign

**159. Uropenia is :**
A. Urinary infection
B. Lack of urinary secretion
C. Brownish discolouration of urine
D. Proteinuria

**160. Maschaladenitis is :**
A. Inflammation of salivary glands
B. Inflammation of lacrimal glands
C. Inflammation of inguinal glands
D. Inflammation of axillary glanus

**161. In thyroid malignancy, due to involvement of artery in malignant process, carotid pulsation is not felt. It is ——— sign.**
A. Berry's B. Milton's
C. Coleman's D. Vermoonten's

**162. Torsion of testis occurs inside the :**
A. Tunica Albuginea B. Tunica vaginalis
C. Cremaster fascia D. Scrotum

**163. In which of the following ureterocele, can the ureteric orifice be normal or even larger in size :**
A. Stenotic B. Sphineteric
C. Sphincterostenotic D. Simple

**164. Which is the most common finding on semen analysis in cases of varicocele :**
A. Stress pattern
B. Decreased sperm count
C. Decreased sperm motility
D. Morphologic abnormalities

| Ans. | | | | | | | | | |
|---|---|---|---|---|---|---|---|---|---|
| 141. C | 142. C | 143. C | 144. C | 145. C | 146. D | 147. D | 148. D | 149. B | 150. B |
| 151. D | 152. C | 153. C | 154. C | 155. D | 156. B | 157. D | 158. B | 159. B | 160. D |
| 161. B | 162. B | 163. B | 164. C | | | | | | |

**165. Carcinoma stomach is least likely to directly extend into which of the following site :**
A. Diaphragm B. Pancreas
C. Duodenum D. Right lobe of liver

**166. The ectopic ureter in males is commonly associated with renal dysgenesis when it opens into the following except :**
A. Vasa B. Ejaculatory duct
C. Seminal vesicles D. Prostatic urethra

**167. Which of the following serves as a specific tumor marker of Ca stomach :**
A. Serum Pepsinogen-I B. Serum pepsinogen-II
C. Tyrosine D. Intrinsic factor

**168. Normal volume of fluid in peritoneal cavity is—— ml.**
A. 60 B. 100
C. 120 D. 200

**169. Length of normal appendix is ——— cm.**
A. 5 B. 7
C. 9 D. 12

**170. Weigert Meyer rule is associated with :**
A. Ectopic ureter
B. Calyceal diverticulum
C. Dysplastic ureter
D. Complete ureteral duplication

**171. On making rectus muscle taut by head lifting or leg raising. If previously palpable abdominal mass is intra abdominal it will disappear, otherwise it is extra abdominal. It is ——— sign.**
A. Fothergill's B. Gifford's
C. Goblet's D. Jowid's

**172. The commonest site of carcinosarcoma of esophagus is :**
A. Upper 1/3
B. Middle 1/3
C. Lower 1/3
D. Gastroesophageal junction

**173. The most common site of vascular leiomyosarcoma is :**
A. IVC B. Abd. aorta
C. Pulmonary artery D. Femoral artery

**174. The most frequent time for development of calf vein thrombosis is :**
A. During operation or within 24 hours
B. 24-72 hours
C. 3-7 days
D. 7-14 days

**175. Prominent superficial epigastric vein or superficial circumflex iliac vein in thin walled patient of femoral hernia suggesting obstructed and/or strangulated hernia is —— sign.**
A. Javid's B. Gaur's
C. Goblet's D. Gofford's

**176. Which of the following is least common in Ca esophagus :**
A. Dysphagia B. Weight loss
C. Regurgitation D. Retrosternal pain

**177. Heart-lung transplantation success is directly related to :**
A. Increase in usage of steroids
B. Monoclonal antibody administration
C. Cyclosporin-A administration
D. Higher concentrations of anti-lymphocytic globulin

**178. Which of the following appears to indicate the poorest prognosis for malignant tumors of the sub maxillary gland :**
A. Nodal metastases B. Soft tissue invasion
C. Mandibular invasion D. Nerve invasion

**179. The incidence of deep vein thrombosis in patients with petrochanteric fracture of femur is ——— %.**
A. 10 B. 25
C. 50 D. 75

**180. Which sign is seen in subclavian steal syndrome :**
A. Harve's B. Javid's
C. Goblet's D. Millon's

**181. Shifting abdominal tenderness seen in acute non-specific mesenteric adenitis or Meckel's diverticulitis is —— sign.**
A. Marion's B. Mallet's guy sign
C. Kelin's D. Rust's

**182. In cases of disc protrusion, compression of internal jugular vein raises intracranial pressure and increases the pain. This is —— test.**
A. Schwartz's B. Cozen's
C. Carnett's D. Naffegier's

**183. Most common radiological type of Ca esophagus is :**
A. Polypoid B. Ulcerating
C. Infiltrating D. Varicoid

**184. Hellmer's sign is seen in :**
A. Appendicitis B. Urethral rupture
C. Pancreatitis D. Ascites

**185. Downward displacement of umbilicus in distended abdomen suggesting presence of ascitis is ——— sign.**
A. Sign-de-dance B. Tanyol's
C. Rust's D. Mose's

**186. Which test is used to determine the nature (cystic or solid) of very small swellings in which fluctuation test can not be used (Centre of cystic swelling is softer than periphery whereas it is firm in solid swelling) :**
A. Schwartz B Paget's
C. Werner's D. Carnett's

| Ans. | | | | | | | | | |
|---|---|---|---|---|---|---|---|---|---|
| 165. C | 166. D | 167. A | 168. B | 169. C | 170. D | 171. A | 172. B | 173. A | 174. A |
| 175. B | 176. C | 177. C | 178. D | 179. D | 180. B | 181. C | 182. D | 183. A | 184. D |
| 185. B | 186. B | | | | | | | | |

**187. Following are predisposing factors for Ca esophagus except :**
A. Tylosis palmaris et plantares
B. Celiac disease
C. Asbestosis
D. Candidiasis

**188. Gardner's syndrome is associated with following except :**
A. Retro-peritoneal leiomyoma
B. Carcinoid
C. Periampullary carcinoma
D. Adenocarcinoma stomach

**189. Splenosis is often seen around the mean age of —— years.**
A. 5 B. 10
C. 25 D. 40

**190. Halo test is used in :**
A. Thyrotoxicosis B. Head injury
C. Ac. appendicitis D. Urethral injury

**191. Tuberculosis of the peritoneum is invariably associated with tuberculosis of the pleura is ——— law.**
A. Kustner's B. Kahler's
C. Gudden D. Godelier

**192. Following position is used for operating Gall bladder is — position.**
A. Elliot B. English
C. Duncan D. Bozeman's

**193. Position used in irrigating a urethra is ——— position.**
A. Jones B. Fowler
C. Kraske D. Valentine

**194. Position in which patient lying supine with a sand bag placed beneath 11th and 12th ribs is used in surgery on biliary tract is ——— position.**
A. Jones B. Robson's
C. Rose's D. Simon's

**195. Secondary neuroblastoma usually metastasized to following except :**
A. Brain B. Skeleton
C. Liver D. Orbit

**196. Lipoma of the brain is most commonly located at :**
A. Tuber cinereum
B. CP angle
C. Genu of corpus callosum
D. Sylvian fissure

**197. In von Hippel-Lindau disease, Lindau tumor is :**
A. Retinal angiomatosis
B. Hemangioblastomas of CNS
C. Craniopharyngioma
D. Calcified hematoma

**198. Glioblastoma multiforme is most common in ——— lobe.**
A. Frontal B. Temporal
C. Parietal D. Occipital

**199. In febrile tachycardia, the pulse beats increase at the rate of about eight per minute to every degree centigrade of temperature is ——— rule.**
A. Lossen's B. Liebermeister
C. Rolleston D. vant's Hoff

**200. Oligodendroglioma is most common in :**
A. Thalamus B. Corpus callosum
C. Frontal lobe D. Temporal lobe

**201. A feeling of pain or discomfort in the epigastric or precordial region while pressing over McBurney's point appendicitis is :**
A. Blumberg sing B. Bikele's sign
C. Aaron sing D. Ahlfeld sign

**202. Abrahams sign is positive in :**
A. Ureteric calculi B. Biliary lithiasis
C. Ac. Pancreatitis D. Crohn's disease

**203. Air cushion sign is present in :**
A. Chronic diverticulitis B. Chronic appendicitis
C. Acid peptic disease D. Ectopic pregnancy

**204. Ballance sign is present in :**
A. Ectopic rupture B. Duodenal perforation
C. Appendix perforation D. Splenic rupture

**205. An ecchymosis behind the ear, indicating a basilar skull fracture is :**
A. Beclard sign B. Becvor sign
C. Battle sign D. Boyce sign

**206. Blumberg sign is indicative of :**
A. Appendicitis B. Cholecystitis
C. Peritonitis D. Pancreatitis

**207. Bouveret sign indicates obstruction in :**
A. Duodenum B. Jejunum
C. Ileum D. Colon

**208. A gurgling sound produced by pressure on the side of the neck, occurring in esophageal diverticulum is —— sign.**
A. Hoover B. Halban
C. Boyce D. Brockenbrough

**209. Brenner's sign is positive in :**
A. Ac. Pancreatitis
B. Kidney rupture
C. Spleen rupture
D. Gastric perforation

| Ans. | | | | | | | | | |
|---|---|---|---|---|---|---|---|---|---|
| 187. D | 188. D | 189. B | 190. B | 191. C | 192. A | 193. D | 194. B | 195. A | 196. C |
| 197. B | 198. A | 199. B | 200. C | 201. C | 202. B | 203. B | 204. D | 205. C | 206. C |
| 207. D | 208. C | 209. D | | | | | | | |

**210. Closed fist sign detects lesion of ——— nerve.**
A. Ulnar B. Median
C. Radial D. All of the above

**211. Caviar sign is detected in :**
A. Int.carotid angiography
B. Lymphangiography
C. Cholecystography
D. Pyelography

**212. Lennhoff's sign is present in :**
A. Hepatocarcinoma
B. Echinococcal liver cyst
C. Amoebic liver abscess
D. Haemangioma liver

**213. With appendiceal adhesions intestinal gas which can be palpated trickling through the ileocaecal valve is known as :**
A. Lichtheim sign B. Loenan sign
C. Lockwood sign D. Lorenzy sign

**214. Prehn sign is positive in :**
A. Appendicular abscess
B. Carcinoid in appendix
C. Epididymo-orchitis
D. Acute diverticulitis

**215. Black hairy tongue is due to :**
A. Benign naevus in the tongue
B. Lingual thyroid
C. Lingual tuberculosis
D. Aspergillus Niger

**216. What is the percentage of neoplasms arising in the parotid gland in comparison to all salivary neoplasms :**
A. 50% B. 60%
C. 70% D. 75%

**217. Of the neoplasms arising in the parotid gland what is the percentage of benign tumours :**
A. 50% B. 60%
C. 70% D. 80%

**218. The treatment of adenocarcinoma of the parotid gland is :**
A. Radioactive needle implantation.
B. Excision of the tumour with wide margin of normal salivary glands.
C. Radical parotidectomy with sacrifice of the facial nerve.
D. Radical excision of the parotid gland with sacrifice of the facial nerve followed by post-operative radiotherapy.

**219. Branchial cyst is a congenital abnormality and mostly found :**
A. In new born babies B. In children
C. In adolescents D. In early adult life

**220. The structures which will lie superficial to the track of the branchial fistula are developed from :**
A. 1st branchial arch B. 2nd branchial arch
C. 3rd branchial arch D. 4th branchial arch

**221. Pizzillo's method is :**
A. Helpful in palpation of each lobe of the thyroid gland.
B. Helpful to detect fixation of the thyroid gland to the trachea and oesophagus.
C. Helpful in inspection of the thyroid for the presence of generalised swelling or isolated swelling of the thyroid gland.
D. Helpful to detect presence of any bruit in the goitre.

**222. Lahey's method is helpful :**
A. In inspection of the thyroid gland for generalised or local enlargement.
B. To detect pulsation of the carotid artery.
C. In palpation of each lobe.
D. In detecting presence of any retrosternal prolongation or not.

**223. Normal range of free thyroxin index (FTI) is :**
A. 1 to 2 B. 2 to 3
C. 3.5 to 8 D. 8.5 to 12

**224. Asymptomatic slight enlargement of the salivary gland is noticed in the following conditions except :**
A. Diabetes mellitus B. Vitamin-D deficiency
C. Cirrhosis of liver D. Kwashiorkar

**225. In case of solitary nodule of the thyroid, his pathological report after lobectomy revealed follicular carcinoma. What more treatment is required :**
A. Near total thyroidectomy.
B. Only radioiodine therapy if there is metastasis.
C. Carefully follow-up and nothing more is advised till appearance of secondaries or recurence.
D. Near total thyroidectomy followed by deep X-ray therapy.

**226. The best treatment of haemothorax with 400 cc blood in the pleural space is :**
A. Thoracotomy and ligation of bleeding vessel.
B. Tube drainage.
C. Needle aspiration.
D. Conservative treatment with antibiotic and no operation is required.

| Ans. | 210. B | 211. B | 212. B | 213. C | 214. C | 215. D | 216. D | 217. D | 218. D | 219. D |
|---|---|---|---|---|---|---|---|---|---|---|
| | 220. B | 221. C | 222. C | 223. C | 224. D | 225. B | 226. C | | | |

**227. Which of the following symptoms is first noticed in case of lung abscess ?**
A. Pleural pain.
B. Dry irritating cough.
C. Expectoration of considerable quantities of offensive blood-stained pus.
D. Influenza-like symptoms without any localising symptoms.

**228. The most effective treatment in case of a small leak in broncho-pleural fistula is :**
A. Immediate thoracotomy and resuturing of the bronchus.
B. Immediate thoracotomy, resuturing of the bronchus and reinforcing the suture line with muscle graft.
C. Repeated aspiration or temporary tube drainage of fluid from the pleural cavity with the patient lying on the affected side.
D. Nothing is to be done except giving antibiotic and the fistula will heal by itself.

**229. The followings are the main histological types of tumours of the thymus except :**
A. Epithelial B. Fibrous
C. Lymph node D. Teratomatous

**230. A few tumours may arise anywhere in the mediastinum. They are as follows except :**
A. Lymphadenopathy B. Lymphogenous cysts
C. Neurogenic tumours D. Lipoma

**231. The treatment of ventricular septal defect is :**
A. That the defect is usually closed by direct suturing as a primary procedure and is never done in two stages.
B. Closure of the defect performed by inserting a patch of dacron graft with the aid of an extracorporeal circulation.
C. To treat over-congestion of the lungs with antibiotics and wait as the defect usually closes by itself
D. Mainly performed for pulmonary hypertension and right ventricular hypertrophy

**232. The treatment of oesophageal cancer :**
A. Should include surgical excision of the tumour in majority of cases
B. Includes radiotherapy in majority of cases
C. Includes chemotherapy in majority of patients
D. Should include gastrostomy to provide palliation for patients with complete dysphagia

**233. Which of the followings is the least frequent site for breast metastasis :**
A. Contralateral breast B. Bone
C. Lung D. Liver

**234. The eczema of the breast :**
A. Is a synonym of Paget's breast.
B. Is mostly seen in the upper and lateral part of the breast.
C. Mainly affects the nipple.
D. Normally does not respond to antieczematous treatment.

**235. Which of the followings may be affected by lymphatic spread in carcinoma of the breast :**
A. Lungs B. Liver
C. Spine D. Ovaries

**236. Involvement of which group of lymph nodes will make the carcinoma of breast a Stage-IV disease:**
A. Supraclavicular group of lymph nodes.
B. Pectoral group of lymph nodes.
C. Brachial group of lymph nodes.
D. Deltopectoral group of lymph nodes.

**237. The sign or symptom which is always present in breast cancer includes :**
A. Pain in the breast.
B. Blood discharge through the nipple.
C. An enlarged and fixed axillary lymph nodes.
D. Skin teethering or nipple retraction.

**238. The prognosis of treated stage I breast cancer :**
A. Is worse if the cancer is discovered during late pregnancy.
B. Is adversely affected by subsequent pregnancy.
C. Is worse in the male.
D. Becomes better when treated by simple mastectomy + radiotherapy.

**239. Seat belt injury may cause the following visceral injuries except :**
A. Detachment of intestine from its mesentery.
B. Injury to the liver.
C. Injury to the spleen
D. Injury to the urinary bladder

**240. The most effective investigation in intraperitoneal rupture of large intestine is :**
A. Selective angiography
B. Presence of small bubbles at the margin of right psoas muscle in straight X-ray
C. Large pneumoperitoneum in straight X-ray
D. X-ray after a thin barium suspension swallow

**241. 'Strangury' may became across in :**
A. Papilloma of urinary bladder
B. Carcinoma of urinary bladder
C. Pelvic peritonitis
D. Carcinoma of rectum involving the bladder

| Ans. | 227. D | 228. C | 229. B | 230. C | 231. B | 232. B | 233. A | 234. C | 235. B | 236. A |
|---|---|---|---|---|---|---|---|---|---|---|
| | 237. D | 238. D | 239. D | 240. C | 241. C | | | | | |

**242. Obturator test is characteristic of :**
A. Pelvic appendicitis
B. Retrocaecal appendicitis
C. Acute cholecystitis
D. Ileal appendicitis

**243. A fall in the serum calcium level is a good index of the severity of acute pancreatitis. Which level should be considered as diagnostic of severe fulminating acute pancreatitis :**
A. 4 mg/100 ml B. 5 mg/100 ml
C. 6 mg/100 ml D. 7 mg/100 ml

**244. In what percentage of cases of acute cholecystitis jaundice may be present :**
A. Nil B. 10% to 20% of cases
C. 20% to 30% of cases D. About 50% of cases

**245. In the third stage of peptic perforation the most characteristic finding in the abdomen is :**
A. Localised rigidity in the epigastrium.
B. Rigidity completely disappears.
C. Abdomen becomes distended in the epigastrium region.
D. Rigidity of the whole of the abdomen will be felt.

**246. Vomiting relieves pain in :**
A. Chronic cholecystitis
B. Gastric ulcer
C. Carcinoma of the stomach
D. Hiatus hernia

**247. The best way to diagnose liver carcinoma is :**
A. Straigh X-ray B. Liver needle biopsy
C. Ultrasound D. Radio-isotope scanning

**248. The complications after gastric operations can be divided into early complications like paralytic ilius, haemorrhage from suture line, stomal obstruction etc. and late complications like recurrent ulcer, gastrojejunocolic fistula, nutritional deficiencies etc. The late complications usually appear :**
A. Later than 1 month of operation
B. Later than 3 months of operation
C. Later than 6 months of operation
D. Later than 1 year of operation

**249. In established portal hypertension, the pressure goes up to :**
A. 25 mm Hg B. 30 mm Hg
C. 35 mm Hg D. 40 mm Hg

**250. The right hemicolectomy means resection of :**
A. Terminal 8 inches of the ilium and whole of the ascending colon.
B. Terminal 8 inches of the ilium, whole of the ascending colon and to the junction of the proximal and middle thirds of the transverse colon.
C. Terminal 8 inches of ilium, whole of the ascending colon and upto the junction of the middle and distal thirds of the transverse colon.
D. Terminal 8 inches of ilium, whole of the ascending colon and whole of the transverse colon.

**Ans. 242. A 243. D 244. C 245. D 246. B 247. D 248. D 249. B 250. B**

# GENERAL SURGERY

## References Quoted

| S.No. | Books |
|---|---|
| 1. | Bailey & Love's **Short Practice of Surgery.** ELBS, London, 1995. |
| 2. | **Current Surgical Diagnosis and Treatment.** Prentice-Hall International, Inc., USA, 1999 |
| 3. | Bhatia's **Quick Medical Text Review Series, General Surgery** CBS Publishers & Distributors Pvt. Ltd., Delhi. |

## Unforgetable Supplement

Bhatia's **Quick Medical Text Review Series** (Quick revision of all the subjects in short time. No need to underline the books (read important points). CBS Publishers & Distributors Pvt. Ltd., Delhi.